ACSM's
Guidelines for
Exercise Testing and Prescription
NINTH EDITION

SENIOR EDITOR

Linda S. Pescatello, PhD, FACSM, FAHA, ACSM-PD, ACSM-ETT
Professor
Department of Kinesiology & Human Performance Laboratory
Neag School of Education
University of Connecticut
Storrs, Connecticut

ASSOCIATE EDITORS

Ross Arena, PhD, PT, FACSM, FAACVPR, FAHA, ACSM-CES
Director and Professor
Physical Therapy Program
Department of Orthopaedics & Rehabilitation
University of New Mexico Health Sciences Center
Albuquerque, New Mexico

Deborah Riebe, PhD, FACSM, ACSM-HFS
Chair and Professor
Department of Kinesiology
University of Rhode Island
Kingston, Rhode Island

Paul D. Thompson, MD, FACSM, FACC
Chief of Cardiology
Hartford Hospital
Hartford, Connecticut

ACSM's
Guidelines for
Exercise Testing and Prescription

NINTH EDITION

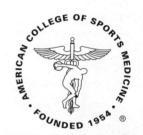

**AMERICAN COLLEGE
OF SPORTS MEDICINE**

Wolters Kluwer | Lippincott Williams & Wilkins
Health

Acquisitions Editor: Emily Lupash
Product Manager: Meredith L. Brittain
Marketing Manager: Sarah Schuessler
Vendor Manager: Marian Bellus
Creative Director: Doug Smock
Compositor: Absolute Service, Inc.

ACSM Committee on Certification and Registry Boards Chair: Deborah Riebe, PhD, FACSM, ACSM-HFS
ACSM Publications Committee Chair: Walter R. Thompson, PhD, FACSM, FAACVPR
ACSM Group Publisher: Kerry O'Rourke
Umbrella Editor: Jonathan K. Ehrman, PhD, FACSM

Ninth Edition

Copyright © 2014, 2010, 2006, 2001 American College of Sports Medicine

351 West Camden Street   Two Commerce Square / 2001 Market Street
Baltimore, MD 21201   Philadelphia, PA 19103

Printed in China

9 8 7 6 5

Library of Congress Cataloging-in-Publication Data

ACSM's guidelines for exercise testing and prescription / American College of Sports Medicine ; senior editor, Linda S. Pescatello ; associate editors, Ross Arena, Deborah Riebe, Paul D. Thompson. — 9th ed.
    p. ; cm.
  Guidelines for exercise testing and prescription
  Includes bibliographical references and index.
  ISBN 978-1-60913-605-5
  I. Pescatello, Linda S. II. American College of Sports Medicine. III. Title: Guidelines for exercise testing and prescription.
  [DNLM: 1. Physical Exertion—Guideline. 2. Exercise Test—standards—Guideline. 3. Exercise Therapy—standards—Guideline. WE 103]

  615.8'2—dc23
                                                                                                2012038784

DISCLAIMER

This book is dedicated to the hundreds of volunteer professionals who have, since 1975, contributed their valuable time and expertise to develop and update the Guidelines. Now in its ninth edition, it is the most widely circulated set of guidelines used by professionals performing exercise testing or exercise programs. Specifically, this edition is dedicated to the editors, contributing authors, and reviewers of this and previous editions, who have not only provided their collective expertise but also their valuable time to ensure the Guidelines meet the highest standards in exercise science and practice.

The American College of Sports Medicine (ACSM) *Guidelines* origins are within the ACSM Committee on Certification and Registry Boards (CCRB, formerly known as the Certification and Education Committee and the Preventive and Rehabilitative Exercise Committee). Today, the *Guidelines* remain under the auspices of the CCRB, and have become *the* primary resource for anyone conducting exercise testing or exercise programs. The *Guidelines* provide the foundation of content for its supporting companion texts produced by ACSM, which include the seventh edition of *ACSM's Resource Manual for Guidelines for Exercise Testing and Prescription*, fourth edition of *ACSM's Certification Review*, fourth edition of *ACSM's Resources for the Personal Trainer*, first edition of *ACSM's Resources for the Health Fitness Specialist*, fourth edition of *ACSM's Health-Related Physical Fitness Assessment Manual*, and second edition of *ACSM's Resources for Clinical Exercise Physiology: Musculoskeletal, Neuromuscular, Neoplastic, Immunologic, and Hematologic Conditions*.

The first edition of the *Guidelines* was published in 1975, with updated editions published approximately every 4 to 6 years. The outstanding scientists and clinicians who have served in leadership positions as chairs and editors of the *Guidelines* since 1975 are:

First Edition, 1975

Karl G. Stoedefalke, PhD, FACSM, Cochair

John A. Faulkner, PhD, FACSM, Cochair

Second Edition, 1980

Anne R. Abbott, PhD, FACSM, Chair

Third Edition, 1986

Steven N. Blair, PED, FACSM, Chair

Fourth Edition, 1991

Russell R. Pate, PhD, FACSM, Chair

Fifth Edition, 1995

Larry W. Kenney, PhD, FACSM, Senior Editor

Reed H. Humphrey, PhD, PT, FACSM, Associate Editor Clinical

Cedric X. Bryant, PhD, FACSM, Associate Editor Fitness

Sixth Edition, 2000

Barry A. Franklin, PhD, FACSM, Senior Editor

Mitchell H. Whaley, PhD, FACSM, Associate Editor Clinical

Edward T. Howley, PhD, FACSM, Associate Editor Fitness

Seventh Edition, 2005

Mitchell H. Whaley, PhD, FACSM, Senior Editor

Peter H. Brubaker, PhD, FACSM, Associate Editor Clinical

Robert M. Otto, PhD, FACSM, Associate Editor Fitness

Eighth Edition, 2009

Walter R. Thompson, PhD, FACSM, Senior Editor

Neil F. Gordon, MD, PhD, FACSM, Associate Editor

Linda S. Pescatello, PhD, FACSM, Associate Editor

Ninth Edition, 2013

Linda S. Pescatello, PhD, FACSM, Senior Editor

Ross Arena, PhD, PT, FACSM, Associate Editor

Deborah Riebe, PhD, FACSM, Associate Editor

Paul D. Thompson, MD, FACSM, Associate Editor

Preface

This edition of *ACSM's Guidelines for Exercise Testing and Prescription* will continue the efforts of the editors and contributing authors of the eighth edition to make the ninth edition a true *guidelines* book rather than a sole and inclusive *resource*. For it was the original intent of the *Guidelines* to be user friendly, easily accessible, and a current primary resource for professionals that conduct exercise testing and exercise programs. To this effect, in this edition, text descriptions have been minimized; more tables, boxes, and figures have been included; summary boxes have been added throughout to highlight important information; and take home messages and key Web sites now conclude each chapter.

The reader of this edition of *ACSM's Guidelines for Exercise Testing and Prescription* will notice several new themes. First and foremost, the ninth edition supports the public health message that all people should adopt a physically active lifestyle by reducing the emphasis on the need for medical evaluation (*i.e.*, medical examination and exercise testing) as part of the preparticipation health screening process prior to initiating a progressive exercise regimen among healthy, asymptomatic persons. This edition of the *Guidelines* seeks to simplify the preparticipaton health screening process in order to remove unnecessary and unproven barriers to adopting a physically active lifestyle. Secondly, we have instituted an automated referencing system that is the beginning of an ACSM evidence-based library that will become available to the membership at some time in the future. We have integrated the most recent guidelines and recommendations available from ACSM position stands and other relevant professional organization's scientific statements so that the *Guidelines* are the most current, primary resource for professionals that conduct exercise testing and exercise programs in academic, corporate, health/fitness, health care, and research settings. It is important for the readership to know these new themes and the more specific innovations of the ninth edition that follow were developed with input from the ACSM membership prior to the initiation of this project via an electronic survey and in-house focus group that asked respondents and participants, respectively, for their suggestions regarding the content of the ninth edition.

More specific, noteworthy innovations of the ninth edition include the following:

- The introduction of the Frequency, Intensity, Time, Type — Volume, and Progression or FITT-VP principle of exercise prescription in *Chapter 7*.
- An expanded number of special populations in *Chapter 10* because more information related to exercise testing, prescription, and special considerations of these new populations has become available since the publication of the eighth edition.
- Inclusion of *Chapter 11*, a new chapter on behavioral change strategies addressing the challenges of exercise adherence.

Several of the appendices have undergone significant changes. *Appendix A*, Common Medications, is now authored by registered pharmacists in academic settings with clinical expertise in the pharmacology of medications likely to be used by patients and clients in exercise testing and programmatic settings. The content of *Appendix B*, Medical Emergency Management, is now based primarily on the fourth edition of *ACSM's Health/Fitness Facility Standards and Guidelines*. The learning objectives have been removed from *Appendix D*, ACSM Certifications, because these are now available via the ACSM Certification link www.acsmcertification.org/exam-content-outlines. *Appendix E*, which lists the contributing authors to the two previous editions of the *Guidelines*, has been added.

Any updates made in this edition of the *Guidelines* after their publication and prior to the publication of the next edition of the *Guidelines*, can be accessed from the ACSM Certification link (www.acsmcertification.org/getp9-updates). Furthermore, the reader is referred to the ACSM Access Public Information Books and Media link for a list of ACSM books (www.acsm.org/access-public-information/books-multimedia), and to the ACSM Get Certified link for a listing of ACSM certifications (www.acsmcertification.org/get-certified).

ACKNOWLEDGMENTS

It is in this preface that the editors of the ninth edition have the opportunity to thank the many people who helped to see this project to completion. To be consistent with the theme of the *Guidelines*, our thanks will remain short, to the point, and without great elaboration.

We thank our families and friends for their understanding of the extensive time commitment we made to this project that encompassed over three years.

We thank our publisher, and in particular Emily Lupash, senior acquisitions editor; Meredith Brittain, senior product manager; Christen Murphy and Sarah Schuessler, marketing managers; and Zachary Shapiro, editorial assistant.

We thank Richard T. Cotton, ACSM National Director of Certification; Traci Sue Rush, ACSM Assistant Director of Certification Programs; Kela Webster, ACSM Certification Coordinator; Robin Ashman and Dru Romanini, ACSM Certification Department Assistants; Angela Chastain, ACSM Editorial Services Office; Kerry O'Rourke, ACSM Director of Publishing; Walter R. Thompson, ACSM Publications Committee Chair; and the extraordinarily hardworking Publications Committee.

We thank the ACSM CCRB for their valuable insights into the content of this edition of the *Guidelines* and counsel on administrative issues related to seeing this project to completion. The ACSM CCRB tirelessly reviewed manuscript drafts to ensure the content of this edition of the *Guidelines* meets the highest standards in exercise science and practice. We thank Dr. David Swain, senior editor of the seventh edition of *ACSM's Resource Manual for Guidelines for Exercise Testing and Prescription*, for his very careful and insightful review of the *Guidelines* and collegial assistance with seeing this project to completion. We thank Dr. Jonathan Ehrman, the umbrella editor of this project, who made it his mission to ensure congruency between the ninth edition of the *Guidelines* and seventh edition of *ACSM's Resource Manual for Guidelines for Exercise Testing and Prescription*. We thank the University of Connecticut Medical Librarian, Jill Livingston, for her patience and guidance with implementing the ACSM evidence-based RefWorks library and teaching the editors and contributing authors how to become proficient in using RefWorks in this edition of the *Guidelines*.

The *Guidelines* review process was extensive, undergoing many layers of expert scrutiny to ensure the highest quality of content. We thank the external and CCRB reviewers of the ninth edition for their careful reviews. These reviewers are listed later in this front matter.

We are in great debt to the contributing authors of the ninth edition of the *Guidelines* for volunteering their expertise and valuable time to ensure the *Guidelines* meet the highest standards in exercise science and practice. The ninth edition contributing authors are listed in the following section.

On a more personal note, I thank my three associate editors — Dr. Ross Arena, Dr. Deborah Riebe, and Dr. Paul D. Thompson — who selflessly devoted their valuable time and expertise to the ninth edition of the *Guidelines*. Their strong sense of selfless commitment to the *Guidelines* emanated from an underlying belief held by the editorial team of the profound importance the *Guidelines* have in informing and directing the work we do in exercise science and practice. Words cannot express the extent of my gratitude to the three of you for your tireless efforts to see this project to completion.

Linda S. Pescatello, PhD, FACSM
Senior Editor

ADDITIONAL RESOURCES

ACSM's Guidelines for Exercise Testing and Prescription, Ninth Edition includes additional resources for instructors that are available on the book's companion Web site at http://thepoint.lww.com/ACSMGETP9e.

INSTRUCTORS

Approved adopting instructors will be given access to the following additional resources:

- Brownstone test generator
- PowerPoint presentations
- Image bank
- WebCT/Angel/Blackboard ready cartridge

In addition, purchasers of the text can access the searchable Full Text Online by going to the *ACSM's Guidelines for Exercise Testing and Prescription, Ninth Edition* Web site at http://thepoint.lww.com/ACSMGETP9e. See the inside front cover of this text for more details, including the passcode you will need to gain access to the Web site.

NOTA BENE

The views and information contained in the ninth edition of *ACSM's Guidelines for Exercise Testing and Prescription* are provided as *guidelines* as opposed to *standards of practice*. This distinction is an important one because specific legal connotations may be attached to standards of practice that are not attached to guidelines. This distinction is critical inasmuch as it gives the professional in exercise testing and programmatic settings the freedom to deviate from these guidelines when necessary and appropriate in the course of using independent and prudent judgment. *ACSM's Guidelines for Exercise Testing and Prescription* presents a framework whereby the professional may certainly — and in some cases has the obligation to — tailor to individual client or patient needs while balancing institutional or legal requirements.

Contributing Authors to the Ninth Edition*

Kelli Allen, PhD
VA Medical Center
Durham, North Carolina
Chapter 10: Exercise Prescription for
    Populations with Other Chronic Diseases
    and Health Conditions

Mark Anderson, PT, PhD
University of Oklahoma Health
    Sciences Center
Oklahoma City, Oklahoma
Chapter 10: Exercise Prescription for
    Populations with Other Chronic Diseases
    and Health Conditions

Gary Balady, MD
Boston University School of Medicine
Boston, Massachusetts
Chapter 9: Exercise Prescription for Patients
    with Cardiovascular and Cerebrovascular
    Disease

Michael Berry, PhD
Wake Forest University
Winston-Salem, North Carolina
Chapter 10: Exercise Prescription for
    Populations with Other Chronic Diseases
    and Health Conditions

Bryan Blissmer, PhD
University of Rhode Island
Kingston, Rhode Island
Chapter 11: Behavioral Theories and
    Strategies for Promoting Exercise

Kim Bonzheim, MSA, FACSM
Genesys Regional Medical Center
Grand Blanc, Michigan
Appendix C: Electrocardiogram Interpretation

Barry Braun, PhD, FACSM
University of Massachusetts
Amherst, Massachusetts
Chapter 10: Exercise Prescription for
    Populations with Other Chronic Diseases
    and Health Conditions

Monthaporn S. Bryant, PT, PhD
Michael E. DeBakey VA Medical Center
Houston, Texas
Chapter 10: Exercise Prescription for
    Populations with Other Chronic Diseases
    and Health Conditions

Thomas Buckley, MPH, RPh
University of Connecticut
Storrs, Connecticut
Appendix A: Common Medications

John Castellani, PhD
United States Army Research Institute of
    Environmental Medicine
Natick, Massachusetts
Chapter 8: Exercise Prescription for Healthy
    Populations with Special Considerations
    and Environmental Considerations

**Dino Costanzo, MA, FACSM, ACSM-RCEP,
ACSM-PD, ACSM-ETT**
The Hospital of Central Connecticut
New Britain, Connecticut
Appendix D: American College of Sports
    Medicine Certifications

Michael Deschenes, PhD, FACSM
The College of William and Mary
Williamsburg, Virginia
Chapter 7: General Principles of Exercise
    Prescription

Joseph E. Donnelly, EdD, FACSM
University of Kansas Medical Center
Kansas City, Kansas
Chapter 10: Exercise Prescription for
    Populations with Other Chronic Diseases
    and Health Conditions

Bo Fernhall, PhD, FACSM
University of Illinois at Chicago
Chicago, Illinois
Chapter 10: Exercise Prescription for
    Populations with Other Chronic Diseases
    and Health Conditions

*See Appendix E for a list of contributing
authors for the previous two editions.

Stephen F. Figoni, PhD, FACSM
VA West Los Angeles Healthcare Center
Los Angeles, California
Chapter 10: Exercise Prescription for
    Populations with Other Chronic Diseases
    and Health Conditions

Nadine Fisher, EdD
University at Buffalo
Buffalo, New York
Chapter 10: Exercise Prescription for
    Populations with Other Chronic Diseases
    and Health Conditions

Charles Fulco, ScD
United States Army Research Institute of
    Environmental Medicine
Natick, Massachusetts
Chapter 8: Exercise Prescription for Healthy
    Populations with Special Considerations
    and Environmental Considerations

**Carol Ewing Garber, PhD, FACSM,
ACSM-RCEP, ACSM-HFS, ACSM-PD**
Columbia University
New York, New York
Chapter 7: General Principles of
    Exercise Prescription

Andrew Gardner, PhD
University of Oklahoma Health Sciences
    Center
Oklahoma City, Oklahoma
Chapter 9: Exercise Prescription for Patients
    with Cardiovascular and Cerebrovascular
    Disease

Neil Gordon, MD, PhD, MPH, FACSM
Intervent International
Savannah, Georgia
Chapter 10: Exercise Prescription for
    Populations with Other Chronic Diseases
    and Health Conditions

Eric Hall, PhD, FACSM
Elon University
Elon, North Carolina
Chapter 11: Behavioral Theories and
    Strategies for Promoting Exercise

Gregory Hand, PhD, MPH, FACSM
University of South Carolina
Columbia, South Carolina
Chapter 10: Exercise Prescription for
    Populations with Other Chronic Diseases
    and Health Conditions

Samuel Headley, PhD, FACSM, ACSM-RCEP
Springfield College
Springfield, Massachusetts
Chapter 10: Exercise Prescription for
    Populations with Other Chronic Diseases
    and Health Conditions

Kurt Jackson, PT, PhD
University of Dayton
Dayton, Ohio
Chapter 10: Exercise Prescription for
    Populations with Other Chronic Diseases
    and Health Conditions

Robert Kenefick, PhD, FACSM
United States Army Research Institute of
    Environmental Medicine
Natick, Massachusetts
Chapter 8: Exercise Prescription for Healthy
    Populations with Special Considerations
    and Environmental Considerations

Christine Kohn, PharmD
University of Connecticut School of
    Pharmacy
Storrs, Connecticut
Appendix A: Common Medications

Wendy Kohrt, PhD, FACSM
University of Colorado—Anschutz Medical
    Campus
Aurora, Colorado
Chapter 10: Exercise Prescription for
    Populations with Other Chronic Diseases
    and Health Conditions

I-Min Lee, MBBS, MPH, ScD
Brigham and Women's Hospital, Harvard
    Medical School
Boston, Massachusetts
Chapter 1: Benefits and Risks Associated with
    Physical Activity

David X. Marquez, PhD, FACSM
University of Illinois at Chicago
Chicago, Illinois
Chapter 11: Behavioral Theories and
    Strategies for Promoting Exercise

Kyle McInnis, ScD, FACSM
Merrimack College
North Andover, Massachusetts
Appendix B: Emergency Risk Management

Miriam Morey, PhD, FACSM
VA and Duke Medical Centers
Durham, North Carolina
Chapter 8: Exercise Prescription for Healthy
    Populations with Special Considerations
    and Environmental Considerations

Michelle Mottola, PhD, FACSM
The University of Western Ontario
London, Ontario, Canada
Chapter 8: Exercise Prescription for Healthy
    Populations with Special Considerations
    and Environmental Considerations

Stephen Muza, PhD, FACSM
United States Army Research Institute of
    Environmental Medicine
Natick, Massachusetts
Chapter 8: Exercise Prescription for Healthy
    Populations with Special Considerations
    and Environmental Considerations

Patricia Nixon, PhD
Wake Forest University
Winston-Salem, North Carolina
Chapter 10: Exercise Prescription for
    Populations with Other Chronic Diseases
    and Health Conditions

Jennifer R. O'Neill, PhD, MPH, ACSM-HFS
University of South Carolina,
Columbia, South Carolina
Chapter 8: Exercise Prescription for Healthy
    Populations with Special Considerations
    and Environmental Considerations

Russell Pate, PhD, FACSM
University of South Carolina
Columbia, South Carolina
Chapter 8: Exercise Prescription for Healthy
    Populations with Special Considerations
    and Environmental Considerations

Richard Preuss, PhD, PT
McGill University
Montreal, Quebec, Canada
Chapter 8: Exercise Prescription for Healthy
    Populations with Special Considerations
    and Environmental Considerations

**Kathryn Schmitz, PhD, MPH, FACSM,
ACSM-HFS**
University of Pennsylvania
Philadelphia, Pennsylvania
Chapter 10: Exercise Prescription for
    Populations with Other Chronic Diseases
    and Health Conditions

Carrie Sharoff, PhD
Arizona State University
Tempe, Arizona
Chapter 10: Exercise Prescription for
    Populations with Other Chronic Diseases
    and Health Conditions

Maureen Simmonds, PhD, PT
University of Texas Health Science Center
San Antonio, Texas
Chapter 8: Exercise Prescription for Healthy
    Populations with Special Considerations
    and Environmental Considerations

Paul D. Thompson, MD, FACSM, FACC
Hartford Hospital
Hartford, Connecticut
Chapter 1: Benefits and Risks Associated with
    Physical Activity
Chapter 2: Preparticipation Health Screening
Chapter 10: Exercise Prescription for
    Populations with Other Chronic Diseases
    and Health Conditions

Reviewers for the Ninth Edition*

Robert Axtell, PhD, FACSM, ACSM-ETT
Southern Connecticut State University
New Haven, Connecticut

*Christopher Berger, PhD, ACSM-HFS
The George Washington University
Washington, District of Columbia

*Clinton A. Brawner, MS, ACSM-RCEP, FACSM
Henry Ford Hospital
Detroit, Michigan

Barbara A. (Kooiker) Bushman, PhD, FACSM, ACSM-PD, ACSM-CES, ACSM-HFS, ACSM-CPT, ACSM-EIM3
Senior Editor of *ACSM's Resources for the Personal Trainer*, Fourth Edition
Missouri State University
Springfield, Missouri

*Brian J. Coyne, MEd, ACSM-RCEP
Duke University Health System
Morrisville, North Carolina

Lance Dalleck, PhD, ACSM-RCEP
University of Auckland
Auckland, New Zealand

*Julie J. Downing, PhD, FACSM, ACSM-HFD, ACSM-CPT
Central Oregon Community College
Bend, Oregon

*Gregory B. Dwyer, PhD, FACSM, ACSM-PD, ACSM-RCEP, ACSM-CES, ACSM-ETT
Senior Editor of *ACSM's Certification Review*, Fourth Edition
East Stroudsburg University
East Stroudsburg, Pennsylvania

Carl Foster, PhD, FACSM
University of Wisconsin-La Crosse
La Crosse, Wisconsin

Patty Freedson, PhD, FACSM
University of Massachusetts
Amherst, Massachusetts

*Denotes reviewers who were also members of the ACSM Committee on Certification and Registry Boards.

Leonard A. Kaminsky, PhD, FACSM, ACSM-PD, ACSM-ETT
Senior Editor of *ACSM's Health-Related Physical Fitness Assessment Manual*, Fourth Edition
Ball State University
Muncie, Indiana

Steven Keteyian, PhD, FACSM
Henry Ford Hospital
Detroit, Michigan

Gary M. Liguori, PhD, FACSM, ACSM-CES, ACSM-HFS
Senior Editor of *ACSM's Resources for the Health Fitness Specialist*, First Edition
North Dakota State University
Fargo, North Dakota

*Randi S. Lite, MA, ACSM-RCEP
Simmons College
Boston, Massachusetts

Claudio Nigg, PhD
University of Hawaii
Honolulu, Hawaii

*Madeline Paternostro-Bayles, PhD, FACSM, ACSM-PD, ACSM-CES
Indiana University of Pennsylvania
Indiana, Pennsylvania

*Peter J. Ronai, MS, FACSM, ACSM-PD, ACSM-RCEP, ACSM-CES, ACSM-ETT, ACSM-HFS
Sacred Heart University
Milford, Connecticut

Robert Sallis, MD, FACSM
Kaiser Permanente Medical Center
Rancho Cucamonga, California

*Jeffrey T. Soukup, PhD, ACSM-CES
Appalachian State University
Boone, North Carolina

Sean Walsh, PhD
Central Connecticut State University
New Britain, Connecticut

David S. Zucker, MD, PhD
Swedish Cancer Institute
Seattle, Washington

Contents

Section III: Exercise Prescription   161

Associate Editor: Deborah Riebe, PhD, FACSM, ACSM-HFS

Abbreviations

AACVPR	American Association of Cardiovascular and Pulmonary Rehabilitation	BMI	body mass index
		BMT	bone marrow transplantation
ABI	ankle-brachial index	BP	blood pressure
ACC	American College of Cardiology	BUN	blood urea nitrogen
		CAAHEP	Commission on Accreditation of Allied Health Education Programs
ACCP	American College of Chest Physicians		
ACE-I	angiotensin-converting enzyme inhibitors	CABG	coronary artery bypass graft
		CAD	coronary artery disease
ACLS	advanced cardiac life support	CCB	calcium channel blocker
		CDC	U.S. Centers for Disease Control and Prevention
ACS	American Cancer Society		
ACSM	American College of Sports Medicine	CEPA	Clinical Exercise Physiology Association
ADL	activities of daily living	CES	ACSM Certified Clinical Exercise Specialist^{SM}
ADP-R	adenosine diphosphate-ribose		
		CHD	coronary heart disease
ADT	androgen deprivation therapy	CHF	congestive heart failure
		CI	chronotropic index
AED	automated external defibrillator	CKD	chronic kidney disease
		CM	cardiomyopathy
AHA	American Heart Association	CNS	central nervous system
AHFS	American Hospital Formulary Service	CO_2	carbon dioxide
		CoAES	Committee on Accreditation for the Exercise Sciences
AIDS	acquired immunodeficiency syndrome		
		COPD	chronic obstructive pulmonary disease
AIT	aerobic interval training		
ALT	alanine transaminase	COX-I	cyclooxygenase inhibitor
AMS	acute mountain sickness	CP	cerebral palsy
APAP	acetaminophen	CP-ISRA	Cerebral Palsy International Sport and Recreation Association
ARB	angiotensin II receptor blocker		
ART	antiretroviral therapy	CPR	cardiopulmonary resuscitation
AST	aspartate transaminase		
ATP	Adult Treatment Panel	CPT	ACSM Certified Personal Trainer®
ATS	American Thoracic Society		
AV	atrioventricular	CPX	cardiopulmonary exercise testing
aVR	augmented voltage right		
BB	beta-blockers	CR	cardiorespiratory
BIA	bioelectrical impedance analysis	CRF	cardiorespiratory fitness
		CSEP	Canadian Society for Exercise Physiology
BLS	basic life support		
BMD	bone mineral density	CT	computed tomography

CV	cardiovascular		GOLD	Global Initiative for Chronic Obstructive Lung Disease
CVD	cardiovascular disease			
DASH	Dietary Approaches to Stop Hypertension		GXT	graded exercise test
			HACE	high altitude cerebral edema
Db	body density		HAPE	high altitude pulmonary edema
DBP	diastolic blood pressure			
DBS	deep brain stimulation		HbA1C	glycosylated hemoglobin
DEXA	dual energy X-ray absorptiometry		HBM	Health Belief Model
			HCTZ	hydrochlorothiazide
DIAD	Detection of Ischemia in Asymptomatic Diabetes		HDL	high-density lipoprotein cholesterol
DM	Diabetes mellitus		HF	heart failure
DNA	deoxyribonucleic acid		HFS	ACSM Certified Health Fitness Specialist^{SM}
DS	Down syndrome			
DVR	Dynamic Variable Resistance		HIPAA	Health Insurance Portability and Accountability Act
EBCT	electron beam computed tomography		HIV	human immunodeficiency virus
ECG	electrocardiogram (electrocardiographic)		HMG-CoA	hydroxymethylglutaryl-CoA
			HR	heart rate
EDSS	expanded disability status scale		HR_{max}	maximal heart rate (maximum heart rate)
EE	energy expenditure		HR_{peak}	peak heart rate
EMG	electromyographic		HRR	heart rate reserve
EMS	emergency medical services		HR_{rest}	resting heart rate
ERS	European Respiratory Society		HSCT	hematopoietic stem cell transplantation
Ex R$_x$	exercise prescription		HTN	hypertension
FBG	fasting blood glucose		HY	Hoehn and Yahr
FC	functional capacity		ICD	implantable cardiac defibrillator
FDA	Food and Drug Administration			
			ID	intellectual disability
$FEV_{1.0}$	forced expiratory volume in one second		IDF	International Diabetes Federation
FFBd	fat-free body density		IDL	intermediate-density lipoprotein
FFM	fat-free mass			
FITT	Frequency, Intensity, Time, and Type		IFG	impaired fasting glucose
			IGT	impaired glucose tolerance
FITT-VP	Frequency, Intensity, Time, and Type, Volume and Progression		ISA	intrinsic sympathomimetic activity
			IVC	obtained on inspiration
FM	fat mass		IVCD	intraventricular conduction delay
FN	false negative			
FP	false positive		JNC7	The Seventh Report of the Joint National Committee on Prevention, Detection, Evaluation, and Treatment of High Blood Pressure
FVC	forced vital capacity			
GEI	ACSM Certified Group Exercise Instructor^{SM}			
GFR	glomerular filtration rate			
GLP-1	glucagon-like peptide 1		JTA	job task analysis

K/DOQI	Kidney Disease Outcomes Quality Initiative
LABS	Longitudinal Assessment of Bariatric Surgery
LBBB	left bundle-branch block
LBP	low back pain
LDL	low-density lipoprotein cholesterol
L-G-L	Lown-Ganong-Levine syndrome
LLN	lower limit of normal
LMWH	low-molecular weight heparin
LV	left ventricular
LVH	left ventricular hypertrophy
MAO-I	monoamine oxidase inhibitor
MET	metabolic equivalent
MI	myocardial infarction
MS	multiple sclerosis
Msyn	metabolic syndrome
MVC	maximum voluntary contraction
$M\dot{V}O_2$	myocardial oxygen consumption
MVV	maximal voluntary ventilation
NCCA	National Commission for Certifying Agencies
NCEP	National Cholesterol Education Program
NCPAD	National Center on Physical Activity and Disability
NHANES	National Health and Nutrition Examination Survey
NHLBI	National Heart, Lung, and Blood Institute
non-DHP	Nondihydropyridines
NOTF	National Obesity Task Force
NPAS	National Physical Activity Society
NSAIDs	nonsteroidal anti-inflammatory drugs
O_2	oxygen
OGTT	oral glucose tolerance test
OSHA	Occupational Safety and Health Administration

P_aCO_2	arterial partial pressure of carbon dioxide (partial pressure of carbon dioxide in arterial blood)
PAC	premature atrial contraction
PAD	peripheral artery disease
PAG	physical activity guideline
P_aO_2	arterial partial pressure of oxygen (partial pressure of oxygen in arterial blood)
PARmed-X	Physical Activity Readiness
PAR-Q	Physical Activity Readiness Questionnaire
PD	Parkinson disease
PDE	phosphodiesterase
PEF	peak expiratory flow
$P_{ET}CO_2$	partial pressure of end-tidal carbon dioxide
PNF	proprioceptive neuromuscular facilitation
PPMS	primary progressive multiple sclerosis
PRMS	progressive relapsing multiple sclerosis
PTCA	percutaneous transluminal coronary angioplasty
PVC	premature ventricular contraction
$\dot{Q}$	cardiac output
QTc	QT corrected for heart rate
RCEP	ACSM Registered Clinical Exercise Physiologist®
RER	respiratory exchange ratio
RHR	resting heart rate
RM	repetition maximum
1-RM	one repetition maximum
ROM	range of motion
RPE	rating of perceived exertion
RPP	rate pressure product
RRMS	relapsing remitting multiple sclerosis
RT	resistance training
RVH	right ventricular hypertrophy
SaO_2	oxygen saturation in arterial blood (arterial oxygen saturation, arterial oxyhemoglobin saturation)

SARI	serotonin antagonist reuptake inhibitor		TPB	theory of planned behavior
			TTM	Transtheoretical Model
SBP	systolic blood pressure		USPSTF	U.S. Preventive Services Task Force
SCA	sudden cardiac arrest			
SCI	spinal cord injury		$\dot{V}CO_2$	carbon dioxide production
SCT	social cognitive theory		$\dot{V}E$	minute ventilation
SD	standard deviation		$\dot{V}E/\dot{V}CO_2$	minute ventilation/carbon dioxide production
SDT	self-determination theory			
SEE	standard error of estimate		$\dot{V}E/\dot{V}O_2$	ventilatory equivalent for oxygen
SET	social ecological theory			
SFT	Senior Fitness Test		$\dot{V}E_{max}$	maximal minute ventilation
SGOT	serum glutamic-oxaloacetic transaminase		$\dot{V}O_2$	oxygen uptake (oxygen consumption)
SGPT	serum glutamic-pyruvic transaminase		$\dot{V}O_{2max}$	maximal volume of oxygen consumed per minute (maximum oxygen consumption, maximal oxygen uptake)
SI	Système International			
SNRI	serotonin-norepinephrine reuptake inhibitor			
SPECT	single-photon emission computed tomography		$\dot{V}O_{2max}/\dot{V}CO_2$	ventilatory equivalent for carbon dioxide
SPMS	secondary progressive multiple sclerosis		$\dot{V}O_{2peak}$	peak oxygen uptake (peak oxygen consumption)
SpO_2	estimation of arterial oxygen saturation		$\dot{V}O_2R$	oxygen uptake reserve (oxygen consumption reserve)
SPPB	Short Physical Performance Battery			
			$\dot{V}O_2R_{max}$	maximal oxygen uptake reserve
SSRI	selective serotonin reuptake inhibitor			
SVC	slow expiration		V_1	chest lead I
SVT	supraventricular tachycardia		VC	vital capacity
			VF	ventricular fibrillation
Tc	technetium		VLDLs	very low-density lipoproteins
TCA	tricyclic antidepressant			
TeCA	tetracyclic antidepressant		VT	ventilatory threshold
THR	target heart rate		WBGT	wet-bulb globe temperature
TLC	total lung capacity		WCT	Wind Chill Temperature Index
TN	true negative			
TOBEC	total body electrical conductivity		WHO	World Health Organization
			WHR	waist-to-hip ratio
TP	true positive		W-P-W	Wolff-Parkinson-White syndrome

Health Appraisal and Risk Assessment

PAUL D. THOMPSON, MD, FACSM, FACC, *Associate Editor*

1

Benefits and Risks Associated with Physical Activity

The purpose of this chapter is to provide current information on the benefits and risks of physical activity and/or exercise. For clarification purposes, key terms used throughout the *Guidelines* related to physical activity and fitness are defined in this chapter. Additional information specific to a disease, disability, or health condition are explained within the context of the chapter in which they are discussed in the *Guidelines*. Physical activity continues to take on an increasingly important role in the prevention and treatment of multiple chronic diseases, health conditions, and their risk factors. Therefore, *Chapter 1* focuses on the public health perspective that forms the basis for the current physical activity recommendations (3,18,23,37,56). *Chapter 1* concludes with recommendations for reducing the incidence and severity of exercise-related complications for primary and secondary prevention programs.

PHYSICAL ACTIVITY AND FITNESS TERMINOLOGY

Physical activity and exercise are often used interchangeably, but these terms are not synonymous. *Physical activity* is defined as any bodily movement produced by the contraction of skeletal muscles that results in a substantial increase in caloric requirements over resting energy expenditure (8,43). *Exercise* is a type of physical activity consisting of planned, structured, and repetitive bodily movement done to improve and/or maintain one or more components of physical fitness. *Physical fitness* is defined as a set of attributes or characteristics individuals have or achieve that relates to their ability to perform physical activity. These characteristics are usually separated into the health-related and skill-related components of physical fitness (see *Box 1.1*).

In addition to defining physical activity, exercise, and physical fitness, it is important to clearly define the wide range of intensities associated with physical activity. Methods for quantifying the relative intensity of physical activity include specifying a percentage of oxygen uptake reserve ($\dot{V}O_2R$), heart rate reserve (HRR), oxygen consumption ($\dot{V}O_2$), heart rate (HR), or metabolic equivalents (METs) (see *Box 7.2*). Each of these methods for describing the intensity of physical activity has strengths and limitations. Although determining the most appropriate method is left to the health/fitness and clinical exercise professional,

BOX 1.1	Health-Related and Skill-Related Components of Physical Fitness

HEALTH-RELATED PHYSICAL FITNESS COMPONENTS
- Cardiorespiratory endurance: The ability of the circulatory and respiratory system to supply oxygen during sustained physical activity.
- Body composition: The relative amounts of muscle, fat, bone, and other vital parts of the body.
- Muscular strength: The ability of muscle to exert force.
- Muscular endurance: The ability of muscle to continue to perform without fatigue.
- Flexibility: The range of motion available at a joint.

SKILL-RELATED PHYSICAL FITNESS COMPONENTS
- Agility: The ability to change the position of the body in space with speed and accuracy.
- Coordination: The ability to use the senses, such as sight and hearing, together with body parts in performing tasks smoothly and accurately.
- Balance: The maintenance of equilibrium while stationary or moving.
- Power: The ability or rate at which one can perform work.
- Reaction time: The time elapsed between stimulation and the beginning of the reaction to it.
- Speed: The ability to perform a movement within a short period of time.

Adapted from (43,55). Available from http://www.fitness.gov/digest_mar2000.htm

Chapter 7 provides the methodology and guidelines for selecting a suitable method.

METs are a useful, convenient, and standarized way to describe the absolute intensity of a variety of physical activities. Light physical activity is defined as requiring <3 METs, moderate as 3–<6 METs, and vigorous as ≥6 METs (42). *Table 1.1* gives specific examples of activities in METs for each of the intensity ranges. A fairly complete list of physical activities and their associated estimates of energy expenditure can be found in the companion book of these *Guidelines, ACSM's Resource Manual for Guidelines for Exercise Testing and Prescription, Seventh Edition* (50).

Maximum aerobic capacity usually declines with age (14,37). For this reason, when older and younger individuals work at the same absolute MET level, the relative exercise intensity (*e.g.*, $\%\dot{V}O_{2max}$) will usually be different. In other words, the older individual will be working at a greater $\%\dot{V}O_{2max}$ than their younger counterpart (see *Chapter 8*). Nonetheless, physically active older adults may have aerobic capacities comparable to or greater than those of sedentary younger adults. *Table 1.2* shows the approximate relationships among relative and absolute exercise intensities for various fitness levels ranging from 6 to 12 METs.

TABLE 1.1. Metabolic Equivalents (METs) Values of Common Physical Activities Classified as Light, Moderate, or Vigorous Intensity

Light (<3 METs)	Moderate (3–<6 METs)	Vigorous (≥6 METs)
Walking	**Walking**	**Walking, jogging, and running**
Walking slowly around home, store, or office = 2.0[a]	Walking 3.0 mi · h^{-1} = 3.0[a]	Walking at very, very brisk pace (4.5 mi · h^{-1}) = 6.3[a]
Household and occupation	Walking at very brisk pace (4 mi · h^{-1}) = 5.0[a]	Walking/hiking at moderate pace and grade with no or light pack (<10 lb) = 7.0
Sitting—using computer, work at desk, using light hand tools = 1.5	**Household and occupation**	Hiking at steep grades and pack 10–42 lb = 7.5–9.0
Standing performing light work, such as making bed, washing dishes, ironing, preparing food, or store clerk = 2.0–2.5	Cleaning, heavy — washing windows, car, clean garage = 3.0	Jogging at 5 mi · h^{-1} = 8.0[a]
Leisure time and sports	Sweeping floors or carpet, vacuuming, mopping = 3.0–3.5	Jogging at 6 mi · h^{-1} = 10.0[a]
Arts and crafts, playing cards = 1.5	Carpentry — general = 3.6	Running at 7 mi · h^{-1} = 11.5[a]
Billiards = 2.5	Carrying and stacking wood = 5.5	**Household and occupation**
Boating — power = 2.5	Mowing lawn — walk power mower = 5.5	Shoveling sand, coal, etc. = 7.0
Croquet = 2.5	**Leisure time and sports**	Carrying heavy loads, such as bricks = 7.5
Darts = 2.5	Badminton — recreational = 4.5	Heavy farming, such as bailing hay = 8.0
Fishing — sitting = 2.5	Basketball — shooting a round = 4.5	Shoveling, digging ditches = 8.5
Playing most musical instruments = 2.0–2.5		**Leisure time and sports** Bicycling on flat — light effort (10–12 mi · h^{-1}) = 6.0
	Dancing — ballroom slow = 3.0; ballroom fast = 4.5	Basketball game = 8.0
	Fishing from riverbank and walking = 4.0	Bicycling on flat — moderate effort (12–14 mi · h^{-1}) = 8 fast (14–16 mi · h^{-1}) = 10
	Golf — walking pulling clubs = 4.3	Skiing cross-country — slow (2.5 mi · h^{-1} = 7.0; fast (5.0–7.9 mi · h^{-1}) = 9.0
	Sailing boat, wind surfing = 3.0	Soccer — casual = 7.0; competitive = 10.0
		Swimming leisurely = 6.0[b] Swimming — moderate/hard = 8–11[b]
	Table tennis = 4.0	Tennis singles = 8.0
	Tennis doubles = 5.0	Volleyball — competitive at gym or beach = 8.0
	Volleyball — noncompetitive = 3.0–4.0	

[a]On flat, hard surface.

[b]MET values can vary substantially from individual to individual during swimming as a result of different strokes and skill levels.

Adapted from (1).

TABLE 1.2. Classification of Physical Activity Intensity

Intensity	Relative Intensity		Absolute Intensity Ranges (METs) Across Fitness Levels			
	$\dot{V}O_2R(\%)$ HRR (%)	Maximal HR (%)	12 METs $\dot{V}O_{2max}$	10 METs $\dot{V}O_{2max}$	8 METs $\dot{V}O_{2max}$	6 METs $\dot{V}O_{2max}$
Very light	<20	<50	<3.2	<2.8	<2.4	<2.0
Light	20–<40	50–<64	3.2–<5.4	2.8–<4.6	2.4–<3.8	2.0–<3.1
Moderate	40–<60	64–<77	5.4–<7.6	4.6–<6.4	3.8–<5.2	3.1–<4.1
Vigorous (hard)	60–<85	77–<94	7.6–<10.3	6.4–<8.7	5.2–<7.0	4.1–<5.3
Vigorous (very hard)	85–<100	94–<100	10.3–<12	8.7–<10	7.0–<8	5.3–<6
Maximal	100	100	12	10	8	6

HR, heart rate; HRR, heart rate reserve; METs, metabolic equivalents (1 MET = 3.5 mL · kg^{-1} · min^{-1}); $\dot{V}O_{2max}$, maximal volume of oxygen consumed per minute; $\dot{V}O_2R$, oxygen uptake reserve.
Adapted from (18,24,55).

PUBLIC HEALTH PERSPECTIVE FOR CURRENT RECOMMENDATIONS

Over 25 yr ago, the American College of Sports Medicine (ACSM) in conjunction with the U.S. Centers for Disease Control and Prevention (CDC) (40), the U.S. Surgeon General (55), and the National Institutes of Health (41) issued landmark publications on physical activity and health. These publications called attention to the health-related benefits of regular physical activity that did not meet traditional criteria for improving fitness levels (*e.g.*, <20 min · session^{-1} of moderate rather than vigorous intensity).

An important goal of these reports was to clarify for public health, health/ fitness, clinical exercise, and health care professionals the amount and intensity of physical activity needed to improve health, lower susceptibility to disease (morbidity), and decrease premature mortality (40,41,55). In addition, these reports documented the dose-response relationship between physical activity and health (*i.e.*, some activity is better than none, and more activity, up to a point, is better than less). Williams (64) performed a meta-analysis of 23 sex-specific cohorts reporting varying levels of physical activity or fitness representing 1,325,004 individual-years of follow-up and showed a dose-response relationship between physical activity or physical fitness and the risks of coronary artery disease (CAD) and cardiovascular disease (CVD) (see *Figure 1.1*). It is clear that greater amounts of physical activity or increased physical fitness levels provide additional health benefits. *Table 1.3* provides the strength of evidence for the dose-response relationships among physical activity and numerous health outcomes.

More recently, the federal government convened an expert panel, the 2008 Physical Activity Guidelines Advisory Committee, to review the scientific evidence on physical activity and health published since the 1996 U.S. Surgeon General's Report (42). This committee found compelling evidence on the

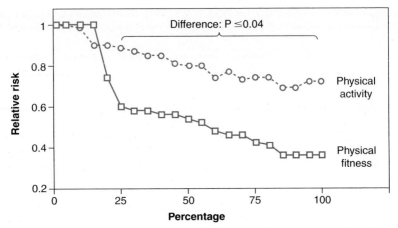

■ FIGURE 1.1. Estimated dose-response curve for the relative risk of atherosclerotic cardiovascular disease (CVD) by sample percentages of fitness and physical activity. Studies weighted by individual-years of experience. Used with permission from (64).

TABLE 1.3. Evidence for Dose-Response Relationship between Physical Activity and Health Outcome

Variable	Evidence for Inverse Dose-Response Relationship	Strength of Evidence[a]
All-cause mortality	Yes	Strong
Cardiorespiratory health	Yes	Strong
Metabolic health	Yes	Moderate
Energy balance:		
Weight maintenance	Insufficient data	Weak
Weight loss	Yes	Strong
Weight maintenance following weight loss	Yes	Moderate
Abdominal obesity	Yes	Moderate
Musculoskeletal health:		
Bone	Yes	Moderate
Joint	Yes	Strong
Muscular	Yes	Strong
Functional health	Yes	Moderate
Colon and breast cancers	Yes	Moderate
Mental health:		
Depression and distress	Yes	Moderate
Well-being Anxiety, cognitive health, and sleep	Insufficient data	Weak

[a]Strength of the evidence was classified as follows:

"Strong" — Strong, consistent across studies and populations

"Moderate" — Moderate or reasonable, reasonably consistent

"Weak" — Weak or limited, inconsistent across studies and populations

Adapted from (42).

benefits of physical activity for health (described in the following section) as well as the presence of a dose-response relationship for many diseases and health conditions.

Two important conclusions from the expert committee that have influenced the development of the recommendations appearing in the *Guidelines* are the following:

- Important health benefits can be obtained by performing a moderate amount of physical activity on most, if not all, days of the week.
- Additional health benefits result from greater amounts of physical activity. Individuals who maintain a regular program of physical activity that is longer in duration and/or of more vigorous intensity are likely to derive greater benefit than those who engage in lesser amounts.

In 1995, the CDC and ACSM issued the recommendation, "every U.S. adult should accumulate 30 minutes or more of moderate physical activity on most, preferably all, days of the week" (40). The intent of this statement was to increase public awareness of the importance of the health-related benefits of moderate intensity, physical activity. Unfortunately, although there is some evidence that leisure time physical inactivity has decreased (9), sedentary behavior remains a major public health concern. Specifically, only 46% of adults in the United States in a recent survey indicated that they met the minimum CDC-ACSM physical activity recommendation of participating in moderate intensity, physical activity for 30 min $\cdot$ d^{-1} on $\geq$5 d $\cdot$ wk^{-1} or vigorous intensity for 20 min $\cdot$ d^{-1} on $\geq$3 d $\cdot$ wk^{-1} (10).

As indicated earlier, the inverse relationship between physical activity and chronic disease and premature mortality is well established. Since the release of the U.S. Surgeon General's Report in 1996 (55), several reports have advocated physical activity levels above the minimum CDC-ACSM physical activity recommendations (14,18,36,46,54). These guidelines and recommendations primarily refer to the volume of physical activity required to prevent weight gain and/or obesity and should not be viewed as contradictory. In other words, physical activity that is sufficient to reduce the risk of developing chronic diseases and delaying mortality is likely insufficient to prevent or reverse weight gain and/or obesity given the typical American lifestyle. Physical activity beyond the minimum recommendations is likely needed in many individuals to manage and/or prevent weight gain and obesity.

Since the original 1995 CDC-ACSM recommendation (40), several large-scale epidemiologic studies have been performed that further document the dose-response relationship between physical activity and CVD and premature mortality (29,31,39,45,51,66). As a result of an increasing awareness of the adverse health effects of sedentary behavior and because of some confusion and misinterpretation of the original physical activity recommendations, the ACSM and American Heart Association (AHA) issued updated recommendations for physical activity and health in 2007 (see *Box 1.2*) (23).

BOX 1.2	The ACSM-AHA Primary Physical Activity Recommendations (23)

- All healthy adults aged 18–65 yr should participate in moderate intensity, aerobic physical activity for a minimum of 30 min on 5 d · wk^{-1} or vigorous intensity, aerobic activity for a minimum of 20 min on 3 d · wk^{-1}.
- Combinations of moderate and vigorous intensity exercise can be performed to meet this recommendation.
- Moderate intensity, aerobic activity can be accumulated to total the 30 min minimum by performing bouts each lasting ≥10 min.
- Every adult should perform activities that maintain or increase muscular strength and endurance for a minimum of 2 d · wk^{-1}.
- Because of the dose-response relationship between physical activity and health, individuals who wish to further improve their fitness, reduce their risk for chronic diseases and disabilities, and/or prevent unhealthy weight gain may benefit by exceeding the minimum recommended amounts of physical activity.

ACSM, American College of Sports Medicine; AHA, American Heart Association.

Similar recommendations have been made in the 2008 federal physical activity guidelines (http://www.health.gov/PAguidelines) (56) based on the *2008 Physical Activity Guidelines Advisory Committee Report* (42) (see *Box 1.3*). Regarding aerobic physical activity, rather than recommending a specific frequency of activity per week, the committee decided the scientific evidence supported a total volume of physical activity per week for health.

BOX 1.3	The Primary Physical Activity Recommendations from the 2008 Physical Activity Guidelines Committee Report (56)

- All Americans should participate in an amount of energy expenditure equivalent to 150 min · wk^{-1} of moderate intensity, aerobic activity; 75 min · wk^{-1} of vigorous intensity, aerobic activity; or a combination of both that generates energy equivalency to either regimen for substantial health benefits.
- These guidelines further specify a dose-response relationship, indicating additional health benefits are obtained with 300 min · wk^{-1} or more of moderate intensity, aerobic activity; 150 min · wk^{-1} or more of vigorous intensity, aerobic activity; or an equivalent combination of moderate and vigorous intensity, aerobic activity.

The 2008 federal physical activity guidelines also recommend breaking the total amount of physical activity into regular sessions during the week (*e.g.*, 30 min on 5 d · wk^{-1} of moderate intensity, aerobic activity) in order to reduce the risk of musculoskeletal injuries.

BENEFITS OF REGULAR PHYSICAL ACTIVITY AND/OR EXERCISE

Evidence to support the inverse relationship between physical activity and premature mortality, CVD/CAD, hypertension, stroke, osteoporosis, Type 2 diabetes mellitus, metabolic syndrome, obesity, colon cancer, breast cancer, depression, functional health, falls, and cognitive function continues to accumulate (42). For many of these diseases and health conditions, there is also strong evidence of a dose-response relationship (see *Table 1.3*). This evidence has resulted from laboratory-based studies as well as large-scale, population-based, observational studies (16,18,23,26,30,55,62).

Since the last edition of the *Guidelines*, additional evidence has strengthened support for these relationships. As stated in the recent ACSM-AHA updated recommendation on physical activity and health (23), "since the 1995 recommendation, several large scale observational epidemiologic studies, enrolling thousands to tens of thousands of individuals, have clearly documented a dose-response relationship between physical activity and risk of cardiovascular disease and premature mortality in men and women, and in ethnically diverse participants" (29,31,38,45,51,66). The 2008 Physical Activity Guidelines Advisory Committee also arrived at similar conclusions (42). It is also important to note aerobic capacity (*i.e.*, cardiorespiratory fitness [CRF]) has an inverse relationship with risk of premature death from all causes and specifically from CVD, and higher levels of CRF are associated with higher levels of habitual physical activity, which in turn are associated with many health benefits (6,7,28,47,61). *Box 1.4* summarizes the benefits of regular physical activity and/or exercise.

Recently, the ACSM and AHA have released statements on "Physical Activity and Public Health in Older Adults" (3,37). In general, these recommendations are similar to the updated guidelines for adults (18,23), but the recommended intensity of aerobic activity is related to the older adult's CRF level. In addition, age-specific recommendations are made concerning the importance of flexibility, neuromotor, and muscle strengthening activities.

In addition, the 2008 federal physical activity guidelines made similar age-specific recommendations targeted at adults (18–64 yr) and older adults (≥65 yr) as well as children and adolescents (6–17 yr) (http://www.health.gov/PAguidelines) (56).

RISKS ASSOCIATED WITH EXERCISE

In general, exercise does not provoke cardiovascular events in healthy individuals with normal cardiovascular systems. The risk of sudden cardiac arrest or myocardial infarction (MI) is very low in apparently healthy individuals performing moderate intensity, physical activity (60,63). However, there is an acute and transient increase in the risk of sudden cardiac death and/or MI in individuals performing vigorous intensity exercise with either diagnosed or occult CVD (20,35,48,52,60,65). Therefore, the risk of these events during exercise increases

BOX 1.4	Benefits of Regular Physical Activity and/or Exercise

IMPROVEMENT IN CARDIOVASCULAR AND RESPIRATORY FUNCTION

- Increased maximal oxygen uptake resulting from both central and peripheral adaptations
- Decreased minute ventilation at a given absolute submaximal intensity
- Decreased myocardial oxygen cost for a given absolute submaximal intensity
- Decreased heart rate and blood pressure at a given submaximal intensity
- Increased capillary density in skeletal muscle
- Increased exercise threshold for the accumulation of lactate in the blood
- Increased exercise threshold for the onset of disease signs or symptoms (*e.g.*, angina pectoris, ischemic ST-segment depression, claudication)

REDUCTION IN CARDIOVASCULAR DISEASE RISK FACTORS

- Reduced resting systolic/diastolic pressure
- Increased serum high-density lipoprotein cholesterol and decreased serum triglycerides
- Reduced total body fat, reduced intra-abdominal fat
- Reduced insulin needs, improved glucose tolerance
- Reduced blood platelet adhesiveness and aggregation
- Reduced inflammation

DECREASED MORBIDITY AND MORTALITY

- Primary prevention (*i.e.*, interventions to prevent the initial occurrence)
- Higher activity and/or fitness levels are associated with lower death rates from coronary artery disease
- Higher activity and/or fitness levels are associated with lower incidence rates for CVD, CAD, stroke, Type 2 diabetes mellitus, metabolic syndrome, osteoporotic fractures, cancer of the colon and breast, and gallbladder disease
- Secondary prevention (*i.e.*, interventions after a cardiac event to prevent another)
- Based on meta-analyses (*i.e.*, pooled data across studies), cardiovascular and all-cause mortality are reduced in patients with post-myocardial infarction (MI) who participate in cardiac rehabilitation exercise training, especially as a component of multifactorial risk factor reduction
- Randomized controlled trials of cardiac rehabilitation exercise training involving patients with post-MI do not support a reduction in the rate of nonfatal reinfarction

OTHER BENEFITS

- Decreased anxiety and depression
- Improved cognitive function

BOX 1.4	Benefits of Regular Physical Activity and/or Exercise *(Continued)*

- Enhanced physical function and independent living in older individuals
- Enhanced feelings of well-being
- Enhanced performance of work, recreational, and sport activities
- Reduced risk of falls and injuries from falls in older individuals
- Prevention or mitigation of functional limitations in older adults
- Effective therapy for many chronic diseases in older adults

CAD, coronary artery disease; CVD, cardiovascular disease.
Adapted from (26,37,55).

with the prevalence of CVD in the population. *Chapter 2* includes the preparticipation health screening guidelines for individuals who wish to be physically active in order to maximize the many health benefits associated with physical activity, while minimizing the risks.

SUDDEN CARDIAC DEATH AMONG YOUNG INDIVIDUALS

The risk of sudden cardiac death in individuals younger than 30–40 yr is very low because of the low prevalence of CVD in this population. In 2007, the AHA released a scientific statement on "Exercise and Acute Cardiovascular Events: Placing the Risks into Perspective" (2). *Table 1.4* (taken from this publication) shows the cardiovascular causes of exercise-related sudden death in young athletes. It is clear from these data that the most common causes of death in young individuals are congenital and hereditary abnormalities including hypertrophic cardiomyopathy, coronary artery abnormalities, and aortic stenosis. The absolute annual risk of exercise-related death among high school and college athletes is one per 133,000 men and 769,000 women (57). It should be noted that these rates, although low, include all sports-related nontraumatic deaths. Of the 136 total identifiable causes of death, 100 were caused by CVD. A more recent estimate places the annual incidence of cardiovascular deaths among young competitive athletes in the United States as one death per 185,000 men and 1.5 million women. (32). Some experts, however, believe the incidence of exercise-related sudden death in young sports participants is as high as one per 50,000 athletes per year. (15). Experts debate on why estimates of the incidence of exercise-related sudden deaths vary among studies. These variances are likely due to differences in (a) the populations studied; (b) estimation of the number of sport participants; and (c) subject and/or incident case assignment.

TABLE 1.4. Cardiovascular Causes of Exercise-Related Sudden Death in Young Athletes[a]

	Van Camp (n = 100)[b] (57)	Maron (n = 134) (33)	Corrado (n = 55)[c] (12)
Hypertrophic CM	51	36	1
Probable hypertrophic CM	5	10	0
Coronary anomalies	18	23	9
Valvular and subvalvular aortic stenosis	8	4	0
Possible myocarditis	7	3	5
Dilated and nonspecific CM	7	3	1
Atherosclerotic CVD	3	2	10
Aortic dissection/rupture	2	5	1
Arrhythmogenic right ventricular CM	1	3	11
Myocardial scarring	0	3	0
Mitral valve prolapse	1	2	6
Other congenital abnormalities	0	1.5	0
Long QT syndrome	0	0.5	0
Wolff-Parkinson-White syndrome	1	0	1
Cardiac conduction disease	0	0	3
Cardiac sarcoidosis	0	0.5	0
Coronary artery aneurysm	1	0	0
Normal heart at necropsy	7	2	1
Pulmonary thromboembolism	0	0	1

[a]Ages ranged from 13 to 24 yr (57), 12 to 40 yr (33), and 12 to 35 yr (12). References (57) and (33) used the same database and include many of the same athletes. All (57), 90% (33), and 89% (12) had symptom onset during or within an hour of training or competition.

[b]Total exceeds 100% because several athletes had multiple abnormalities.

[c]Includes some athletes whose deaths were not associated with recent exertion. Includes aberrant artery origin and course, tunneled arteries, and other abnormalities.

CM, cardiomyopathy; CVD, cardiovascular disease.

Used with permission from (2).

EXERCISE-RELATED CARDIAC EVENTS IN ADULTS

The risk of sudden cardiac death or acute MI is higher in middle-aged and older adults than in younger individuals. This is due to the higher prevalence of CVD in the older population. The absolute risk of sudden cardiac death during vigorous intensity, physical activity has been estimated at one per year for every 15,000–18,000 previously asymptomatic individuals (48,53). Although these rates are low, more recent available research has confirmed the increased rate of sudden cardiac death and acute MI among adults performing vigorous intensity exercise when compared with their younger counterparts (20,35,48,53,65). In addition, the rates of sudden cardiac death and acute MI are disproportionately higher in the most sedentary individuals when they perform unaccustomed or infrequent exercise (2).

Health/fitness and clinical exercise professionals should understand that although there is an increased risk of sudden cardiac death and acute MI with vigorous intensity exercise, the physically active or fit adult has about 30%–40% lower risk of developing CVD compared to those who are inactive (56). The exact mechanism of sudden cardiac death during vigorous intensity exercise with asymptomatic adults is not completely understood. However, evidence exists that the increased frequency of cardiac contraction and excursion of the coronary arteries produces bending and flexing of the coronary arteries may be the underlying cause. This response may cause cracking of the atherosclerotic plaque with resulting platelet aggregation and possible acute thrombosis and has been documented angiographically in individuals with exercise-induced cardiac events (5,11,21).

EXERCISE TESTING AND THE RISK OF CARDIAC EVENTS

As with vigorous intensity exercise, the risk of cardiac events during exercise testing varies directly with the prevalence of diagnosed or occult CVD in the study population. Several studies have documented the risks of exercise testing (4,19,25,27,34,44,49). _Table 1.5_ summarizes the risks of various cardiac events including acute MI, ventricular fibrillation, hospitalization, and death. These data indicate in a mixed population the risk of exercise testing is low with approximately six cardiac events per 10,000 tests. One of these studies includes data for which the exercise testing was supervised by nonphysicians (27). In addition, the majority of these studies used symptom-limited exercise tests. Therefore, it would be expected that the risk of submaximal testing in a similar population would be lower.

TABLE 1.5. Cardiac Complications during Exercise Testing[a]

Reference	Year	Site	No. of Tests	MI	VF	Death	Hospitalization	Comment
Rochmis (44)	1971	73 U.S. centers	170,000	NA	NA	1	3	34% of tests were symptom limited; 50% of deaths in 8 h; 50% over the next 4 d
Irving (25)	1977	15 Seattle facilities	10,700	NA	4.67	0	NR	
McHenry (34)	1977	Hospital	12,000	0	0	0	0	
Atterhog (4)	1979	20 Swedish centers	50,000	0.8	0.8	6.4	5.2	
Stuart (49)	1980	1,375 U.S. centers	518,448	3.58	4.78	0.5	NR	VF includes other dysrhythmias requiring treatment
Gibbons (19)	1989	Cooper Clinic	71,914	0.56	0.29	0	NR	Only 4% of men and 2% of women had CVD
Knight (27)	1995	Geisinger Cardiology Service	28,133	1.42	1.77	0	NR	25% were inpatient tests supervised by non-MDs

[a]Events are per 10,000 tests.

CVD, cardiovascular disease; MD, medical doctor; MI, myocardial infarction; NA, not applicable; NR, not reported; VF, ventricular fibrillation.

RISKS OF CARDIAC EVENTS DURING CARDIAC REHABILITATION

The highest risk of cardiovascular events occurs in those individuals with diagnosed CAD. In one survey, there was one nonfatal complication per 34,673 h and one fatal cardiovascular complication per 116,402 h of cardiac rehabilitation (22). More recent studies have found a lower rate, one cardiac arrest per 116,906 patient-hours, one MI per 219,970 patient-hours, one fatality per 752,365 patient-hours, and one major complication per 81,670 patient-hours (13,17,58,59). These studies are presented in *Table 1.6* (2). Although these complication rates are low, it should be noted that patients were screened and exercised in medically supervised settings equipped to handle cardiac emergencies. The mortality rate appears to be six times higher when patients exercised in facilities without the ability to successfully manage cardiac arrest (2,13,17,58,59). Interestingly, however, a review of home-based cardiac rehabilitation programs found no increase in cardiovascular complications versus formal center-based exercise programs (62).

PREVENTION OF EXERCISE-RELATED CARDIAC EVENTS

Because of the low incidence of cardiac events related to vigorous intensity exercise, it is very difficult to test the effectiveness of strategies to reduce the occurrence of these events. According to a recent statement by the ACSM and AHA, "Physicians should not overestimate the risks of exercise because the benefits of habitual physical activity substantially outweigh the risks." This report also recommends several strategies to reduce these cardiac events during vigorous intensity exercise (2):

- Health care professionals should know the pathologic conditions associated with exercise-related events so that physically active children and adults can be appropriately evaluated.

TABLE 1.6. Summary of Contemporary Exercise-Based Cardiac Rehabilitation Program Complication Rates

Investigator	Year	Patient Exercise Hours	Cardiac Arrest	Myocardial Infarction	Fatal Events	Major Complications[a]
Van Camp (58)	1980–1984	2,351,916	1/111,996[b]	1/293,990	1/783,972	1/81,101
Digenio (13)	1982–1988	480,000	1/120,000[c]		1/160,000	1/120,000
Vongvanich (59)	1986–1995	268,503	1/89,501[d]	1/268,503[d]	0/268,503	1/67,126
Franklin (17)	1982–1998	292,254	1/146,127[d]	1/97,418[d]	0/292,254	1/58,451
Average			1/116,906	1/219,970	1/752,365	1/81,670

[a]Myocardial infarction and cardiac arrest.
[b]Fatal 14%.
[c]Fatal 75%.
[d]Fatal 0%.
Used with permission from (2).

- Physically active individuals should know the nature of cardiac prodromal symptoms (*e.g.*, excessive, unusual fatigue and pain in the chest and/or upper back) and seek prompt medical care if such symptoms develop (see *Table 2.1*).
- High school and college athletes should undergo preparticipation screening by qualified professionals.
- Athletes with known cardiac conditions or a family history should be evaluated prior to competition using established guidelines.
- Health care facilities should ensure their staff is trained in managing cardiac emergencies and have a specified plan and appropriate resuscitation equipment (see *Appendix B*).
- Physically active individuals should modify their exercise program in response to variations in their exercise capacity, habitual activity level, and the environment (see *Chapters 7* and *8*).

Although strategies for reducing the number of cardiovascular events during vigorous intensity exercise have not been systematically studied, it is incumbent on the health/fitness and clinical exercise professional to take reasonable precautions when working with individuals who wish to become more physically active/fit and/or increase their physical activity/fitness levels. These precautions are particularly true when the exercise program will be of vigorous intensity. Although many sedentary individuals can safely begin a light-to-moderate intensity, physical activity program, individuals of all ages should undergo risk classification to determine the need for further medical evaluation and/or clearance, need for and type of exercise testing (maximal or submaximal), and need for medical supervision during testing (see *Chapter 2*).

Sedentary individuals or those who exercise infrequently should begin their programs at lower intensities and progress at a slower rate because a disproportionate number of cardiac events occur in this population. Individuals with known or suspected cardiovascular, pulmonary, metabolic, or renal disease should obtain medical clearance before beginning a vigorous intensity exercise program. Health/fitness and clinical exercise professionals who supervise vigorous intensity exercise programs should have current training in basic and/or advanced cardiac life support and emergency procedures. These emergency procedures should be reviewed and practiced at regular intervals (see *Appendix B*). Finally, individuals should be educated on the signs and symptoms of CVD and should be referred to a physician for further evaluation should these symptoms occur.

THE BOTTOM LINE

- A large body of scientific evidence supports the role of physical activity in delaying premature mortality and reducing the risks of many chronic diseases and health conditions. There is also clear evidence for a dose-response relationship between physical activity and health. Thus, any amount of physical activity should be encouraged.
- Ideally, an initial target should be 150 min $\cdot$ wk^{-1} of moderate intensity, aerobic activity; 75 min $\cdot$ wk^{-1} of vigorous intensity, aerobic activity; or an equivalent

combination of moderate and vigorous intensity, aerobic activity. To minimize musculoskeletal injuries, physical activity bouts should be broken up during the week (*e.g.*, 30 min of moderate intensity, aerobic activity on 5 d · wk^{-1}).

- Additional health benefits result from greater amounts of physical activity. Individuals who maintain a regular program of physical activity that is longer in duration and/or is more vigorous in intensity are likely to derive greater benefit than those who do lesser amounts.

- Although the risks associated with exercise transiently increase while exercising, especially exercising at vigorous intensity, the benefits of habitual physical activity substantially outweigh the risks. In addition, the transient increase in risk is of lesser magnitude among individuals who are regularly physically active compared with those who are inactive.

Online Resources

American College of Sports Medicine Position Stand on the Quantity and Quality of Exercise:
http://www.acsm.org

2008 Physical Activity Guidelines for All Americans:
http://www.health.gov/PAguidelines

REFERENCES

1. Ainsworth BE, Haskell WL, Whitt MC, et al. Compendium of physical activities: an update of activity codes and MET intensities. *Med Sci Sports Exerc*. 2000;32(9 Suppl):S498–504.
2. American College of Sports Medicine, American Heart Association. Exercise and acute cardiovascular events: placing the risks into perspective. *Med Sci Sports Exerc*. 2007;39(5):886–97.
3. American College of Sports Medicine, Chodzko-Zajko WJ, Proctor DN, et al. American College of Sports Medicine position stand. Exercise and physical activity for older adults. *Med Sci Sports Exerc*. 2009;41(7):1510–30.
4. Atterhog JH, Jonsson B, Samuelsson R. Exercise testing: a prospective study of complication rates. *Am Heart J*. 1979;98(5):572–9.
5. Black A, Black MM, Gensini G. Exertion and acute coronary artery injury. *Angiology*. 1975;26(11):759–83.
6. Blair SN, Kohl HW,3rd, Barlow CE, Paffenbarger RS,Jr, Gibbons LW, Macera CA. Changes in physical fitness and all-cause mortality. A prospective study of healthy and unhealthy men. *JAMA*. 1995;273(14):1093–8.
7. Blair SN, Kohl HW,3rd, Paffenbarger RS,Jr, Clark DG, Cooper KH, Gibbons LW. Physical fitness and all-cause mortality. A prospective study of healthy men and women. *JAMA*. 1989;262(17):2395–401.
8. Caspersen CJ, Powell KE, Christenson GM. Physical activity, exercise, and physical fitness: definitions and distinctions for health-related research. *Public Health Rep*. 1985;100(2):126–31.
9. Centers for Disease Control and Prevention. Adult participation in recommended levels of physical activity—United States, 2001 and 2003. *MMWR Morb Mortal Wkly Rep*. 2005;54(47):1208–12.
10. Centers for Disease Control and Prevention. Trends in leisure-time physical inactivity by age, sex, and race/ethnicity—United States, 1994–2004. *MMWR Morb Mortal Wkly Rep*. 2005;54(39):991–4.
11. Ciampricotti R, Deckers JW, Taverne R, el Gamal M, Relik-van Wely L, Pool J. Characteristics of conditioned and sedentary men with acute coronary syndromes. *Am J Cardiol*. 1994;73(4):219–22.
12. Corrado D, Basso C, Rizzoli G, Schiavon M, Thiene G. Does sports activity enhance the risk of sudden death in adolescents and young adults? *J Am Coll Cardiol*. 2003;42(11):1959–63.
13. Digenio AG, Sim JG, Dowdeswell RJ, Morris R. Exercise-related cardiac arrest in cardiac rehabilitation. The Johannesburg experience. *S Afr Med J*. 1991;79(4):188–91.
14. Donnelly JE, Blair SN, Jakicic JM, et al. American College of Sports Medicine Position Stand. Appropriate physical activity intervention strategies for weight loss and prevention of weight regain for adults. *Med Sci Sports Exerc*. 2009;41(2):459–71.

15. Drezner JA, Chun JS, Harmon KG, Derminer L. Survival trends in the United States following exercise-related sudden cardiac arrest in the youth: 2000–2006. *Heart Rhythm.* 2008;5(6):794–9.
16. Feskanich D, Willett W, Colditz G. Walking and leisure-time activity and risk of hip fracture in postmenopausal women. *JAMA.* 2002;288(18):2300–6.
17. Franklin BA, Bonzheim K, Gordon S, Timmis GC. Safety of medically supervised outpatient cardiac rehabilitation exercise therapy: a 16-year follow-up. *Chest.* 1998;114(3):902–6.
18. Garber CE, Blissmer B, Deschenes MR, et al. American College of Sports Medicine Position Stand. The quantity and quality of exercise for developing and maintaining cardiorespiratory, musculoskeletal, and neuromotor fitness in apparently healthy adults: guidance for prescribing exercise. *Med Sci Sports Exerc.* 2011;43(7):1334–559.
19. Gibbons L, Blair SN, Kohl HW, Cooper K. The safety of maximal exercise testing. *Circulation.* 1989;80(4):846–52.
20. Giri S, Thompson PD, Kiernan FJ, et al. Clinical and angiographic characteristics of exertion-related acute myocardial infarction. *JAMA.* 1999;282(18):1731–6.
21. Hammoudeh AJ, Haft JI. Coronary-plaque rupture in acute coronary syndromes triggered by snow shoveling. *N Engl J Med.* 1996;335(26):2001.
22. Haskell WL. Cardiovascular complications during exercise training of cardiac patients. *Circulation.* 1978;57(5):920–4.
23. Haskell WL, Lee IM, Pate RR, et al. Physical activity and public health: updated recommendation for adults from the American College of Sports Medicine and the American Heart Association. *Med Sci Sports Exerc.* 2007;39(8):1423–34.
24. Howley ET. Type of activity: resistance, aerobic and leisure versus occupational physical activity. *Med Sci Sports Exerc.* 2001;33(6 Suppl):S364,S369; discussion S419–20.
25. Irving JB, Bruce RA, DeRouen TA. Variations in and significance of systolic pressure during maximal exercise (treadmill) testing. *Am J Cardiol.* 1977;39(6):841–8.
26. Kesaniemi YK, Danforth E,Jr, Jensen MD, Kopelman PG, Lefebvre P, Reeder BA. Dose-response issues concerning physical activity and health: an evidence-based symposium. *Med Sci Sports Exerc.* 2001;33(6 Suppl):S351–8.
27. Knight JA, Laubach CA,Jr, Butcher RJ, Menapace FJ. Supervision of clinical exercise testing by exercise physiologists. *Am J Cardiol.* 1995;75(5):390–1.
28. Kodama S, Saito K, Tanaka S, et al. Cardiorespiratory fitness as a quantitative predictor of all-cause mortality and cardiovascular events in healthy men and women: a meta-analysis. *JAMA.* 2009;301(19):2024–35.
29. Lee IM, Rexrode KM, Cook NR, Manson JE, Buring JE. Physical activity and coronary heart disease in women: is "no pain, no gain" passe? *JAMA.* 2001;285(11):1447–54.
30. Leitzmann MF, Rimm EB, Willett WC, et al. Recreational physical activity and the risk of cholecystectomy in women. *N Engl J Med.* 1999;341(11):777–84.
31. Manson JE, Greenland P, LaCroix AZ, et al. Walking compared with vigorous exercise for the prevention of cardiovascular events in women. *N Engl J Med.* 2002;347(10):716–25.
32. Maron BJ, Doerer JJ, Haas TS, Tierney DM, Mueller FO. Sudden deaths in young competitive athletes: analysis of 1866 deaths in the United States, 1980–2006. *Circulation.* 2009;119(8):1085–92.
33. Maron BJ, Shirani J, Poliac LC, Mathenge R, Roberts WC, Mueller FO. Sudden death in young competitive athletes. Clinical, demographic, and pathological profiles. *JAMA.* 1996;276(3):199–204.
34. McHenry PL. Risks of graded exercise testing. *Am J Cardiol.* 1977;39(6):935–7.
35. Mittleman MA, Maclure M, Tofler GH, Sherwood JB, Goldberg RJ, Muller JE. Triggering of acute myocardial infarction by heavy physical exertion. Protection against triggering by regular exertion. Determinants of Myocardial Infarction Onset Study Investigators. *N Engl J Med.* 1993;329(23):1677–83.
36. National Research Council (U.S.). *Dietary Reference Intakes for Energy, Carbohydrates, Fiber, Fat, Protein, and Amino Acids.* Washington (DC): National Academies; 2003. 1331 p.
37. Nelson ME, Rejeski WJ, Blair SN, et al. Physical activity and public health in older adults: recommendation from the American College of Sports Medicine and the American Heart Association. *Med Sci Sports Exerc.* 2007;39(8):1435–45.
38. Paffenbarger RS,Jr, Hyde RT, Wing AL, Lee IM, Jung DL, Kampert JB. The association of changes in physical-activity level and other lifestyle characteristics with mortality among men. *N Engl J Med.* 1993;328(8):538–45.
39. Paffenbarger RS,Jr, Lee IM. Smoking, physical activity, and active life expectancy. *Clin J Sport Med.* 1999;9(4):244.
40. Pate RR, Pratt M, Blair SN, et al. Physical activity and public health. A recommendation from the Centers for Disease Control and Prevention and the American College of Sports Medicine. *JAMA.* 1995;273(5):402–7.
41. Physical activity and cardiovascular health. NIH Consensus Development Panel on Physical Activity and Cardiovascular Health. *JAMA.* 1996;276(3):241–6.

42. *Physical Activity Guidelines Advisory Committee Report, 2008. To the Secretary of Health and Human Services* [Internet]. Washington (DC): U.S. Department of Health and Human Services; 2008 [cited 2010 Aug 11]. 683 p. Available from: http://www.health.gov/paguidelines/committeereport.aspx; http://www.health.gov/paguidelines/Report/pdf/CommitteeReport.pdf

43. The President's Council on Physical Fitness and Sports. *Definitions—Health, Fitness, and Physical Activity* [Internet]. Washington (DC): President's Council on Physical Fitness and Sports; 2000 [cited 2012 Jan 7]. 11 p. Available from: http://purl.access.gpo.gov/GPO/LPS21074

44. Rochmis P, Blackburn H. Exercise tests. A survey of procedures, safety, and litigation experience in approximately 170,000 tests. *JAMA.* 1971;217(8):1061–6.

45. Rockhill B, Willett WC, Manson JE, et al. Physical activity and mortality: a prospective study among women. *Am J Public Health.* 2001;91(4):578–83.

46. Saris WH, Blair SN, van Baak MA, et al. How much physical activity is enough to prevent unhealthy weight gain? Outcome of the IASO 1st Stock Conference and consensus statement. *Obes Rev.* 2003;4(2):101–14.

47. Sesso HD, Paffenbarger RS Jr, Lee IM. Physical activity and coronary heart disease in men: The Harvard Alumni Health Study. *Circulation.* 2000;102(9):975–80.

48. Siscovick DS, Weiss NS, Fletcher RH, Lasky T. The incidence of primary cardiac arrest during vigorous exercise. *N Engl J Med.* 1984;311(14):874–7.

49. Stuart RJ Jr, Ellestad MH. National survey of exercise stress testing facilities. *Chest.* 1980;77(1):94–7.

50. Swain DP, American College of Sports Medicine. *ACSM's Resource Manual for Guidelines for Exercise Testing and Prescription.* 7th ed. Baltimore (MD): Lippincott Williams & Wilkins; 2014.

51. Tanasescu M, Leitzmann MF, Rimm EB, Willett WC, Stampfer MJ, Hu FB. Exercise type and intensity in relation to coronary heart disease in men. *JAMA.* 2002;288(16):1994–2000.

52. Thompson PD, Funk EJ, Carleton RA, Sturner WQ. Incidence of death during jogging in Rhode Island from 1975 through 1980. *JAMA.* 1982;247(18):2535–8.

53. Thompson PD, Stern MP, Williams P, Duncan K, Haskell WL, Wood PD. Death during jogging or running. A study of 18 cases. *JAMA.* 1979;242(12):1265–7.

54. U.S. Department of Agriculture, U.S. Department of Health and Human Services. *Dietary Guidelines for Americans, 2010.* 7th ed. Washington (DC): U.S. Government Printing Office; 2010. 112 p.

55. U.S. Department of Health and Human Services. *Physical Activity and Health: A Report of the Surgeon General.* Atlanta, GA: U.S. Department of Health and Human Services, Public Health Service, CDC, National Center for Chronic Disease Prevention and Health Promotion; 1996. 278 p.

56. U.S. Department of Health and Human Services. *2008 Physical Activity Guidelines for Americans* [Internet]. Rockville (MD): Office of Disease Prevention & Health Promotion, U.S. Department of Health and Human Services; 2008 [cited 2012 Jan 7]. 76 p. Available from: http://www.health.gov/paguidelines

57. Van Camp SP, Bloor CM, Mueller FO, Cantu RC, Olson HG. Nontraumatic sports death in high school and college athletes. *Med Sci Sports Exerc.* 1995;27(5):641–7.

58. Van Camp SP, Peterson RA. Cardiovascular complications of outpatient cardiac rehabilitation programs. *JAMA.* 1986;256(9):1160–3.

59. Vongvanich P, Paul-Labrador MJ, Merz CN. Safety of medically supervised exercise in a cardiac rehabilitation center. *Am J Cardiol.* 1996;77(15):1383–5.

60. Vuori I. The cardiovascular risks of physical activity. *Acta Med Scand Suppl.* 1986;711:205–14.

61. Wang CY, Haskell WL, Farrell SW, et al. Cardiorespiratory fitness levels among US adults 20-49 years of age: findings from the 1999-2004 National Health and Nutrition Examination Survey. *Am J Epidemiol.* 2010;171(4):426–35.

62. Wenger NK, Froelicher ES, Smith LK, et al. Cardiac rehabilitation as secondary prevention. Agency for Health Care Policy and Research and National Heart, Lung, and Blood Institute. *Clin Pract Guidel Quick Ref Guide Clin.* 1995;(17):1–23.

63. Whang W, Manson JE, Hu FB, et al. Physical exertion, exercise, and sudden cardiac death in women. *JAMA.* 2006;295(12):1399–403.

64. Williams PT. Physical fitness and activity as separate heart disease risk factors: a meta–analysis. *Med Sci Sports Exerc.* 2001;33(5):754–61.

65. Willich SN, Lewis M, Lowel H, Arntz HR, Schubert F, Schroder R. Physical exertion as a trigger of acute myocardial infarction. Triggers and Mechanisms of Myocardial Infarction Study Group. *N Engl J Med.* 1993;329(23):1684–90.

66. Yu S, Yarnell JW, Sweetnam PM, Murray L, Caerphilly study. What level of physical activity protects against premature cardiovascular death? The Caerphilly study. *Heart.* 2003;89(5):502–6.

2

Preparticipation Health Screening

The previous versions of *Chapter 2* have recommended cardiovascular disease (CVD) risk assessment and stratification of all individuals, and a medical examination and symptom-limited exercise testing as part of the preparticipation health screening prior to initiating vigorous intensity, physical activity in individuals at increased risk for occult CVD. Individuals at increased risk in these recommendations were men ≥45 and women ≥55 yr, those with two or more major CVD risk factors, individuals with signs and symptoms of CVD, and those with known cardiac, pulmonary, or metabolic disease. These recommendations were designed to avoid exposing physically unfit individuals to the documented risks of exercise including sudden cardiac death and acute myocardial infarction (MI) as discussed in *Chapter 1*.

Compared to previous editions of the *Guidelines*, the present version of *Chapter 2* regarding the preparticipation health screening process:

- Reduces the emphasis on the need for medical evaluation (*i.e.*, medical examination and exercise testing) as part of the preparticipation health screening process prior to initiating a progressive exercise regimen in healthy, asymptomatic individuals.
- Uses the term *risk classification* to group individuals as low, moderate, or high risk based on the presence or absence of CVD risk factors, signs and symptoms, and/or known cardiovascular, pulmonary, renal, or metabolic disease.
- Emphasizes identifying those with known disease because they are at greatest risk for an exercise-related cardiac event.
- Adopts the American Association of Cardiovascular and Pulmonary Rehabilitation (AACVPR) risk stratification scheme for individuals with known CVD because it considers overall patient prognosis and potential for rehabilitation (32) (see *Chapter 9*).
- Supports the public health message that all individuals should adopt a physically active lifestyle.

This edition of the *Guidelines* continues to encourage atherosclerotic CVD risk factor assessment because such measurements are an important part of the preparticipation health screening process and good medical care, but does seek to simplify the preparticipation health screening process in order to remove unnecessary and unproven barriers to adopting a physically active lifestyle (24). This edition of the *Guidelines* also recommends health/fitness and clinical exercise professionals consult with their medical colleagues when there are questions about patients with known disease and their ability to participate in exercise programs.

There are multiple considerations that have prompted these different points of emphasis in the present version of *Chapter 2*. The risk of a cardiovascular event is increased during vigorous intensity exercise relative to rest, but the absolute risk of a cardiac event is low in healthy individuals (see *Chapter 1*). Recommending a medical examination and/or stress test as part of the preparticipation health screening process for all individuals at moderate to high risk prior to initiating light-to-moderate intensity exercise programs implies being physically active confers greater risk than a sedentary lifestyle (7). Yet, the cardiovascular health benefits of regular exercise far outweigh the risks of exercise for the general population (28,29). There is also an increased appreciation that exercise testing is a poor predictor of CVD events in asymptomatic individuals probably because such testing detects flow-limiting coronary lesions, whereas sudden cardiac death and acute MI are usually produced by the rapid progression of a previously nonobstructive lesion (29).

Furthermore, there is lack of consensus regarding the extent of the medical evaluation (*i.e.*, medical examination, stress testing) needed as part of the preparticipation health screening process prior to initiating an exercise program even if it is of vigorous intensity. The American College of Cardiology (ACC)/American Heart Association (AHA) recommend exercise testing prior to moderate or vigorous intensity exercise programs when the risk of CVD is increased but recognize these recommendations are based on conflicting evidence and divergent opinions (12). The U.S. Preventive Services Task Force (USPSTF) concluded that there is an insufficient evidence to evaluate the benefits and harm of exercise testing before initiating a physical activity program and did not make a specific recommendation regarding the need for exercise testing (31). The *2008 Physical Activity Guidelines Advisory Committee Report* to the Secretary of Health and Human Services (24) states that even "symptomatic persons or those with cardiovascular disease, diabetes, or other active chronic conditions who want to begin engaging in *vigorous* physical activity and who have not already developed a physical activity plan with their health care provider may wish to do so," but does not mandate such medical contact. There is also evidence from decision analysis modeling routine screening that using exercise testing prior to initiating an exercise program is not warranted regardless of baseline individual risk (16). These considerations form the basis for the present American College of Sports Medicine (ACSM) recommendations made in *Chapter 2* of this edition of the *Guidelines*.

The present version of *Chapter 2* does not recommend abandoning all medical evaluation as part of the preparticipation health screening process, as implied by the *Physical Activity Guidelines Advisory Committee Report* (24). Such changes would be a radical departure from prior editions of the *Guidelines*. In addition, individuals at highest risk and those with possible CVD symptoms may benefit from an evaluation by a health care provider.

The present chapter provides guidance for:

- Identifying individuals with unstable symptoms of CVD who could benefit from medical evaluation and treatment (see *Table 2.1*).

TABLE 2.1. Major Signs or Symptoms Suggestive of Cardiovascular, Pulmonary, or Metabolic Disease[a]

Signs or Symptoms	Clarification/Significance
Pain; discomfort (or other anginal equivalent) in the chest, neck, jaw, arms, or other areas that may result from ischemia	One of the cardinal manifestations of cardiac disease, in particular coronary artery disease Key features *favoring an ischemic origin* include the following: • *Character*: constricting, squeezing, burning, "heaviness," or "heavy feeling" • *Location*: substernal, across midthorax, anteriorly; in one or both arms, shoulders; in neck, cheeks, teeth; in forearms, fingers in interscapular region • *Provoking factors*: exercise or exertion, excitement, other forms of stress, cold weather, occurrence after meals Key features *against an ischemic origin* include the following: • *Character*: dull ache; "knifelike," sharp, stabbing; "jabs" aggravated by respiration • *Location*: in left submammary area; in left hemithorax • *Provoking factors*: after completion of exercise, provoked by a specific body motion
Shortness of breath at rest or with mild exertion	Dyspnea (defined as an abnormally uncomfortable awareness of breathing) is one of the principal symptoms of cardiac and pulmonary disease. It commonly occurs during strenuous exertion in healthy, well-trained individuals and during moderate exertion in healthy, untrained individuals. However, it should be regarded as abnormal when it occurs at a level of exertion that is not expected to evoke this symptom in a given individual. Abnormal exertional dyspnea suggests the presence of cardiopulmonary disorders, in particular left ventricular dysfunction or chronic obstructive pulmonary disease.
Dizziness or syncope	Syncope (defined as a loss of consciousness) is most commonly caused by a reduced perfusion of the brain. Dizziness and, in particular, syncope *during* exercise may result from cardiac disorders that prevent the normal rise (or an actual fall) in cardiac output. Such cardiac disorders are potentially life threatening and include severe coronary artery disease, hypertrophic cardiomyopathy, aortic stenosis, and malignant ventricular dysrhythmias. Although dizziness or syncope shortly *after* cessation of exercise should not be ignored, these symptoms may occur even in healthy individuals as a result of a reduction in venous return to the heart.
Orthopnea or paroxysmal nocturnal dyspnea	Orthopnea refers to dyspnea occurring at rest in the recumbent position that is relieved promptly by sitting upright or standing. Paroxysmal nocturnal dyspnea refers to dyspnea, beginning usually 2–5 h after the onset of sleep, which may be relieved by sitting on the side of the bed or getting out of bed. Both are symptoms of left ventricular dysfunction. Although nocturnal dyspnea may occur in individuals with chronic obstructive pulmonary disease, it differs in that it is usually relieved after the individual relieves himself or herself of secretions rather than specifically by sitting up.
Ankle edema	Bilateral ankle edema that is most evident at night is a characteristic sign of heart failure or bilateral chronic venous insufficiency. Unilateral edema of a limb often results from venous thrombosis or lymphatic blockage in the limb. Generalized edema (known as anasarca) occurs in individuals with the nephrotic syndrome, severe heart failure, or hepatic cirrhosis.

(continued)

TABLE 2.1. Major Signs or Symptoms Suggestive of Cardiovascular, Pulmonary, or Metabolic Disease[a] (*Continued*)

Signs or Symptoms	Clarification/Significance
Palpitations or tachycardia	Palpitations (defined as an unpleasant awareness of the forceful or rapid beating of the heart) may be induced by various disorders of cardiac rhythm. These include tachycardia, bradycardia of sudden onset, ectopic beats, compensatory pauses, and accentuated stroke volume resulting from valvular regurgitation. Palpitations also often result from anxiety states and high cardiac output (or hyperkinetic) states, such as anemia, fever, thyrotoxicosis, arteriovenous fistula, and the so-called idiopathic hyperkinetic heart syndrome.
Intermittent claudication	Intermittent claudication refers to the pain that occurs in a muscle with an inadequate blood supply (usually as a result of atherosclerosis) that is stressed by exercise. The pain does not occur with standing or sitting, is reproducible from day to day, is more severe when walking upstairs or up a hill, and is often described as a cramp, which disappears within 1–2 min after stopping exercise. Coronary artery disease is more prevalent in individuals with intermittent claudication. Patients with diabetes are at increased risk for this condition.
Known heart murmur	Although some may be innocent, heart murmurs may indicate valvular or other cardiovascular disease. From an exercise safety standpoint, it is especially important to exclude hypertrophic cardiomyopathy and aortic stenosis as underlying causes because these are among the more common causes of exertion-related sudden cardiac death.
Unusual fatigue or shortness of breath with usual activities	Although there may be benign origins for these symptoms, they also may signal the onset of or change in the status of cardiovascular, pulmonary, or metabolic disease.

[a]These signs or symptoms must be interpreted within the clinical context in which they appear because they are not all specific for cardiovascular, pulmonary, or metabolic disease.

Modified from (14).

- Identifying those with diagnosed disease who could benefit from a medical evaluation that includes an exercise test.
- Providing appropriate recommendations regarding the initiation, continuation, or progression of an individual's physical activity program to minimize the potential for catastrophic cardiac events.

Potential participants should be screened for the presence of risk factors for various cardiovascular, pulmonary, and metabolic diseases as well as other health conditions (*e.g.*, pregnancy, orthopedic limitations) that require special attention (14,17,18) to (a) optimize safety during exercise testing; and (b) aid in the development of a safe and effective exercise prescription (Ex R_x).

The purposes of the preparticipation health screening include the following:

- Identification of individuals with medical contraindications that require exclusion from exercise programs until those conditions have been abated or controlled.
- Recognition of individuals with clinically significant disease(s) or conditions who should participate in a medically supervised exercise program.

- Detection of individuals who should undergo a medical evaluation and/or exercise testing as part of the preparticipation health screening process before initiating an exercise program or increasing the frequency and intensity of their current program.

PREPARTICIPATION HEALTH SCREENING

Preparticipation health screening before initiating physical activity or an exercise program is a multistage process that may include

1. Self-guided methods such as the Physical Activity Readiness Questionnaire (PAR-Q) (8) (see *Figure 2.1*) or the modified AHA/ACSM Health/Fitness Facility Preparticipation Screening Questionnaire (4) (see *Figure 2.2*);
2. CVD risk factor assessment and classification by qualified health/fitness, clinical exercise, or health care professionals; and
3. Medical evaluation including a physical examination and stress test by a qualified health care provider.

Preparticipation health screening before initiating an exercise program should be distinguished from a periodic medical examination (24). A periodic health examination or a similar contact with a health care provider should be encouraged as part of routine health maintenance and to detect medical conditions unrelated to exercise.

SELF-GUIDED METHODS

Preparticipation health screening by self-reported medical history or health risk appraisal should be done for all individuals wishing to initiate a physical activity program. These self-guided methods can be easily accomplished by using such instruments as the PAR-Q (8) (see *Figure 2.1*) or an adaptation of the AHA/ACSM Health/Fitness Facility Preparticipation Screening Questionnaire (4) (see *Figure 2.2*). Patients with cardiac symptoms often perceive chest discomfort rather than pain. The AHA/ACSM Health/Fitness Facility Preparticipation Screening Questionnaire may be more useful in these situations because it inquires about "chest discomfort" rather than "chest pain" as does the PAR-Q.

ATHEROSCLEROTIC CARDIOVASCULAR DISEASE RISK FACTOR ASSESSMENT

ACSM risk classification as delineated in *Figure 2.3* is based in part on the presence or absence of the CVD risk factors listed in *Table 2.2* (5,9,12,21,22,26,30,31). The completed PAR-Q or AHA/ACSM Health/Fitness Facility Preparticipation Screening Questionnaire should be reviewed by a qualified health/fitness, clinical exercise, or health care professional to determine if the individual meets any of the criteria for positive CVD risk factors shown in *Table 2.2*. If the presence or absence

Physical Activity Readiness
Questionnaire - PAR-Q
(revised 2002)

PAR-Q & YOU

(A Questionnaire for People Aged 15 to 69)

Regular physical activity is fun and healthy, and increasingly more people are starting to become more active every day. Being more active is very safe for most people. However, some people should check with their doctor before they start becoming much more physically active.

If you are planning to become much more physically active than you are now, start by answering the seven questions in the box below. If you are between the ages of 15 and 69, the PAR-Q will tell you if you should check with your doctor before you start. If you are over 69 years of age, and you are not used to being very active, check with your doctor.

Common sense is your best guide when you answer these questions. Please read the questions carefully and answer each one honestly: check YES or NO.

YES	NO		
☐	☐	**1.**	**Has your doctor ever said that you have a heart condition <u>and</u> that you should only do physical activity recommended by a doctor?**
☐	☐	**2.**	**Do you feel pain in your chest when you do physical activity?**
☐	☐	**3.**	**In the past month, have you had chest pain when you were not doing physical activity?**
☐	☐	**4.**	**Do you lose your balance because of dizziness or do you ever lose consciousness?**
☐	☐	**5.**	**Do you have a bone or joint problem (for example, back, knee or hip) that could be made worse by a change in your physical activity?**
☐	☐	**6.**	**Is your doctor currently prescribing drugs (for example, water pills) for your blood pressure or heart condition?**
☐	☐	**7.**	**Do you know of <u>any other reason</u> why you should not do physical activity?**

If you answered

YES to one or more questions

Talk with your doctor by phone or in person BEFORE you start becoming much more physically active or BEFORE you have a fitness appraisal. Tell your doctor about the PAR-Q and which questions you answered YES.

- You may be able to do any activity you want — as long as you start slowly and build up gradually. Or, you may need to restrict your activities to those which are safe for you. Talk with your doctor about the kinds of activities you wish to participate in and follow his/her advice.
- Find out which community programs are safe and helpful for you.

NO to all questions

If you answered NO honestly to <u>all</u> PAR-Q questions, you can be reasonably sure that you can:
- start becoming much more physically active — begin slowly and build up gradually. This is the safest and easiest way to go.
- take part in a fitness appraisal — this is an excellent way to determine your basic fitness so that you can plan the best way for you to live actively. It is also highly recommended that you have your blood pressure evaluated. If your reading is over 144/94, talk with your doctor before you start becoming much more physically active.

→

DELAY BECOMING MUCH MORE ACTIVE:
- if you are not feeling well because of a temporary illness such as a cold or a fever — wait until you feel better; or
- if you are or may be pregnant — talk to your doctor before you start becoming more active.

PLEASE NOTE: If your health changes so that you then answer YES to any of the above questions, tell your fitness or health professional. Ask whether you should change your physical activity plan.

<u>Informed Use of the PAR-Q:</u> The Canadian Society for Exercise Physiology, Health Canada, and their agents assume no liability for persons who undertake physical activity, and if in doubt after completing this questionnaire, consult your doctor prior to physical activity.

No changes permitted. You are encouraged to photocopy the PAR-Q but only if you use the entire form.

NOTE: If the PAR-Q is being given to a person before he or she participates in a physical activity program or a fitness appraisal, this section may be used for legal or administrative purposes.

"I have read, understood and completed this questionnaire. Any questions I had were answered to my full satisfaction."

NAME _____

SIGNATURE _____   DATE_____

SIGNATURE OF PARENT _____   WITNESS _____
or GUARDIAN (for participants under the age of majority)

Note: This physical activity clearance is valid for a maximum of 12 months from the date it is completed and becomes invalid if your condition changes so that you would answer YES to any of the seven questions.

CSEP
SCPE © Canadian Society for Exercise Physiology   Supported by: [Canada flag] Health   Santé
                                                                        Canada   Canada   continued on other side...

■ **FIGURE 2.1.** Physical Activity Readiness Questionnaire (PAR-Q) form. Reprinted from (8), with permission from the Canadian Society for Exercise Physiology, http://www.csep.ca. © 2002.

Assess your health status by marking all *true* statements

History
You have had:
____ a heart attack
____ heart surgery
____ cardiac catheterization
____ coronary angioplasty (PTCA)
____ pacemaker/implantable cardiac
      defibrillator/rhythm disturbance
____ heart valve disease
____ heart failure
____ heart transplantation
____ congenital heart disease

*If you marked any of these statements in this section, consult your physician or other appropriate health care provider before engaging in exercise. You may need to use a facility with a **medically qualified staff**.*

Symptoms
____ You experience chest discomfort with exertion
____ You experience unreasonable breathlessness
____ You experience dizziness, fainting, or blackouts
____ You experience ankle swelling
____ You experience unpleasant awareness of a forceful
      or rapid heart rate
____ You take heart medications

Other health issues
____ You have diabetes
____ You have asthma or other lung disease
____ You have burning or cramping sensation in your
      lower legs when walking short distance
____ You have musculoskeletal problems that limit your
      physical activity
____ You have concerns about the safety of exercise
____ You take prescription medications
____ You are pregnant

Cardiovascular risk factors
____ You are a man ≥45 yr
____ You are a woman ≥55 yr
____ You smoke or quit smoking within the previous 6 mo
____ Your blood pressure is ≥140/90 mm Hg
____ You do not know your blood pressure
____ You take blood pressure medication
____ Your blood cholesterol level is ≥200 mg · dL^{-1}
____ You do not know your cholesterol level
____ You have a close blood relative who had a
      heart attack or heart surgery before age
      55 (father or brother) or age 65 (mother or sister)
____ You are physically inactive (*i.e.*, you get <30 min of
      physical activity on at least 3 d per week)
____ You have a body mass index ≥30 kg · m^{-2}
____ You have prediabetes
____ You do not know if you have prediabetes

*If you marked two or more of the statements in this section you should consult your physician or other appropriate health care provider as part of good medical care and progress gradually with your exercise program. You might benefit from using a facility with a **professionally qualified exercise staff**[a] to guide your exercise program.*

____ None of the above

You should be able to exercise safely without consulting your physician or other appropriate health care provider in a self-guide program or almost any facility that meets your exercise program needs.

[a]Professionally qualified exercise staff refers to appropriately trained individuals who possess academic training, practical and clinical knowledge, skills, and abilities commensurate with the credentials defined in *Appendix D*.

■ **FIGURE 2.2.** AHA/ACSM Health/Fitness Facility Preparticipation Screening Questionnaire. Individuals with multiple CVD risk factors (see *Table 2.2*) should be encouraged to consult with their physician prior to initiating a vigorous intensity exercise program as part of good medical care and should progress gradually with their exercise program of any exercise intensity. ACSM, American College of Sports Medicine; AHA, American Heart Association; CVD, cardiovascular disease, PTCA, percutaneous transluminal coronary angioplasty. Modified from (4).

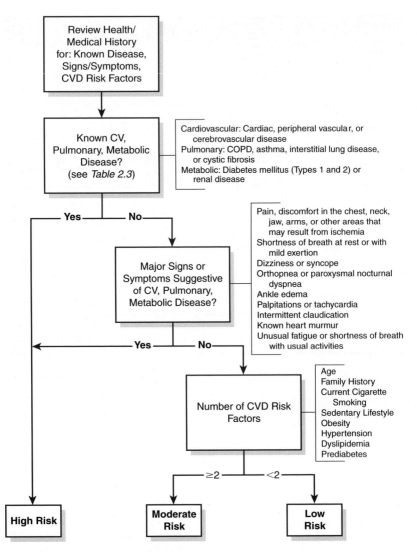

■ FIGURE 2.3. Logic model for classification of risk. CV, cardiovascular; CVD, cardiovascular disease.

of a CVD risk factor is not disclosed or is not available, that CVD risk factor should be counted as a risk factor except for prediabetes. If the prediabetes criteria are missing or unknown, prediabetes should be counted as a risk factor for those (a) ≥45 yr, especially for those with a body mass index (BMI) ≥25 kg · m^{-2}; and (b) <45 yr with a BMI ≥25 kg · m^{-2} and additional CVD risk factors for prediabetes (*e.g.,* family history of diabetes mellitus). The number of positive risk factors is

TABLE 2.2. Atherosclerotic Cardiovascular Disease (CVD) Risk Factors and Defining Criteria (26,31)

Risk Factors	Defining Criteria
Age	Men ≥45 yr; women ≥55 yr (12)
Family history	Myocardial infarction, coronary revascularization, or sudden death before 55 yr in father or other male first-degree relative or before 65 yr in mother or other female first-degree relative
Cigarette smoking	Current cigarette smoker or those who quit within the previous 6 mo or exposure to environmental tobacco smoke
Sedentary lifestyle	Not participating in at least 30 min of moderate intensity, physical activity (40%–<60% $\dot{V}O_2R$) on at least 3 d of the week for at least 3 mo (22,30)
Obesity	Body mass index ≥30 kg · m^{-2} *or* waist girth >102 cm (40 in) for men and >88 cm (35 in) for women (10)
Hypertension	Systolic blood pressure ≥140 mm Hg and/or diastolic ≥90 mm Hg, confirmed by measurements on at least two separate occasions, *or* on antihypertensive medication (9)
Dyslipidemia	Low-density lipoprotein (LDL) cholesterol ≥130 mg · dL^{-1} (3.37 mmol · L^{-1}) *or* high-density lipoprotein[b] (HDL) cholesterol <40 mg · dL^{-1} (1.04 mmol · L^{-1}) *or* on lipid-lowering medication. If total serum cholesterol is all that is available, use ≥200 mg · dL^{-1} (5.18 mmol · L^{-1}) (21)
Prediabetes[a]	Impaired fasting glucose (IFG) = fasting plasma glucose ≥100 mg · dL^{-1} (5.55 mmol · L^{-1}) and ≤125 mg · dL^{-1} (6.94 mmol · L^{-1}) *or* impaired glucose tolerance (IGT) = 2 h values in oral glucose tolerance test (OGTT) ≥140 mg · dL^{-1} (7.77 mmol · L^{-1}) and ≤199 mg · dL^{-1} (11.04 mmol · L^{-1}) confirmed by measurements on at least two separate occasions (5)
Negative Risk Factors	**Defining Criteria**
High-density lipoprotein (HDL) cholesterol	≥60 mg · dL^{-1} (1.55 mmol · L^{-1})

[a]If the presence or absence of a CVD risk factor is not disclosed or is not available, that CVD risk factor should be counted as a risk factor except for prediabetes. If the prediabetes criteria are missing or unknown, prediabetes should be counted as a risk factor for those ≥45 yr, especially for those with a body mass index (BMI) ≥25 kg · m^{-2}, and those <45 yr with a BMI ≥25 kg · m^{-2} and additional CVD risk factors for prediabetes. The number of positive risk factors is then summed.

[b]High HDL is considered a negative risk factor. For individuals having high HDL ≥60 mg · dL^{-1} (1.55 mmol · L^{-1}), for these individuals one positive risk factor is subtracted from the sum of positive risk factors.

$\dot{V}O_2R$, oxygen uptake reserve.

then summed. Because of the cardioprotective effect of high-density lipoprotein cholesterol (HDL), HDL is considered a negative CVD risk factor. For individuals having HDL ≥60 mg · dL^{-1} (1.55 mmol · L^{-1}), one positive CVD risk factor is subtracted from the sum of positive CVD risk factors.

CVD risk factor assessment provides the health/fitness, clinical exercise, and health care professionals with important information for the development of a client or patient's Ex R$_x$. CVD risk factor assessment in combination with the determination of the presence of various cardiovascular, pulmonary, renal, and metabolic diseases is important when making decisions about (a) the level of medical clearance; (b) the need for exercise testing; and (c) the level of supervision for exercise testing and exercise program participation (see *Figures 2.3* and *2.4*). Please refer to the case studies in *Box 2.1* that provide a framework for conducting CVD risk factor assessment and classification.

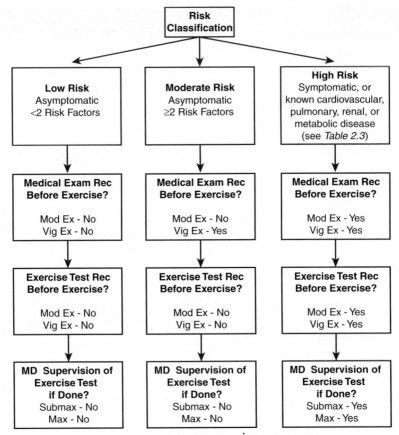

Mod Ex: Moderate intensity exercise; 40%–<60% $\dot{V}O_2R$; 3–<6 METs
"An intensity that causes noticeable increases in HR and breathing."

Vig Ex: Vigorous intensity exercise; ≥60% $\dot{V}O_2R$; ≥6 METs
"An intensity that causes substantial increases in HR and breathing."

Not Rec: Reflects the notion a medical examination, exercise test, and physician supervision of exercise testing are not recommended in the preparticipation screening; however, they may be considered when there are concerns about risk, more information is needed for the Ex R_x, and/or are requested by the patient or client.

Rec: Reflects the notion a medical examination, exercise test, and physician supervision are recommended in the preparticipation health screening process.

■ **FIGURE 2.4.** Medical examination, exercise testing, and supervision of exercise testing preparticipation recommendations based on classification of risk. Ex R_x, exercise prescription; HR, heart rate; METs, metabolic equivalents; $\dot{V}O_2R$, oxygen uptake reserve.

BOX 2.1	Case Studies to Conduct Cardiovascular Disease (CVD) Risk Factor Assessment and Determine Risk Classification

CASE STUDY I

Female, age 21 yr, smokes socially on weekends (~10–20 cigarettes). Drinks alcohol one or two nights a week, usually on weekends. Height = 63 in (160 cm), weight = 124 lb (56.4 kg), BMI = 22.0 kg $\cdot$ m^{-2}. RHR = 76 beats $\cdot$ min^{-1}, resting BP = 118/72 mm Hg. Total cholesterol = 178 mg $\cdot$ dL^{-1} (4.61 mmol $\cdot$ L^{-1}), LDL = 98 mg $\cdot$ dL^{-1} (2.54 mmol $\cdot$ L^{-1}), HDL = 57 mg $\cdot$ dL^{-1} (1.48 mmol $\cdot$ L^{-1}), FBG unknown. Currently taking oral contraceptives. Attends group exercise class two to three times a week. Reports no symptoms. Both parents living and in good health.

CASE STUDY II

Man, age 54 yr, nonsmoker. Height = 72 in (182.9 cm), weight = 168 lb (76.4 kg), BMI = 22.8 kg $\cdot$ m^{-2}. RHR = 64 beats $\cdot$ min^{-1}, resting BP = 124/78 mm Hg. Total cholesterol = 187 mg $\cdot$ dL^{-1} (4.84 mmol $\cdot$ L^{-1}), LDL = 103 mg $\cdot$ L^{-1} (2.67 mmol $\cdot$ L^{-1}), HDL = 52 mg $\cdot$ dL^{-1} (1.35 mmol $\cdot$ L^{-1}), FBG = 88 mg $\cdot$ dL^{-1} (4.84 mmol $\cdot$ L^{-1}). Recreationally competitive runner, runs 4–7 d $\cdot$ wk^{-1}, completes one to two marathons and numerous other road races every year. No medications other than over-the-counter ibuprofen as needed. Reports no symptoms. Father died at age 77 yr of a heart attack, mother died at age 81 yr of cancer.

CASE STUDY III

Man, age 44 yr, nonsmoker. Height = 70 in (177.8 cm), weight = 216 lb (98.2 kg), BMI = 31.0 kg $\cdot$ m^{-2}. RHR = 62 beats $\cdot$ min^{-1}, resting BP = 128/84 mm Hg. Total serum cholesterol = 184 mg $\cdot$ dL^{-1} (4.77 mmol $\cdot$ L^{-1}), LDL = 106 mg $\cdot$ dL^{-1} (2.75 mmol $\cdot$ L^{-1}), HDL = 44 mg $\cdot$ dL^{-1} (1.14 mmol $\cdot$ L^{-1}), FBG unknown. Walks 2–3 mi two to three times a week. Father had Type 2 diabetes and died at age 67 yr of a heart attack; mother living, no CVD. No medications; reports no symptoms.

CASE STUDY IV

Women, age 36 yr, nonsmoker. Height = 64 in (162.6 cm), weight = 108 lb (49.1 kg), BMI = 18.5 kg $\cdot$ m^{-2}. RHR = 61 beats $\cdot$ min^{-1}, resting BP = 114/62 mm Hg. Total cholesterol = 174 mg $\cdot$ dL^{-1} (4.51 mmol $\cdot$ L^{-1}), blood glucose normal with insulin injections. Type 1 diabetes diagnosed at age 7 yr. Teaches dance aerobic classes three times a week, walks approximately 45 min four times a week. Reports no symptoms. Both parents in good health with no history of CVD.

(continued)

BOX 2.1	Case Studies to Conduct Cardiovascular Disease (CVD) Risk Factor Assessment and Determine Risk Classification (*Continued*)

	Case Study I	Case Study II	Case Study III	Case Study IV
Known cardiovascular, pulmonary, and/or metabolic disease?	No	No	No	Yes — diagnosed Type 1 diabetes
Major signs or symptoms?	No	No	No	Yes
CVD risk factors:				
Age?	No	Yes	No	No
Family history?	No	No	No	No
Current cigarette smoking?	Yes	No	No	No
Sedentary lifestyle?	No	No	No	No
Obesity?	No	No	Yes — BMI >30 kg · m^{-2}	No
Hypertension?	No	No	No	No
Hypercholesterolemia?	No	No	No	No
Prediabetes?	Unknown — count as No in absence of age or obesity as risk factors	No	Unknown — count as Yes in presence of obesity	Diagnosed Type 1 diabetes
Summary	No known disease, no major signs or symptoms, one CVD risk factor	No known disease, no major signs or symptoms, one CVD risk factor	No known disease, no major signs or symptoms, two CVD risk factors	Diagnosed metabolic disease with major signs and symptoms
At low, moderate, or high risk?^{a}	Low	Low	Moderate	High

^{a}See *Figure 2.4* for medical examination, exercise testing, and supervision of exercise testing preparticipation recommendations based on classification of risk.

BMI, body mass index; BP, blood pressure; CVD, cardiovascular disease; FBG, fasting blood glucose; HDL, high-density lipoprotein cholesterol; LDL, low-density lipoprotein cholesterol; RHR, resting heart rate.

All individuals wanting to initiate a physical activity program should be screened at minimum by a self-reported medical history or health risk appraisal questionnaire such as the PAR-Q (8) (see *Figure 2.1*) or the modified AHA/ACSM Health/Fitness Facility Preparticipation Screening Questionnaire (4) (see *Figure 2.2*) for the presence of risk factors for various cardiovascular, pulmonary, renal, and metabolic diseases as well as other conditions (*e.g.*, pregnancy, orthopedic injury) that require special attention when developing the Ex R_x (14,17,18). The answers to the self-guided methods of the preparticipation health screening process then determine the need for and degree of follow-up by a qualified health/fitness, clinical exercise, or health care provider before initiating physical activity or an exercise program. The ACSM recommendations regarding the need for and degree of follow-up are detailed in the following sections.

RECOMMENDATIONS FOR A MEDICAL EXAMINATION PRIOR TO INITIATING PHYSICAL ACTIVITY

The risk of an exercise-related event such as sudden cardiac death (27) or acute MI (13,19,27) is greatest in those individuals performing unaccustomed physical activity and is greatest during vigorous intensity, physical activity. However, the CVD risk of light-to-moderate intensity, physical activity approximates that at rest (33). Consequently, physically unfit individuals initiating a physical activity program should start with light-to-moderate intensity levels of exercise and progress gradually as their fitness improves. Moderate intensity in most studies of exercise-related CVD events is defined as activity requiring 3 to <6 metabolic equivalents (METs), but the relative intensity of any specific activity varies with the fitness and age of the subject. Moderate intensity, physical activity can also be defined as that requiring 40% to <60% oxygen uptake reserve ($\dot{V}O_2R$). This physical exertion level can be estimated without exercise testing and direct measurement of maximal oxygen consumption ($\dot{V}O_{2max}$) by instructing subjects to use a rating of perceived exertion scale (see *Chapter 7*) or by exercising to the point of developing moderate shortness of breath or dyspnea but still able to talk comfortably (6,23).

The present ACSM recommendations (see *Box 2.2*) are based on the observations that the absolute risk of an exercise-related CVD event is low especially for

| BOX 2.2 | Recommendations for a Medical Examination Prior to Initiating Physical Activity |

- Individuals at moderate risk with two or more CVD risk factors (see *Table 2.2* and *Figure 2.3*) should be encouraged to consult with their physician prior to initiating a vigorous intensity exercise program as part of good medical care and should progress gradually with their exercise program of any exercise intensity (see *Figure 2.4*). Although medical evaluation is taking place for the initiation of vigorous intensity exercise, the majority of these individuals can begin light-to-moderate intensity exercise programs such as walking without consulting a physician.
- Individuals at high risk with symptoms or diagnosed disease (see *Table 2.1*) should consult with their physician prior to initiating an exercise program (see *Figure 2.4*).

CVD, cardiovascular disease.

individuals willing to initiate light-to-moderate intensity exercise and to progress gradually. The exceptions to these observations are individuals with diagnosed disease, with unstable symptoms, or at extremely high risk for occult disease (see *Table 2.1*).

RECOMMENDATIONS FOR EXERCISE TESTING PRIOR TO INITIATING PHYSICAL ACTIVITY

See *Table 2.3* for recommendations for exercise testing prior to initiating physical activity.

No set of guidelines for exercise testing prior to initiation of physical activity covers all situations. Local circumstances and policies vary, and specific program procedures are also properly diverse. To provide guidance on the need for a medical examination and exercise test before participation in a moderate-to-vigorous intensity exercise program, ACSM suggests the recommendations presented in *Figure 2.4* for determining when a medical examination and exercise test are appropriate and when physician supervision of exercise testing is recommended.

Exercise testing before initiating a physical activity program is not routinely recommended except for individuals at high risk as defined earlier (see *Tables 2.1* and *2.3*). Nevertheless, the information gathered from an exercise test may be useful in establishing a safe and effective Ex R_x for lower risk individuals. Recommending an exercise test for lower risk individuals may be considered if the purpose of the test is to design an effective Ex R_x. The exercise testing recommendations found in *Figure 2.4* reflect the notion that the risk of cardiovascular events increases as a direct function of exercise intensity (*i.e.*, vigorous > moderate > light intensity exercise) and the number of CVD risk factors (see *Table 2.2*

TABLE 2.3. New ACSM Recommendations for Exercise Testing Prior to Exercise-Diagnosed Cardiovascular Disease

Unstable or new or possible symptoms of cardiovascular disease (see *Table 2.1*)
Diabetes mellitus and at least one of the following:
Age >35 yr OR
Type 2 diabetes mellitus >10-yr duration OR
Type 1 diabetes mellitus >15-yr duration OR
Hypercholesterolemia (total cholesterol ≥240 mg · L^{-1}) (6.62 mmol · L^{-1}) OR
Hypertension (systolic blood pressure ≥140 or diastolic ≥90 mm Hg) OR
Smoking OR
Family history of CAD in first-degree relative <60 yr OR
Presence of microvascular disease OR
Peripheral artery disease OR
Autonomic neuropathy
End-stage renal disease
Patients with symptomatic or diagnosed pulmonary disease including chronic obstructive pulmonary disease (COPD), asthma, interstitial lung disease, or cystic fibrosis.

ACSM, American College of Sports Medicine; CAD, coronary artery disease.

and *Figure 2.3*). Although *Figure 2.4* provides both absolute (METs) and relative (%$\dot{V}O_{2max}$) thresholds for moderate and vigorous intensity exercise, health/fitness and clinical exercise professionals should choose the most appropriate absolute or relative intensity threshold for their setting and population when making decisions about the level of preparticipation health screening needed before initiating an exercise program.

RECOMMENDATIONS FOR SUPERVISION OF EXERCISE TESTING

The degree of medical supervision of exercise testing varies appropriately from physician-supervised tests to situations in which there is no physician present (11). It is important to distinguish between patients who require an exercise test before exercise participation and patients who require a physician to supervise the exercise test. Exercise tests as part of the preparticipation health screening for individuals at moderate to high risk are often maximal tests done in those without prior exercise training. Both factors probably increase the risk of a cardiac event. Furthermore, there are legal implications for the testing facility if a complication occurs during testing and the testing is not physician or professionally supervised.

There is consensus that exercise testing of all patient risk groups can be supervised by nonphysician health care professionals if the professional is specially trained in clinical exercise testing and a physician is immediately available if needed (20). There is also general agreement that such testing in patients at low risk can be supervised by nonphysicians without a physician being immediately available. There is no consensus whether or not nonphysicians should supervise exercise testing in patients at moderate risk without a physician immediately available. Having a physician available for testing of patients at moderate risk is recommended, but whether or not a physician must be immediately available for exercise testing of patients at moderate risk will depend on local policies and circumstances, the health status of the patients, and the training and experience of the laboratory staff. See *Box 2.3* for a summary of these recommendations.

BOX 2.3	Recommendations for Supervision of Exercise Testing

Exercise testing of individuals at high risk can be supervised by nonphysician health care professionals if the professional is specially trained in clinical exercise testing with a physician immediately available if needed. Exercise testing of individuals at moderate risk can be supervised by nonphysician health care professionals if the professional is specially trained in clinical exercise testing, but whether or not a physician must be immediately available for exercise testing is dependent on local policies and circumstances, the health status of the patients, and the training and experience of the laboratory staff.

Physicians responsible for supervising exercise testing should meet or exceed the minimal competencies for supervision and interpretation of results as established by the AHA (25). In all situations in which exercise testing is performed, site personnel should at least be certified at a level of basic life support (cardiopulmonary resuscitation [CPR]) and have automated external defibrillator (AED) training. Preferably, one or more staff members should also be certified in first aid and advanced cardiac life support (ACLS) (15). All exercise testing facilities with or without physician supervision (a) should also have a written medical emergency response plan with procedures and contact numbers; (b) should practice this plan at least quarterly; and (c) be equipped with a defibrillator or an AED depending on staffing competencies (20).

RISK STRATIFICATION FOR PATIENTS WITH CARDIOVASCULAR DISEASE

Patients with CVD may be further stratified regarding safety during exercise using published guidelines (2). Risk stratification criteria from the AACVPR are presented in *Box 2.4* (2).

BOX 2.4	American Association of Cardiovascular and Pulmonary Rehabilitation (AACVPR) Risk Stratification Criteria for Patients with Cardiovascular Disease

LOWEST RISK

Characteristics of patients at lowest risk for exercise participation (all characteristics listed must be present for patients to remain at lowest risk)

- Absence of complex ventricular dysrhythmias during exercise testing and recovery
- Absence of angina or other significant symptoms (*e.g.*, unusual shortness of breath, light-headedness, or dizziness, during exercise testing and recovery)
- Presence of normal hemodynamics during exercise testing and recovery (*i.e.*, appropriate increases and decreases in heart rate and systolic blood pressure with increasing workloads and recovery)
- Functional capacity ≥7 metabolic equivalents (METs)

Nonexercise Testing Findings
- Resting ejection fraction ≥50%
- Uncomplicated myocardial infarction or revascularization procedure
- Absence of complicated ventricular dysrhythmias at rest
- Absence of congestive heart failure
- Absence of signs or symptoms of postevent/postprocedure ischemia
- Absence of clinical depression

BOX 2.4	American Association of Cardiovascular and Pulmonary Rehabilitation (AACVPR) Risk Stratification Criteria for Patients with Cardiovascular Disease (*Continued*)

MODERATE RISK

Characteristics of patients at moderate risk for exercise participation (any one or combination of these findings places a patient at moderate risk)

- Presence of angina or other significant symptoms (*e.g.*, unusual shortness of breath, light-headedness, or dizziness occurring only at high levels of exertion [$\geq$7 METs])
- Mild to moderate level of silent ischemia during exercise testing or recovery (ST-segment depression <2 mm from baseline)
- Functional capacity <5 METs

Nonexercise Testing Findings
- Rest ejection fraction 40% to 49%

HIGHEST RISK

Characteristics of patients at high risk for exercise participation (any one or combination of these findings places a patient at high risk)

- Presence of complex ventricular dysrhythmias during exercise testing or recovery
- Presence of angina or other significant symptoms (*e.g.*, unusual shortness of breath, light-headedness, or dizziness at low levels of exertion [<5 METs] or during recovery)
- High level of silent ischemia (ST-segment depression $\geq$2 mm from baseline) during exercise testing or recovery
- Presence of abnormal hemodynamics with exercise testing (*i.e.*, chronotropic incompetence or flat or decreasing systolic BP with increasing workloads) or recovery (*i.e.*, severe postexercise hypotension)

Nonexercise Testing Findings
- Rest ejection fraction <40%
- History of cardiac arrest or sudden death
- Complex dysrhythmias at rest
- Complicated myocardial infarction or revascularization procedure
- Presence of congestive heart failure
- Presence of signs or symptoms of postevent/postprocedure ischemia
- Presence of clinical depression

Reprinted from (32), with permission from Elsevier.

The AACVPR guidelines provide recommendations for participant and/or patient monitoring and supervision and for activity restriction. Clinical exercise professionals should recognize the AACVPR guidelines do not consider comorbidities (*e.g.*, Type 2 diabetes mellitus, morbid obesity, severe pulmonary disease, debilitating neurologic, orthopedic conditions) that could result in modification of the recommendations for monitoring and supervision during exercise training.

THE BOTTOM LINE

The ACSM Preparticipation Health Screening Recommendations are the following:

- All individuals wishing to initiate a physical activity program should be screened at minimum by a self-reported medical history or health risk appraisal questionnaire. The need and degree of follow-up is determined by the answers to these self-guided methods.
- Individuals at moderate risk with two or more CVD risk factors (see *Table 2.2* and *Figures* 2.3 and 2.4) should be encouraged to consult with their physician prior to initiating a vigorous intensity, physical activity program. Although medical evaluation is taking place, the majority of these individuals can begin light-to-moderate intensity exercise programs such as walking without consulting their physician.
- Individuals at high risk with symptoms or diagnosed disease (see *Table 2.1*) should consult with their physician prior to initiating a physical activity program (see *Figure 2.4*).
- Routine exercise testing is recommended only for individuals at high risk (see *Table 2.3* and *Figures* 2.3 and 2.4) including those with diagnosed CVD, symptoms suggestive of new or changing CVD, diabetes mellitus, and additional CVD risk factors, end-stage renal disease, and specified lung disease.
- Exercise testing of individuals at high risk can be supervised by nonphysician health care professionals if the professional is specially trained in clinical exercise testing with a physician immediately available if needed. Exercise testing of individuals at moderate risk can be supervised by nonphysician health care professionals if the professional is specially trained in clinical exercise testing, but whether or not a physician must be immediately available for exercise testing is dependent on a variety of considerations.

These recommendations are made to reduce barriers to the adoption of a physically active lifestyle because (a) much of the risk associated with exercise can be mitigated by adopting a progressive exercise training regimen; and (b) there is an overall low risk of participation in physical activity programs (24).

Online Resources

REFERENCES

1. *2008 Physical Activity Guidelines for Americans* [Internet]. Rockville (MD): Office of Disease Prevention & Health Promotion, U.S. Department of Health and Human Services; 2008 [cited 2010 Sep 22]. 76 p. Available from: http://www.health.gov/paguidelines

2. American Association of Cardiovascular and Pulmonary Rehabilitation. *Guidelines for Cardiac Rehabilitation and Secondary Prevention Programs.* 4th ed. Champaign (IL): Human Kinetics; 2004. 280 p.

3. American Association of Cardiovascular and Pulmonary Rehabilitation. *Guidelines for Pulmonary Rehabilitation Programs.* 3rd ed. Champaign (IL): Human Kinetics; 2004. 188 p.

4. American College of Sports Medicine Position Stand, American Heart Association. Recommendations for cardiovascular screening, staffing, and emergency policies at health/fitness facilities. *Med Sci Sports Exerc.* 1998;30(6):1009–18.

5. American Diabetes Association. Diagnosis and classification of diabetes mellitus. *Diabetes Care.* 2007;30 Suppl 1:S42–7.

6. Brawner CA, Vanzant MA, Ehrman JK, et al. Guiding exercise using the talk test among patients with coronary artery disease. *J Cardiopulm Rehabil.* 2006;26(2):72–5; quiz 76–7.

7. Buchner DM. Physical activity to prevent or reverse disability in sedentary older adults. *Am J Prev Med.* 2003;25(3 Suppl 2):214–5.

8. *Canada's Physical Activity Guide to Healthy Active Living* [Internet]. Ontario (Canada): Public Health Agency of Canada; [cited 2007 Jun 15]. Available from: http://www.phac-aspc.gc.ca/pau-uap/paguide/index.html

9. Chobanian AV, Bakris GL, Black HR, et al. The seventh report of the Joint National Committee on Prevention, Detection, Evaluation, and Treatment of High Blood Pressure: the JNC 7 report. *JAMA.* 2003;289(19):2560–72.

10. Executive summary of the clinical guidelines on the identification, evaluation, and treatment of overweight and obesity in adults. *Arch Intern Med.* 1998;158(17):1855–67.

11. Fletcher GF, Balady GJ, Amsterdam EA, et al. Exercise standards for testing and training: a statement for healthcare professionals from the American Heart Association. *Circulation.* 2001; 104(14):1694–740.

12. Gibbons RJ, Balady GJ, Bricker JT, et al. ACC/AHA 2002 guideline update for exercise testing: summary article. A report of the American College of Cardiology/American Heart Association Task Force on Practice Guidelines (Committee to Update the 1997 Exercise Testing Guidelines). *J Am Coll Cardiol.* 2002;40(8):1531–40.

13. Giri S, Thompson PD, Kiernan FJ, et al. Clinical and angiographic characteristics of exertion-related acute myocardial infarction. *JAMA.* 1999;282(18):1731–6.

14. Gordon SMBS. Health appraisal in the non-medical setting. In: Durstine JL, editor. *ACSM's Resource Manual for Guidelines for Exercise Testing and Prescription.* 2nd ed. Philadelphia: Williams & Wilkins; 1993. p. 219–28.

15. Kern KB, Halperin HR, Field J. New guidelines for cardiopulmonary resuscitation and emergency cardiac care: changes in the management of cardiac arrest. *JAMA.* 2001;285(10):1267–9.

16. Lahav D, Leshno M, Brezis M. Is an exercise tolerance test indicated before beginning regular exercise? A decision analysis. *J Gen Intern Med.* 2009;24(8):934–8.

17. Maron BJ, Araujo CG, Thompson PD, et al. Recommendations for preparticipation screening and the assessment of cardiovascular disease in masters athletes: an advisory for healthcare professionals from the working groups of the World Heart Federation, the International Federation of Sports Medicine, and the American Heart Association Committee on Exercise, Cardiac Rehabilitation, and Prevention. *Circulation.* 2001;103(2):327–34.

18. Maron BJ, Thompson PD, Puffer JC, et al. Cardiovascular preparticipation screening of competitive athletes. A statement for health professionals from the Sudden Death Committee (clinical cardiology) and Congenital Cardiac Defects Committee (cardiovascular disease in the young), American Heart Association. *Circulation*. 1996;94(4):850–6.

19. Mittleman MA, Maclure M, Tofler GH, et al. Triggering of acute myocardial infarction by heavy physical exertion. Protection against triggering by regular exertion. Determinants of Myocardial Infarction Onset Study Investigators. *N Engl J Med*. 1993;329(23):1677–83.

20. Myers J, Arena R, Franklin B, et al. Recommendations for clinical exercise laboratories: a scientific statement from the American Heart Association. *Circulation*. 2009;119(24):3144–61.

21. National Cholesterol Education Program (NCEP) Expert Panel on Detection, Evaluation, and Treatment of High Blood Cholesterol in Adults (Adult Treatment Panel III). Third Report of the National Cholesterol Education Program (NCEP) Expert Panel on Detection, Evaluation, and Treatment of High Blood Cholesterol in Adults (Adult Treatment Panel III) final report. *Circulation*. 2002;106(25):3143–421.

22. Pate RR, Pratt M, Blair SN, et al. Physical activity and public health. A recommendation from the Centers for Disease Control and Prevention and the American College of Sports Medicine. *JAMA*. 1995;273(5):402–7.

23. Persinger R, Foster C, Gibson M, Fater DC, Porcari JP. Consistency of the talk test for exercise prescription. *Med Sci Sports Exerc*. 2004;36(9):1632–6.

24. *Physical Activity Guidelines Advisory Committee Report, 2008* [Internet]. Washington (DC): U.S. Department of Health and Human Services; 2008 [cited 2011 Jan 6]. 683 p. Available from: http://www.health.gov/paguidelines/Report/pdf/CommitteeReport.pdf

25. Rodgers GP, Ayanian JZ, Balady G, et al. American College of Cardiology/American Heart Association clinical competence statement on stress testing. A report of the American College of Cardiology/American Heart Association/American College of Physicians-American Society of Internal Medicine Task Force on Clinical Competence. *Circulation*. 2000;102(14):1726–38.

26. Roger VL, Go AS, Lloyd-Jones DM, et al. Heart Disease and Stroke Statistics—2012 Update: a report from the American Heart Association. *Circulation*. 2012;125(1):e2–220.

27. Siscovick DS, Weiss NS, Fletcher RH, Lasky T. The incidence of primary cardiac arrest during vigorous exercise. *N Engl J Med*. 1984;311(14):874–7.

28. Thompson PD, Buchner D, Pina IL, et al. Exercise and physical activity in the prevention and treatment of atherosclerotic cardiovascular disease: a statement from the Council on Clinical Cardiology (Subcommittee on Exercise, Rehabilitation, and Prevention) and the Council on Nutrition, Physical Activity, and Metabolism (Subcommittee on Physical Activity). *Circulation*. 2003;107(24):3109–16.

29. Thompson PD, Franklin BA, Balady GJ, et al. Exercise and acute cardiovascular events placing the risks into perspective: a scientific statement from the American Heart Association Council on Nutrition, Physical Activity, and Metabolism and the Council on Clinical Cardiology. *Circulation*. 2007;115(17):2358–68.

30. U.S. Department of Health and Human Services. *Physical Activity and Health: A Report of the Surgeon General*. Atlanta, GA: U.S. Department of Health and Human Services, Public Health Service, CDC, National Center for Chronic Disease Prevention and Health Promotion; 1996. 278 p.

31. U.S. Preventive Services Task Force. Screening for coronary heart disease: recommendation statement. *Ann Intern Med*. 2004;140(7):569–72.

32. Williams MA. Exercise testing in cardiac rehabilitation. Exercise prescription and beyond. *Cardiol Clin*. 2001;19(3):415–31.

33. Willich SN, Lewis M, Lowel H, Arntz HR, Schubert F, Schroder R. Physical exertion as a trigger of acute myocardial infarction. Triggers and Mechanisms of Myocardial Infarction Study Group. *N Engl J Med*. 1993;329(23):1684–90.

Exercise Testing

ROSS ARENA, PHD, PT, FACSM, FAACVPR, FAHA, ACSM-CES, *Associate Editor*

3

Preexercise Evaluation

This chapter contains information related to the preexercise evaluation and serves as a bridge among the preparticipation health screening concepts presented in *Chapter 2*, the fitness assessment in *Chapter 4*, and the clinical exercise testing concepts in *Chapters 5* and *6*. Although *Chapter 3* contents (*e.g.*, medical history, physical examination, identification of exercise contraindications, informed consent procedures) relate to health/fitness and clinical exercise settings, lower risk populations typically encountered in health/fitness settings will allow for a less sophisticated approach to the preexercise evaluation. Therefore, abbreviated versions of the preexercise evaluation described within this chapter are appropriate for low- and moderate-risk individuals wishing to engage in light-to-moderate intensity exercise within health/fitness settings. However, high-risk individuals whether in health/fitness or clinical settings will require a more intensive medical evaluation prior to initiating an exercise program (see *Chapter 2*).

The extent of the preexercise evaluation depends on the assessment of risk as outlined in *Chapter 2* and the proposed exercise intensity of the physical activity program. For individuals at high risk (see *Tables 2.1* and *2.3*), a physical examination and exercise test are recommended as part of the preexercise evaluation by a qualified health care professional to develop a safe and effective exercise prescription (Ex R_x). For individuals at low and moderate risk wishing to perform light-to-moderate intensity exercise such as walking, a preexercise evaluation that includes an exercise test is generally not recommended (see *Figures 2.3* and *2.4*). Nonetheless, a preexercise evaluation that includes a physical examination, an exercise test, and/or laboratory tests may be warranted for these lower risk individuals whenever the health/fitness and clinical exercise professional has concerns about an individual's cardiovascular disease (CVD) risk, requires additional information to design an Ex R_x, or when the exercise participant has concerns about starting an exercise program of any intensity without such a medical evaluation.

A comprehensive preexercise test evaluation in the clinical setting generally includes a medical history, physical examination, and laboratory tests, the results of which should be documented in the client's or patient's file. The goal of *Chapter 3* is not to be totally inclusive or to supplant more specific considerations that may surround the exercise participant, but rather to provide a concise set of guidelines for the various components of the preexercise evaluation.

MEDICAL HISTORY, PHYSICAL EXAMINATION, AND LABORATORY TESTS

The preexercise medical history should be thorough and include past and current information. Appropriate components of the medical history are presented in *Box 3.1*. A preliminary physical examination should be performed by a physician or other qualified health care professional before exercise testing individuals at high risk as outlined in *Chapter 2*. Appropriate components of the physical examination specific to subsequent exercise testing are presented in *Box 3.2*. An expanded discussion and alternatives can be found in *ACSM's Resource Manual for Guidelines for Exercise Testing and Prescription, Seventh Edition* (26).

Identification and risk stratification of individuals with CVD and those at high risk of developing CVD are facilitated by review of previous test results such as coronary angiography, nuclear imaging, echocardiography, or coronary artery calcium score studies (13) (see *Box 2.2*). Additional testing may include ambulatory electrocardiogram (ECG) or Holter monitoring and pharmacologic stress testing to further clarify the need for and extent of intervention, assess response to treatment such as medical therapies and revascularization procedures, or determine the need for additional assessment. As outlined in *Box 3.3*, other laboratory tests may be warranted based on the level of risk and clinical status of the patient, especially for those with diabetes mellitus. These laboratory tests may include, but are not limited to, serum chemistries, complete blood count, serum lipids and lipoproteins, inflammatory markers, fasting plasma glucose, hemoglobin A1C, and pulmonary function. Detailed exercise testing/training guidelines for a number of chronic diseases can be found in *Chapters 5, 6, 9*, and *10* within the *Guidelines*.

Although a detailed description of all the physical examination procedures listed in *Box 3.2* and the recommended laboratory tests listed in *Box 3.3* are beyond the scope of the *Guidelines*, additional basic information related to assessment of blood pressure (BP), lipids and lipoproteins, other blood chemistries, and pulmonary function are provided in the following section. For more detailed descriptions of these assessments, the reader is referred to the work of Bickley (7).

BLOOD PRESSURE

Measurement of resting BP is an integral component of the preexercise evaluation. Subsequent decisions should be based on the average of two or more properly measured, seated BP readings recorded during each of two or more office visits (21). Specific techniques for measuring BP are critical to accuracy and detection of high BP and are presented in *Box 3.4*. In addition to high BP readings, unusually low readings should also be evaluated for clinical significance. The *Seventh Report of the Joint National Committee on Prevention, Detection, Evaluation, and Treatment of High Blood Pressure* (JNC7) provides guidelines for hypertension

BOX 3.1   Components of the Medical History

Appropriate components of the medical history may include the following:

- Medical diagnosis. Cardiovascular disease risk factors including hypertension, obesity, dyslipidemia, diabetes, and metabolic syndrome; cardiovascular disease including heart failure, valvular dysfunction (*e.g.*, aortic stenosis/mitral valve disease), myocardial infarction, and other acute coronary syndromes; percutaneous coronary interventions including angioplasty and coronary stent(s), coronary artery bypass surgery, and other cardiac surgeries such as valvular surgery(s); cardiac transplantation; pacemaker and/or implantable cardioverter defibrillator; ablation procedures for dysrhythmias; peripheral vascular disease; pulmonary disease including asthma, emphysema, and bronchitis; cerebrovascular disease including stroke and transient ischemic attacks; anemia and other blood dyscrasias (*e.g.*, lupus erythematosus); phlebitis, deep vein thrombosis, or emboli; cancer; pregnancy; osteoporosis; musculoskeletal disorders; emotional disorders; and eating disorders.
- Previous physical examination findings. Murmurs, clicks, gallop rhythms, other abnormal heart sounds, and other unusual cardiac and vascular findings; abnormal pulmonary findings (*e.g.*, wheezes, rales, crackles); plasma glucose, hemoglobin A1C, high sensitivity C-reactive protein, serum lipids and lipoproteins, or other significant laboratory abnormalities; high blood pressure; and edema.
- History of symptoms. Discomfort (*e.g.*, pressure, tingling sensation, pain, heaviness, burning, tightness, squeezing, numbness) in the chest, jaw, neck, back, or arms; light-headedness, dizziness, or fainting; temporary loss of visual acuity or speech; transient unilateral numbness or weakness; shortness of breath; rapid heartbeat or palpitations, especially if associated with physical activity, eating a large meal, emotional upset, or exposure to cold (or any combination of these activities).
- Recent illness, hospitalization, new medical diagnoses, or surgical procedures.
- Orthopedic problems including arthritis, joint swelling, and any condition that would make ambulation or use of certain test modalities difficult.
- Medication use (including dietary/nutritional supplements) and drug allergies.
- Other habits including caffeine, alcohol, tobacco, or recreational (illicit) drug use.
- Exercise history. Information on readiness for change and habitual level of activity: frequency, duration or time, type, and intensity or FITT of exercise.
- Work history with emphasis on current or expected physical demands, noting upper and lower extremity requirements.
- Family history of cardiac, pulmonary, or metabolic disease, stroke, or sudden death.

FITT, *F*requency, *I*ntensity, *T*ime, and *T*ype.
Adapted from (7).

BOX 3.2	Components of the Preparticipation Symptom-Limited Exercise Test Physical Examination (7)

Appropriate components of the physical examination may include the following:

- Body weight; in many instances determination of body mass index, waist girth, and/or body composition (percent body fat) is desirable
- Apical pulse rate and rhythm
- Resting blood pressure: seated, supine, and standing
- Auscultation of the lungs with specific attention to uniformity of breath sounds in all areas (absence of rales, wheezes, and other breathing sounds)
- Palpation of the cardiac apical impulse and point of maximal impulse
- Auscultation of the heart with specific attention to murmurs, gallops, clicks, and rubs
- Palpation and auscultation of carotid, abdominal, and femoral arteries
- Evaluation of the abdomen for bowel sounds, masses, visceromegaly, and tenderness
- Palpation and inspection of lower extremities for edema and presence of arterial pulses
- Absence or presence of tendon xanthoma and skin xanthelasma
- Follow-up examination related to orthopedic or other medical conditions that would limit exercise testing
- Tests of neurologic function including reflexes and cognition (as indicated)
- Inspection of the skin, especially of the lower extremities in known patients with diabetes mellitus

Adapted from (7).

detection and management (23). *Table 3.1* summarizes the JNC7 recommendations for the classification and management of BP for adults.

The relationship between BP and risk for cardiovascular events is continuous, consistent, and independent of other risk factors. For individuals 40–70 yr, each increment of 20 mm Hg in systolic BP (SBP) or 10 mm Hg in diastolic BP (DBP) doubles the risk of CVD across the entire BP range of 115/75 to 185/115 mm Hg. According to JNC7, individuals with a SBP of 120–139 mm Hg and/or a DBP of 80–89 mm Hg have prehypertension and require health-promoting lifestyle modifications to prevent the development of hypertension (4,23).

Lifestyle modification including physical activity, weight reduction, a Dietary Approaches to Stop Hypertension (DASH) eating plan (*i.e.*, a diet rich in fruits, vegetables, low-fat dairy products with a reduced content of saturated and total fat), dietary sodium reduction (no more than 100 mmol or 2.4 g sodium $\cdot$ d^{-1}), and moderation of alcohol consumption remains the cornerstone of antihypertensive therapy (4,23). However, JNC7 emphasizes the fact that most patients with hypertension who require drug therapy in addition to lifestyle modification

| BOX 3.3 | Recommended Laboratory Tests by Level of Risk and Clinical Assessment |

INDIVIDUALS AT LOW-TO-MODERATE RISK

- Fasting serum total cholesterol, LDL cholesterol, HDL cholesterol, and triglycerides
- Fasting plasma glucose, especially in individuals ≥45 yr and younger individuals who are overweight (body mass index ≥25 kg · m^{-2}) and have one or more of the following risk factors for Type 2 diabetes mellitus: a first-degree relative with diabetes, member of a high-risk ethnic population (*e.g.*, African American, Latino, Native American, Asian American, Pacific Islander), delivered a baby weighing >9 lb (4.08 kg) or history of gestational diabetes, hypertension (BP ≥140/90 mm Hg in adults), HDL cholesterol <40 mg · dL^{-1} (<1.04 mmol · L^{-1}) and/or triglycerides ≥150 mg · dL^{-1} (≥1.69 mmol · L^{-1}), previously identified impaired glucose tolerance or impaired fasting glucose (fasting glucose ≥100 mg · dL^{-1}; ≥5.55 mmol · L^{-1}), habitual physical inactivity, polycystic ovary disease, and history of vascular disease
- Thyroid function, as a screening evaluation especially if dyslipidemia is present

INDIVIDUALS AT HIGH RISK

- Preceding tests plus pertinent previous cardiovascular laboratory tests (*e.g.*, resting 12-lead ECG, Holter monitoring, coronary angiography, radionuclide or echocardiography studies, previous exercise tests)
- Carotid ultrasound and other peripheral vascular studies
- Consider measures of lipoprotein(a), high sensitivity C-reactive protein, LDL particle size and number, and HDL subspecies (especially in young individuals with a strong family history of premature CVD and in those individuals without traditional CVD risk factors)
- Chest radiograph, if heart failure is present or suspected
- Comprehensive blood chemistry panel and complete blood count as indicated by history and physical examination (see *Table 3.4*)

PATIENTS WITH PULMONARY DISEASE

- Chest radiograph
- Pulmonary function tests (see *Table 3.5*)
- Carbon monoxide diffusing capacity
- Other specialized pulmonary studies (*e.g.*, oximetry or blood gas analysis)

BP, blood pressure; CVD, cardiovascular disease; ECG, electrocardiogram; HDL, high-density lipoprotein cholesterol; LDL, low-density lipoprotein cholesterol.

| BOX 3.4 | Procedures for Assessment of Resting Blood Pressure |

1. Patients should be seated quietly for at least 5 min in a chair with back support (rather than on an examination table) with their feet on the floor and their arms supported at heart level. Patients should refrain from smoking cigarettes or ingesting caffeine for at least 30 min preceding the measurement.
2. Measuring supine and standing values may be indicated under special circumstances.
3. Wrap cuff firmly around upper arm at heart level; align cuff with brachial artery.
4. The appropriate cuff size must be used to ensure accurate measurement. The bladder within the cuff should encircle at least 80% of the upper arm. Many adults require a large adult cuff.
5. Place stethoscope chest piece below the antecubital space over the brachial artery. Bell and diaphragm side of chest piece appear equally effective in assessing BP (15).
6. Quickly inflate cuff pressure to 20 mm Hg above first Korotkoff sound.
7. Slowly release pressure at rate equal to 2–5 mm Hg $\cdot$ s^{-1}.
8. SBP is the point at which the first of two or more Korotkoff sounds is heard (phase 1), and DBP is the point before the disappearance of Korotkoff sounds (phase 5).
9. At least two measurements should be made (minimum of 1 min apart) and the average should be taken.
10. BP should be measured in both arms during the first examination. Higher pressure should be used when there is consistent interarm difference.
11. Provide to patients, verbally and in writing, their specific BP numbers and BP goals.

BP, blood pressure; DBP; diastolic blood pressure; SBP, systolic blood pressure.
Modified from (23). For additional, more detailed recommendations, see (21).

require two or more antihypertensive medications to achieve the goal BP (*i.e.*, <140/90 mm Hg or <130/80 mm Hg for patients with diabetes mellitus or chronic kidney disease) (23).

LIPIDS AND LIPOPROTEINS

The *Third Report of the Expert Panel on Detection, Evaluation, and Treatment of High Blood Cholesterol in Adults* (*Adult Treatment Panel III* or *ATP III*) outlines the National Cholesterol Education Program's (NCEP) recommendations for cholesterol testing and management (see *Table 3.2*) (27). ATP III and subsequent updates by the National Heart, Lung, and Blood Institute (NHLBI), American

TABLE 3.1. Classification and Management of Blood Pressure for Adults[a]

BP Classification	SBP (mm Hg)	DBP (mm Hg)	Lifestyle Modification	Initial Drug Therapy Without Compelling Indication	Initial Drug Therapy With Compelling Indications
Normal	<120	And <80	Encourage		
Prehypertension	120–139	Or 80–89	Yes	No antihypertensive drug indicated	Drug(s) for compelling indications[b]
Stage 1 hypertension	140–159	Or 90–99	Yes	Antihypertensive drug(s) indicated	Drug(s) for compelling indications[b] Other antihypertensive drugs, as needed
Stage 2 hypertension	≥160	Or ≥100	Yes	Antihypertensive drug(s) indicated Two-drug combination for most[c]	

[a]Treatment determined by highest BP category.

[b]Compelling indications include heart failure, postmyocardial infarction, high coronary heart disease risk, diabetes mellitus, chronic kidney disease, and recurrent stroke prevention. Treat patients with chronic kidney disease or diabetes mellitus to BP goal of <130/80 mm Hg.

[c]Initial combined therapy should be used cautiously in those at risk for orthostatic hypotension.

BP, blood pressure; DBP, diastolic blood pressure; SBP, systolic blood pressure.

Adapted from (23).

TABLE 3.2. ATP III Classification of LDL, Total, and HDL Cholesterol (mg · dL^{-1})

LDL Cholesterol	
<100[a]	Optimal
100–129	Near optimal/above optimal
130–159	Borderline high
160–189	High
≥190	Very high
Total Cholesterol	
<200	Desirable
200–239	Borderline high
≥240	High
HDL Cholesterol	
<40	Low
≥60	High
Triglycerides	
<150	Normal
150–199	Borderline high
200–499	High
≥500	Very high

[a]According to the American Heart Association/American College of Cardiology 2006 update (endorsed by the National Heart, Lung, and Blood Institute), it is reasonable to treat LDL cholesterol to <70 mg · dL^{-1} (<1.81 mmol · L^{-1}) in patients with coronary and other atherosclerotic vascular disease (24).

NOTE: To convert LDL, total cholesterol, and HDL from mg · dL^{-1} to mmol · L^{-1}, multiply by 0.0259. To convert triglycerides from mg · dL^{-1} to mmol · L^{-1}, multiply by 0.0113.

ATP III, Adult Treatment Panel III; HDL, high-density lipoprotein cholesterol; LDL, low-density lipoprotein cholesterol.

Adapted from (27).

Heart Association (AHA), and American College of Cardiology (ACC) identify low-density lipoprotein (LDL) cholesterol as the primary target for cholesterol-lowering therapy (12,24,27). This designation is based on a wide variety of evidence indicating elevated LDL cholesterol is a powerful risk factor for CVD, and lowering of LDL cholesterol results in a striking reduction in the incidence of CVD. *Table 3.2* summarizes the ATP III classifications of LDL, total, and high-density lipoprotein (HDL) cholesterol, and triglycerides.

According to ATP III, a low HDL cholesterol, defined as <40 mg $\cdot$ dL^{-1}, is strongly and inversely associated with CVD risk. Clinical trials provide suggestive evidence that raising HDL cholesterol reduces CVD risk. However, the mechanism explaining the role of low serum HDL cholesterol in accelerating the CVD process remains unclear. Moreover, it remains uncertain whether raising HDL cholesterol *per se*, independent of other changes in lipid and/or nonlipid risk factors, always reduces the risk for CVD. In view of this, ATP III does not identify a specific HDL cholesterol goal level to achieve with therapy. Rather, ATP III encourages nondrug and drug therapies that raise HDL cholesterol and are part of the management of other lipid and nonlipid risk factors.

There is growing evidence of a strong association between elevated triglycerides and CVD risk. Recent studies suggest some species of triglyceride-rich lipoproteins, notably small very low-density lipoproteins (VLDLs) and intermediate-density lipoproteins (IDLs), promote atherosclerosis and predispose to CVD. Because VLDL and IDL appear to have atherogenic potential similar to that of LDL cholesterol, ATP III recommends non-HDL cholesterol (*i.e.*, VLDL plus LDL cholesterol) as a secondary target of therapy for individuals with elevated triglycerides (triglycerides ≥ 200 mg $\cdot$ dL^{-1}).

The metabolic syndrome is characterized by a constellation of metabolic risk factors in one individual. Abdominal obesity, atherogenic dyslipidemia (*i.e.*, elevated triglycerides, small LDL cholesterol particles, and reduced HDL cholesterol), elevated BP, insulin resistance, prothrombotic state (*i.e.*, increased risk for thrombus formation), and proinflammatory state (*i.e.*, elevated C-reactive protein and interleukin-6) generally are accepted as being characteristic of the metabolic syndrome. Although the primary cause is debatable, the root causes of the metabolic syndrome are overweight/obesity, physical inactivity, insulin resistance, and genetic factors. Because the metabolic syndrome has emerged as an important contributor to CVD, ATP III places emphasis on the metabolic syndrome as a risk enhancer. However, ATP III recognized that there are no well-established criteria for diagnosing the metabolic syndrome. *Table 3.3* lists different professional organizations' proposed metabolic syndrome criteria including the recommendations put forth by ATP III (27).

ATP III designates hypertension, cigarette smoking, diabetes mellitus, overweight and obesity, physical inactivity, and an atherogenic diet as modifiable nonlipid risk factors, whereas age, male gender, and family history of premature CVD are nonmodifiable nonlipid risk factors for CVD. Triglycerides, lipoprotein remnants, lipoprotein(a), small LDL particles, HDL subspecies, apolipoproteins B

TABLE 3.3. Metabolic Syndrome Criteria: NCEP/ATP III, IDF, and WHO

Criteria	NCEP/ATP III (8)	IDF (14)	WHO (1)[a]
Body Weight	Waist circumference[a,c]	Required[b]	Waist-to-hip ratio and/or BMI of >30 kg · m^{-2}
Men	>102 cm (>40 in)	≥94 cm (≥37 in)	>0.9 ratio
Women	>88 cm (>35 in)	≥80 cm (≥31.5 in)	>0.85 ratio
Insulin Resistance/ Glucose	≥110 mg · dL^{-1d}	≥100 mg · dL^{-1} or previously diagnosed Type 2 diabetes	Required[e]
Dyslipidemia		Specific treatment or	
HDL	Men: <40 mg · dL^{-1} Women: <50 mg · dL^{-1}	Men: <40 mg · dL^{-1} Women: <50 mg · dL^{-1f}	Men: <35 mg · dL^{-1} Women: <39 mg · dL^{-1f}
Triglycerides	≥150 mg · dL^{-1}	≥150 mg · dL^{-1}	≥150 mg · dL^{-1}
Elevated Blood Pressure	≥130 or ≥85 mm Hg	≥130 or ≥85 mm Hg or treatment of previously diagnosed hypertension	Antihypertensive medication and/or a BP of ≥140 or ≥90 mm Hg
Other	N/A	N/A	Urinary albumin excretion rate ≥20 µg · min^{-1} or albumin:creatinine ratio ≥30 mg · g^{-1}

[a]Overweight and obesity are associated with insulin resistance and the metabolic syndrome (Msyn). However, the presence of abdominal obesity is more highly correlated with these metabolic risk factors than is elevated BMI. Therefore, the simple measure of waist circumference is recommended to identify the body weight component of the Msyn.

[b]Defined as waist circumference ≥94 cm (≥37 in) for Europid men and ≥80 cm (≥31.2 in) for Europid women, with ethnicity-specific values for other groups.

[c]Some men develop multiple metabolic risk factors when the waist circumference is only marginally increased (94–102 cm [37–39 in]). Such patients may have a strong genetic contribution to insulin resistance. They should benefit from changes in life habits, similarly to men with categorical increases in waist circumference.

[d]The American Diabetes Association has established a cut point of ≥100 mg · dL^{-1}, above which individuals have either prediabetes (impaired fasting glucose) or diabetes mellitus (2). This cut point should be applicable for identifying the lower boundary to define an elevated glucose as one criterion for metabolic syndrome.

[e]A required criteria of one of the following: Type 2 diabetes mellitus, impaired fasting glucose, impaired glucose tolerance, or for those with normal fasting glucose levels (<110 mg · dL^{-1}), glucose uptake below the lowest quartile for background populations under investigation under hyperinsulinemic and euglycemic conditions.

[f]These values have been updated from those originally presented to ensure consistence with ATP III cut points.

NOTE: To convert glucose from mg · dL^{-1} to mmol · L^{-1}, multiply by 0.0555. To convert HDL from mg · dL^{-1} to mmol · L^{-1}, multiply by 0.0259. To convert triglycerides from mg · dL^{-1} to mmol · L^{-1}, multiply by 0.0113.

ATP III, Adult Treatment Panel III; BMI, body mass index; BP, blood pressure; HDL, high-density lipoprotein cholesterol; IDF, International Diabetes Federation; NCEP, National Cholesterol Education Program; WHO, World Health Organization.

and A1, and the total cholesterol-to-HDL cholesterol ratio are designated by ATP III as emerging lipid risk factors. Thrombogenic and hemostatic factors, inflammatory markers (*e.g.*, high sensitivity C-reactive protein), impaired fasting glucose, and homocysteine are designated by ATP III as emerging nonlipid risk factors. Nevertheless, recent studies suggest that homocysteine-lowering therapy does not result in a reduction in CVD risk.

The guiding principle of ATP III and subsequent updates by the NHLBI, AHA, and ACC is that the intensity of LDL-lowering therapy should be adjusted to the individual's absolute risk for CVD (6,8,12,13,24,27). The ATP III treatment guidelines and subsequent updates by the NHLBI, AHA, and ACC are summarized in *ACSM's Resource Manual for Guidelines for Exercise Testing and Prescription, Seventh Edition* (26).

BLOOD PROFILE ANALYSES

Multiple analyses of blood profiles are commonly evaluated in clinical exercise programs. Such profiles may provide useful information about an individual's overall health status and ability to exercise and may help to explain certain ECG abnormalities. Because of varied methods of assaying blood samples, some caution is advised when comparing blood chemistries from different laboratories. *Table 3.4* gives normal ranges for selected blood chemistries, derived from a variety of sources. For many patients with CVD, medications for dyslipidemia and hypertension are common. Many of these medications act in the liver to lower blood cholesterol and in the kidneys to lower BP (see *Appendix A*). One should pay particular attention to liver function tests such as alanine transaminase (ALT), aspartate transaminase (AST), and bilirubin as well as to renal (kidney) function tests such as creatinine, glomerular filtration rate, blood urea nitrogen (BUN), and BUN/creatinine ratio in patients on such medications. Indication of volume depletion and potassium abnormalities can be seen in the sodium and potassium measurements.

PULMONARY FUNCTION

Pulmonary function testing with spirometry is recommended for all smokers >45 yr and in any individual presenting with dyspnea (*i.e.*, shortness of breath), chronic cough, wheezing, or excessive mucus production (9). Spirometry is a simple and noninvasive test that can be performed easily. Indications for spirometry are listed in *Table 3.5*. When performing spirometry, standards for the performance of the test should be followed (16).

Although many measurements can be made from a spirometric test, the most commonly used include the forced vital capacity (FVC), forced expiratory volume in one second ($FEV_{1.0}$), $FEV_{1.0}$/FVC ratio, and peak expiratory flow (PEF). Results from these measurements can help to identify the presence of restrictive or obstructive respiratory abnormalities, sometimes before symptoms or signs of disease are present. The $FEV_{1.0}$/FVC is diminished with obstructive airway diseases (*e.g.*, asthma, chronic bronchitis, emphysema, chronic obstructive pulmonary disease [COPD]) but remains normal with restrictive disorders (*e.g.*, kyphoscoliosis, neuromuscular disease, pulmonary fibrosis, other interstitial lung diseases).

The Global Initiative for Chronic Obstructive Lung Disease classifies the presence and severity of COPD as seen in *Table 3.5* (22). The term COPD can be used when chronic bronchitis, emphysema, or both are present, and spirometry documents an obstructive defect. A different approach for classifying the severity of obstructive and restrictive defects is that of the American Thoracic Society (ATS) and European Respiratory Society (ERS) Task Force on Standardization of Lung Function Testing as presented in *Table 3.5* (20). This ATS/ERS Task Force prefers to use the largest available vital capacity (VC), whether it is obtained on

TABLE 3.4. Typical Ranges of Normal Values for Selected Blood Variables in Adults[a]

Variable	Men	Neutral	Women	SI Conversion Factor
Hemoglobin (g · dL^{-1})	13.5–17.5		11.5–15.5	10 (g · L^{-1})
Hematocrit (%)	40–52		36–48	0.01 (proportion of 1)
Red cell count (×10^6 · µL^{-1})	4.5–6.5 million		3.9–5.6 million	1 (×10^{12} · L^{-1})
Hemoglobin (whole blood) Mass concentration (g · dL^{-1})		30–35		10 (g · L^{-1})
White blood cell count (×10^3 · µL^{-1})		4–11 thousand		1 (×10^9 · L^{-1})
Platelet count (×10^3 · µL^{-1})		150–450 thousand		1 (×10^9 · L^{-1})
Fasting glucose[b] (mg · dL^{-1})		60–99		0.0555 (mmol · L^{-1})
Hemoglobin A1C		≤6%		N/A
Blood urea nitrogen (BUN; mg · dL^{-1})		4–24		0.357 (mmol · L^{-1})
Creatinine (mg · dL^{-1})		0.3–1.4		88.4 (µmol · L^{-1})
BUN/creatinine ratio		7–27		
Uric acid (mg · dL^{-1})		3.6–8.3		59.48 (µmol · L^{-1})
Sodium (mEq · dL^{-1})		135–150		1.0 (mmol · L^{-1})
Potassium (mEq · dL^{-1})		3.5–5.5		1.0 (mmol · L^{-1})
Chloride (mEq · dL^{-1})		98–110		1.0 (mmol · L^{-1})
Osmolality (mOsm · kg^{-1})		278–302		1.0 (mmol · kg^{-1})
Calcium (mg · dL^{-1})		8.5–10.5		0.25 (mmol · L^{-1})
Calcium, ion (mg · dL^{-1})		4.0–5.0		0.25 (mmol · L^{-1})
Phosphorus (mg · dL^{-1})		2.5–4.5		0.323 (mmol · L^{-1})
Protein, total (g · dL^{-1})		6.0–8.5		10 (g · L^{-1})
Albumin (g · dL^{-1})		3.0–5.5		10 (g · L^{-1})
Globulin (g · dL^{-1})		2.0–4.0		10 (g · L^{-1})
A/G ratio		1.0–2.2		10
Iron, total (µg · dL^{-1})		40–190	35–180	0.179 (µmol · L^{-1})
Liver Function Tests				
Bilirubin (mg · dL^{-1})		<1.5		17.1 (µmol · L^{-1})
SGOT (AST; U · L^{-1})	8–46		7–34	1 (U · L^{-1})
SGPT (ALT; U · L^{-1})	7–46		4–35	1 (U · L^{-1})

[a]Certain variables must be interpreted in relation to the normal range of the issuing laboratory.

[b]Fasting blood glucose 100–125 mg · dL^{-1} is considered impaired fasting glucose or prediabetes.

NOTE: For a complete list of Système International (SI) conversion factors, please see http://jama.ama-assn.org/content/vol295/issue1/images/data/103/DC6/JAMA_auinst_si.dtl

ALT, alanine transaminase (formerly SGPT); AST, aspartate transaminase (formerly SGOT); SGOT, serum glutamic-oxaloacetic transaminase; SGPT, serum glutamic-pyruvic transaminase.

TABLE 3.5. Indications for Spirometry

A. Indications for Spirometry

Diagnosis

To evaluate symptoms, signs, or abnormal laboratory tests

To measure the effect of disease on pulmonary function

To screen individuals at risk of having pulmonary disease

To assess preoperative risk

To assess prognosis

To assess health status before beginning strenuous physical activity programs

Monitoring

To assess therapeutic intervention

To describe the course of diseases that affect lung function

To monitor individuals exposed to injurious agents

To monitor for adverse reactions to drugs with known pulmonary toxicity

Disability/Impairment Evaluations

To assess patients as part of a rehabilitation program

To assess risks as part of an insurance evaluation

To assess individuals for legal reasons

Public Health

Epidemiologic surveys

Derivation of reference equations

Clinical research

B. The Global Initiative for Chronic Obstructive Lung Disease Spirometric Classification of COPD Severity Based on Postbronchodilator $FEV_{1.0}$

Stage I	Mild	$FEV_{1.0}/FVC$ <0.70
		$FEV_{1.0}$ ≥80% of predicted
Stage II	Moderate	$FEV_{1.0}/FVC$ <0.70
		50% ≤ $FEV_{1.0}$ <80% predicted
Stage III	Severe	$FEV_{1.0}/FVC$ <0.70
		30% ≤ $FEV_{1.0}$ <50% predicted
Stage IV	Very severe	$FEV_{1.0}/FVC$ <0.70
		$FEV_{1.0}$ <30% predicted or $FEV_{1.0}$ <50% predicted plus chronic respiratory failure

C. The American Thoracic Society and European Respiratory Society Classification of Severity of Any Spirometric Abnormality Based on $FEV_{1.0}$

Degree of Severity	$FEV_{1.0}$ % Predicted
Mild	Less than the LLN but ≥70
Moderate	60–69
Moderately severe	50–59
Severe	35–49
Very severe	<35

COPD, chronic obstructive pulmonary disease; $FEV_{1.0}$, forced expiratory volume in one second; FVC, forced vital capacity; respiratory failure defined as arterial partial pressure of oxygen (PaO_2) <8.0 kPa (60 mm Hg) with or without arterial partial pressure of CO_2 (P_aCO_2) >6.7 kPa (50 mm Hg) while breathing air at sea level; LLN, lower limit of normal.

Modified from (20,22).

inspiration (IVC), slow expiration (SVC), or forced expiration (FVC). An obstructive defect is defined by a reduced $FEV_{1.0}/FVC$ ratio below the fifth percentile of the predicted value. The use of the fifth percentile of the predicted value as the lower limit of normal does not lead to an overestimation of the presence of an obstructive defect in older individuals, which is more likely when a fixed value for $FEV_{1.0}/FVC$ or a $FEV_{1.0}/FVC$ of 0.7 is used as the dividing line between normal and abnormal (17). A restrictive defect is characterized by a reduction in the total lung capacity (TLC), as measured on a lung volume study, below the fifth percentile of the predicted value, and a normal $FEV_{1.0}/VC$ (17).

The spirometric classification of lung disease is useful in predicting health status, use of health resources, and mortality. Abnormal spirometry can also be indicative of an increased risk for lung cancer, heart attack, and stroke and can be used to identify patients in which interventions such as smoking cessation and use of pharmacologic agents would be most beneficial. Spirometric testing is also valuable in identifying patients with chronic disease (i.e., COPD and heart failure) that have diminished pulmonary function that may benefit from an inspiratory muscle training program (6,19).

The determination of the maximal voluntary ventilation (MVV) should also be obtained during routine spirometric testing (16,20). MVV can be used to estimate breathing reserve during maximal exercise. The MVV should ideally be measured rather than estimated by multiplying the $FEV_{1.0}$ by a constant value as is often done in practice (20).

CONTRAINDICATIONS TO EXERCISE TESTING

For certain individuals, the risks of exercise testing outweigh the potential benefits. For these patients, it is important to carefully assess risk versus benefit when deciding whether the exercise test should be performed. Box 3.5 outlines both absolute and relative contraindications to exercise testing (10). Performing the preexercise evaluation with a careful review of prior medical history, as described earlier in Chapter 3, helps identify potential contraindications and increases the safety of the exercise test. Patients with absolute contraindications should not perform exercise tests until such conditions are stabilized or adequately treated. Patients with relative contraindications may be tested only after careful evaluation of the risk–benefit ratio. However, it should be emphasized that contraindications might not apply in certain specific clinical situations such as soon after acute myocardial infarction, revascularization procedure, or bypass surgery or to determine the need for or benefit of drug therapy. Finally, conditions exist that preclude reliable diagnostic ECG information from exercise testing (e.g., left bundle-branch block, digitalis therapy). The exercise test may still provide useful information regarding exercise capacity, subjective symptomatology, pulmonary function, dysrhythmias, and hemodynamics. In these conditions, additional evaluative techniques such as ventilatory expired gas analysis, echocardiography, or nuclear imaging can be added to the exercise test to improve sensitivity, specificity, and diagnostic capabilities.

BOX 3.5	Contraindications to Exercise Testing

ABSOLUTE
- A recent significant change in the resting electrocardiogram (ECG) suggesting significant ischemia, recent myocardial infarction (within 2 d), or other acute cardiac event
- Unstable angina
- Uncontrolled cardiac dysrhythmias causing symptoms or hemodynamic compromise
- Symptomatic severe aortic stenosis
- Uncontrolled symptomatic heart failure
- Acute pulmonary embolus or pulmonary infarction
- Acute myocarditis or pericarditis
- Suspected or known dissecting aneurysm
- Acute systemic infection, accompanied by fever, body aches, or swollen lymph glands

RELATIVE[a]
- Left main coronary stenosis
- Moderate stenotic valvular heart disease
- Electrolyte abnormalities (*e.g.*, hypokalemia or hypomagnesemia)
- Severe arterial hypertension (*i.e.*, systolic blood pressure [SBP] of >200 mm Hg and/or a diastolic BP [DBP] of >110 mm Hg) at rest
- Tachydysrhythmia or bradydysrhythmia
- Hypertrophic cardiomyopathy and other forms of outflow tract obstruction
- Neuromotor, musculoskeletal, or rheumatoid disorders that are exacerbated by exercise
- High-degree atrioventricular block
- Ventricular aneurysm
- Uncontrolled metabolic disease (*e.g.*, diabetes, thyrotoxicosis, or myxedema)
- Chronic infectious disease (*e.g.*, HIV)
- Mental or physical impairment leading to inability to exercise adequately

[a]Relative contraindications can be superseded if benefits outweigh the risks of exercise. In some instances, these individuals can be exercised with caution and/or using low-level endpoints, especially if they are asymptomatic at rest.
Modified from (11) cited 2007 June 15. Available from: http://www.ncbi.nlm.nih.gov/pubmed/12356646

Emergency departments may perform a symptom-limited exercise test on patients who present with chest pain (*i.e.*, 8–12 h after initial evaluation) and meet the indications outlined in *Table 3.6* (3,25). This practice (a) appears to be safe in appropriately screened patients; (b) may improve diagnostic accuracy; and (c) may reduce cost of care. Generally, these patients include those who are no

TABLE 3.6. Indications and Contraindications for Exercise ECG Testing in the Emergency Department Setting

Requirements before exercise ECG testing that should be considered in the emergency department setting
- 2 Sets of cardiac enzymes at 4-h intervals should be normal
- ECG at the time of presentation, and preexercise 12-lead ECG shows no significant change
- Absence of rest ECG abnormalities that would preclude accurate assessment of the exercise ECG
- From admission to the time results are available from the second set of cardiac enzymes: patient asymptomatic, lessening chest pain symptoms, or persistent atypical symptoms
- Absence of ischemic chest pain at the time of exercise testing

Contraindications to exercise ECG testing in the emergency department setting
- New or evolving ECG abnormalities on the rest tracing
- Abnormal cardiac enzymes
- Inability to perform exercise
- Worsening or persistent ischemic chest pain symptoms from admission to the time of exercise testing
- Clinical risk profiling indicating imminent coronary angiography is likely

ECG, electrocardiogram.
Reprinted with permission from (25).

longer symptomatic and who have unremarkable ECGs and no change in serial cardiac enzymes. Exercise testing in this setting should be performed only as part of a carefully constructed patient management protocol, what is now commonly referred to as a chest pain unit, and only after patients have been screened for high-risk features or other indicators for hospital admission (3).

INFORMED CONSENT

Obtaining adequate informed consent from participants before exercise testing in health/fitness or clinical settings is an important ethical and legal consideration. Although the content and extent of consent forms may vary, enough information must be present in the informed consent process to ensure that the participant knows and understands the purposes and risks associated with the test or exercise program in health/fitness or clinical settings. The consent form should be verbally explained and include a statement indicating the client or patient has been given an opportunity to ask questions about the procedure and has sufficient information to give informed consent. Note specific questions from the participant on the form along with the responses provided. The consent form must indicate the participant is free to withdraw from the procedure at any time. If the participant is a minor, a legal guardian or parent must sign the consent form. It is advisable to check with authoritative bodies (*e.g.*, hospital risk management, institutional review boards, facility legal counsel) to determine what is appropriate for an acceptable informed consent process. Also, all reasonable efforts must be made to protect the privacy of the patient's health information (*e.g.*, medical history, test results) as described in the Health Insurance Portability and Accountability Act (HIPAA) of 1996. A sample consent form for exercise testing is provided in *Figure 3.1*. No sample form should be adopted for a specific test

Informed Consent for an Exercise Test

1. **Purpose and Explanation of the Test**
   You will perform an exercise test on a cycle ergometer or a motor-driven treadmill. The exercise intensity will begin at a low level and will be advanced in stages depending on your fitness level. We may stop the test at any time because of signs of fatigue or changes in your heart rate, electrocardiogram, or blood pressure, or symptoms you may experience. It is important for you to realize that you may stop when you wish because of feelings of fatigue or any other discomfort.

2. **Attendant Risks and Discomforts**
   There exists the possibility of certain changes occurring during the test. These include abnormal blood pressure; fainting; irregular, fast, or slow heart rhythm; and, in rare instances, heart attack, stroke, or death. Every effort will be made to minimize these risks by evaluation of preliminary information relating to your health and fitness and by careful observations during testing. Emergency equipment and trained personnel are available to deal with unusual situations that may arise.

3. **Responsibilities of the Participant**
   Information you possess about your health status or previous experiences of heart-related symptoms (*e.g.*, shortness of breath with low-level activity; pain; pressure; tightness; heaviness in the chest, neck, jaw, back, and/or arms) with physical effort may affect the safety of your exercise test. Your prompt reporting of these and any other unusual feelings with effort during the exercise test itself is very important. You are responsible for fully disclosing your medical history as well as symptoms that may occur during the test. You are also expected to report all medications (including nonprescription) taken recently and, in particular, those taken today to the testing staff.

4. **Benefits To Be Expected**
   The results obtained from the exercise test may assist in the diagnosis of your illness, in evaluating the effect of your medications, or in evaluating what type of physical activities you might do with low risk.

5. **Inquiries**
   Any questions about the procedures used in the exercise test or the results of your test are encouraged. If you have any concerns or questions, please ask us for further explanations.

6. **Use of Medical Records**
   The information that is obtained during exercise testing will be treated as privileged and confidential as described in the Health Insurance Portability and Accountability Act of 1996. It is not to be released or revealed to any individual except your referring physician without your written consent. However, the information obtained may be used for statistical analysis or scientific purposes with your right to privacy retained.

7. **Freedom of Consent**
   I hereby consent to voluntarily engage in an exercise test to determine my exercise capacity and state of cardiovascular health. My permission to perform this exercise test is given voluntarily. I understand that I am free to stop the test at any point if I so desire.

I have read this form, and I understand the test procedures that I will perform and the attendant risks and discomforts. Knowing these risks and discomforts, and having had an opportunity to ask questions that have been answered to my satisfaction, I consent to participate in this test.

Date	Signature of Patient
Date	Signature of Witness
Date	Signature of Physician or Authorized Delegate

■ **FIGURE 3.1.** Sample of informed consent form for a symptom-limited exercise test.

or program unless approved by local legal counsel and/or the appropriate institutional review board.

When the exercise test is for purposes other than diagnosis or Ex R$_x$ (*i.e.*, for experimental purposes), this should be indicated during the consent process and reflected on the *Informed Consent Form* and applicable policies for the testing of human subjects must be implemented. Health care professionals and scientists should obtain approval from their institutional review board when conducting an exercise test for research purposes.

Because most consent forms include the statement "emergency procedures and equipment are available," the program must ensure available personnel are appropriately trained and authorized to carry out emergency procedures that use such equipment. Written emergency policies and procedures should be in place, and emergency drills should be practiced at least once every 3 mo or more often when there is a change in staff (18). See *Appendix B* for more information on emergency management.

PARTICIPANT INSTRUCTIONS

Explicit instructions for participants before exercise testing increase test validity and data accuracy. Whenever possible, written instructions along with a description of the preexercise evaluation should be provided well in advance of the appointment so the client or patient can prepare adequately. When serial testing is performed, every effort should be made to ensure exercise testing procedures are consistent between/among assessments (5). The following points should be considered for inclusion in such preliminary instructions; however, specific instructions vary with test type and purpose:

- At a minimum, participants should refrain from ingesting food, alcohol, or caffeine or using tobacco products within 3 h of testing.
- Participants should be rested for the assessment, avoiding significant exertion or exercise on the day of the assessment.
- Clothing should permit freedom of movement and include walking or running shoes. Women should bring a loose fitting, short-sleeved blouse that buttons down the front, and should avoid restrictive undergarments.
- If the evaluation is on an outpatient basis, participants should be made aware that the exercise test may be fatiguing, and they may wish to have someone accompany them to the assessment to drive home afterward.
- If the exercise test is for diagnostic purposes, it may be helpful for patients to discontinue prescribed cardiovascular medications, but only with physician approval. Currently, prescribed antianginal agents alter the hemodynamic response to exercise and significantly reduce the sensitivity of ECG changes for ischemia. Patients taking intermediate or high dose β-blocking agents may be asked to taper their medication over a 2- to 4-d period to minimize hyperadrenergic withdrawal responses (see *Appendix A*).

- If the exercise test is for functional or Ex R$_x$ purposes, *patients should continue their medication regimen* on their usual schedule so that the exercise responses will be consistent with responses expected during exercise training.
- Participants should bring a list of their medications including dosage and frequency of administration to the assessment and should report the last actual dose taken. As an alternative, participants may wish to bring their medications with them for the exercise testing staff to record.
- Drink ample fluids over the 24-h period preceding the exercise test to ensure normal hydration before testing.

THE BOTTOM LINE

The ACSM Exercise Testing Summary Statements are the following:

- The preexercise evaluation is vital to ensuring exercise training can be safely initiated.
- Regardless of whether or not an exercise test is indicated prior to starting a physical activity program, identifying known CVD risk factors (see *Table* 2.2) is important for patient management.
- Exercise testing information can be used to counsel an individual regarding the risk for developing CVD, tayloring the lifestyle intervention program (*i.e.*, exercise, diet, and weight loss) to potentially ameliorate CVD risk factors, and when appropriate, refer to the appropriate health care professional for additional assessment.
- In those individuals who require exercise testing, absolute and relative contraindications must be considered before initiating the assessment (see *Box* 3.5).
- Individuals undergoing an exercise test should receive detailed instructions regarding the procedure and complete an informed consent document.

Online Resources

American College of Sports Medicine Exercise is Medicine:
http://exerciseismedicine.org

American Heart Association:
http://www.americanheart.org

National Heart, Lung, and Blood Institute Health Information for Professionals:
http://www.nhlbi.nih.gov/health/indexpro.htm

Physical Activity Guidelines for Americans (28):
http://www.health.gov/PAguidelines

REFERENCES

1. Alberti KG, Zimmet PZ. Definition, diagnosis and classification of diabetes mellitus and its complications. Part 1: diagnosis and classification of diabetes mellitus provisional report of a WHO consultation. *Diabet Med.* 1998;15(7):539–53.
2. American Diabetes Association. Diagnosis and classification of diabetes mellitus. *Diabetes Care.* 2007;30 Suppl 1:S42–7.
3. Amsterdam EA, Kirk JD, Bluemke DA, et al. Testing of low-risk patients presenting to the emergency department with chest pain: a scientific statement from the American Heart Association. *Circulation.* 2010;122(17):1756–76.
4. Appel LJ, Brands MW, Daniels SR, et al. Dietary approaches to prevent and treat hypertension: a scientific statement from the American Heart Association. *Hypertension.* 2006;47(2):296–308.
5. Arena R, Myers J, Williams MA, et al. Assessment of functional capacity in clinical and research settings: a scientific statement from the American Heart Association Committee on Exercise, Rehabilitation, and Prevention of the Council on Clinical Cardiology and the Council on Cardiovascular Nursing. *Circulation.* 2007;116(3):329–43.
6. Arena R, Pinkstaff S, Wheeler E, Peberdy MA, Guazzi M, Myers J. Neuromuscular electrical stimulation and inspiratory muscle training as potential adjunctive rehabilitation options for patients with heart failure. *J Cardiopulm Rehabil Prev.* 2010;30(4):209–23.
7. Bickley LS, Bates B. *Bates' Pocket Guide to Physical Examination and History Taking.* Baltimore (MD): Lippincott Williams & Wilkins; 2008. 416 p.
8. Expert Panel on Detection, Evaluation, and Treatment of High Blood Cholesterol in Adults. Executive Summary of the Third Report of the National Cholesterol Education Program (NCEP) Expert Panel on Detection, Evaluation, and Treatment of High Blood Cholesterol in Adults (Adult Treatment Panel III). *JAMA.* 2001;285(19):2486–97.
9. Ferguson GT, Enright PL, Buist AS, et al. Office spirometry for lung health assessment in adults: a consensus statement from the National Lung Health Education Program. *Chest.* 2000;117(4):1146–61.
10. Gibbons RJ, Abrams J, Chatterjee K, et al. Committee on the management of patients with chronic stable angina. ACC/AHA 2002 guideline update for the management of patients with chronic stable angina—summary article: a report of the American College of Cardiology/American Heart Association Task Force on practice guidelines (Committee on the Management of Patients with Chronic Stable Angina). *Circulation.* 2003;107(1):149–58.
11. Gibbons RJ, Balady GJ, Bricker JT, et al. Committee to Update the 1997 Exercise Testing Guidelines. ACC/AHA 2002 guideline update for exercise testing: summary article. A report of the American College of Cardiology/American Heart Association Task Force on Practice Guidelines (Committee to Update the 1997 Exercise Testing Guidelines). *J Am Coll Cardiol.* 2002;40(8):1531–40.
12. Grundy SM, Cleeman JI, Merz CN, et al. Implications of recent clinical trials for the National Cholesterol Education Program Adult Treatment Panel III Guidelines. *J Am Coll Cardiol.* 2004; 44(3):720–32.
13. Hendel RC, Berman DS, Di Carli MF, et al. ACCF/ASNC/ACR/AHA/ASE/SCCT/SCMR/SNM 2009 appropriate use criteria for cardiac radionuclide imaging: a report of the American College of Cardiology Foundation Appropriate Use Criteria Task Force, the American Society of Nuclear Cardiology, the American College of Radiology, the American Heart Association, the American Society of Echocardiography, the Society of Cardiovascular Computed Tomography, the Society for Cardiovascular Magnetic Resonance, and the Society of Nuclear Medicine. *Circulation.* 2009;119(22):e561–87.
14. *The IDF Consensus Worldwide Definition of the Metabolic Syndrome* [Internet]. Brussels (Belgium): International Diabetes Federation; 2006 [cited 2008 Jul 23]. 24 p. Available from: http://www.idf.org/webdata/docs/IDF_Meta_def_final.pdf
15. Kantola I, Vesalainen R, Kangassalo K, Kariluoto A. Bell or diaphragm in the measurement of blood pressure? *J Hypertens.* 2005;23(3):499–503.
16. Miller MR, Hankinson J, Brusasco V, et al. Standardisation of spirometry. *Eur Respir J.* 2005; 26(2):319–38.
17. Miller MR, Quanjer PH, Swanney MP, Ruppel G, Enright PL. Interpreting lung function data using 80 percent of predicted and fixed thresholds misclassifies over 20% of patients. *Chest.* 2010.
18. Myers J, Arena R, Franklin B, et al. Recommendations for clinical exercise laboratories: a scientific statement from the American Heart Association. *Circulation.* 2009;119(24):3144–61.
19. Nici L, Donner C, Wouters E, et al. American Thoracic Society/European Respiratory Society statement on pulmonary rehabilitation. *Am J Respir Crit Care Med.* 2006;173(12):1390–413.
20. Pellegrino R, Viegi G, Brusasco V, et al. Interpretative strategies for lung function tests. *Eur Respir J.* 2005;26(5):948–68.

21. Pickering TG, Hall JE, Appel LJ, et al. Recommendations for blood pressure measurement in humans and experimental animals: Part 1: blood pressure measurement in humans: a statement for professionals from the Subcommittee of Professional and Public Education of the American Heart Association Council on High Blood Pressure Research. *Hypertension.* 2005;45(1):142–61.

22. Rabe KF, Hurd S, Anzueto A, et al. Global strategy for the diagnosis, management, and prevention of chronic obstructive pulmonary disease: GOLD executive summary. *Am J Respir Crit Care Med.* 2007;176(6):532–55.

23. *The Seventh Report of the Joint National Committee on Prevention, Detection, Evaluation, and Treatment of High Blood Pressure (JNC7)* [Internet]. Bethesda, (MD): National High Blood Pressure Education Program; 2004 [cited 2012 Jan 7]. 104 p. Available from: http://www.nhlbi.nih.gov/guidelines/hypertension

24. Smith SC,Jr, Allen J, Blair SN, et al. AHA/ACC guidelines for secondary prevention for patients with coronary and other atherosclerotic vascular disease: 2006 update: endorsed by the National Heart, Lung, and Blood Institute. *Circulation.* 2006;113(19):2363–72.

25. Stein RA, Chaitman BR, Balady GJ, et al. Safety and utility of exercise testing in emergency room chest pain centers: an advisory from the Committee on Exercise, Rehabilitation, and Prevention, Council on Clinical Cardiology, American Heart Association. *Circulation.* 2000;102(12):1463–7.

26. Swain DP, American College of Sports Medicine. *ACSM's Resource Manual for Guidelines for Exercise Testing and Prescription.* 7th ed. Baltimore (MD): Lippincott Williams & Wilkins; 2014.

27. *Third Report of the National Cholesterol Education Program (NCEP) Expert Panel on Detection, Evaluation, and Treatment of High Blood Cholesterol in Adults (Adult Treatment Panel III)* [Internet]. Bethesda (MD): National Cholesterol Education Program; 2004 [cited Mar 19]. 284 p. Available from: http://www.nhlbi.nih.gov/guidelines/cholesterol/index.htm

28. U.S. Department of Health and Human Services. *2008 Physical Activity Guidelines for Americans* [Internet]. Rockville (MD): Office of Disease Prevention & Health Promotion, U.S. Department of Health and Human Services; 2008 [cited 2012 Jan 7]. 76 p. Available from: http://www.health.gov/paguidelines

Health-Related Physical Fitness Testing and Interpretation

Evidence as outlined in *Chapter 1* now clearly supports the numerous health benefits that result from regular participation in physical activity and structured exercise programs including enhancement of aerobic capacity (*i.e.,* cardio-respiratory fitness [CRF]). The health-related components of physical fitness have a strong relationship with overall health, are characterized by an ability to perform activities of daily living with vigor, and are associated with a lower prevalence of chronic disease and health conditions and their risk factors (29). Measures of health-related physical fitness and CRF are closely allied with disease prevention and health promotion and can be modified through regular participation in physical activity and structured exercise programs. A fundamental goal of primary and secondary prevention and rehabilitative programs should be the promotion of health; therefore, exercise programs should focus on enhancement of the health-related components of physical fitness including CRF. Accordingly, the focus of this chapter is on the health-related components of physical fitness rather than the skill-related components for the general population (46).

PURPOSES OF HEALTH-RELATED PHYSICAL FITNESS TESTING

Measurement of physical fitness is a common and appropriate practice in preventive and rehabilitative exercise programs. The purposes of health/fitness testing in such exercise programs include the following:

- Educating participants about their present health/fitness status relative to health-related standards and age and sex matched norms.
- Providing data that are helpful in development of individualized exercise prescriptions (Ex R$_x$) to address all health/fitness components.
- Collecting baseline and follow-up data that allow evaluation of progress by exercise program participants.
- Motivating participants by establishing reasonable and attainable health/fitness goals (see *Chapter 11*).

BASIC PRINCIPLES AND GUIDELINES

The information obtained from health-related physical fitness testing, in combination with the individual's health and medical information, is used by the health/fitness and clinical exercise professional to enable an individual to achieve specific health/fitness goals. An ideal health-related physical fitness test is reliable, valid, relatively inexpensive, and easy to administer. The test should yield results that are indicative of the current state of physical fitness, reflect positive changes in health status from participation in a physical activity or exercise intervention, and be directly comparable to normative data.

PRETEST INSTRUCTIONS

All pretest instructions should be provided and adhered to prior to arrival at the testing facility (see *Chapter 3*). Certain steps should be taken to ensure client safety and comfort before administering a health-related physical fitness test. A minimal recommendation is that individuals complete a self-guided questionnaire such as the Physical Activity Readiness Questionnaire (PAR-Q) (see *Figure 2.1*) (89) or the American Heart Association (AHA)/American College of Sports Medicine (ACSM) Health/Fitness Facility Preparticipation Screening Questionnaire (see *Figure 2.2*) (3,102). A listing of preliminary testing instructions for all clients can be found in *Chapter 3* under "Participant Instructions." These instructions may be modified to meet specific needs and circumstances.

TEST ORGANIZATION

The following should be accomplished before the client/patient arrives at the test site:

- Assure all forms, score sheets, tables, graphs, and other testing documents are organized in the client's or patient's file and available for the test's administration.
- Calibrate all equipment (*e.g.*, metronome, cycle ergometer, treadmill, sphygmomanometer, skinfold calipers) at least monthly, or more frequently based on use; certain equipment such as ventilatory expired gas analysis systems should be calibrated prior to each test according to manufacturers' specifications; and document equipment calibration in a designated folder.
- Organize equipment so that tests can follow in sequence without stressing the same muscle group repeatedly.
- Provide an informed consent form and allow time for the individual undergoing assessment to have all questions adequately addressed (see *Figure 3.1*).
- Maintain room temperature between 68° F and 72° F (20° C and 22° C) and humidity of less than 60% with adequate airflow.

When multiple tests are to be administered, the organization of the testing session can be very important, depending on what physical fitness components are to be evaluated. Resting measurements such as heart rate (HR), blood pressure (BP), height, weight, and body composition should be obtained first. Research has not established an optimal testing order for multiple health-related components of fitness (*i.e.*, cardiorespiratory [CR] endurance, muscular fitness, body composition, and flexibility), but sufficient time should be allowed for HR and BP to return to baseline between tests conducted serially. Because certain medications, such as β-blockers which lower HR, will affect some physical fitness test results, use of these medications should be noted (see *Appendix A*).

TEST ENVIRONMENT

The environment is important for test validity and reliability. Test anxiety, emotional problems, room temperature, and ventilation should be controlled as much as possible. To minimize subject anxiety, the test procedures should be explained adequately, and the test environment should be quiet and private. The room should be equipped with a comfortable seat and/or examination table to be used for resting BP and HR and/or electrocardiographic (ECG) recordings. The demeanor of personnel should be one of relaxed confidence to put the subject at ease. Testing procedures should not be rushed, and all procedures must be explained clearly prior to initiating the process.

BODY COMPOSITION

It is well established that excess body fat, particularly when located centrally around the abdomen, is associated with hypertension, metabolic syndrome, Type 2 diabetes mellitus, stroke, cardiovascular disease (CVD), and dyslipidemia (95). Approximately two-thirds of American adults are classified as overweight (body mass index [BMI] ≥25 kg $\cdot$ m^{-2}), and about 33% of these are classified as obese (BMI ≥30 kg $\cdot$ m^{-2}). Although the prevalence of obesity has steadily risen over the last three decades, recent data indicate a plateau in obesity trends, particularly in women (23,38). Perhaps more troubling are the statistics relating to children that indicate (a) approximately 32% of children aged 2–19 yr are overweight or obese; and (b) over the past three decades, the percentage of children aged 6–11 yr who are considered obese has increased from approximately 4% to more than 17% (95). Moreover, 2006 data indicate race and sex differences in overweight/obesity, with Black and Hispanic women continuing to have the highest prevalence (95). The troubling data on overweight/obesity prevalence among the adult and pediatric populations and its health implications have precipitated an increased awareness in the value of identifying and treating individuals with excess body weight (26,33,64,105).

Basic body composition can be expressed as the relative percentage of body mass that is fat and fat-free tissue using a two-compartment model. Body composition can be estimated with laboratory and field techniques that vary in terms of complexity, cost, and accuracy (34,65). Different assessment techniques are briefly reviewed in this section, but details associated with obtaining measurements and calculating estimates of body fat for all of these techniques are beyond the scope of the *Guidelines*. For more detailed information, see *ACSM's Resource Manual for Guidelines for Exercise Testing and Prescription, Seventh Edition* (101) and elsewhere (48,51,60). Before collecting data for body composition assessment, the technician must be trained, experienced in the techniques, and already have demonstrated reliability in his or her measurements, independent of the technique being used. Experience can be accrued under the direct supervision of a highly qualified mentor in a controlled testing environment.

ANTHROPOMETRIC METHODS

Body Mass Index

BMI or the Quetelet index is used to assess weight relative to height and is calculated by dividing body weight in kilograms by height in meters squared ($kg \cdot m^{-2}$). For most individuals, obesity-related health problems increase beyond a BMI of 25.0 $kg \cdot m^{-2}$. The *Expert Panel on the Identification, Evaluation, and Treatment of Overweight and Obesity in Adults* (35) defines a BMI of $25.0–29.9$ $kg \cdot m^{-2}$ as overweight and BMI of ≥ 30.0 $kg \cdot m^{-2}$ as obese. BMI fails to distinguish between body fat, muscle mass, or bone. Nevertheless, an increased risk of hypertension, sleep apnea, Type 2 diabetes mellitus, certain cancers, CVD, and mortality are associated with a BMI ≥ 30.0 $kg \cdot m^{-2}$ (*Table 4.1*) (86). Interestingly, there is compelling evidence to indicate patients diagnosed with congestive heart failure (CHF) actually have improved survival when BMI is ≥ 30.0 $kg \cdot m^{-2}$, a phenomenon known as the "obesity paradox" (79), for reasons that are not clear (4).

Compared to individuals classified as obese, the link between a BMI in the overweight range ($25.0–29.9$ $kg \cdot m^{-2}$) and higher mortality risk is less clear. However, a BMI of $25.0–29.9$ $kg \cdot m^{-2}$, similar to a BMI ≥ 30.0 $kg \cdot m^{-2}$, is more convincingly linked to an increased risk for other health issues such as Type 2 diabetes mellitus, dyslipidemia, hypertension, and certain cancers (68). A BMI of <18.5 $kg \cdot m^{-2}$

TABLE 4.1. Classification of Disease Risk Based on Body Mass Index (BMI) and Waist Circumference

	BMI ($kg \cdot m^{-2}$)	Disease Risk[a] Relative to Normal Weight and Waist Circumference	
		Men, ≤ 102 cm Women, ≤ 88 cm	Men, >102 cm Women, >88 cm
Underweight	<18.5	—	—
Normal	$18.5–24.9$	—	—
Overweight	$25.0–29.9$	Increased	High
Obesity, class			
I	$30.0–34.9$	High	Very high
II	$35.0–39.9$	Very high	Very high
III	≥ 40.0	Extremely high	Extremely high

[a]Disease risk for Type 2 diabetes, hypertension, and cardiovascular disease. Dashes (—) indicate that no additional risk at these levels of BMI was assigned. Increased waist circumference can also be a marker for increased risk even in individuals of normal weight.

Modified from (35).

TABLE 4.2. Predicted Body Fat Percentage Based on Body Mass Index (BMI) for African American and White Adults[a]

BMI (kg · m⁻²)	Health Risk	20–39 yr	40–59 yr	60–79 yr
Men				
<18.5	Elevated	<8%	<11%	<13%
18.6–24.9	Average	8%–19%	11%–21%	13%–24%
25.0–29.9	Elevated	20%–24%	22%–27%	25%–29%
>30	High	≥25%	≥28%	≥30%
Women				
<18.5	Elevated	<21%	<23%	<24%
18.6–24.9	Average	21%–32%	23%–33%	24%–35%
25.0–29.9	Elevated	33%–38%	34%–39%	36%–41%
>30	High	≥39%	≥40%	≥42%

[a]Standard error of estimate is ±5% for predicting percent body fat from BMI (based on a four compartment estimate of body fat percentage).

Reprinted with permission from (41).

also increases mortality risk and is responsible for the lower portion of the J-shaped curve when plotting risk on the y-axis and BMI on the x-axis (39). The use of specific BMI values to predict percent body fat and health risk can be found in *Table 4.2* (41). Because of the relatively large standard error of estimating percent body fat from BMI (±5% fat) (34), other methods of body composition assessment should be used to estimate percent body fat during a physical fitness assessment.

Circumferences

The pattern of body fat distribution is recognized as an important indicator of health and prognosis (28,90). Android obesity that is characterized by more fat on the trunk (*i.e.*, abdominal fat) increases the risk of hypertension, metabolic syndrome, Type 2 diabetes mellitus, dyslipidemia, CVD, and premature death compared with individuals who demonstrate gynoid or gynecoid obesity (*i.e.*, fat distributed in the hip and thigh) (85). Moreover, among individuals with increased abdominal fat, higher levels in the visceral compartment confer a higher risk for development of the metabolic syndrome compared to a similar distribution of fat within the subcutaneous compartment (40).

Circumference (or girth) measurements may be used to provide a general representation of body composition, and equations are available for both sexes and a range of age groups (103,104). The accuracy may be within 2.5%–4.0% of the actual body composition if the subject possesses similar characteristics to the original validation population and the girth measurements are precise. A cloth tape measure with a spring-loaded handle (*e.g.*, Gulick tape measure) reduces skin compression and improves consistency of measurement. Duplicate measurements are recommended at each site and should be obtained in a rotational instead of a consecutive order (*i.e.*, take measurements of all sites being assessed and then repeat the sequence). The average of the two measures is used provided they do not differ by more than 5 mm. *Box 4.1* contains a description of the common measurement sites.

The waist-to-hip ratio (WHR) is the circumference of the waist (above the iliac crest) divided by the circumference of the hips (see *Box 4.1* for buttocks/hips

BOX 4.1	Standardized Description of Circumference Sites and Procedures

Abdomen: With the subject standing upright and relaxed, a horizontal measure taken at the height of the iliac crest, usually at the level of the umbilicus.

Arm: With the subject standing erect and arms hanging freely at the sides with hands facing the thigh, a horizontal measure midway between the acromion and olecranon processes.

Buttocks/Hips: With the subject standing erect and feet together, a horizontal measure is taken at the maximal circumference of buttocks. This measure is used for the hip measure in a waist/hip measure.

Calf: With the subject standing erect (feet apart ~20 cm), a horizontal measure taken at the level of the maximum circumference between the knee and the ankle, perpendicular to the long axis.

Forearm: With the subject standing, arms hanging downward but slightly away from the trunk and palms facing anteriorly, a measure is taken perpendicular to the long axis at the maximal circumference.

Hips/Thigh: With the subject standing, legs slightly apart (~10 cm), a horizontal measure is taken at the maximal circumference of the hip/proximal thigh, just below the gluteal fold.

Mid-Thigh With the subject standing and one foot on a bench so the knee is flexed at 90 degrees, a measure is taken midway between the inguinal crease and the proximal border of the patella, perpendicular to the long axis.

Waist: With the subject standing, arms at the sides, feet together, and abdomen relaxed, a horizontal measure is taken at the narrowest part of the torso (above the umbilicus and below the xiphoid process). The National Obesity Task Force (NOTF) suggests obtaining a horizontal measure directly above the iliac crest as a method to enhance standardization. Unfortunately, current formulae are not predicated on the NOTF suggested site.

| BOX 4.1 | Standardized Description of Circumference Sites and Procedures (*Continued*) |

Procedures
- All measurements should be made with a flexible yet inelastic tape measure.
- The tape should be placed on the skin surface without compressing the subcutaneous adipose tissue.
- If a Gulick spring-loaded handle is used, the handle should be extended to the same marking with each trial.
- Take duplicate measures at each site and retest if duplicate measurements are not within 5 mm.
- Rotate through measurement sites or allow time for skin to regain normal texture.

Modified from (18).

measure) and has traditionally been used as a simple method for assessing body fat distribution and identifying individuals with higher and more detrimental amounts of abdominal fat (34,85). Health risk increases as WHR increases, and the standards for risk vary with age and sex. For example, health risk is *very high* for young men when WHR is >0.95 and for young women when WHR is >0.86. For individuals aged 60–69 yr, the WHR cutoff values are >1.03 for men and >0.90 for women for the same high-risk classification as young adults (51).

The waist circumference may also be used as an indicator of health risk because abdominal obesity is the primary issue (20,28). The Expert Panel on the Identification, Evaluation, and Treatment of Overweight and Obesity in Adults provides a classification of disease risk based on both BMI and waist circumference as shown in *Table 4.1* (35). Previous research has demonstrated that the waist circumference thresholds shown in *Table 4.1* effectively identify individuals at increased health risk across the different BMI categories (56). Furthermore, a newer risk stratification scheme for adults based on waist circumference has been proposed (see *Table 4.3*) (14). Several methods for waist circumference measurement involving different anatomical sites are available. Evidence indicates that all currently available waist circumference measurement techniques

TABLE 4.3. Risk Criteria for Waist Circumference in Adults

	Waist Circumference cm (in)	
Risk Category	Women	Men
Very low	<70 cm (<28.5 in)	<80 cm (31.5 in)
Low	70–89 (28.5–35.0)	80–99 (31.5–39.0)
High	90–110 (35.5–43.0)	100–120 (39.5–47.0)
Very high	>110 (>43.5)	>120 (>47.0)

Reprinted with permission from (14).

are equally reliable and effective in identifying individuals at increased health risk (96,108).

Measurement of Waist Circumference

Measurement of waist circumference immediately above the iliac crest, as proposed by National Institutes of Health guidelines, may be the preferable circumference method to assess health risk given the ease by which this anatomical landmark is identified (25).

Skinfold Measurements

Body composition determined from skinfold thickness measurements correlates well ($r = 0.70$–0.90) with body composition determined by hydrodensitometry (48). The principle behind skinfold measurements is that the amount of subcutaneous fat is proportional to the total amount of body fat. It is assumed that close to one-third of the total fat is located subcutaneously. The exact proportion of subcutaneous to total fat varies with sex, age, and race (94). Therefore, regression equations used to convert sum of skinfolds to percent body fat should consider these variables for greatest accuracy. *Box 4.2* presents a standardized description of skinfold sites and procedures. Refer to *ACSM's Resource Manual for Guidelines for Exercise Testing and Prescription, Seventh Edition* (101) for additional descriptions of skinfold sites. Skinfold assessment of body composition is very dependent on the expertise of the technician, so proper training (*i.e.*, knowledge of anatomical landmarks) and ample practice of the technique is necessary to obtain accurate measurements. The accuracy of predicting percent body fat from skinfolds is approximately ±3.5%, assuming appropriate techniques and equations have been used (51).

Factors that may contribute to measurement error within skinfold assessment include poor technique and/or an inexperienced evaluator, an extremely obese or extremely lean subject, and an improperly calibrated caliper (*i.e.*, tension should be set at ~12 g $\cdot$ mm^{-2}) (49). Various regression equations have been developed to predict body density or percent body fat from skinfold measurements. For example, *Box 4.3* lists generalized equations that allow calculation of body density without a loss in prediction accuracy for a wide range of individuals (49,54). Other equations have been published that are sex, age, race, fat, and sport specific (50). At a minimum, simple anthropometric measurements should be included in the health assessment of all individuals.

Anthropometric Measurements

Although limited in the ability to provide highly precise estimates of percent body fat, anthropometric measurements (*i.e.*, BMI, WHR, waist circumference, and skinfolds) provide valuable information on general health and risk stratification. As such, inclusion of these easily obtainable variables during a comprehensive health/fitness assessment is beneficial.

| BOX 4.2 | Standardized Description of Skinfold Sites and Procedures |

SKINFOLD SITE

Abdominal — Vertical fold; 2 cm to the right side of the umbilicus

Triceps — Vertical fold; on the posterior midline of the upper arm, halfway between the acromion and olecranon processes, with the arm held freely to the side of the body

Biceps — Vertical fold; on the anterior aspect of the arm over the belly of the biceps muscle, 1 cm above the level used to mark the triceps site

Chest/Pectoral — Diagonal fold; one-half the distance between the anterior axillary line and the nipple (men), or one-third of the distance between the anterior axillary line and the nipple (women)

Medial calf — Vertical fold; at the maximum circumference of the calf on the midline of its medial border

Midaxillary — Vertical fold; on the midaxillary line at the level of the xiphoid process of the sternum. An alternate method is a horizontal fold taken at the level of the xiphoid/sternal border in the midaxillary line

Subscapular — Diagonal fold (at a 45-degree angle); 1–2 cm below the inferior angle of the scapula

Suprailiac — Diagonal fold; in line with the natural angle of the iliac crest taken in the anterior axillary line immediately superior to the iliac crest

Thigh — Vertical fold; on the anterior midline of the thigh, midway between the proximal border of the patella and the inguinal crease (hip)

Procedures
- All measurements should be made on the right side of the body with the subject standing upright
- Caliper should be placed directly on the skin surface, 1 cm away from the thumb and finger, perpendicular to the skinfold, and halfway between the crest and the base of the fold
- Pinch should be maintained while reading the caliper
- Wait 1–2 s (not longer) before reading caliper
- Take duplicate measures at each site and retest if duplicate measurements are not within 1–2 mm
- Rotate through measurement sites or allow time for skin to regain normal texture and thickness

BOX 4.3	Generalized Skinfold Equations

MEN

- **Seven-Site Formula** (chest, midaxillary, triceps, subscapular, abdomen, suprailiac, thigh)
  Body density = 1.112 − 0.00043499 (sum of seven skinfolds)
      + 0.00000055 (sum of seven skinfolds)^2
      − 0.00028826 (age) *[SEE 0.008 or ~3.5% fat]*

- **Three-Site Formula** (chest, abdomen, thigh)
  Body density = 1.10938 − 0.0008267 (sum of three skinfolds)
      + 0.0000016 (sum of three skinfolds)^2 − 0.0002574 (age)
      [SEE 0.008 or ~3.4% fat]

- **Three-Site Formula** (chest, triceps, subscapular)
  Body density = 1.1125025 − 0.0013125 (sum of three skinfolds)
      + 0.0000055 (sum of three skinfolds)^2 − 0.000244 (age)
      [SEE 0.008 or ~3.6% fat]

WOMEN

- **Seven-Site Formula** (chest, midaxillary, triceps, subscapular, abdomen, suprailiac, thigh)
  Body density = 1.097 − 0.00046971 (sum of seven skinfolds)
      + 0.00000056 (sum of seven skinfolds)^2 − 0.00012828
      (age) *[SEE 0.008 or ~3.8% fat]*

- **Three-Site Formula** (triceps, suprailiac, thigh)
  Body density = 1.099421 − 0.0009929 (sum of three skinfolds)
      + 0.0000023 (sum of three skinfolds)^2 − 0.0001392 (age)
      [SEE 0.009 or ~3.9% fat]

- **Three-Site Formula** (triceps, suprailiac, abdominal)
  Body density = 1.089733 − 0.0009245 (sum of three skinfolds)
      + 0.0000025 (sum of three skinfolds)^2 − 0.0000979 (age)
      [SEE 0.009 or ~3.9% fat]

SEE, standard error of estimate.
Adapted from (55,87).

DENSITOMETRY

Body composition can be estimated from a measurement of whole-body density using the ratio of body mass to body volume. Densitometry has been used as a reference or criterion standard for assessing body composition for many years. The limiting factor in the measurement of body density is the accuracy of the body volume measurement because body mass is measured simply as body weight. Body volume can be measured by hydrodensitometry (underwater) weighing and by plethysmography.

Hydrodensitometry (Underwater) Weighing

This technique of measuring body composition is based on Archimedes' principle that states when a body is immersed in water, it is buoyed by a counterforce equal to the weight of the water displaced. This loss of weight in water allows for calculation of body volume. Bone and muscle tissue are denser than water, whereas fat tissue is less dense. Therefore, an individual with more fat-free mass (FFM) for the same total body mass weighs more in water and has a higher body density and lower percentage of body fat. Although hydrostatic weighing is a standard method for measuring body volume and hence, body composition, it requires special equipment, the accurate measurement of residual volume, population-specific formulas, and significant cooperation by the subject (44). For a more detailed explanation of the technique, see *ACSM's Resource Manual for Guidelines for Exercise Testing and Prescription, Seventh Edition* (101).

Plethysmography

Body volume also can be measured by air rather than water displacement. One commercial system uses a dual-chamber plethysmograph that measures body volume by changes in pressure in a closed chamber. This technology is now well established and generally reduces the anxiety associated with the technique of hydrodensitometry (31,44,70). For a more detailed explanation of the technique, see *ACSM's Resource Manual for Guidelines for Exercise Testing and Prescription, Seventh Edition* (101).

Conversion of Body Density to Body Composition

Percent body fat can be estimated once body density has been determined. Two of the most common prediction equations used to estimate percent body fat from body density are derived from the two-component model of body composition (15,100):

$$\% \text{ fat} = \frac{457}{\text{Body Density}} - 414.2$$

$$\% \text{ fat} = \frac{495}{\text{Body Density}} - 450$$

Each method assumes a slightly different density of fat mass (FM) and FFM. Several population-specific, two-component model conversion formulas are also available (see *Table 4.4*). Currently, three to six component model conversion formulas are available and are increasingly more precise in calculating percent body fat compared to two-component models (34,51).

TABLE 4.4. Population-Specific Formulas for Conversion of Body Density to Percent Body Fat

	Population	Age	Gender	%BF	FFBd[a] (g · cm^{-3})
ETHNICITY		9–17	Women	(5.24 / Db) − 4.82	1.088
	African American	19–45	Men	(4.86 / Db) − 4.39	1.106
		24–79	Women	(4.86 / Db) − 4.39	1.106
	American Indian	18–62	Men	(4.97 / Db) − 4.52	1.099
		18–60	Women	(4.81 / Db) − 4.34	1.108
		18–48	Men	(4.97 / Db) − 4.52	1.099
	Asian Japanese Native		Women	(4.76 / Db) − 4.28	1.111
		61–78	Men	(4.87 / Db) − 4.41	1.105
			Women	(4.95 / Db) − 4.50	1.100
	Singaporean (Chinese, Indian, Malay)		Men	(4.94 / Db) − 4.48	1.102
			Women	(4.84 / Db) − 4.37	1.107
		8–12	Men	(5.27 / Db) − 4.85	1.086
			Women	(5.27 / Db) − 4.85	1.086
		13–17	Men	(5.12 / Db) − 4.69	1.092
	Caucasian		Women	(5.19 / Db) − 4.76	1.090
		18–59	Men	(4.95 / Db) − 4.50	1.100
			Women	(4.96 / Db) − 4.51	1.101
		60–90	Men	(4.97 / Db) − 4.52	1.099
			Women	(5.02 / Db) − 4.57	1.098
	Hispanic		Men	NA	NA
		20–40	Women	(4.87 / Db) − 4.41	1.105
ATHLETES	Resistance trained	24 ± 4	Men	(5.21 / Db) − 4.78	1.089
		35 ± 6	Women	(4.97 / Db) − 4.52	1.099
	Endurance trained	21 ± 2	Men	(5.03 / Db) − 4.59	1.097
		21 ± 4	Women	(4.95 / Db) − 4.50	1.100
	All sports	18–22	Men	(5.12 / Db) − 4.68	1.093
		18–22	Women	(4.97 / Db) − 4.52	1.099
CLINICAL POPULATIONS[b]	Anorexia nervosa	15–44	Women	(4.96 / Db) − 4.51	1.101
	Cirrhosis				
	Childs A			(5.33 / Db) − 4.91	1.084
	Childs B			(5.48 / Db) − 5.08	1.078
	Childs C			(5.69 / Db) − 5.32	1.070
	Obesity	17–62	Women	(4.95 / Db) − 4.50	1.100
	Spinal cord injury (paraplegic/quadriplegic)	18–73	Men	(4.67 / Db) − 4.18	1.116
		18–73	Women	(4.70 / Db) − 4.22	1.114

[a]FFBd, fat-free body density based on average values reported in selected research articles.

[b]There are insufficient multicomponent model data to estimate the average FFBd of the following clinical populations: coronary artery disease, heart/lung transplants, chronic obstructive pulmonary disease, cystic fibrosis, diabetes mellitus, thyroid disease, HIV/AIDS, cancer, kidney failure (dialysis), multiple sclerosis, and muscular dystrophy.

%BF, percentage of body fat; Db, body density; NA, no data available for this population subgroup.

Adapted with permission from (51).

OTHER TECHNIQUES

Additional reliable and accurate body composition assessment techniques include dual-energy X-ray absorptiometry (DEXA) and total body electrical conductivity (TOBEC), but these techniques have limited applicability in routine health/fitness testing because of cost and the need for highly trained personnel (48). Rather, bioelectrical impedance analysis (BIA) and near-infrared interactance are used as assessment techniques in routine health/fitness testing. Generally, the accuracy of BIA is similar to skinfolds, as long as stringent protocol adherence (e.g., assurance of normal hydration status) is followed, and the equations programmed into the analyzer are valid and accurate for the populations being tested (30,47). It should be noted, however, that the ability of BIA to provide an accurate assessment of percent body fat in obese individuals may be limited secondary to differences in body water distribution compared to those who are in the normal weight range (34). Near-infrared interactance requires additional research to substantiate the validity and accuracy for body composition assessment (58,73). Detailed explanations of these techniques are found in *ACSM's Resource Manual for Guidelines for Exercise Testing and Prescription, Seventh Edition* (101).

BODY COMPOSITION NORMS

There are no universally accepted norms for body composition; however, *Tables 4.5* and *4.6*, which are based on selected populations, provide percentile values for percent body fat in men and women, respectively. A consensus opinion for an exact percent body fat value associated with optimal health risk has yet to be defined; however, a range of 10%–22% and 20%–32% for men and women, respectively, has long been viewed as satisfactory for health (70). More recent data support this range although age and race, in addition to sex, impact what may be construed as a healthy percent body fat (41).

CARDIORESPIRATORY FITNESS

CRF is related to the ability to perform large muscle, dynamic, moderate-to-vigorous intensity exercise for prolonged periods of time. Performance of exercise at this level of physical exertion depends on the integrated physiologic and functional state of the respiratory, cardiovascular, and musculoskeletal systems. CRF is considered a health-related component of physical fitness because (a) low levels of CRF have been associated with a markedly increased risk of premature death from all causes and specifically from CVD; (b) increases in CRF are associated with a reduction in death from all causes; and (c) high levels of CRF are associated with higher levels of habitual physical activity, which in turn are associated with many health benefits (10,11,63,98,107). As such, the assessment of CRF is an important part of any primary or secondary prevention and rehabilitative programs.

TABLE 4.5. Fitness Categories for Body Composition (% Body Fat) for Men by Age

%		Age (year)					
		20–29	30–39	40–49	50–59	60–69	70–79
99	Very lean[a]	4.2	7.3	9.5	11.0	11.9	13.6
95		6.4	10.3	12.9	14.8	16.2	15.5
90	Excellent	7.9	12.4	15.0	17.0	18.1	17.5
85		9.1	13.7	16.4	18.3	19.2	19.0
80		10.5	14.9	17.5	19.4	20.2	20.1
75	Good	11.5	15.9	18.5	20.2	21.0	21.0
70		12.6	16.8	19.3	21.0	21.7	21.6
65		13.8	17.7	20.1	21.7	22.4	22.3
60		14.8	18.4	20.8	22.3	23.0	22.9
55	Fair	15.8	19.2	21.4	23.0	23.6	23.7
50		16.6	20.0	22.1	23.6	24.2	24.1
45		17.5	20.7	22.8	24.2	24.9	24.7
40		18.6	21.6	23.5	24.9	25.6	25.3
35	Poor	19.7	22.4	24.2	25.6	26.4	25.8
30		20.7	23.2	24.9	26.3	27.0	26.5
25		22.0	24.1	25.7	27.1	27.9	27.1
20		23.3	25.1	26.6	28.1	28.8	28.4
15	Very poor	24.9	26.4	27.8	29.2	29.8	29.4
10		26.6	27.8	29.2	30.6	31.2	30.7
5		29.2	30.2	31.3	32.7	33.3	32.9
1		33.4	34.4	35.2	36.4	36.8	37.2
n =		1,844	10,099	15,073	9,255	2,851	522

Total *n* = 39,644

[a]Very lean, no less than 3% body fat is recommended for men.

Adapted with permission from *Physical Fitness Assessments and Norms for Adults and Law Enforcement.* The Cooper Institute, Dallas, Texas. 2009. For more information: www.cooperinstitute.org

THE CONCEPT OF MAXIMAL OXYGEN UPTAKE

Maximal oxygen uptake ($\dot{V}O_{2max}$) is accepted as the criterion measure of CRF. This variable is typically expressed clinically in relative (mL $\cdot$ kg^{-1} $\cdot$ min^{-1}) as opposed to absolute (mL $\cdot$ min^{-1}) terms, allowing for meaningful comparisons between/among individuals with differing body weight. $\dot{V}O_{2max}$ is the product of the maximal cardiac output $\dot{Q}$ (L blood $\cdot$ min^{-1}) and arterial-venous oxygen difference (mL O_2 $\cdot$ L blood^{-1}). Significant variation in $\dot{V}O_{2max}$ across populations and fitness levels results primarily from differences in $\dot{Q}$ in individuals without pulmonary disease; therefore, $\dot{V}O_{2max}$ is closely related to the functional capacity of the heart. The designation of $\dot{V}O_{2max}$ implies an individual's true physiologic limit has been reached and a plateau in $\dot{V}O_2$ may be observed between the final two work rates of a progressive exercise test. This plateau is rarely observed in individuals with CVD or pulmonary disease. Therefore, peak $\dot{V}O_2$ is commonly used to describe CRF in these and other populations with chronic diseases and health conditions (5).

Open circuit spirometry is used to measure $\dot{V}O_{2max}$. In this procedure, the subject breathes through a low-resistance valve with her or his nose occluded

TABLE 4.6. Fitness Categories for Body Composition (% Body Fat) for Women by Age

%		Age (year)					
		20–29	30–39	40–49	50–59	60–69	70–79
99	Very lean[a]	11.4	11.2	12.1	13.9	13.9	11.7
95		14.0	13.9	15.2	16.9	17.7	16.4
90	Excellent	15.1	15.5	16.8	19.1	20.2	18.3
85		16.1	16.5	18.3	20.8	22.0	21.2
80		16.8	17.5	19.5	22.3	23.3	22.5
75	Good	17.6	18.3	20.6	23.6	24.6	23.7
70		18.4	19.2	21.7	24.8	25.7	24.8
65		19.0	20.1	22.7	25.8	26.7	25.7
60		19.8	21.0	23.7	26.7	27.5	26.6
55	Fair	20.6	22.0	24.6	27.6	28.3	27.6
50		21.5	22.8	25.5	28.4	29.2	28.2
45		22.2	23.7	26.4	29.3	30.1	28.9
40		23.4	24.8	27.5	30.1	30.8	30.5
35	Poor	24.2	25.8	28.4	30.8	31.5	31.0
30		25.5	26.9	29.5	31.8	32.6	31.9
25		26.7	28.1	30.7	32.9	33.3	32.9
20		28.2	29.6	31.9	33.9	34.4	34.0
15	Very poor	30.5	31.5	33.4	35.0	35.6	35.3
10		33.5	33.6	35.1	36.1	36.6	36.4
5		36.6	36.2	37.1	37.6	38.2	38.1
1		38.6	39.0	39.1	39.8	40.3	40.2
n =		1,250	4,130	5,902	4,118	1,450	295

Total n = 17,145

[a]Very lean, no less than 10%–13% body fat is recommended for women.

Adapted with permission from *Physical Fitness Assessments and Norms for Adults and Law Enforcement.* The Cooper Institute, Dallas, Texas. 2009. For more information: www.cooperinstitute.org

(or through a nonlatex mask) while pulmonary ventilation and expired fractions of oxygen (O_2) and carbon dioxide (CO_2) are measured. Modern automated systems provide ease of use and a detailed printout of test results that save time and effort (27). However, system calibration is still essential to obtain accurate results (76). Administration of the test and interpretation of results should be reserved for professional personnel with a thorough understanding of exercise science. Because of costs associated with the equipment, space, and personnel needed to carry out these tests, direct measurement of $\dot{V}O_{2max}$ generally is reserved for research or clinical settings.

When direct measurement of $\dot{V}O_{2max}$ is not feasible, a variety of submaximal and maximal exercise tests can be used to estimate $\dot{V}O_{2max}$. These tests have been validated by examining (a) the correlation between directly measured $\dot{V}O_{2max}$ and the $\dot{V}O_{2max}$ estimated from physiologic responses to submaximal exercise (*e.g.*, HR at a specified power output); or (b) the correlation between directly measured $\dot{V}O_{2max}$ and test performance (*e.g.*, time to run 1 or 1.5 mi [1.6 or 2.4 km]), or time to volitional fatigue using a standard graded exercise test protocol. It should be noted that there is the potential for a significant overestimation of directly measured $\dot{V}O_{2max}$ by these types of indirect measurement techniques. Overestimation is more likely to occur when (a) the exercise protocol chosen for testing is too aggressive for a given individual (*i.e.*, Bruce treadmill protocol in patients with CHF); or (b) when treadmill testing is employed and the individual heavily relies on handrail support (5). Every effort should therefore be taken to choose the appropriate exercise protocol given an individual's characteristics and minimize handrail use during testing on a treadmill (76).

MAXIMAL VERSUS SUBMAXIMAL EXERCISE TESTING

The decision to use a maximal or submaximal exercise test depends largely on the reasons for the test, risk level of the client/patient, and availability of appropriate equipment and personnel. $\dot{V}O_{2max}$ can be estimated using conventional exercise test protocols by considering test duration at a given workload on an ergometer and using the prediction equations found in *Chapter 7*. The user should consider the population being tested and standard error of the associated equation. Maximal tests require participants to exercise to the point of volitional fatigue, which might entail the need for medical supervision as detailed in *Chapter 2* and/ or emergency equipment (see *Appendix B*). However, maximal exercise testing offers increased sensitivity in the diagnosis of CVD in asymptomatic individuals and provides a better estimate of $\dot{V}O_{2max}$ (see "Indications and Purposes" section in *Chapter 5*). In addition, the use of open circuit spirometry during maximal exercise testing may allow for the accurate assessment of anaerobic/ventilatory threshold and direct measurement of $\dot{V}O_{2max} / \dot{V}O_{2peak}$.

Practitioners commonly rely on submaximal exercise tests to assess CRF because maximal exercise testing is not always feasible in the health/fitness setting. Submaximal exercise testing is also recommended in stable patients 4–7 d post-myocardial infarction (MI) to assess efficacy of medical therapy prior to hospital discharge among other clinical indices (43). In the health/ fitness setting, the basic aim of submaximal exercise testing is to determine the HR response to one or more submaximal work rates and use the results to predict $\dot{V}O_{2max}$. Although the primary purpose of the test has traditionally been to predict $\dot{V}O_{2max}$ from the HR workload relationship, it is important to obtain additional indices of the client's response to exercise. The practitioner should use the various submaximal measures of HR, BP, workload, rating of perceived exertion (RPE), and other subjective indices as valuable information regarding one's functional response to exercise. This information can be used to evaluate submaximal exercise responses over time in a controlled environment and appropriately determine the Ex R_x.

The most accurate estimate of $\dot{V}O_{2max}$ is achieved from the HR response to submaximal exercise tests if all of the following assumptions are achieved:

- A steady state HR is obtained for each exercise work rate.
- A linear relationship exists between HR and work rate.
- The difference between actual and predicted maximal HR is minimal.
- Mechanical efficiency (*i.e.*, $\dot{V}O_2$ at a given work rate) is the same for everyone.

- The subject is not on medications, using high quantities of caffeine, under large amounts of stress, ill, or in a high temperature environment, all of which may alter HR.

MODES OF TESTING

Commonly used modes for exercise testing include treadmills, cycle ergometers, steps, and field tests. The mode of exercise testing used is dependent on the setting, equipment available, and training of personnel. Medical supervision is recommended for high-risk individuals as detailed in *Chapter 2* regardless of mode (see *Figure 2.4* and *Table 2.3*).

There are advantages and disadvantages of each exercise testing mode:

- **Field tests** consist of walking or running in a predetermined time or distance (*i.e.*, 12-min and 1.5-mi [2.4 km] walk/run tests, and the 1-mi and 6-min walk test). The advantages of field tests are they are easy to administer to large numbers of individuals at one time and little equipment (*e.g.*, a stopwatch) is needed. The disadvantages are some tests can be maximal for some individuals, particularly in individuals with low aerobic fitness, and potentially be unmonitored for BP and HR. An individual's level of motivation and pacing ability also can have a profound impact on test results. These all-out run tests may be inappropriate for sedentary individuals or individuals at increased risk for cardiovascular and/or musculoskeletal complications. Nevertheless, $\dot{V}O_{2max}$ can be estimated from the test results.
- **Motor-driven treadmills** can be used for submaximal and maximal testing and are often employed for diagnostic testing in the United States (5). They provide a familiar form of exercise and, if the correct protocol is chosen (*i.e.*, aggressive vs. conservative adjustments in workload), can accommodate the least physically fit to the fittest individuals across the continuum of walking to running speeds. Nevertheless, a practice session might be necessary in some cases to permit habituation and reduce anxiety. On the other hand, treadmills usually are expensive, not easily transportable, and potentially make some measurements (*e.g.*, BP, ECG) more difficult, particularly while an individual is running. Treadmills must be calibrated to ensure the accuracy of the test (76). In addition, holding on to the support rail(s) should be discouraged to ensure accuracy of metabolic work output, particularly when $\dot{V}O_2$ is estimated as opposed to directly measured. Extensive handrail use often leads to significant overestimation of $\dot{V}O_2$ compared to actual values.
- **Mechanically braked cycle ergometers** are also a viable test modality for submaximal and maximal testing and are frequently used for diagnostic testing, particularly in European laboratories (76). Advantages of this exercise mode include lower equipment expense, transportability, and greater ease in obtaining BP and ECG (if appropriate) measurements. Cycle ergometers also provide a non–weight-bearing test modality in which work rates are easily adjusted in small increments. The main disadvantage is cycling is a less familiar mode of exercise to individuals in the United States, often resulting

in limiting localized muscle fatigue and an underestimation of $\dot{V}O_2$. The cycle ergometer must be calibrated, and the subject must maintain the proper pedal rate because most tests require HR to be measured at specific work rates (76). Electronic cycle ergometers can deliver the same work rate across a range of pedal rates (*i.e.*, revolutions $\cdot$ min^{-1}, rpm), but calibration might require special equipment not available in some laboratories. Some electronic fitness cycles cannot be calibrated and should not be used for testing.

- **Step testing** is an inexpensive modality for predicting CRF by measuring the HR response to stepping at a fixed rate and/or a fixed step height or by measuring postexercise recovery HR. Step tests require little or no equipment, steps are easily transportable, stepping skill requires little practice, the test usually is of short duration, and stepping is advantageous for mass testing (22,72). Postexercise (recovery) HR decreases with improved CRF, and test results are easy to explain to participants (59). Special precautions may be needed for those who have balance problems or are extremely deconditioned. Some single-stage step tests require an energy cost of 7–9 metabolic equivalents (METs), which may exceed the maximal capacity of the participant (6). Therefore, the protocol chosen must be appropriate for the physical fitness level of the client. In addition, inadequate compliance to the step cadence and excessive fatigue in the lead limb may diminish the value of a step test. Most tests do not monitor HR and BP while stepping because of the difficulty of measuring HR and BP.

Field Tests

Two of the most widely used walk/run (based on subject preference) tests for assessing CRF are the Cooper 12-min test and the 1.5-mi (2.4 km) test for time. The objective of the 12-min test is to cover the greatest distance in the allotted time period and for the 1.5-mi (2.4 km) test to run the distance in the shortest period of time. $\dot{V}O_{2max}$ can be estimated from the equations in *Chapter 7*.

The Rockport One-Mile Fitness Walking Test is another well-recognized field test for estimating CRF. In this test, an individual walks 1 mi (1.6 km) as fast as possible, preferably on a track or a level surface, and HR is obtained in the final minute. An alternative is to measure a 10 s HR immediately on completion of the 1 mi (1.6 km) walk, but this may overestimate the $\dot{V}O_{2max}$ compared to when HR is measured during the walk. $\dot{V}O_{2max}$ is estimated from a regression equation found in *Chapter 7* based on weight, age, sex, walk time, and HR (62).

In addition to independently predicting morbidity and mortality (21,97), the 6-min walk test has been used to evaluate CRF in older adults and some clinical patient populations (*e.g.*, individuals with CHF or pulmonary disease). The American Thoracic Society has published guidelines on 6-min walk test procedures and interpretation (8). Even though the test is considered submaximal, it may result in near-maximal performance for those with low physical fitness levels or disease (57). Clients and patients completing less than 300 m (~984 ft) during the 6-min walk demonstrate a poorer short-term survival compared to those surpassing this threshold (16). Several multivariate equations are available to predict $\dot{V}O_{2\ peak}$ from the 6-min walk; however, the following equation requires minimal clinical information (16):

- $\dot{V}O_{2peak} = \dot{V}O_2$ mL $\cdot$ kg^{-1} $\cdot$ min^{-1} = (0.02 × distance [m]) − (0.191 × age [yr]) − (0.07 × weight [kg]) + (0.09 × height [cm]) + (0.26 × RPP [× 10^{-3}]) + 2.45

  Where m = distance in meters; yr = year; kg = kilogram; cm = centimeter; RPP = rate pressure product (HR × systolic BP [SBP] in mm Hg)

- For the aforementioned equation: R^2 = 0.65 and SEE = 2.68 (R^2 = coefficient of determination; SEE = standard error of estimate)

Submaximal Exercise Tests

Single-stage and multistage submaximal exercise tests are available to estimate $\dot{V}O_{2max}$ from simple HR measurements. Accurate measurement of HR is critical for valid testing. Although HR obtained by palpation is commonly used, the accuracy of this method depends on the experience and technique of the evaluator. It is recommended that an ECG, HR monitor, or a stethoscope be used to determine HR. The use of a relatively inexpensive HR monitor can reduce a significant source of error in the test. The submaximal HR response is easily altered by a number of environmental (*e.g.*, heat, humidity, see *Chapter 8*), dietary (*e.g.*, caffeine, time since last meal), and behavioral (*e.g.*, anxiety, smoking, previous physical activity) factors. These variables must be controlled to have a valid estimate that can be used as a reference point in an individual's fitness program. In addition, the test mode (*e.g.*, cycle, treadmill, step) should be consistent with the primary exercise modality used by the participant to address specificity of training issues. Standardized procedures for submaximal testing are presented in *Box 4.4*. Although there are no specific submaximal protocols for treadmill testing, several stages from any of the treadmill protocols found in *Chapter 5* can be used to assess submaximal exercise responses. Preexercise test instructions are presented in *Chapter 3*.

Cycle Ergometer Tests

The Astrand-Ryhming cycle ergometer test is a single-stage test lasting 6 min (7). For the population studied, these researchers observed at 50% $\dot{V}O_{2max}$, the average HR was 128 and 138 beats $\cdot$ min^{-1} for men and women, respectively. If a woman was working at a $\dot{V}O_2$ of 1.5 L $\cdot$ min^{-1} and her HR was 138 beats $\cdot$ min^{-1}, then her $\dot{V}O_{2max}$ was estimated to be 3.0 L $\cdot$ min^{-1}. The suggested work rate is based on sex and an individual's fitness status as follows:

men, unconditioned:	300 or 600 kg $\cdot$ m $\cdot$ min^{-1} (50 or 100 W)
men, conditioned:	600 or 900 kg $\cdot$ m $\cdot$ min^{-1} (100 or 150 W)
women, unconditioned:	300 or 450 kg $\cdot$ m $\cdot$ min^{-1} (50 or 75 W)
women, conditioned:	450 or 600 kg $\cdot$ m $\cdot$ min^{-1} (75 or 100 W)

BOX 4.4	General Procedures for Submaximal Testing of Cardiorespiratory Fitness

1. Obtain resting HR and BP immediately prior to exercise in the exercise posture.
2. The client should be familiarized with the ergometer. If using a cycle ergometer, properly position the client on the ergometer (*i.e.*, upright posture, ~25-degree bend in the knee at maximal leg extension, and hands in proper position on handlebars) (81–83).
3. The exercise test should begin with a 2–3 min warm-up to acquaint the client with the cycle ergometer and prepare him or her for the exercise intensity in the first stage of the test.
4. A specific protocol should consist of 2- or 3-min stages with appropriate increments in work rate.
5. HR should be monitored at least two times during each stage, near the end of the second and third minutes of each stage. If HR is >110 beats $\cdot$ min^{-1}, steady state HR (*i.e.*, two HRs within 5 beats $\cdot$ min^{-1}) should be reached before the workload is increased.
6. BP should be monitored in the last minute of each stage and repeated (verified) in the event of a hypotensive or hypertensive response.
7. RPE (using either the Borg category or category-ratio scale [see *Table 4.7*]) and additional rating scales should be monitored near the end of the last minute of each stage.
8. Client's appearance and symptoms should be monitored and recorded regularly.
9. The test should be terminated when the subject reaches 70% heart rate reserve (85% of age-predicted HR$_{max}$), fails to conform to the exercise test protocol, experiences adverse signs or symptoms, requests to stop, or experiences an emergency situation.
10. An appropriate cool-down/recovery period should be initiated consisting of either
    a. continued exercise at a work rate equivalent to that of the first stage of the exercise test protocol or lower or
    b. a passive cool-down if the subject experiences signs of discomfort or an emergency situation occurs
11. All physiologic observations (*e.g.*, HR, BP, signs and symptoms) should be continued for at least 5 min of recovery unless abnormal responses occur, which would warrant a longer posttest surveillance period. Continue low-level exercise until HR and BP stabilize, but not necessarily until they reach preexercise levels.

BP, blood pressure; HR, heart rate; HR$_{max}$, maximal heart rate; RPE, rating of perceived exertion.

TABLE 4.7. The Borg Rating of Perceived Exertion Scale

6	No exertion at all
7	
8	Extremely light
9	Very light
10	
11	Light
12	
13	Somewhat hard
14	
15	Hard (heavy)
16	
17	Very hard
18	
19	Extremely hard
20	Maximal exertion

From (13). © Gunnar Borg. Reproduced with permission. The scale with correct instructions can be obtained from Borg Perception, Radisvagen 124, 16573 Hasselby, Sweden. See also the home page: http://www.borgperception.se/index.html.

The pedal rate is set at 50 rpm. The goal is to obtain HR values between 125 and 170 beats · min^{-1}, with HR measured during the fifth and sixth minute of work. The average of the two HRs is then used to estimate $\dot{V}O_{2max}$ from a nomogram (see *Figure 4.1*). This value must then be adjusted for age because HR$_{max}$ decreases with age by multiplying the $\dot{V}O_{2max}$ value by the following correction factors (6):

AGE	CORRECTION FACTOR
15	1.10
25	1.00
35	0.87
40	0.83
45	0.78
50	0.75
55	0.71
60	0.68
65	0.65

In contrast to the Astrand-Ryhming cycle ergometer single-stage test, Maritz et al. (71) measured HR at a series of submaximal work rates and extrapolated the response to the subject's age-predicted HR$_{max}$. This multistage method is a well-known assessment technique to estimate $\dot{V}O_{2max}$, and the YMCA test is a good example (111). The YMCA protocol uses two to four 3-min stages of continuous exercise (see *Figure 4.2*). The test is designed to raise the steady state HR of the subject to between 110 beats · min^{-1} and 70% heart rate reserve (HRR) (or 85% of the age-predicted HR$_{max}$) for at least two consecutive stages. It is important to remember that two consecutive HR measurements must be obtained within this HR range to predict $\dot{V}O_{2max}$.

In the YMCA protocol, each work rate is performed for at least 3 min, and HR is recorded during the final 15–30 s of the second and third minutes. The work

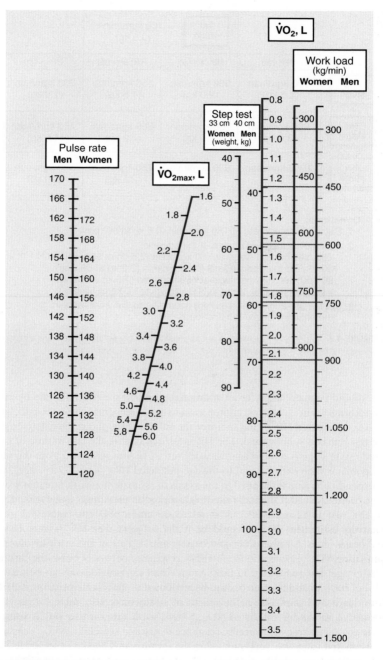

■ **FIGURE 4.1.** Modified Astrand-Ryhming nomogram. Used with permission from (7).

	1st stage	150 kgm/min (0.5 kg)		
	HR: <80	HR: 80–89	HR: 90–100	HR: >100
2nd stage	750 kgm/min (2.5 kg)*	600 kgm/min (2.0 kg)	450 kgm/min (1.5 kg)	300 kgm/min (1.0 kg)
3rd stage	900 kgm/min (3.0 kg)	750 kgm/min (2.5 kg)	600 kgm/min (2.0 kg)	450 kgm/min (1.5 kg)
4th stage	1050 kgm/min (3.5 kg)	900 kgm/min (3.0 kg)	750 kgm/min (2.5 kg)	600 kgm/min (2.0 kg)

Directions:
1 Set the 1st work rate at 150 kgm/min (0.5 kg at 50 rpm)
2 If the HR in the third minute of the stage is:
  <80, set the 2nd stage at 750 kgm/min (2.5 kg at 50 rpm)
  80-89, set the 2nd stage at 600 kgm/min (2.0 kg at 50 rpm)
  90-100, set the 2nd stage at 450 kgm/min (1.5 kg at 50 rpm)
  >100, set the 2nd stage at 300 kgm/min (1.0 kg at 50 rpm)
3 Set the 3rd and 4th (if required) according to the work rates in the columns below the 2nd loads

■ **FIGURE 4.2.** YMCA cycle ergometry protocol. Resistance settings shown here are appropriate for an ergometer with a flywheel of 6 m · rev^{-1} (111).

rate should be maintained for an additional minute if the two HRs vary by more than 5 beats · min^{-1}. The test administrator should recognize the error associated with age-predicted HR$_{max}$ and monitor the subject throughout the test to ensure the test remains submaximal. The HR measured during the last minute of each steady state stage is plotted against work rate. The line generated from the plotted points is then extrapolated to the age-predicted HR$_{max}$ (e.g., 220 − age), and a perpendicular line is dropped to the x-axis to estimate the work rate that would have been achieved if the individual had worked to maximum (see *Figure 4.3*).

The two lines noted as ±1 standard deviation (SD) in *Figure 4.3* show what the estimated $\dot{V}O_{2max}$ would be if the subject's true HR$_{max}$ were 168 or 192 beats · min^{-1}, rather than 180 beats · min^{-1}. Part of the error involved in estimating $\dot{V}O_{2max}$ from submaximal HR responses occurs because the formula "220 − age" has an SD of ±12 beats · min^{-1} and can provide only an estimate of HR$_{max}$ (106). In addition, errors can be attributed to inaccurate pedaling cadence (workload) and imprecise achievement of steady state HR. *Table 4.8* provides normative values for estimated $\dot{V}O_{2max}$ from work rate on the YMCA submax cycle ergometer test with specific reference to age and sex (111). $\dot{V}O_{2max}$ can also be estimated from the work rate using the formula in *Chapter 7* (see *Table 7.3*). This equation is valid to estimate $\dot{V}O_2$ at submaximal steady state workloads

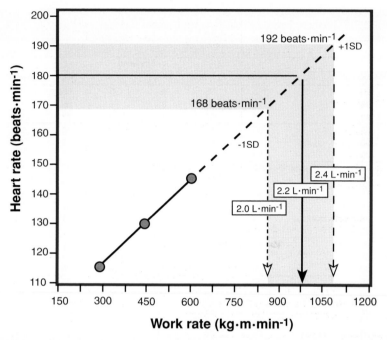

■ **FIGURE 4.3.** Heart rate responses to three submaximal work rates for a sedentary woman 40 yr of age weighing 64 kg. $\dot{V}O_{2max}$ was estimated by extrapolating the heart rate (HR) response to the age-predicted HR_{max} of 180 beats · min⁻¹ (based on 220 − age). The work rate that would have been achieved at that HR was determined by dropping a line from that HR value to the x-axis. $\dot{V}O_{2max}$ estimated using the formula in *Chapter 7* and expressed in L · min⁻¹ was 2.2 L · min⁻¹. The other two lines estimate what the $\dot{V}O_{2max}$ would have been if the subject's true HR_{max} was ±1 standard deviation (SD) from the 180 beats · min⁻¹ value.

(from 300 to 1,200 kg · m · min⁻¹) (49.0 W to 196.1 W); therefore, caution must be used if extrapolating to workloads outside of this range.

Treadmill Tests

The primary exercise modality for submaximal exercise testing traditionally has been the cycle ergometer, although treadmills are used in many settings. The same endpoint (70% HRR or 85% of age-predicted HR_{max}) is used, and the stages of the test should be 3 min or longer to ensure a steady state HR response at each stage. The HR values are extrapolated to age-predicted HR_{max}, and $\dot{V}O_{2max}$ is estimated using the formula in *Chapter 7* from the highest speed and/or grade that would have been achieved if the individual had worked to maximum. Most common treadmill protocols presented in *Chapter 5* can be used, but the duration of each stage should be at least 3 min.

TABLE 4.8. Fitness Categories for Estimated $\dot{V}O_{2max}$ from the YMCA Submaximal Cycle Ergometer Test by Age and Sex

% Ranking		Norms for Max $\dot{V}O_2$ (mL/kg) — MEN Age (year)					
		18–25	26–35	36–45	46–55	56–65	Over 65
100		100	95	90	83	65	53
95	Excellent	75	66	61	55	50	42
90		65	60	55	49	43	38
85		60	55	49	45	40	34
80	Good	56	52	47	43	38	33
75		53	50	45	40	37	32
70	Above average	50	48	43	39	35	31
65		49	45	41	38	34	30
60		48	44	40	36	33	29
55	Average	45	42	38	35	32	28
50		44	40	37	33	31	27
45		43	39	36	32	30	26
40	Below average	42	38	35	31	28	25
35		39	37	33	30	27	24
30		38	34	31	29	26	23
25		36	33	30	27	25	22
20	Poor	35	32	29	26	23	21
15		32	30	27	25	22	20
10		30	27	24	24	21	18
5	Very poor	26	24	21	20	18	16
0		20	15	14	13	12	10

% Ranking		Norms for Max $\dot{V}O_2$ (mL/kg) — WOMEN Age (year)					
		18–25	26–35	36–45	46–55	56–65	Over 65
100		95	95	75	72	58	55
95	Excellent	69	65	56	51	44	48
90		59	58	50	45	40	34
85		56	53	46	41	36	31
80	Good	52	51	44	39	35	30
75		50	48	42	36	33	29
70	Above average	47	45	41	35	32	28
65		45	44	38	34	31	27
60		44	43	37	32	30	26
55	Average	42	41	36	31	28	25
50		40	40	34	30	27	24
45		39	37	33	29	26	23
40	Below average	38	36	32	28	25	22
35		37	35	30	27	24	21
30		35	34	29	26	23	20
25		33	32	28	25	22	19
20	Poor	32	30	26	23	20	18
15		30	28	25	22	19	17
10		27	25	24	20	18	16
5	Very poor	24	22	20	18	15	14
0		15	14	12	11	10	10

Step Tests

Step tests are also used to estimate $\dot{V}O_{2max}$. Astrand and Ryhming (7) used a single-step height of 33 cm (13 in) for women and 40 cm (15.7 in) for men at a rate of 22.5 steps $\cdot$ min^{-1}. These tests require $\dot{V}O_2$ of about 25.8 and 29.5 mL $\cdot$ kg^{-1} $\cdot$ min^{-1}, respectively. HR is measured as described for the cycle test, and $\dot{V}O_{2max}$ is estimated from the nomogram (see *Figure 4.1*). In contrast, Maritz et al. (71) used a single-step height of 12 in (30.5 cm) and four step rates to systematically increase the work rate. A steady state HR is measured for each step rate, and a line formed from these HR values are extrapolated to age-predicted HR$_{max}$. The maximal work rate is determined as described for the YMCA cycle test. $\dot{V}O_{2max}$ can be estimated from the formula for stepping in *Chapter 7*. Such step tests should be modified to suit the population being tested. The Canadian Home Fitness Test has demonstrated that such testing can be performed on a large scale and at low cost (99).

Instead of estimating $\dot{V}O_{2max}$ from HR responses to several submaximal work rates, a wide variety of step tests have been developed to categorize CRF based on an individual's recovery HR following a standardized step test. The 3-Minute YMCA Step Test is a good example of such a test. This test uses a 12-in (30.5 cm) bench, with a stepping rate of 24 steps $\cdot$ min^{-1} (estimated $\dot{V}O_2$ of 25.8 mL $\cdot$ kg^{-1} $\cdot$ min^{-1}). After stepping is completed, the subject immediately sits down and HR is counted for 1 min. Counting must start within 5 s at the end of exercise. HR values are used to obtain a qualitative rating of fitness from published normative tables (111).

CARDIORESPIRATORY TEST SEQUENCE AND MEASURES

A minimum of HR, BP, and subjective symptoms (*i.e.*, RPE, dyspnea, and angina) should be measured during exercise tests. After the initial screening process, selected baseline measurements should be obtained prior to the start of the exercise test. Taking a resting ECG prior to exercise testing requires that trained personnel are available to interpret the ECG and provide medical guidance. An ECG is not considered necessary when diagnostic testing is not being done. The sequence of measures is listed in *Table 5.2*.

HR can be determined using several techniques including radial pulse palpation, auscultation with a stethoscope, or the use of HR monitors. The pulse palpation technique involves "feeling" the pulse by placing the second and third fingers (*i.e.*, index and middle fingers) most typically over the radial artery, located near the thumb side of the wrist. The pulse is typically counted for 15 s, and then multiplied by 4, to determine the HR for 1 min. For the auscultation method, the bell of the stethoscope should be placed to the left of the sternum just above the level of the nipple. The auscultation method is most accurate when the heart sounds are clearly audible, and the subject's torso is relatively stable. HR telemetry monitors with chest electrodes or radio telemetry have proven to be accurate and reliable, provided there is no outside electrical interference (*e.g.*, emissions from the display consoles of computerized exercise equipment) (66). Many electronic cycles and treadmills have embedded HR telemetry monitoring into the equipment.

BP should be measured at heart level with the subject's arm relaxed and not grasping a handrail (treadmill) or handlebar (cycle ergometer). To help ensure accurate readings, the use of an appropriate-sized BP cuff is important. The rubber bladder of the BP cuff should encircle at least 80% of the subject's upper arm. If the subject's arm is large, a normal size adult cuff will be too small, thus resulting in an erroneous elevated reading; whereas if the cuff is too large for the subject's arm, the resultant reading will be erroneously low. BP measurements should be taken with a recently calibrated aneroid sphygmomanometer. Systolic (SBP) and diastolic (DBP) BP measurements can be used as indicators for stopping an exercise test (see next section of *Chapter 4*). To obtain accurate BP measures during exercise, follow the guidelines in *Chapter 3* (see *Box 3.4*) for resting BP; however, BP will be obtained in the exercise position. If an automated BP system is used during exercise testing, calibration checks with manual BP measurements must be routinely performed to confirm accuracy of the automated readings (76).

RPE can be a valuable indicator for monitoring an individual's exercise tolerance. Although RPEs correlate with exercise HRs and work rates, large interindividual variability in RPE with healthy individuals as well as patient populations mandates caution in the universal application of RPE scales (109). Borg's RPE scale was developed to allow the exerciser to subjectively rate her or his feelings during exercise, taking into account personal physical fitness level and general fatigue levels (77). Ratings can be influenced by psychological factors, mood states, environmental conditions (13), exercise modes, and age reducing its utility (93). Currently, two RPE scales are widely used: (a) the original Borg or category scale, which rates exercise intensity from 6 to 20 (see *Table 4.7*); and (b) the category-ratio scale of 0–10. Both RPE scales are appropriate subjective tools (13,43).

During exercise testing, the RPE can be used as an indication of impending fatigue. Most apparently, healthy subjects reach their subjective limit of fatigue at an RPE of 18–19 (very, very hard) on the category Borg scale, or 9–10 (very, very strong) on the category-ratio scale; therefore, RPE can be used to monitor progress toward maximal exertion during exercise testing (75).

The development of dyspnea and/or angina during exercise is also important to subjectively quantify. In particular, exercise limited by dyspnea as opposed to other subjective symptoms appears to indicate an increased risk for future adverse events (2,12). Four level scales for perceived dyspnea and angina during exercise are available through the current AHA scientific statements on recommendations for clinical exercise laboratories (76).

TEST TERMINATION CRITERIA

Graded exercise test (GXT), whether maximal or submaximal, is a safe procedure when subject screening and testing guidelines as outlined in *Chapter 2* are adhered to. Occasionally, for safety reasons, the test may have to be terminated prior to the subject reaching a measured $\dot{V}O_{2max}/\dot{V}O_{2peak}$, volitional fatigue, or a predetermined endpoint (i.e., 50%–70% HRR or 70%–85% age-predicted HR_{max}). Because of the individual variation in HR_{max}, the upper limit of 85% of an estimated HR_{max} may

BOX 4.5	General Indications for Stopping an Exercise Test[a]

- Onset of angina or angina-like symptoms
- Drop in SBP of ≥10 mm Hg with an increase in work rate or if SBP decreases below the value obtained in the same position prior to testing
- Excessive rise in BP: systolic pressure >250 mm Hg and/or diastolic pressure >115 mm Hg
- Shortness of breath, wheezing, leg cramps, or claudication
- Signs of poor perfusion: light-headedness, confusion, ataxia, pallor, cyanosis, nausea, or cold and clammy skin
- Failure of HR to increase with increased exercise intensity
- Noticeable change in heart rhythm by palpation or auscultation
- Subject requests to stop
- Physical or verbal manifestations of severe fatigue
- Failure of the testing equipment

[a]Assumes that testing is nondiagnostic and is being performed without direct physician involvement or ECG monitoring. For clinical testing, *Box 5.2* provides more definitive and specific termination criteria. BP, blood pressure; ECG, electrocardiogram; HR, heart rate; SBP, systolic blood pressure.

result in a maximal effort for some individuals and submaximal effort in others. General indications — those that do not rely on physician involvement or ECG monitoring — for stopping an exercise test are outlined in *Box 4.5*. More specific termination criteria for clinical or diagnostic testing are provided in *Chapter 5*.

INTERPRETATION OF RESULTS

Table 4.9 provides normative values for $\dot{V}O_{2max}$ (in mL $\cdot$ kg^{-1} $\cdot$ min^{-1}) estimated from treadmill speed and grade with specific reference to age and sex. Research suggests a $\dot{V}O_{2max}$ below the 20th percentile for age and sex, that is often indicative of a sedentary lifestyle, is associated with an increased risk of death from all causes (10). Several regression equations for estimating CRF according to age and sex are also available. These equations produce a single expected aerobic capacity value for comparison to a measured response as opposed to percentiles. Of the available regression equations, research indicates prediction formulas derived from a Veterans Affairs cohort (Predicted METs = 18 − 0.15*age) and the St. James Take Heart project (Predicted METs = 14.7 − 0.13*age) may provide somewhat better prognostic information in men and women, respectively (61).

Although percent predicted aerobic capacity appears to be prognostic (*i.e.*, lower percent predicted = worse prognosis), an individual's age has a significant influence on predictive characteristics in men and women. Specifically, in younger individuals (~40–60 yr), percent predicted aerobic capacity may have to decrease below 60%–70% before indicating poor prognosis, after which the

TABLE 4.9. Fitness Categories for Maximal Aerobic Power for Men and Women by Age

MEN

%		Age 20-29				Age 30-39			
		Balke Treadmill (time)	Max $\dot{V}O_2$ (mL/kg/min)	12-Min Run (miles)	1.5-Mi Run (time)	Balke Treadmill (time)	Max $\dot{V}O_2$ (mL/kg/min)	12-Min Run (miles)	1.5-Mi Run (time)
99	Superior	31:30	60.5	2.00	8:29	30:00	58.3	1.94	8:49
95		28:05	55.5	1.86	9:17	27:03	54.1	1.82	9:33
90		27:00	54.0	1.81	9:34	25:25	51.7	1.75	10:01
85	Excellent	25:30	51.8	1.75	10:00	24:13	50.0	1.70	10:24
80		25:00	51.1	1.73	10:09	23:06	48.3	1.66	10:46
75		23:13	48.5	1.66	10:43	22:10	47.0	1.62	11:06
70	Good	22:30	47.5	1.63	10:59	21:30	46.0	1.59	11:22
65		22:00	46.8	1.61	11:10	21:00	45.3	1.57	11:33
60		21:10	45.6	1.58	11:29	20:09	44.1	1.54	11:54
55		21:40	44.8	1.56	11:41	20:00	43.9	1.53	11:58
50	Fair	20:00	43.9	1.53	11:58	19:00	42.4	1.49	12:24
45		19:08	42.6	1.50	12:20	18:07	41.2	1.46	12:50
40		18:30	41.7	1.47	12:38	17:49	40.7	1.44	12:58
35		18:00	41.0	1.45	12:53	17:00	39.5	1.41	13:24
30	Poor	17:17	39.9	1.42	13:15	16:24	38.7	1.39	13:44
25		16:38	39.0	1.40	13:36	15:46	37.8	1.36	14:05
20		15:56	38.0	1.37	14:00	15:00	36.7	1.33	14:34
15		15:00	36.7	1.33	14:34	14:02	35.2	1.29	15:13
10	Very poor	13:37	34.7	1.28	15:30	13:00	33.8	1.25	15:57
5		11:38	31.8	1.20	17:04	11:15	31.2	1.18	17:25
1		8:00	26.5	1.05	20:58	8:00	26.5	1.05	20:58

$n = 2,328$ $n = 12,730$

Total $n = 15,058$

		Age 40-49				Age 50-59			
MEN									
%		Balke Treadmill (time)	Max VO$_2$ (mL/kg/min)	12-Min Run (miles)	1.5-Mi Run (time)	Balke Treadmill (time)	Max VO$_2$ (mL/kg/min)	12-Min Run (miles)	1.5-Mi Run (time)
99	Superior	28:30	56.1	1.87	9:10	27:00	54.0	1.81	9:34
95		26:00	52.5	1.77	9:51	23:32	49.0	1.68	10:37
90		24:00	49.6	1.69	10:28	22:00	46.8	1.61	11:10
85	Excellent	23:00	48.2	1.65	10:48	20:30	44.6	1.55	11:45
80		21:45	46.4	1.60	11:15	19:37	43.3	1.52	12:08
75		20:42	44.9	1.56	11:40	18:35	41.8	1.48	12:36
70	Good	20:01	43.9	1.53	11:58	18:00	41.0	1.45	12:53
65		19:30	43.1	1.51	12:11	17:08	39.7	1.42	13:20
60		19:00	42.4	1.49	12:24	16:39	39.0	1.40	13:35
55		18:00	41.0	1.45	12:53	16:00	38.1	1.37	13:58
50	Fair	17:22	40.1	1.43	13:12	15:18	37.1	1.34	14:23
45		17:00	39.5	1.41	13:24	15:00	36.7	1.33	14:34
40		16:14	38.4	1.38	13:50	14:12	35.5	1.30	15:06
35		15:38	37.6	1.36	14:11	13:43	34.8	1.28	15:26
30	Poor	15:00	36.7	1.33	14:34	13:00	33.8	1.25	15:58
25		14:30	35.9	1.31	14:53	12:21	32.8	1.23	16:28
20		13:45	34.8	1.28	15:24	11:45	32.0	1.20	16:58
15		13:00	33.8	1.25	15:58	11:00	30.9	1.17	17:38
10	Very poor	12:00	32.3	1.21	16:46	10:00	29.4	1.13	18:37
5		10:01	29.4	1.13	18:48	8:15	26.9	1.06	20:38
1		7:00	25.1	1.01	22:22	5:25	22.8	0.95	25:00
		$n = 18,104$				$n = 10,627$			

Total $n = 28,731$

(continued)

TABLE 4.9. Fitness Categories for Maximal Aerobic Power for Men and Women by Age *(Continued)*

MEN

%		Age 60-69				Age 70-79			
		Balke Treadmill (time)	Max V̇O₂ (mL/kg/min)	12-Min Run (miles)	1.5-Mi Run (time)	Balke Treadmill (time)	Max V̇O₂ (mL/kg/min)	12-Min Run (miles)	1.5-Mi Run (time)
99	Superior	25:00	51.1	1.73	10:09	24:00	49.6	1.69	10:28
95		21:18	45.7	1.59	11:26	20:00	43.9	1.53	11:58
90		19:10	42.7	1.50	12:20	17:00	39.5	1.41	13:24
85	Excellent	18:01	41.0	1.45	12:53	16:00	38.1	1.37	13:58
80		17:01	39.6	1.41	13:23	15:00	36.7	1.33	14:34
75		16:09	38.3	1.38	13:52	14:01	35.2	1.29	15:14
70	Good	15:30	37.4	1.35	14:16	13:05	33.9	1.26	15:54
65		15:00	36.7	1.33	14:34	12:32	33.1	1.23	16:19
60		14:15	35.6	1.30	15:04	12:03	32.4	1.21	16:43
55		13:47	34.9	1.28	15:23	11:29	31.6	1.19	17:12
50	Fair	13:02	33.8	1.25	15:56	11:00	30.9	1.17	17:38
45		12:30	33.0	1.23	16:21	10:26	30.1	1.15	18:11
40		12:00	32.3	1.21	16:46	10:00	29.4	1.13	18:38
35		11:30	31.6	1.19	17:11	9:17	28.4	1.10	19:24
30	Poor	10:57	30.8	1.17	17:41	9:00	28.0	1.09	19:43
25		10:04	29.5	1.13	18:33	8:17	26.9	1.06	20:36
20		9:30	28.7	1.11	19:10	7:24	25.7	1.03	21:47
15		8:30	27.3	1.07	20:19	6:40	24.6	1.00	22:52
10	Very poor	7:21	25.6	1.03	21:51	5:31	23.0	0.95	24:49
5		5:57	23.6	0.97	24:03	4:00	20.8	0.89	27:58
1		3:16	19.7	0.86	29:47	2:15	18.2	0.82	32:46
		n = 2,971				*n* = 417			

Total *n* = 3,388

		WOMEN							
		Age 20-29				Age 30-39			
%		Balke Treadmill (time)	Max $\dot{V}O_2$ (mL/kg/min)	12-Min Run (miles)	1.5-Mi Run (time)	Balke Treadmill (time)	Max $\dot{V}O_2$ (mL/kg/min)	12-Min Run (miles)	1.5-Mi Run (time)
99	Superior	27:23	54.5	1.83	9:30	25:37	52.0	1.76	9:58
95	Superior	24:00	49.6	1.69	10:28	22:26	47.4	1.63	11:00
90		22:00	46.8	1.61	11:10	21:00	45.3	1.57	11:33
85	Excellent	21:00	45.3	1.57	11:33	20:00	43.9	1.53	11:58
80	Excellent	20:01	43.9	1.53	11:58	19:00	42.4	1.49	12:24
75		19:00	42.4	1.49	12:24	18:02	41.0	1.45	12:53
70	Good	18:04	41.1	1.46	12:51	17:01	39.6	1.41	13:24
65	Good	18:00	41.0	1.45	12:53	16:18	38.5	1.38	13:47
60		17:00	39.5	1.41	13:24	15:43	377	1.36	14:08
55		16:17	38.5	1.38	13:48	15:10	36.9	1.34	14:28
50	Fair	15:50	378	1.37	14:04	15:00	36.7	1.33	14:34
45	Fair	15:00	36.7	1.33	14:34	14:00	35.2	1.29	15:14
40		14:36	36.1	1.32	14:50	13:20	34.2	1.27	15:43
35		14:00	35.2	1.29	15:14	13:00	33.8	1.25	15:58
30	Poor	13:15	34.1	1.26	15:46	12:03	32.4	1.21	16:42
25	Poor	12:30	33.0	1.23	16:21	11:47	32.0	1.20	16:56
20		12:00	32.3	1.21	16:46	11:00	30.9	1.17	17:38
15		11:01	30.9	1.17	17:38	10:00	29.4	1.13	18:37
10	Very poor	10:04	29.5	1.13	18:33	9:00	28.0	1.09	19:43
5	Very poor	8:43	27.6	1.08	20:03	7:33	25.9	1.03	21:34
1		6:00	23.7	0.97	23:58	5:27	22.9	0.95	24:56
		$n = 1,280$				$n = 4,257$			

Total $n = 5,537$

(continued)

TABLE 4.9. Fitness Categories for Maximal Aerobic Power for Men and Women by Age (Continued)

WOMEN

%		Age 40-49				Age 50-59			
		Balke Treadmill (time)	Max VO₂ (mL/kg/min)	12-Min Run (miles)	1.5-Mi Run (time)	Balke Treadmill (time)	Max VO₂ (mL/kg/min)	12-Min Run (miles)	1.5-Mi Run (time)
99	Superior	25:00	51.1	1.73	10:09	21:31	46.1	1.59	11:20
95		21:00	45.3	1.57	11:33	18:01	41.0	1.45	12:53
90		19:30	43.1	1.51	12:11	16:30	38.8	1.39	13:40
85	Excellent	18:02	41.0	1.45	12:53	15:16	37.0	1.34	14:24
80		17:02	39.6	1.41	13:23	15:00	36.7	1.33	14:34
75		16:22	38.6	1.39	13:45	14:02	35.2	1.29	15:13
70	Good	16:00	38.1	1.37	13:58	13:20	34.2	1.27	15:43
65		15:01	36.7	1.33	14:34	12:40	33.3	1.24	16:13
60		14:30	35.9	1.31	14:53	12:13	32.6	1.22	16:35
55		14:01	35.2	1.29	15:13	12:00	32.3	1.21	16:46
50	Fair	13:32	34.5	1.27	15:34	11:21	31.4	1.19	17:19
45		13:00	33.8	1.25	15:58	11:00	30.9	1.17	17:38
40		12:18	32.8	1.22	16:31	10:19	29.9	1.14	18:18
35		12:00	32.3	1.21	16:46	10:00	29.4	1.13	18:37
30	Poor	11:10	31.1	1.18	17:29	9:30	28.7	1.11	19:10
25		10:32	30.2	1.15	18:05	9:00	28.0	1.09	19:43
20		10:00	29.4	1.13	18:37	8:10	26.8	1.06	20:44
15		9:07	28.2	1.10	19:35	7:30	25.8	1.03	21:38
10	Very poor	8:04	26.6	1.05	20:52	6:40	24.6	1.00	22:52
5		7:00	25.1	1.01	22:22	5:33	23.0	0.95	24:46
1		5:00	22.2	0.93	25:49	3:31	20.1	0.87	29:09

n = 5,908

n = 3,923

Total n = 9,831

	%	Balke Treadmill (time)	Max $\dot{V}O_2$ (mL/kg/min)	12-Min Run (miles)	1.5-Mi Run (time)	Balke Treadmill (time)	Max $\dot{V}O_2$ (mL/kg/min)	12-Min Run (miles)	1.5-Mi Run (time)
			WOMEN						
		Age 60–69				Age 70–79			
Superior	99	19:00	42.4	1.49	12:24	19:00	42.4	1.49	12:24
	95	15:46	37.8	1.36	14:05	15:21	37.2	1.35	14:21
	90	14:30	35.9	1.31	14:53	12:06	32.5	1.22	16:40
Excellent	85	13:17	34.2	1.26	15:45	12:00	32.3	1.21	16:46
	80	12:15	32.7	1.22	16:33	10:47	30.6	1.16	17:51
	75	12:00	32.3	1.21	16:46	10:16	29.8	1.14	18:21
Good	70	11:09	31.1	1.18	17:30	10:01	29.4	1.13	18:37
	65	11:00	30.9	1.17	17:38	10:00	29.4	1.13	18:37
	60	10:10	29.7	1.14	18:27	9:06	28.1	1.10	19:36
	55	10:00	29.4	1.13	18:37	9:00	28.0	1.09	19:43
Fair	50	9:35	28.8	1.12	19:04	8:44	27.6	1.08	20:02
	45	9:07	28.2	1.10	19:35	8:05	26.7	1.05	20:52
	40	8:33	27.3	1.07	20:16	7:35	25.9	1.03	21:31
	35	8:04	26.6	1.05	20:52	7:07	25.3	1.02	22:07
Poor	30	7:32	25.9	1.03	21:36	6:44	24.7	1.00	22:46
	25	7:01	25.1	1.01	22:21	6:23	24.2	0.99	23:20
	20	6:39	24.6	1.00	22:52	5:55	23.5	0.97	24:06
	15	6:12	23.9	0.98	23:37	5:00	22.2	0.93	25:49
Very poor	10	5:32	23.0	0.95	24:48	4:30	21.5	0.91	26:51
	5	4:45	21.8	0.92	26:19	3:12	19.6	0.86	30:00
	1	3:07	19.5	0.86	30:12	1:17	16.8	0.78	36:13
		$n = 1,131$				$n = 155$			

Total $n = 1,286$

Adapted with permission from *Physical Fitness Assessments and Norms for Adults and Law Enforcement*. The Cooper Institute, Dallas, Texas. 2009.
For more information: www.cooperinstitute.org

increase in mortality risk becomes rather steep. In older individuals ($>$60 yr), there appears to be a more linear relationship between percent predicted aerobic capacity and mortality risk across the range of potential values as opposed to a single threshold. In a comparison of the physical fitness status of any one individual to published norms, the accuracy of the classification is dependent on the similarities between the populations and methodology (*e.g.*, estimated vs. measured $\dot{V}O_{2max}$, maximal vs. submaximal).

Although submaximal exercise testing is not as precise as maximal exercise testing, it provides a general reflection of an individual's physical fitness at a lower cost, potentially reduced risk for adverse events, and requires less time and effort on the part of the subject. Some of the assumptions inherent in a submaximal test are more easily met (*e.g.*, steady state HR can be verified), whereas others (*e.g.*, estimated HR_{max}) introduce unknown errors into the prediction of $\dot{V}O_{2max}$. When an individual is given repeated submaximal exercise tests over a period of weeks or months and the HR response to a fixed work rate decreases over time, it is likely that the individual's CRF has improved, independent of the accuracy of the $\dot{V}O_{2max}$ prediction. Despite differences in test accuracy and methodology, virtually all evaluations can establish a baseline and be used to track relative progress.

MUSCULAR STRENGTH AND MUSCULAR ENDURANCE

Muscular strength and endurance are health-related fitness components that may improve or maintain the following (110):

- Bone mass, which is related to osteoporosis.
- Glucose tolerance, which is pertinent in both the prediabetic and diabetic state.
- Musculotendinous integrity, which is related to a lower risk of injury including low back pain.
- The ability to carry out the activities of daily living, which is related to perceived quality of life and self-efficacy among other indicators of mental health.
- The FFM and resting metabolic rate, which are related to weight management.

The ACSM has melded the terms muscular strength, endurance, and power into a category termed "muscular fitness" and included it as an integral portion of total health-related fitness in the position stand on the quantity and quality of exercise for developing and maintaining fitness (42). Muscular strength refers to *the muscle's ability to exert force*, muscular endurance is *the muscle's ability to continue to perform successive exertions or many repetitions*, and muscular power is *the muscle's ability to exert force per unit of time* (*i.e.*, rate) (29). Traditionally, tests allowing few ($<$3) repetitions of a task prior to reaching momentary muscular fatigue have been considered strength measures, whereas those in which numerous repetitions ($>$12) are performed prior to momentary muscular fatigue were considered measures of muscular endurance. However, the performance of a maximal repetition range (*i.e.*, 4, 6, or 8 repetitions at a given resistance) also can be used to assess strength.

RATIONALE

Physical fitness tests of muscular strength and muscular endurance before commencing exercise training or as part of a health/fitness screening evaluation can provide valuable information on a client's baseline physical fitness level. For example, muscular fitness test results can be compared to established standards and can be helpful in identifying weaknesses in certain muscle groups or muscle imbalances that could be targeted in exercise training programs. The information obtained during baseline muscular fitness assessments can also serve as a basis for designing individualized exercise training programs. An equally useful application of physical fitness testing is to show a client's progressive improvements over time as a result of the training program, and thus provide feedback that is often beneficial in promoting long-term exercise adherence.

PRINCIPLES

Muscle function tests are very specific to the muscle group tested, the type of muscle action, velocity of muscle movement, type of equipment, and joint range of motion (ROM). Results of any one test are specific to the procedures used, and no single test exists for evaluating total body muscular endurance or strength. Individuals should participate in familiarization/practice sessions with test equipment and adhere to a specific protocol including a predetermined repetition duration and ROM in order to obtain a reliable score that can be used to track true physiologic adaptations over time. Moreover, warm-up consisting of 5–10 min of light intensity, aerobic exercise (*i.e.*, treadmill or cycle ergometer), static stretching, and several light intensity repetitions of the specific testing exercise should precede muscular fitness testing. These warm-up activities increase muscle temperature and localized blood flow and promotes appropriate cardiovascular responses to exercise. A summary of standardized conditions include the following:

- Strict posture.
- Consistent repetition duration (movement speed).
- Full ROM.
- Use of spotters (when necessary).
- Equipment familiarization.
- Warm-up.

Change in muscular fitness over time can be based on the absolute value of the external load or resistance (*e.g.*, newtons, kilograms [kg], or pounds [lb]), but when comparisons are made between individuals, the values should be expressed as relative values (per kilogram of body weight [$kg \cdot kg^{-1}$]). In both cases, caution must be used in the interpretation of the scores because the norms may not include a representative sample of the individual being measured, a standardized protocol may be absent, or the exact test being used (*e.g.*, free weight vs. machine weight) may differ. In addition, the biomechanics for a given resistance exercise may differ significantly when using equipment from different manufactures, further impacting *generalizability*.

MUSCULAR STRENGTH

Although muscular strength refers to the external force (properly expressed in newtons, although kilograms and pounds are commonly used as well) that can be generated by a specific muscle or muscle group, it is commonly expressed in terms of resistance met or overcome. Strength can be assessed either statically (i.e., no overt muscular movement at a given joint or group of joints) or dynamically (i.e., movement of an external load or body part in which the muscle changes length). Static or isometric strength can be measured conveniently using a variety of devices including cable tensiometers and handgrip dynamometers. In certain instances, measures of static strength are specific to the muscle group and joint angle involved in testing; therefore, their utility in describing overall muscular strength may be limited. Peak force development in such tests is commonly referred to as the maximum voluntary contraction (MVC).

Traditionally, the one repetition maximum (1-RM), the greatest resistance that can be moved through the full ROM in a controlled manner with good posture, has been the standard for dynamic strength assessment. With appropriate testing familiarization, 1-RM is a reliable indicator of muscle strength (67,84). A multiple RM, such as 4- or 8-RM, can be used as a measure of muscular strength. For example, if one were training with 6- to 8-RM, the performance of a 6-RM to momentary muscular fatigue would provide an index of strength changes over time, independent of the true 1-RM. Reynolds et al. (91) have demonstrated multiple repetition tests in the 4- to 8-RM range provide a reasonably accurate estimate of 1-RM.

In addition, a conservative approach to assessing maximal muscle strength should be considered in patients at high risk for or with known CVD, pulmonary, and metabolic diseases and health conditions. For these groups, assessment of 10- to 15-RM that approximates training recommendations may be prudent (110). Valid measures of general upper body strength include the 1-RM values for bench press or shoulder press. Corresponding indices of lower body strength include 1-RM values for the leg press or leg extension. Norms based on resistance lifted divided by body mass for the bench press and leg press are provided in *Tables 4.10* and *4.11*, respectively. The following represents the basic steps in 1-RM (or any multiple RM) testing following familiarization/practice sessions (69):

1. The subject should warm up by completing a number of submaximal repetitions of the specific exercise that will be used to determine the 1-RM.
2. Determine the 1-RM (or any multiple of 1-RM) within four trials with rest periods of 3–5 min between trials.
3. Select an initial weight that is within the subject's perceived capacity (~50%–70% of capacity).
4. Resistance is progressively increased by 2.5–20.0 kg (5.5–44.0 lb) until the subject cannot complete the selected repetition(s); all repetitions should be performed at the same speed of movement and ROM to instill consistency between trials.
5. The final weight lifted successfully is recorded as the absolute 1-RM or multiple RM.

TABLE 4.10. Fitness Categories for Upper Body Strength[a] for Men and Women by Age

Bench Press Weight Ratio = $\dfrac{\text{weight pushed in lbs}}{\text{body weight in lbs}}$

		\<20	20–29	30–39	40–49	50–59	60+
MEN							
				Age			
%		**\<20**	**20–29**	**30–39**	**40–49**	**50–59**	**60+**
99	Superior	>1.76	>1.63	>1.35	>1.20	>1.05	>0.94
95		1.76	1.63	1.35	1.20	1.05	0.94
90		1.46	1.48	1.24	1.10	0.97	0.89
85	Excellent	1.38	1.37	1.17	1.04	0.93	0.84
80		1.34	1.32	1.12	1.00	0.90	0.82
75		1.29	1.26	1.08	0.96	0.87	0.79
70	Good	1.24	1.22	1.04	0.93	0.84	0.77
65		1.23	1.18	1.01	0.90	0.81	0.74
60		1.19	1.14	0.98	0.88	0.79	0.72
55		1.16	1.10	0.96	0.86	0.77	0.70
50	Fair	1.13	1.06	0.93	0.84	0.75	0.68
45		1.10	1.03	0.90	0.82	0.73	0.67
40		1.06	0.99	0.88	0.80	0.71	0.66
35		1.01	0.96	0.86	0.78	0.70	0.65
30	Poor	0.96	0.93	0.83	0.76	0.68	0.63
25		0.93	0.90	0.81	0.74	0.66	0.60
20		0.89	0.88	0.78	0.72	0.63	0.57
15		0.86	0.84	0.75	0.69	0.60	0.56
10	Very poor	0.81	0.80	0.71	0.65	0.57	0.53
5		0.76	0.72	0.65	0.59	0.53	0.49
1		\<0.76	\<0.72	\<0.65	\<0.59	\<0.53	\<0.49
n		60	425	1,909	2,090	1,279	343

Total *n* = 6,106

		\<20	20–29	30–39	40–49	50–59	60+
WOMEN							
99	Superior	>0.88	>1.01	>0.82	>0.77	>0.68	>0.72
95		0.88	1.01	0.82	0.77	0.68	0.72
90		0.83	0.90	0.76	0.71	0.61	0.64
85	Excellent	0.81	0.83	0.72	0.66	0.57	0.59
80		0.77	0.80	0.70	0.62	0.55	0.54
75		0.76	0.77	0.65	0.60	0.53	0.53
70	Good	0.74	0.74	0.63	0.57	0.52	0.51
65		0.70	0.72	0.62	0.55	0.50	0.48
60		0.65	0.70	0.60	0.54	0.48	0.47
55		0.64	0.68	0.58	0.53	0.47	0.46
50	Fair	0.63	0.65	0.57	0.52	0.46	0.45
45		0.60	0.63	0.55	0.51	0.45	0.44
40		0.58	0.59	0.53	0.50	0.44	0.43
35		0.57	0.58	0.52	0.48	0.43	0.41
30	Poor	0.56	0.56	0.51	0.47	0.42	0.40
25		0.55	0.53	0.49	0.45	0.41	0.39
20		0.53	0.51	0.47	0.43	0.39	0.38

(continued)

TABLE 4.10. Fitness Categories for Upper Body Strength[a] for Men and Women by Age (*Continued*)

Bench Press Weight Ratio $= \dfrac{\text{weight pushed in lbs}}{\text{body weight in lbs}}$

		WOMEN					
		Age					
%		<20	20–29	30–39	40–49	50–59	60+
15		0.52	0.50	0.45	0.42	0.38	0.36
10	Very poor	0.50	0.48	0.42	0.38	0.37	0.33
5		0.41	0.44	0.39	0.35	0.31	0.26
1		<0.41	<0.44	<0.39	<0.35	<0.31	<0.26
n		20	191	379	333	189	42

Total *n* = 1,154

[a]One repetition maximum bench press, with bench press weight ratio = weight pushed in pounds per body weight in pounds.

Adapted with permission from *Physical Fitness Assessments and Norms for Adults and Law Enforcement*. The Cooper Institute, Dallas, Texas. 2009. For more information: www.cooperinstitute.org

TABLE 4.11. Fitness Categories for Leg Strength by Age and Sex[a]

Percentile		Age (year)				
		20–29	30–39	40–49	50–59	60+
		Men				
90	Well above average	2.27	2.07	1.92	1.80	1.73
80	Above average	2.13	1.93	1.82	1.71	1.62
70		2.05	1.85	1.74	1.64	1.56
60	Average	1.97	1.77	1.68	1.58	1.49
50		1.91	1.71	1.62	1.52	1.43
40	Below average	1.83	1.65	1.57	1.46	1.38
30		1.74	1.59	1.51	1.39	1.30
20	Well below average	1.63	1.52	1.44	1.32	1.25
10		1.51	1.43	1.35	1.22	1.16
		Women				
90	Well above average	1.82	1.61	1.48	1.37	1.32
80	Above average	1.68	1.47	1.37	1.25	1.18
70		1.58	1.39	1.29	1.17	1.13
60	Average	1.50	1.33	1.23	1.10	1.04
50		1.44	1.27	1.18	1.05	0.99
40	Below average	1.37	1.21	1.13	0.99	0.93
30		1.27	1.15	1.08	0.95	0.88
20	Well below average	1.22	1.09	1.02	0.88	0.85
10		1.14	1.00	0.94	0.78	0.72

[a]One repetition maximum leg press with leg press weight ratio = weight pushed per body weight.

Adapted from Institute for Aerobics Research, Dallas, 1994. Study population for the data set was predominantly white and college educated. A Universal Dynamic Variable Resistance (DVR) machine was used to measure the 1-repetition maximum (RM).

Isokinetic testing involves the assessment of maximal muscle tension throughout a ROM set at a constant angular velocity (*e.g.*, 60 angles · s^{-1}). Equipment that allows control of the speed of joint rotation (degrees · s^{-1}) as well as the ability to test movement around various joints (*e.g.*, knee, hip, shoulder, elbow) is available from commercial sources. Such devices measure peak rotational force or torque, but an important drawback is that this equipment is substantially more expensive compared to other strength testing modalities (45).

MUSCULAR ENDURANCE

Muscular endurance is the ability of a muscle group to execute repeated muscle actions over a period of time sufficient to cause muscular fatigue or to maintain a specific percentage of the 1-RM for a prolonged period of time. If the total number of repetitions at a given amount of resistance is measured, the result is termed absolute muscular endurance. If the number of repetitions performed at a percentage of the 1-RM (*e.g.*, 70%) is used pretesting and posttesting, the result is termed relative muscular endurance. Simple field tests such as a curl-up (crunch) test (19,45) or the maximum number of push-ups that can be performed without rest (19) may be used to evaluate the endurance of the abdominal muscle groups and upper body muscles, respectively. Procedures for conducting the push-up and curl-up (crunch) muscular endurance tests are given in *Box 4.6*, and physical fitness categories are provided in *Tables 4.12* and *4.13*, respectively.

Resistance training equipment also can be adapted to measure muscular endurance by selecting an appropriate submaximal level of resistance and measuring the number of repetitions or the duration of static muscle action before fatigue. For example, the YMCA bench press test involves performing standardized repetitions at a rate of 30 lifts or reps · min^{-1}. Men are tested using a 36.3-kg (80 lb) barbell and women using a 15.9-kg (35 lb) barbell. Subjects are scored by the number of successful repetitions completed (111). The YMCA test is an excellent example of a test that attempts to control for repetition duration and posture alignment, thus possessing high reliability. Normative data for the YMCA bench press test are presented in *Table 4.14*.

SPECIAL CONSIDERATIONS IN MUSCULAR FITNESS

Older Adults

The number of older adults in the United States is expected to increase exponentially over the next several decades as described in *Chapter 8*. As individuals are living longer, it is becoming increasingly more important to find ways to extend active and independent life expectancy. Assessing muscular strength and endurance, neuromotor fitness, and other aspects of health-related physical fitness among older adults can aid in detecting physical limitations and yield important information used to design exercise programs that improve muscular fitness before serious functional limitations or injuries occur. The Senior Fitness Test (SFT) was developed in response to a need for improved health/fitness

BOX 4.6	Push-up and Curl-up (Crunch) Test Procedures for Measurement of Muscular Endurance

PUSH-UP

1. The push-up test is administered with men starting in the standard "down" position (hands pointing forward and under the shoulder, back straight, head up, using the toes as the pivotal point) and women in the modified "knee push-up" position (legs together, lower leg in contact with mat with ankles plantar-flexed, back straight, hands shoulder width apart, head up, using the knees as the pivotal point).
2. The client/patient must raise the body by straightening the elbows and return to the "down" position, until the chin touches the mat. The stomach should not touch the mat.
3. For both men and women, the subject's back must be straight at all times and the subject must push up to a straight arm position.
4. The maximal number of push-ups performed consecutively without rest is counted as the score.
5. The test is stopped when the client strains forcibly or unable to maintain the appropriate technique within two repetitions.

CURL-UP (CRUNCH)†

1. Two strips of masking tape are to be placed on a mat on the floor at a distance of 12 cm apart (for clients/patients <45 yr) or 8 cm apart (for clients/patients ≥45 yr).
2. Subjects are to lie in a supine position across the tape, knees bent at 90° with feet on the floor and arms extended to their sides, such that their fingertips touch the nearest strip. This is the bottom position. To reach the top position, subjects are to flex their spines to 30°, reaching their hands forward until their fingers touch the second strip of tape.
3. A metronome is to be set at 40 beats · min^{-1}. At the first beep, the subject begins the curl-up, reaching the top position at the second beep, returning to the starting position at the third, top position at the fourth, etc.
4. Repetitions are counted each time the subject reaches the bottom position. The test is concluded either when the subject reaches 75 curl-ups, or the cadence is broken.
5. Every subject will be allowed several practice repetitions prior to the start of the test.

†Alternatives include: 1) having the hands held across the chest with the head activating a counter when the trunk reaches a 30° position (32) and placing the hands on the thighs and curling up until the hands reach the knee caps (37). Elevation of the trunk to 30° is the important aspect of the movement. Reprinted with permission from (19). ©2003. Used with permission from the Canadian Society for Exercise Physiology www.csep.ca

TABLE 4.12. Fitness Categories for the Push-Up by Age and Sex

	Age (year)									
Category	**20–29**		**30–39**		**40–49**		**50–59**		**60–69**	
Sex	**M**	**W**	**M**	**W**	**M**	**W**	**M**	**W**	**M**	**W**
Excellent	36	30	30	27	25	24	21	21	18	17
Very good	35	29	29	26	24	23	20	20	17	16
	29	21	22	20	17	15	13	11	11	12
Good	28	20	21	19	16	14	12	10	10	11
	22	15	17	13	13	11	10	7	8	5
Fair	21	14	16	12	12	10	9	6	7	4
	17	10	12	8	10	5	7	2	5	2
Needs improvement	16	9	11	7	9	4	6	1	4	1

M, men; W, women.

Reprinted with permission from (19). ©2003. Used with permission from the Canadian Society for Exercise Physiology www.csep.ca

assessment tools for older individuals (92). The test was designed to assess the key physiologic parameters (*e.g.*, strength, endurance, agility, balance) needed to perform common everyday physical activities that are often difficult to perform in later years. One aspect of the SFT is the 30-s chair stand test. This test, and others of the SFT, meets scientific standards for reliability and validity, is simple and easy to administer in the "field" setting, and has accompanying performance norms for older men and women 60–94 yr based on a study of over 7,000 older Americans (92). This test has been shown to correlate well with other muscular fitness tests such as the 1-RM. Two specific tests included in the SFT — the 30-s chair stand and single-arm curl — can be used by the health/fitness and clinical exercise professionals to safely and effectively assess muscular strength and endurance in most older adults.

TABLE 4.13. Fitness Categories for the Partial Curl-Up by Age and Sex

		Age (year)									
Percentile		**20–29**		**30–39**		**40–49**		**50–59**		**60–69**	
Gender		**M**	**W**	**M**	**W**	**M**	**W**	**M**	**W**	**M**	**W**
90	Well above average	75	70	75	55	75	55	74	48	53	50
80	Above average	56	45	69	43	75	42	60	30	33	30
70		41	37	46	34	67	33	45	23	26	24
60	Average	31	32	36	28	51	28	35	16	19	19
50		27	27	31	21	39	25	27	9	16	13
40	Below average	24	21	26	15	31	20	23	2	9	9
30		20	17	19	12	26	14	19	0	6	3
20	Well below average	13	12	13	0	21	5	13	0	0	0
10		4	5	0	0	13	0	0	0	0	0

M, men; W, women.

Adapted from (37).

TABLE 4.14. Fitness Categories for the YMCA Bench Press Test (Total Lifts) by Age and Sex

Category		Age (year)									
		18–25		26–35		36–45		46–55		56–65		>65
Sex	M	W	M	W	M	W	M	W	M	W	M	W
Excellent	64	66	61	62	55	57	47	50	41	42	36	30
	44	42	41	40	36	33	28	29	24	24	20	18
Good	41	38	37	34	32	30	25	24	21	21	16	16
	34	30	30	29	26	26	21	20	17	17	12	12
Above average	33	28	29	28	25	24	20	18	14	14	10	10
	29	25	26	24	22	21	16	14	12	12	9	8
Average	28	22	24	22	21	20	14	13	11	10	8	7
	24	20	21	18	18	16	12	10	9	8	7	5
Below average	22	18	20	17	17	14	11	9	8	6	6	4
	20	16	17	14	14	12	9	7	5	5	4	3
Poor	17	13	16	13	12	10	8	6	4	4	3	2
	13	9	12	9	9	6	5	2	2	2	2	0
Very poor	<10	6	9	6	6	4	2	1	1	1	1	0

M, men; W, women.

Reprinted with permission from (111). © 2000 by YMCA of the USA, Chicago. All rights reserved.

Coronary Prone Clients

Moderate intensity resistance training performed 2–3 d · wk^{-1} is effective for improving muscular fitness, preventing and managing a variety of chronic medical conditions, modifying CVD risk factors, and enhancing psychosocial well-being for individuals with and without CVD. Consequently, authoritative professional health organizations including the ACSM and AHA support the inclusion of resistance training as an adjunct to aerobic exercise in their current recommendations and guidelines on exercise for individuals with CVD (see *Chapter 9*) (110).

The absence of anginal symptoms, ischemic ST-segment changes on the ECG, abnormal hemodynamics, and complex ventricular dysrhythmias suggests moderate intensity (*e.g.*, performance of 10–15 repetitions) resistance testing and training can be performed safely by patients with CVD deemed "low risk" (*e.g.*, individuals without resting or exercise-induced evidence of myocardial ischemia, severe left ventricular dysfunction, or complex ventricular dysrhythmias, and with normal or near normal CRF [see *Chapter 2*]). Moreover, despite concerns that resistance exercise elicits abnormal cardiovascular "pressor responses" in patients with CVD and/or controlled hypertension, studies have found strength testing and resistance training in these patients elicit HR and BP responses that appear to fall within clinically acceptable limits (110). Resistance training in moderate-to-high risk patients with CVD may be deemed appropriate following a thorough clinical assessment by an experienced health care professional. Furthermore, moderate-to-high risk patients with CVD who do participate in a resistance training program should be closely monitored (110). Absolute and relative contraindications to resistance testing and training are provided in *Box 4.7*.

BOX 4.7	Absolute and Relative Contraindications to Resistance Training and Testing

ABSOLUTE

Unstable CHD

Decompensated HF

Uncontrolled arrhythmias

Severe pulmonary hypertension (mean pulmonary arterial pressure >55 mm Hg)

Severe and symptomatic aortic stenosis

Acute myocarditis, endocarditis, or pericarditis

Uncontrolled hypertension (>180/110 mm Hg)

Aortic dissection

Marfan syndrome

High intensity RT (80% to 100% of 1-RM) in patients with active proliferative retinopathy or moderate or worse nonproliferative diabetic retinopathy

RELATIVE (SHOULD CONSULT A PHYSICIAN BEFORE PARTICIPATION)

Major risk factors for CHD

Diabetes at any age

Uncontrolled hypertension (>160/100 mm Hg)

Low functional capacity (<4 METs)

Musculoskeletal limitations

Individuals who have implanted pacemakers or defibrillators

CHD, Coronary heart disease; HF, Heart failure; METs, Metabolic equivalents; RM, Repetition maximum; RT, Resistance training.
Reprinted with permission from (110). ©2007, American Heart Association, Inc.

Children and Adolescents

Along with CRF, flexibility, and body composition, muscular fitness is recognized as an important component of health-related fitness in children and adolescents (see *Chapter 8*) (9,36). The benefits of enhancing muscular strength and endurance in youth include developing proper posture, reducing the risk of injury, improving body composition, enhancing motor performance skills such as sprinting and jumping, and enhancing self-confidence and self-esteem. As a general guide, children who are ready to begin participation in sport activities (~7–8 yr) may also be ready to initiate a resistance training program (36).

Assessing muscular strength and endurance with the push-up and abdominal curl-up is common practice in most physical education programs, YMCA/YWCA recreation programs, and youth sport centers. Use of resistance training equipment commonly available in fitness facilities is also appropriate for the assessment of muscle strength and endurance. When properly administered, different muscular fitness measures can be used to assess a child's strengths and weaknesses, develop a personalized fitness program, track progress, and motivate participants. Conversely, unsupervised or poorly administered muscular fitness assessments may not only discourage youth from participating in fitness activities, but may also result in injury. Qualified health/fitness and clinical exercise professionals should demonstrate proper performance of each skill, provide an opportunity for each child to practice a few repetitions of each skill, and offer guidance and instruction when necessary. In addition, it is important and usually required to obtain informed consent from the parent or legal guardian prior to initiating muscular testing. The informed consent includes information on potential benefits and risks, the right to withdraw at any time, and issues regarding confidentiality. General guidelines for resistance training in children and adolescents are listed in *Box 4.8* (see *Chapter 8*).

BOX 4.8   Guidelines for Resistance Training in Children and Adolescents

- Ensure appropriate training for individual providing training instruction and supervision
- Provide a safe exercise environment
- Start training session with a 5- to 10-min dynamic warm-up
- Initiate training program two to three times per week on nonconsecutive days, with light resistance, and ensure exercise technique is correct
- General training session guidelines: one to three sets of 6–15 repetitions with combination of upper and lower body exercise
- Incorporate exercises specifically focusing on trunk
- Training program should induce symmetrical and balanced muscular development
- Individualized exercise progression based on goals and skill
- Gradual increase (~5%–10%) in training resistance as gains are made
- Use calisthenics and/or stretching postresistance training session
- Be aware of individual needs/concerns during each session
- Consider use of an individualized exercise log
- Continually alter training program to maintain interest and avoid training plateaus
- Ensure proper nutrition, hydration, and sleep
- Instructor and parents should be supportive and encouraging to help maintain interest

Adapted from (36).

FLEXIBILITY

Flexibility is the ability to move a joint through its complete ROM. It is important in athletic performance (*e.g.*, ballet, gymnastics) and in the ability to carry out activities of daily living. Consequently, maintaining flexibility of all joints facilitates movement; in contrast, when an activity moves the structures of a joint beyond its full ROM, tissue damage can occur.

Flexibility depends on a number of specific variables including distensibility of the joint capsule, adequate warm-up, and muscle viscosity. In addition, compliance (*i.e.*, tightness) of various other tissues such as ligaments and tendons affects the ROM. Just as muscular strength and endurance is specific to the muscles involved, flexibility is joint specific; therefore, no single flexibility test can be used to evaluate total body flexibility. Laboratory tests usually quantify flexibility in terms of ROM expressed in degrees. Common devices for this purpose include goniometers, electrogoniometers, the Leighton flexometer, inclinometers, and tape measures. Comprehensive instructions are available for the evaluation of flexibility of most anatomic joints (24,80). Visual estimates of ROM can be useful in fitness screening but are inaccurate relative to directly measured ROM. These estimates can include neck and trunk flexibility, hip flexibility, lower extremity flexibility, shoulder flexibility, and postural assessment.

A more precise measurement of joint ROM can be assessed at most anatomic joints following strict procedures (24,80) and the proper use of a goniometer. Accurate measurements require in-depth knowledge of bone, muscle, and joint anatomy as well as experience in administering the evaluation. *Table 4.15*

TABLE 4.15. Range of Motion of Select Single Joint Movements in Degrees

	Degrees		Degrees
Shoulder Girdle Movement			
Flexion	90–120	Extension	20–60
Abduction	80–100		
Horizontal abduction	30–45	Horizontal adduction	90–135
Medial rotation	70–90	Lateral rotation	70–90
Elbow Movement			
Flexion	135–160		
Supination	75–90	Pronation	75–90
Trunk Movement			
Flexion	120–150	Extension	20–45
Lateral flexion	10–35	Rotation	20–40
Hip Movement			
Flexion	90–135	Extension	10–30
Abduction	30–50	Adduction	10–30
Medial rotation	30–45	Lateral rotation	45–60
Knee Movement			
Flexion	130–140	Extension	5–10
Ankle Movement			
Dorsiflexion	15–20	Plantarflexion	30–50
Inversion	10–30	Eversion	10–20

Adapted from (78).

provides normative ROM values for select anatomic joints. Additional information can be found in the *ACSM's Resource Manual for Guidelines for Exercise Testing and Prescription, Seventh Edition* (101).

The sit-and-reach test has been used commonly to assess low back and hamstring flexibility; however, its relationship to predict the incidence of low back pain is limited (54). The sit-and-reach test is suggested to be a better measure of hamstring flexibility than low back flexibility (53). The relative importance of hamstring flexibility to activities of daily living and sports performance, therefore, supports the inclusion of the sit-and-reach test for health-related fitness testing until a criterion measure evaluation of low back flexibility is available. Although limb and torso length disparity may impact sit-and-reach scoring, modified testing that establishes an individual zero point for each participant has not enhanced the predictive index for low back flexibility or low back pain (17,52,74).

Poor lower back and hip flexibility, in conjunction with poor abdominal strength and endurance or other causative factors, may contribute to development of muscular low back pain; however, this hypothesis remains to be substantiated (88). Methods for administering the sit-and-reach test are presented in *Box 4.9*. Normative data for two sit-and-reach tests are presented in *Tables 4.16* and *4.17*.

BOX 4.9   Trunk Flexion (Sit-and-Reach) Test Procedures

Pretest: Clients/Patients should perform a short warm-up prior to this test and include some stretches (*e.g.*, modified hurdler's stretch). It is also recommended that the participant refrain from fast, jerky movements, which may increase the possibility of an injury. The participant's shoes should be removed.

1. For the Canadian Trunk Forward Flexion test, the client sits without shoes and the soles of the feet flat against the flexometer (sit-and-reach box) at the 26 cm mark. Inner edges of the soles are placed within 2 cm of the measuring scale. For the YMCA sit-and-reach test, a yardstick is placed on the floor and tape is placed across it at a right angle to the 15 in mark. The client/patient sits with the yardstick between the legs, with legs extended at right angles to the taped line on the floor. Heels of the feet should touch the edge of the taped line and be about 10 to 12 in apart. (Note the zero point at the foot/box interface and use the appropriate norms.)

2. The client/patient should slowly reach forward with both hands as far as possible, holding this position approximately 2 s. Be sure that the participant keeps the hands parallel and does not lead with one hand. Fingertips can be overlapped and should be in contact with the measuring portion or yardstick of the sit-and-reach box.

BOX 4.9	Trunk Flexion (Sit-and-Reach) Test Procedures (*Continued*)

3. The score is the most distant point (cm or in) reached with the fingertips. The best of two trials should be recorded. To assist with the best attempt, the client/patient should exhale and drop the head between the arms when reaching. Testers should ensure that the knees of the participant stay extended; however, the participant's knees should not be pressed down. The client/patient should breathe normally during the test and should not hold her/his breath at any time. Norms for the Canadian test are presented in *Table 4.16*. Note that these norms use a sit-and-reach box in which the "zero" point is set at the 26 cm mark. If a box is used in which the zero point is set at 23 cm (*e.g.*, Fitnessgram), subtract 3 cm from each value in this table. The norms for the YMCA test are presented in *Table 4.17*.

Reprinted with permission from (19) and (111).

A COMPREHENSIVE HEALTH FITNESS EVALUATION

A comprehensive health/fitness assessment includes the following:

- Prescreening/risk classification.
- Resting HR, BP, height, weight, BMI, and ECG (if appropriate).
- Body composition.
  - Waist circumference.
  - Skinfold assessment.

TABLE 4.16. Fitness Categories for Trunk Forward Flexion Using a Sit-and-Reach Box (cm)[a] by Age and Sex

Category	Age (year)									
	20–29		30–39		40–49		50–59		60–69	
Sex	M	W	M	W	M	W	M	W	M	W
Excellent	40	41	38	41	35	38	35	39	33	35
Very good	39	40	37	40	34	37	34	38	32	34
	34	37	33	36	29	34	28	33	25	31
Good	33	36	32	35	28	33	27	32	24	30
	30	33	28	32	24	30	24	30	20	27
Fair	29	32	27	31	23	29	23	29	19	26
	25	28	23	27	18	25	16	25	15	23
Needs improvement	24	27	22	26	17	24	15	24	14	22

[a]These norms are based on a sit-and-reach box in which the "zero" point is set at 26 cm. When using a box in which the zero point is set at 23 cm, subtract 3 cm from each value in this table.

M, men; W, women.

Reprinted with permission from (19). ©2003. Used with permission from the Canadian Society for Exercise Physiology www.csep.ca

TABLE 4.17. Fitness Categories for the YMCA Sit-and-Reach Test (in) by Age and Sex

Percentile		Age (year)										
		18–25		26–35		36–45		46–55		56–65		>65	
Gender		M	W	M	W	M	W	M	W	M	W	M	W
90	Well above average	22	24	21	23	21	22	19	21	17	20	17	20
80	Above	20	22	19	21	19	21	17	20	15	19	15	18
70	average	19	21	17	20	17	19	15	18	13	17	13	17
60	Average	18	20	17	20	16	18	14	17	13	16	12	17
50		17	19	15	19	15	17	13	16	11	15	10	15
40	Below	15	18	14	17	13	16	11	14	9	14	9	14
30	average	14	17	13	16	13	15	10	14	9	13	8	13
20	Well below	13	16	11	15	11	14	9	12	7	11	7	11
10	average	11	14	9	13	7	12	6	10	5	9	4	9

M, men; W, women.

- Cardiorespiratory fitness.
  - Submaximal or maximal test typically on a cycle ergometer or treadmill.
- Muscular strength.
  - 1- to multiple-RM upper body (bench press) and lower body (leg press).
- Muscular endurance.
  - Curl-up test.
  - Push-up test.
  - Specific motion using appropriate equipment to fatigue (*i.e.*, bench press).
- Flexibility.
  - Sit-and-reach test or goniometric measures of isolated anatomic joints.

Additional evaluations may be administered; however, the components of a health/fitness evaluation listed earlier represent a comprehensive assessment that can be performed within 1 d. The data accrued from the evaluation should be interpreted by a competent health/fitness or clinical exercise professional and conveyed to the client/patient. This information is central to the development of a client's/patient's short- and long-term goals as well as forming the basis for the initial Ex R_x and subsequent evaluations to monitor progress.

THE BOTTOM LINE

The ACSM Health-Related Fitness Testing and Interpretation Summary Statements.

- Health/fitness assessments provide a wealth of information regarding an individual's health and functional status. A comprehensive assessment includes an evaluation of body composition, CRF, muscle strength/endurance, and flexibility.

- Each component of the assessment can be performed through several approaches to accommodate availability of equipment, the facility, training of personnel, and health/fitness status of the individual undergoing testing.
- Adherence to the recommendations for the health/fitness assessments provided in *Chapter 4* allows for an individualized and safe approach.
- When available, results from each component of the health/fitness assessment should be compared to normative data provided in *Chapter 4*.

Online Resources

ACSM Exercise is Medicine:
http://exerciseismedicine.org

American Heart Association:
http://www.americanheart.org

Clinical Guidelines on the Identification, Evaluation, and Treatment of Overweight and Obesity in Adults: The Evidence Report:
http://www.nhlbi.nih.gov/guidelines/obesity/ob_gdlns.htm

The Cooper Institute:
http://www.cooperinstitute.org

National Heart, Lung, and Blood Institute Health Information for Professionals:
http://www.nhlbi.nih.gov/health/indexpro.htm

2008 Physical Activity Guidelines for Americans (1):
http://www.health.gov/PAguidelines

REFERENCES

1. *2008 Physical Activity Guidelines for Americans* [Internet]. Rockville (MD): Office of Disease Prevention & Health Promotion, U.S. Department of Health and Human Services. 2008 [cited 2012 Jan 7]. 76 p. Available from: http://www.health.gov/paguidelines
2. Abidov A, Rozanski A, Hachamovitch R, et al. Prognostic significance of dyspnea in patients referred for cardiac stress testing. *N Engl J Med.* 2005;353(18):1889–98.
3. American College of Sports Medicine Position Stand, American Heart Association. Recommendations for cardiovascular screening, staffing, and emergency policies at health/fitness facilities. *Med Sci Sports Exerc.* 1998;30(6):1009–18.
4. Arena R, Lavie CJ. The obesity paradox and outcome in heart failure: is excess bodyweight truly protective? *Future Cardiol.* 2010;6(1):1–6.
5. Arena R, Myers J, Williams MA, et al. Assessment of functional capacity in clinical and research settings: a scientific statement from the American Heart Association Committee on Exercise, Rehabilitation, and Prevention of the Council on Clinical Cardiology and the Council on Cardiovascular Nursing. *Circulation.* 2007;116(3):329–43.
6. Astrand PO. Aerobic work capacity in men and women with special reference to age. *Acta Physiol Scand.* 1960;49(Supplement 169):45–60.
7. Astrand PO, Ryhming I. A nomogram for calculation of aerobic capacity (physical fitness) from pulse rate during sub-maximal work. *J Appl Physiol.* 1954;7(2):218–21.
8. ATS Committee on Proficiency Standards for Clinical Pulmonary Function Laboratories. ATS statement: guidelines for the six-minute walk test. *Am J Respir Crit Care Med.* 2002;166(1):111–7.
9. Behm DG, Faigenbaum AD, Falk B, Klentrou P. Canadian Society for Exercise Physiology position paper: resistance training in children and adolescents. *Appl Physiol Nutr Metab.* 2008;33(3):547–61.
10. Blair SN, Kohl HW,3rd, Barlow CE, Paffenbarger RS,Jr, Gibbons LW, Macera CA. Changes in physical fitness and all-cause mortality. A prospective study of healthy and unhealthy men. *JAMA.* 1995;273(14):1093–8.

11. Blair SN, Kohl HW,3rd, Paffenbarger RS,Jr, Clark DG, Cooper KH, Gibbons LW. Physical fitness and all-cause mortality. A prospective study of healthy men and women. *JAMA*. 1989;262(17):2395–401.
12. Bodegard J, Erikssen G, Bjornholt JV, Gjesdal K, Liestol K, Erikssen J. Reasons for terminating an exercise test provide independent prognostic information: 2014 apparently healthy men followed for 26 years. *Eur Heart J*. 2005;26(14):1394–401.
13. Borg G. *Borg's Perceived Exertion and Pain Scales*. Champaign (IL): Human Kinetics; 1998. 104 p.
14. Bray GA. Don't throw the baby out with the bath water. *Am J Clin Nutr*. 2004;79(3):347–9.
15. Brozek J, Grande F, Anderson JT, Keys A. Densitometric analysis of body composition: revision of some quantitative assumptions. *Ann N Y Acad Sci*. 1963;110:113–40.
16. Cahalin LP, Mathier MA, Semigran MJ, Dec GW, DiSalvo TG. The six-minute walk test predicts peak oxygen uptake and survival in patients with advanced heart failure. *Chest*. 1996;110(2):325–32.
17. Cailliet R. *Low Back Pain Syndrome*. 4th ed. Philadelphia (PA): F.A. Davis; 1988. 341 p.
18. Callaway CW, Chumlea WC, Bouchard C, Himes JH, Lohman TG, Martin AD. Circumferences. In: Lohman TG, Roche AF, Martorell R, editors. *Anthropometric Standardization Reference Manual*. Champaign: Human Kinetics; 1988. p. 39–80.
19. Canadian Society for Exercise Physiology. *The Canadian Physical Activity, Fitness & Lifestyle Approach (CPAFLA): CSEP—Health & Fitness Program's Health-Related Appraisal and Counselling Strategy*. 3rd ed. Ottawa (Ontario): Canadian Society for Exercise Physiology; 2003. 300 p.
20. Canoy D. Distribution of body fat and risk of coronary heart disease in men and women. *Curr Opin Cardiol*. 2008;23(6):591–8.
21. Casanova C, Cote C, Marin JM, et al. Distance and oxygen desaturation during the 6-min walk test as predictors of long-term mortality in patients with COPD. *Chest*. 2008;134(4):746–52.
22. Castellani JW, Young AJ, Ducharme MB, et al. American College of Sports Medicine position stand: prevention of cold injuries during exercise. *Med Sci Sports Exerc*. 2006;38(11):2012–29.
23. Ciampricotti R, Deckers JW, Taverne R, el Gamal M, Relik-van Wely L, Pool J. Characteristics of conditioned and sedentary men with acute coronary syndromes. *Am J Cardiol*. 1994;73(4):219–22.
24. Clarkson HM. *Musculoskeletal Assessment: Joint Range of Motion and Manual Muscle Strength*. 2nd ed. Baltimore (MD): Lippincott Williams & Wilkins; 2000. 432 p.
25. *Clinical Guidelines on the Identification, Evaluation, and Treatment of Overweight and Obesity in Adults: The Evidence Report* [Internet]. Bethesda (MD): National Institutes of Health, National Heart, Lung, and Blood Institute. 1998 [cited 2011 Apr 27]. 266 p. Available from: http://www.nhlbi.nih.gov/guidelines/obesity/ob_gdlns.htm
26. Daniels SR, Jacobson MS, McCrindle BW, Eckel RH, Sanner BM. American Heart Association Childhood Obesity Research Summit Report. *Circulation*. 2009;119(15):e489–517.
27. Davis JA. Direct determination of aerobic power. In: Maud PJ, editor. *Physiological Assessment of Human Fitness*. Champaign: Human Kinetics; 1995. p. 9–17.
28. de Koning L, Merchant AT, Pogue J, Anand SS. Waist circumference and waist-to-hip ratio as predictors of cardiovascular events: meta-regression analysis of prospective studies. *Eur Heart J*. 2007; 28(7):850–6.
29. *Definitions—Health, Fitness, and Physical Activity* [Internet]. Washington (DC): President's Council on Physical Fitness and Sports. 2000 [cited 2012 Jan 7]. 11 p. Available from: http://purl.access.gpo.gov/GPO/LPS21074
30. Dehghan M, Merchant AT. Is bioelectrical impedance accurate for use in large epidemiological studies? *Nutr J*. 2008;7:26.
31. Dempster P, Aitkens S. A new air displacement method for the determination of human body composition. *Med Sci Sports Exerc*. 1995;27(12):1692–7.
32. Diener MH, Golding LA, Diener D. Validity and reliability of a one-minute half sit-up test of abdominal strength and endurance. *Sports Med Training Rehab*. 1995;6:105–19.
33. Donnelly JE, Blair SN, Jakicic JM, et al. American College of Sports Medicine Position Stand. Appropriate physical activity intervention strategies for weight loss and prevention of weight regain for adults. *Med Sci Sports Exerc*. 2009;41(2):459–71.
34. Duren DL, Sherwood RJ, Czerwinski SA, et al. Body composition methods: comparisons and interpretation. *J Diabetes Sci Technol*. 2008;2(6):1139–46.
35. Executive summary of the clinical guidelines on the identification, evaluation, and treatment of overweight and obesity in adults. *Arch Intern Med*. 1998;158(17):1855–67.
36. Faigenbaum AD, Kraemer WJ, Blimkie CJ, et al. Youth resistance training: updated position statement paper from the national strength and conditioning association. *J Strength Cond Res*. 2009;23 (5 Suppl):S60–79.
37. Faulkner RA, Sprigings EJ, McQuarrie A, Bell RD. A partial curl-up protocol for adults based on an analysis of two procedures. *Can J Sport Sci*. 1989;14(3):135–41.
38. Flegal KM, Carroll MD, Ogden CL, Curtin LR. Prevalence and trends in obesity among US adults, 1999–2008. *JAMA*. 2010;303(3):235–41.

39. Flegal KM, Graubard BI, Williamson DF, Gail MH. Excess deaths associated with underweight, overweight, and obesity. *JAMA*. 2005;293(15):1861–7.
40. Fox CS, Massaro JM, Hoffmann U, et al. Abdominal visceral and subcutaneous adipose tissue compartments: association with metabolic risk factors in the Framingham Heart Study. *Circulation*. 2007;116(1):39–48.
41. Gallagher D, Heymsfield SB, Heo M, Jebb SA, Murgatroyd PR, Sakamoto Y. Healthy percentage body fat ranges: an approach for developing guidelines based on body mass index. *Am J Clin Nutr*. 2000;72(3):694–701.
42. Garber CE, Blissmer B, Deschenes MR, et al. American College of Sports Medicine Position Stand. The quantity and quality of exercise for developing and maintaining cardiorespiratory, musculoskeletal, and neuromotor fitness in apparently healthy adults: guidance for prescribing exercise. *Med Sci Sports Exerc*. 2011;43(7):1334–559.
43. Gibbons RJ, Balady GJ, Bricker JT, et al. ACC/AHA 2002 guideline update for exercise testing: summary article. A report of the American College of Cardiology/American Heart Association Task Force on Practice Guidelines (Committee to Update the 1997 Exercise Testing Guidelines). *J Am Coll Cardiol*. 2002;40(8):1531–40.
44. Going BS. Densitometry. In: Roche AF, editor. *Human Body Composition*. Champaign: Human Kinetics; 1996. p. 3–23.
45. Graves JE, Pollock ML, Bryant CX. Assessment of muscular strength and endurance. In: Roitman JL, editor. *ACSM's Resource Manual for Guidelines for Exercise Testing and Prescription*. 4th ed. Baltimore: Lippincott Williams & Wilkins; 2001. p. 376–80.
46. Haskell WL, Lee IM, Pate RR, et al. Physical activity and public health: updated recommendation for adults from the American College of Sports Medicine and the American Heart Association. *Circulation*. 2007;116(9):1081–93.
47. Hendel HW, Gotfredsen A, Hojgaard L, Andersen T, Hilsted J. Change in fat-free mass assessed by bioelectrical impedance, total body potassium and dual energy X-ray absorptiometry during prolonged weight loss. *Scand J Clin Lab Invest*. 1996;56(8):671–9.
48. Heymsfield S. *Human Body Composition*. 2nd ed. Champaign (IL): Human Kinetics; 2005. 523 p.
49. Heyward VH. Practical body composition assessment for children, adults, and older adults. *Int J Sport Nutr*. 1998;8(3):285–307.
50. Heyward VH, Stolarczyk LM. *Applied Body Composition Assessment*. Champaign (IL): Human Kinetics; 1996. 221 p.
51. Heyward VH, Wagner DR. *Applied Body Composition Assessment*. 2nd ed. Champaign (IL): Human Kinetics; 2004. 268 p.
52. Hoeger WW, Hopkins DR. A comparison of the sit and reach and the modified sit and reach in the measurement of flexibility in women. *Res Q Exerc Sport*. 1992;63(2):191–5.
53. Jackson AW, Baker AA. The relationship of the sit and reach test to criterion measures of hamstring and back flexibility in young females. *Res Q Exerc Sport*. 1986;57(3):183–6.
54. Jackson AW, Morrow JR,Jr, Brill PA, Kohl HW,3rd, Gordon NF, Blair SN. Relations of sit-up and sit-and-reach tests to low back pain in adults. *J Orthop Sports Phys Ther*. 1998;27(1):22–6.
55. Jackson AW, Pollock ML. Practical assessment of body composition. *Phys Sportsmed*. 1985;13(5):76, 80, 82–90.
56. Janssen I, Katzmarzyk PT, Ross R. Body mass index, waist circumference, and health risk: evidence in support of current National Institutes of Health guidelines. *Arch Intern Med*. 2002;162(18): 2074–9.
57. Jehn M, Halle M, Schuster T, et al. The 6-min walk test in heart failure: is it a max or sub-maximum exercise test? *Eur J Appl Physiol*. 2009;107(3):317–23.
58. Jennings CL, Micklesfield LK, Lambert MI, Lambert EV, Collins M, Goedecke JH. Comparison of body fatness measurements by near-infrared reactance and dual-energy X-ray absorptiometry in normal-weight and obese black and white women. *Br J Nutr*. 2010;103(7):1065–9.
59. Jette M, Campbell J, Mongeon J, Routhier R. The Canadian Home Fitness Test as a predictor for aerobic capacity. *Can Med Assoc J*. 1976;114(8):680–2.
60. Kaminsky LA, American College of Sports Medicine. *ACSM's Resource Manual for Guidelines for Exercise Testing and Prescription*. 5th ed. Baltimore (MD): Lippincott Williams & Wilkins; 2005. 749 p.
61. Kim ES, Ishwaran H, Blackstone E, Lauer MS. External prognostic validations and comparisons of age- and gender-adjusted exercise capacity predictions. *J Am Coll Cardiol*. 2007;50(19):1867–75.
62. Kline GM, Porcari JP, Hintermeister R. Estimation of VO2max from a one-mile track walk, gender, age, and body weight. *Med Sci Sports Exerc*. 1987;19(3):253–9.
63. Kodama S, Saito K, Tanaka S, et al. Cardiorespiratory fitness as a quantitative predictor of all-cause mortality and cardiovascular events in healthy men and women: a meta-analysis. *JAMA*. 2009; 301(19):2024–35.

64. Kumanyika SK, Obarzanek E, Stettler N, et al. Population-based prevention of obesity: the need for comprehensive promotion of healthful eating, physical activity, and energy balance: a scientific statement from American Heart Association Council on Epidemiology and Prevention, Interdisciplinary Committee for Prevention (formerly the expert panel on population and prevention science). *Circulation.* 2008;118(4):428–64.

65. Lee SY, Gallagher D. Assessment methods in human body composition. *Curr Opin Clin Nutr Metab Care.* 2008;11(5):566–72.

66. Leger L, Thivierge M. Heart rate monitors: validity, stability, and functionality. *Phys Sportsmed.* 1988; 16(5):143,146,148,149,151.

67. Levinger I, Goodman C, Hare DL, Jerums G, Toia D, Selig S. The reliability of the 1RM strength test for untrained middle-aged individuals. *J Sci Med Sport.* 2009;12(2):310–6.

68. Lewis CE, McTigue KM, Burke LE, et al. Mortality, health outcomes, and body mass index in the overweight range: a science advisory from the American Heart Association. *Circulation.* 2009; 119(25):3263–71.

69. Logan P, Fornasiero D, Abernathy P. Protocols for the assessment of isoinertial strength. In: Gore CJ, editor. *Physiological Tests for Elite Athletes.* Champaign: Human Kinetics; 2000. p. 200–21.

70. Lohman TG. Body composition methodology in sports medicine. *Phys Sportsmed.* 1982;10(12):46–7.

71. Maritz JS, Morrison JF, Peter J. A practical method of estimating an individual's maximal oxygen uptake. *Ergonomics.* 1961;4:97–122.

72. McConnell TR. Cardiorespiratory assessment of apparently healthy populations. In: American College of Sports Medicine, editor. *ACSM's Resource Manual for Guidelines for Exercise Testing and Prescription.* Baltimore: Lippincott Williams & Wilkins; 2009. p. 361–75.

73. McLean KP, Skinner JS. Validity of Futrex-5000 for body composition determination. *Med Sci Sports Exerc.* 1992;24(2):253–8.

74. Minkler S, Patterson P. The validity of the modified sit-and-reach test in college-age students. *Res Q Exerc Sport.* 1994;65(2):189–92.

75. Morgan W, Borg GA. Perception of effort in the prescription of physical activity. In: Nelson T, editor. *Mental Health and Emotional Aspects of Sports.* Chicago: American Medical Association; 1976. p. 126–9.

76. Myers J, Arena R, Franklin B, et al. Recommendations for clinical exercise laboratories: a scientific statement from the American Heart Association. *Circulation.* 2009;119(24):3144–61.

77. Noble BJ, Borg GA, Jacobs I, Ceci R, Kaiser P. A category-ratio perceived exertion scale: relationship to blood and muscle lactates and heart rate. *Med Sci Sports Exerc.* 1983;15(6):523–8.

78. Norkin CC, Levangie PK. *Joint Structure & Function: A Comprehensive Analysis.* 2nd ed. Philadelphia (PA): Davis; 1992. 512 p.

79. Oreopoulos A, Padwal R, Kalantar-Zadeh K, Fonarow GC, Norris CM, McAlister FA. Body mass index and mortality in heart failure: a meta-analysis. *Am Heart J.* 2008;156(1):13–22.

80. Palmer ML, Epler ME. *Fundamentals of Musculoskeletal Assessment Techniques.* 2nd ed. Baltimore (MD): Lippincott Williams & Wilkins; 1998. 415 p.

81. Peveler WW. Effects of saddle height on economy in cycling. *J Strength Cond Res.* 2008;22(4): 1355–9.

82. Peveler WW, Green JM. Effects of saddle height on economy and anaerobic power in well-trained cyclists. *J Strength Cond Res.* 2011;25(3):633.

83. Peveler WW, Pounders JD, Bishop PA. Effects of saddle height on anaerobic power production in cycling. *J Strength Cond Res.* 2007;21(4):1023–7.

84. Phillips WT, Batterham AM, Valenzuela JE, Burkett LN. Reliability of maximal strength testing in older adults. *Arch Phys Med Rehabil.* 2004;85(2):329–34.

85. Pi-Sunyer FX. The epidemiology of central fat distribution in relation to disease. *Nutr Rev.* 2004; 62(7 Pt 2):S120–6.

86. Poirier P, Giles TD, Bray GA, et al. Obesity and cardiovascular disease: pathophysiology, evaluation, and effect of weight loss: an update of the 1997 American Heart Association Scientific Statement on Obesity and Heart Disease from the Obesity Committee of the Council on Nutrition, Physical Activity, and Metabolism. *Circulation.* 2006;113(6):898–918.

87. Pollack ML, Schmidt DH, Jackson AS. Measurement of cardiorespiratory fitness and body composition in the clinical setting. *Compr Ther.* 1980;6(9):12–27.

88. Protas EJ. Flexibility and range of motion. In: Roitman JL, editor. *ACSM's Resource Manual for Guidelines for Exercise Testing and Prescription.* 4th ed. Baltimore: Lippincott Williams & Wilkins; 2001. p. 381–90.

89. Public Health Agency of Canada, Canadian Society for Exercise Physiology. Physical Activity Readiness Questionnaire (PAR-Q). 2007.

90. Reis JP, Macera CA, Araneta MR, Lindsay SP, Marshall SJ, Wingard DL. Comparison of overall obesity and body fat distribution in predicting risk of mortality. *Obesity (Silver Spring)*. 2009; 17(6):1232–9.

91. Reynolds JM, Gordon TJ, Robergs RA. Prediction of one repetition maximum strength from multiple repetition maximum testing and anthropometry. *J Strength Cond Res*. 2006;20(3):584–92.

92. Rikli RE, Jones CJ. *Senior Fitness Test Manual*. Champaign (IL): Human Kinetics; 2001. 161 p.

93. Robertson RJ, Noble BJ. Perception of physical exertion: methods, mediators, and applications. *Exerc Sport Sci Rev*. 1997;25:407–52.

94. Roche AF. Anthropometry and ultrasound. In: Roche AF, Heymsfield S, Lohman T, editors. *Human Body Composition*. Champaign: Human Kinetics; 1996. p. 167–89.

95. Roger VL, Go AS, Lloyd-Jones DM, et al. Heart Disease and Stroke Statistics—2012 update: a report from the American Heart Association. *Circulation*. 2012;125(1):e2–220.

96. Ross R, Berentzen T, Bradshaw AJ, et al. Does the relationship between waist circumference, morbidity and mortality depend on measurement protocol for waist circumference? *Obes Rev*. 2008;9(4):312–25.

97. Salzman SH. The 6-min walk test: clinical and research role, technique, coding, and reimbursement. *Chest*. 2009;135(5):1345–52.

98. Sesso HD, Paffenbarger RS,Jr, Lee IM. Physical activity and coronary heart disease in men: The Harvard Alumni Health Study. *Circulation*. 2000;102(9):975–80.

99. Shephard RJ, Thomas S, Weller I. The Canadian Home Fitness Test. 1991 update. *Sports Med*. 1991;11(6):358–66.

100. Siri WE. Body composition from fluid spaces and density: analysis of methods. *Nutrition*. 1961; 9(5):480,491; discussion 480,492.

101. Swain DP, American College of Sports Medicine. *ACSM's Resource Manual for Guidelines for Exercise Testing and Prescription*. 7th ed. Baltimore (MD): Lippincott Williams & Wilkins; 2014.

102. Tharrett SJ, Peterson JA, American College of Sports Medicine. *ACSM's Health/Fitness Facility Standards and Guidelines*. 4th ed. Champaign (IL): Human Kinetics; 2012. 256 p.

103. Tran ZV, Weltman A. Generalized equation for predicting body density of women from girth measurements. *Med Sci Sports Exerc*. 1989;21(1):101–4.

104. Tran ZV, Weltman A. Predicting body composition of men from girth measurements. *Hum Biol*. 1988;60(1):167–75.

105. U.S. Preventive Services Task Force, Barton M. Screening for obesity in children and adolescents: US Preventive Services Task Force recommendation statement. *Pediatrics*. 2010;125(2):361–7.

106. Wallace J. Principles of cardiorespiratory endurance programming. In: Kaminsky LA, editor. *ACSM's Resource Manual for Guidelines for Exercise Testing and Prescription*. 5th ed. Baltimore: Lippincott Williams & Wilkins; 2006. p. 336–349.

107. Wang CY, Haskell WL, Farrell SW, et al. Cardiorespiratory fitness levels among US adults 20–49 years of age: findings from the 1999–2004 National Health and Nutrition Examination Survey. *Am J Epidemiol*. 2010;171(4):426–35.

108. Wang J, Thornton JC, Bari S, et al. Comparisons of waist circumferences measured at 4 sites. *Am J Clin Nutr*. 2003;77(2):379–84.

109. Whaley MH, Brubaker PH, Kaminsky LA, Miller CR. Validity of rating of perceived exertion during graded exercise testing in apparently healthy adults and cardiac patients. *J Cardiopulm Rehabil*. 1997;17(4):261–7.

110. Williams MA, Haskell WL, Ades PA, et al. Resistance exercise in individuals with and without cardiovascular disease: 2007 update: a scientific statement from the American Heart Association Council on Clinical Cardiology and Council on Nutrition, Physical Activity, and Metabolism. *Circulation*. 2007;116(5):572–84.

111. YMCA of the USA, Golding LA. *YMCA Fitness Testing and Assessment Manual*. 4th ed. Champaign (IL): Human Kinetics; 2000.

Clinical Exercise Testing

Standard graded exercise tests (GXT) are used clinically to assess a patient's ability to tolerate increasing intensities of aerobic exercise. Electrocardiographic (ECG), hemodynamic, and symptomatic responses are monitored during the GXT for manifestations of myocardial ischemia, hemodynamic/electrical instability, or other exertion-related signs or symptoms. Ventilatory expired gas analysis may also be performed during the GXT, particularly in patients with congestive heart failure (CHF), suspected/confirmed pulmonary limitations, and/or unexplained dyspnea upon exertion.

INDICATIONS AND PURPOSES

The exercise test may be used for diagnostic (*i.e.*, identify abnormal physiologic responses), prognostic (*i.e.*, identify adverse events), and therapeutic (*i.e.*, gauge impact of a given intervention) purposes as well as for physical activity counseling and to design an exercise prescription (Ex R$_x$) (see *Chapters* 7 and 9). However, the recommendations for conducting the GXT as part of the preparticipation health screening for purposes of initiating or maintaining an exercise program (see *Chapter 2*), especially a program of vigorous intensity, may differ from those regarding the use of the GXT to gain information for clinical decision making and management that may include an exercise program.

DIAGNOSTIC EXERCISE TESTING

Determining appropriateness for diagnostic exercise testing to assess for angiographically significant cardiovascular disease (CVD) is influenced by age, sex, and symptomatolgy as outlined in *Table 5.1*. Asymptomatic men and women have a very low (<5% probability) to low (<10% probability) likelihood of angiographically significant CVD across the third to the sixth decade of life. Conversely, the presence of definite angina pectoris increases the likelihood of angiographically significant CVD, although the probability is modulated by sex. Specifically, men with definite angina pectoris have a high (>90% probability) likelihood of angiographically significant CVD from the fourth to the sixth decade of life, whereas women have an intermediate (10%–90% probability) likelihood from the fourth to the fifth decade and high likelihood in the sixth decade onward.

TABLE 5.1. Pretest Likelihood of Atherosclerotic Cardiovascular Disease (CVD)[a]

Age	Sex	Typical/Definite Angina Pectoris	Atypical/Probable Angina Pectoris	Nonanginal Chest Pain	Asymptomatic
30 to 39 yr	Men	Intermediate	Intermediate	Low	Very low
	Women	Intermediate	Very low	Very low	Very low
40 to 49 yr	Men	High	Intermediate	Intermediate	Low
	Women	Intermediate	Low	Very low	Very low
50 to 59 yr	Men	High	Intermediate	Intermediate	Low
	Women	Intermediate	Intermediate	Low	Very low
60 to 69 yr	Men	High	Intermediate	Intermediate	Low
	Women	High	Intermediate	Intermediate	Low

[a]No data exist for patients who are <30 or >69 yr, but it can be assumed that prevalence of CVD increases with age. In a few cases, patients with ages at the extremes of the decades listed may have probabilities slightly outside the high or low range. High indicates >90%; intermediate, 10% to 90%; low, <10%; and very low, <5%.

Reprinted with permission from (25).

It is widely believed the diagnostic GXT has the greatest use in patients with an intermediate pretest probability of angiographically significant CVD. The reason for this belief is the dramatic impact the exercise response has on posttest probability of disease. This concept is illustrated in *Figure 5.1*. From this graph, it is clear that a positive GXT (*i.e.*, ST-segment depression suggestive of CVD) improves the probability of angiographically significant CVD to the greatest level in the subject with intermediate pretest likelihood (*i.e.*, third bar from left; probability increases from ~10% pretest to >60% posttest).

The same exercise testing procedures and concepts are also used when more advanced diagnostic techniques are employed such as nuclear perfusion scanning. Asymptomatic individuals generally represent those with a low likelihood (*i.e.*, <10%) of significant CVD. Therefore, diagnostic GXT in asymptomatic individuals generally is not indicated but may be useful to ensure a normal physiologic response (*i.e.*, hemodynamics, ECG, and symptomatology) when multiple CVD risk factors are present (25) (see *Table 2.2*), indicating at least a moderate risk of experiencing a serious cardiovascular event within 5 yr (72). Among asymptomatic men, ST-segment depression, failure to reach 85% of the predicted maximal heart rate (HR_{max}), and a diminished exercise capacity during peak or symptom-limited treadmill testing provide additional prognostic information in age and Framingham risk score adjusted models, particularly among those in the highest risk group (10 yr predicted coronary risk ≥20%) (13). A diagnostic GXT may be indicated in selected individuals that are about to start a vigorous intensity, exercise program (see *Chapter 2*), or those involved in occupations in which acute cardiovascular events may affect public safety.

In general, patients with a high probability of disease (*e.g.*, typical angina, prior coronary revascularization, myocardial infarction [MI]) are tested to assess residual myocardial ischemia, threatening ventricular arrhythmias, and prognosis rather than for diagnostic purposes. Exercise electrocardiography for diagnostic purposes is less accurate in women largely because of a greater number of false positive responses. Although differences in test accuracy between men

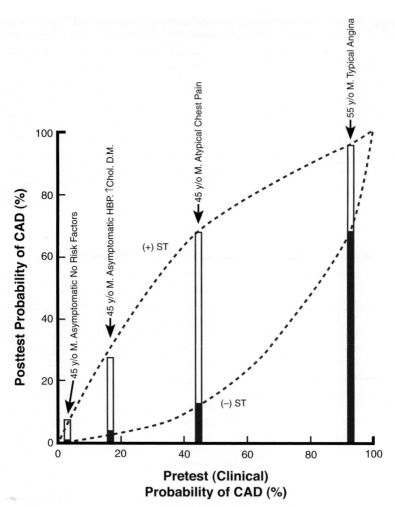

FIGURE 5.1. Impact of positive or negative ST-segment response during GXT on the posttest probability of angiographically significant CVD in subjects with different pretest probabilities. CAD, coronary artery disease. Reprinted with permission from (63).

and women may approximate 10% on average, the standard GXT is considered the initial diagnostic evaluation of choice, regardless of sex (25). A truly positive exercise test requires a hemodynamically significant coronary lesion (*e.g.*, >75% stenosis) (3), yet nearly 90% of acute MIs occur at the site of previously nonobstructive atherosclerotic plaque(s) (36).

The use of maximal or sign/symptom-limited GXT has expanded greatly to help guide decisions regarding medical management and surgical therapy in a broad spectrum of patients. For example, immediate exercise testing of selected low-risk patients (*i.e.*, no hemodynamic abnormalities and arrhythmias, near normal/normal ECG, and negative initial biomarkers for cardiac injury) presenting to the emergency department with signs/symptoms of acute coronary syndrome is becoming increasingly recognized as a valuable tool in making decisions regarding which patients require additional diagnostic studies before hospital discharge (4,5,43,46,71). The use of exercise testing in this capacity has been found to be safe and reduces both length of hospital stay and cost. Patients initially screened to be at low risk subsequently demonstrate a preserved exercise capacity (*i.e.*, ≥7 metabolic equivalents [METs]) and no hemodynamic/ECG abnormalities during testing have a low likelihood of acute coronary syndrome and subsequent events (4). In patients with chronic conditions such as CHF and pulmonary hypertension, exercise testing may also prove valuable in guiding treatment decisions as several variables obtained from this assessment respond favorably to numerous pharmacologic and surgical interventions (6,8,27).

EXERCISE TESTING FOR DISEASE SEVERITY AND PROGNOSIS

Exercise testing is useful for the evaluation of disease severity among individuals with known or suspected CVD. The magnitude of ischemia caused by a coronary lesion generally is (a) directly proportional to the degree of ST-segment depression, the number of ECG leads involved, and the duration of ST-segment depression in recovery; and (b) inversely proportional to the ST slope, the rate pressure product (RPP) (*i.e.*, heart rate [HR] × systolic blood pressure [SBP]) at which the ST-segment depression occurs, and the HR_{max}, SBP, and METs achieved.

The exercise testing response is likewise an important gauge of disease severity in patients with chronic conditions such as CHF, pulmonary hypertension, and chronic obstructive pulmonary disease (COPD) (9). A progressively diminished aerobic capacity is universally reflective of increasing disease severity in these chronic conditions. Data exclusively obtained from ventilatory expired gas analysis and reflective of abnormalities in ventilation perfusion matching (*i.e.*, minute ventilation/carbon dioxide production [$\dot{V}E/\dot{V}CO_2$] slope, and partial pressure of end-tidal carbon dioxide [$P_{ET}CO_2$]) also provide insight into disease severity, especially among patients with CHF, pulmonary hypertension, and COPD. The prognostic value of exercise testing appears to be consistent in all individuals regardless of their health status when there is a progressively diminishing aerobic capacity that is a warning of worsening prognosis (9). In addition, several other HR, hemodynamic, and ventilatory expired gas variables obtained from exercise testing provide robust prognostic information in certain populations such as heart failure. Several numeric indices of prognosis have been proposed and are discussed in *Chapter 6* (11,47).

EXERCISE TESTING AFTER MYOCARDIAL INFARCTION

Exercise testing after MI can be performed before or soon after hospital discharge for prognostic assessment, Ex R_x, and evaluation of medical therapy or interventions including coronary revascularization (25). Submaximal exercise tests are currently recommended before hospital discharge at 4–6 d after acute MI. Submaximal exercise testing provides sufficient data to assess the effectiveness of current pharmacologic management (*e.g.*, hemodynamic response to physical exertion on antihypertensive medication) (see *Appendix A*) as well as activities of daily living and early ambulatory exercise therapy recommendations. Symptom-limited GXTs are considered safe and appropriate early after discharge (~14–21 d) for Ex R$_x$ and physical activity counseling and further assessment of pharmacologic management efficacy (25). Patients who have not undergone coronary revascularization and are unable to undergo exercise testing appear to have a poor prognosis. Other indicators of adverse prognosis in the post-MI patient include ischemic ST-segment depression at a low level of exercise (particularly if accompanied by reduced left ventricular systolic function), functional capacity of <5 METs, and a hypotensive SBP response to exercise (see *Box 6.1*).

FUNCTIONAL EXERCISE TESTING

Exercise testing is useful to determine functional capacity. This information can be valuable for physical activity counseling, Ex R$_x$, disability assessment, and to help estimate prognosis. Exercise testing may also provide valuable information as part of a return to work evaluation if the patient's occupation requires aerobic activity.

Functional capacity can be evaluated based on percentile ranking (based on apparently healthy men and women) as presented in *Table 4.9*. Exercise capacity also may be reported as the percentage of expected METs for age using one of several established nomograms with 100% considered normal (see *Figure 5.2*) (25,51). Separate nomograms are provided in *Figure 5.2* for men with suspected CVD and healthy men, and for asymptomatic healthy and sedentary women. Normal standards for exercise capacity based on directly measured maximal oxygen consumption ($\dot{V}O_{2max}$) are also available for men and women (59). When using a particular regression equation for estimating percentage of normal exercise capacity achieved, factors such as population specificity, exercise mode, and whether exercise capacity was measured directly or estimated should be considered. Lastly, recent investigations have found that percent predicted aerobic capacity is prognostic in patients with CVD and CHF (7,39).

Data supporting the prognostic ability of aerobic capacity in apparently healthy, high-risk individuals for the development of CVD, and known CVD cohorts are convincing (9). Kodama et al. (42) performed a meta-analysis that collectively included 33 studies totaling more than 100,000 subjects and 6,000 all-cause mortality and 4,000 cardiovascular events. They found estimated aerobic capacity from treadmill speed and grade or ergometer workload was a consistent prognostic marker in apparently healthy men and women. Each 1 MET increase in aerobic capacity reflected a 13% decrease in all-cause mortality and 15% decrease in cardiovascular events (42). Myers et al. (55) examined a large cohort of >3,000 men with variable CVD risk factors with and without confirmed disease and found aerobic capacity was a superior predictor of mortality when compared to tobacco use, hypertension, elevated lipids, and diabetes mellitus. Subjects with CVD and

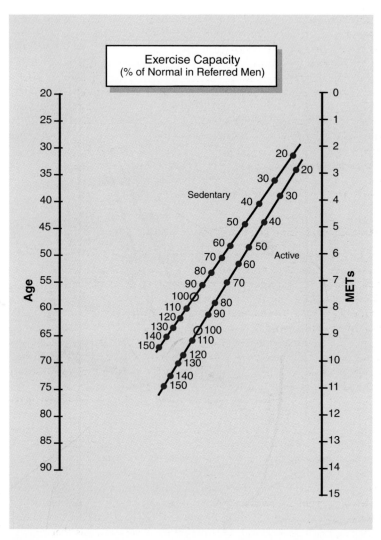

■ FIGURE 5.2. Nomograms of percent normal exercise capacity in men with suspected coronary artery disease who were referred for clinical exercise testing and in apparently healthy men and women. METs, metabolic equivalents. Reprinted with permission from (51) and (28). (*continued*)

an exercise capacity ≤4.9 METs had a relative risk of death 4.1 times greater compared to those with an exercise capacity ≥10.7 METs over a mean follow-up of 6.2 yr. For every 1 MET increase in exercise capacity, there was a 12% improvement in survival. Similarly, findings from the National Exercise and Heart Disease Project among post-MI patients demonstrated that every 1 MET increase after the

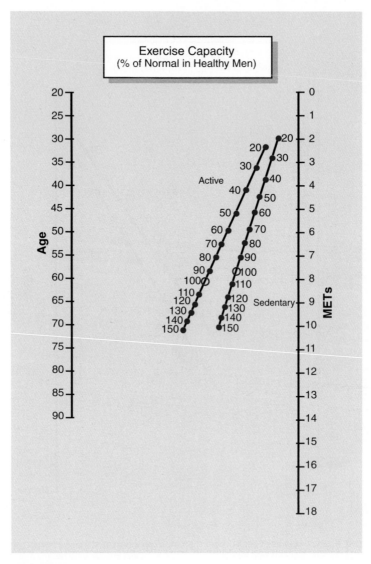

■ **FIGURE 5.2.** (*Continued*)

exercise training program conferred an approximate 10% reduction in mortality from any cause over 19 yr of follow-up, regardless of study group assignment (21).

Kavanagh et al. (37,38) investigated two large cohorts of men and women with confirmed CVD who were referred to cardiac rehabilitation and found directly measured peak oxygen uptake ($\dot{V}O_{2peak}$) during a progressive cycle ergometer test

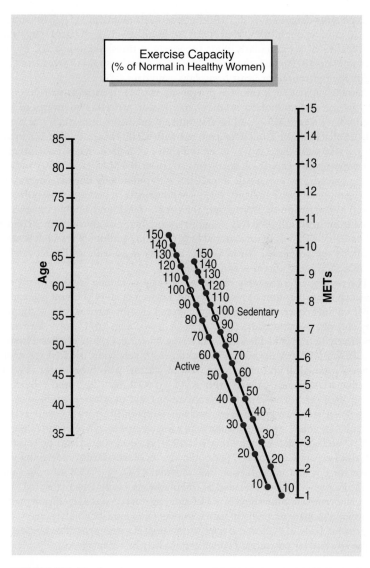

FIGURE 5.2. (*Continued*)

to exhaustion at program entry was a powerful predictor of cardiovascular and all-cause mortality. The cutoff points above which there was a marked survival benefit were 13 mL · kg · min^{-1} (3.7 METs) in women and 15 mL · kg · min^{-1} (4.3 METs) in men. For each 1 mL · kg · min^{-1} increase in aerobic capacity, there was a 9% and 10% reduction in cardiac mortality in men and women, respectively.

In patients diagnosed with CHF, the prognostic ability of $\dot{V}O_{2peak}$ is supported by ~20 yr of research (8). O'Neil et al. (59) found a $\dot{V}O_{2peak}$ <10 mL · kg · min^{-1} is indicative of a particularly poor prognosis, a threshold supported by other investigations (8). In fact, the use of $\dot{V}O_{2peak}$ at this threshold is considered a key acceptable indication for heart transplant candidacy (25).

Aerobic capacity is a valuable prognostic marker in patients with interstitial lung disease and pulmonary arterial hypertension as well. Two groups of investigators have found $\dot{V}O_{2peak}$ to be a significant predictor of mortality in patients with COPD (32,60). Similar to patients with CHF, Hiraga et al. (32) found a $\dot{V}O_{2peak}$ <10 mL · kg · min^{-1} to be indicative of a particularly poor prognosis in a cohort with COPD. A small investigation by Miki et al. (50) indicated $\dot{V}O_{2peak}$ may also be prognostic in patients with pulmonary fibrosis. Several small investigations likewise indicate $\dot{V}O_{2peak}$ is prognostic in patients with pulmonary arterial hypertension (6). Moreover, Shah et al. (69) found aerobic capacity estimated from treadmill time was a significant predictor of mortality in a cohort of 603 patients with pulmonary arterial hypertension. Additional research is needed to solidify the prognostic use of aerobic capacity in patients with interstitial and vascular pulmonary diseases and conditions.

The presurgical assessment of aerobic capacity is gaining increased recognition as an important indicator of poor outcome. Loewen et al. (45) found patients with suspected lung cancer are at significantly greater risk for surgical complications and poor outcome postprocedure if $\dot{V}O_{2peak}$ falls lower than 16–15 mL · kg · min^{-1}, respectively. Recent guidelines put forth by the American College of Chest Physicians (ACCP) support the use of exercise testing with ventilatory expired gas analysis to assess presurgical and postsurgical risk in patients with lung cancer (19). This guideline recommends patients with a $\dot{V}O_{2peak}$ <10 mL · kg · min^{-1} be considered at high risk for postsurgical complications and mortality, regardless of other characteristics such as pulmonary function. Additionally, patients with a $\dot{V}O_{2peak}$ <15 mL · kg · min^{-1} in combination with a forced expiratory volume in one second (FEV$_{1.0}$) and diffusion capacity that is <40% predicted should also be considered high risk for complications and poor outcome. In older patients undergoing gastric bypass surgery, McCullough et al. (48) reported a $\dot{V}O_{2peak}$ <15.8 mL · kg · min^{-1} signified a higher risk for postsurgical complications. Lastly, Older et al. (61) found a $\dot{V}O_2$ at a ventilatory threshold of <11.0 mL · kg · min^{-1} was a significant predictor of cardiopulmonary mortality in patients undergoing intraabdominal surgery. Given the growing body of evidence, it appears presurgical assessment of aerobic capacity to quantify risk for postsurgical complications may be advantageous.

EXERCISE TEST MODALITIES

The treadmill is the most common exercise testing mode used in the United States. Treadmills in clinical exercise laboratories should be electronically driven, allow for a wide range of speed (1–8 mph or 1.61–12.8 km · h^{-1}) and grade (0%–20%), and be able to support a body weight of at least 350 lb (159.1 kg). The treadmill should have handrails for balance and stability; but given the negative impact tight gripping of the handrails can have on both the accuracy of estimated exercise capacity (i.e., estimated $\dot{V}O_{2peak}$ with handrail gripping is greater than measured $\dot{V}O_{2peak}$) and the quality of the ECG recording, handrail use should be discouraged or minimized to the lowest level possible when maintaining balance is a concern. An emergency stop button should be readily visible and available to both the subject undergoing testing and supervising staff (52).

Cycle ergometers are the most common exercise testing modes used in many European countries. Cycle ergometry is less expensive and requires less space than treadmill testing and is a viable alternative to treadmill testing in individuals with obesity and those who have orthopedic, peripheral vascular, and/or neurologic limitations. The cycle ergometer must include handlebars and an adjustable seat, allowing for the knee to be flexed ~25 degrees of full extension in a given subject (64–66). Incremental work rates on an electronically braked cycle ergometer are more sensitive than mechanically braked ergometers because the work rate can be maintained over a wide range of pedal rates. Because there is less movement of the patient's arms and thorax during cycling, it is easier to obtain better quality ECG recordings and blood pressure (BP) measurements. However, stationary cycling is an unfamiliar method of exercise for many and is highly dependent on patient motivation. Thus, the test may end prematurely (i.e., because of localized leg fatigue) before a cardiopulmonary endpoint has been achieved. Lower values for $\dot{V}O_{2max}/\dot{V}O_{2peak}$ during cycle ergometer testing (vs. treadmill testing) can range from 5% to 25%, depending on the participant's habitual activity, physical conditioning, leg strength, and familiarity with cycling (30,54,67).

Arm ergometry is an alternative method of exercise testing for patients who cannot perform leg exercise. Because a smaller muscle mass is used during arm ergometry, $\dot{V}O_{2max}/\dot{V}O_{2peak}$ during arm exercise is generally 20%–30% lower than that obtained during treadmill testing (24). Although this test has diagnostic use (14), it has been largely replaced by the nonexercise pharmacologic stress techniques that are described later in this chapter. Arm ergometer tests can be used for physical activity counseling and Ex R_x for certain disabled populations (e.g., spinal cord injury) and individuals who perform primarily dynamic upper body work during occupational or leisure time activities.

Routine calibration procedures should be followed for all exercise testing modes (i.e., treadmill, lower extremity, and upper extremity ergometry). Specific calibration procedures are usually provided by the manufacturer. A description of general calibration procedures for the treadmill and cycle and arm ergometers are available from Myers et al. (52).

EXERCISE PROTOCOLS

The protocol employed during an exercise test should consider the purpose of the evaluation, the specific outcomes desired, and the characteristics of the individual being tested (e.g., age, symptomatology). Some of the most common exercise protocols and the predicted $\dot{V}O_2$ for each stage are illustrated in *Figure 5.3*. The Bruce treadmill test remains one of the most commonly used protocols,

FUNCTIONAL CLASS	CLINICAL STATUS		O₂ COST ml/kg/min	METS	BICYCLE ERGOMETER	BRUCE		RAMP	
						3 MIN STAGES MPH / %AGR			
			73.5	21					
			70	20		5.5	20		
			66.5	19	FOR 70 KG BODY WEIGHT Kpm/min (WATTS)				
			63	18					
			59.5	17		5.0	18		
			56.0	16					
NORMAL AND I	HEALTHY, DEPENDENT ON AGE, ACTIVITY		52.5	15					
			49.0	14	1500 (246)	4.2	16	PER 30 SEC MPH / %GR	
			45.5	13				3.0	25.0
								3.0	24.0
			42.0	12	1350 (221)			3.0	23.0
								3.0	22.0
			38.5	11	1200 (197)			3.0	21.0
								3.0	20.0
								3.0	19.0
			35.0	10	1050 (172)	3.4	14	3.0	18.0
								3.0	17.0
			31.5	9				3.0	16.0
	SEDENTARY HEALTHY				900 (148)			3.0	15.0
			28.0	8				3.0	14.0
					750 (123)			3.0	13.0
			24.5	7		2.5	12	3.0	12.0
					600 (98)			3.0	11.0
			21.0	6				3.0	10.0
II					450 (74)			3.0	9.0
			17.5	5				3.0	8.0
		LIMITED				1.7	10	3.0	7.0
			14.0	4	300 (49)			3.0	6.0
		SYMPTOMATIC						3.0	5.0
III			10.5	3	150 (24)			3.0	4.0
								3.0	3.0
			7.0	2				3.0	2.0
								3.0	1.0
								3.0	0
								2.5	0
								2.0	0
								1.5	0
IV			3.5	1				1.0	0
								0.5	0

■ **FIGURE 5.3.** Common exercise protocols and associated metabolic costs of each stage.

TREADMILL PROTOCOLS

BRUCE RAMP (PER MIN, MPH / %GR)		BALKE-WARE	USAFSAM (MPH / %GR)		"SLOW" USAFSAM (MPH / %GR)		MODIFIED BALKE (MPH / %GR)		ACIP (MPH / %GR)		MOD. NAUGHTON (CHF) (MPH / %GR)		METS
5.8	20												21
5.6	19	%GRADE AT 3.3 MPH											20
		1 MIN STAGES											19
5.3	18												18
5.0	18												17
4.8	17												16
		26 / 25 / 24	3.3	25					3.4	24.0			15
4.5	16	23					3.0	25	3.1	24.0	3.0	25	14
4.2	16	22 / 21											13
4.1	15	20	3.3	20			3.0	22.5			3.0	22.5	
		19 / 18					3.0	20	3.0	21.0	3.0	20	12
3.8	14	17 / 16											11
		15	3.3	15			3.0	17.5	3.0	17.5	3.0	17.5	10
3.4	14	14 / 13			2	25	3.0	15			3.0	15	9
		12							3.0	14.0	3.0	12.5	
3.1	13	11					3.0	12.5					8
		10	3.3	10	2	20	3.0	10	3.0	10.5	3.0	10	
2.8	12	9											7
2.5	12	8			2	15	3.0	7.5			3.0	7.5	
2.3	11	7							3.0	7.0			6
2.1	10	6 / 5	3.3	5	2	10	3.0	5			2.0	10.5	
		4											5
1.7	10	3					3.0	2.5	3.0	3.0	2.0	7.0	4
		2			2	5			2.5	2.0			
		1	3.3	0			3.0	0			2.0	3.5	3
1.3	5		2.0	0	2	0	2.0	0	2.0	0.0			
											1.5	0	2
1.0	0										1.0	0	1

particularly in cardiac stress testing centers (56). However, the Bruce protocol employs relatively large incremental workload adjustments (*i.e.*, 2–3 METs per stage) every 3 min. Consequently, changes in physiologic responses tend to be less uniform, and exercise capacity may be markedly overestimated when it is predicted from exercise time or workload, which is particularly true with hand-rail use.

Recent evidence indicates ischemic thresholds are observed at similar RPP when comparing the Bruce protocol to a more conservative treadmill protocol (57). However, it does appear the RPP corresponding to an ischemic threshold is significantly different for a given patient with CVD when performing an exercise test on a treadmill compared to a cycle ergometer (57,58). Specifically, the RPP corresponding to an ischemic threshold and maximal ST-segment depression is significantly lower during cycle ergometry compared to treadmill testing. In general, protocols with larger incremental workload adjustments such as the Bruce or Ellestad are better suited for screening younger and/or physically active individuals; whereas protocols with smaller increments such as the Naughton or Balke-Ware (*i.e.*, ≤1 MET per stage) are preferable for older or deconditioned individuals and patients with chronic diseases. If serial testing is performed, the mode of testing and exercise protocol should be consistent across all assessments.

Ramping protocols, which increase work rate in a constant and continuous manner, are an alternative approach to incremental exercise testing that has gained in popularity (10). Individualized (53) and standardized ramp tests, such as the Ball State University/Bruce ramp (35), have been used to improve patient tolerance and test quality. The former test individualizes the rate of increase in intensity based on the subject. The latter standardized ramp test matches work rates to equivalent periods on the Bruce protocol while increasing the work rates in ramp fashion.

Advantages of ramp protocols include the following (54):

- Avoidance of large and unequal increments in workload.
- Uniform increase in hemodynamic and physiologic responses.
- More accurate estimates of exercise capacity and ventilatory threshold.
- Individualized test protocol (ramp rate).
- Targeted test duration (applies only to individualized ramp protocols).

Whichever exercise protocol is chosen, it should be individualized so that the treadmill speed and increments in grade are based on the subject's perceived functional capacity. Ideally, increments in work rate should be chosen so that the total test time ranges between 8 and 12 min (10), assuming the endpoint is volitional fatigue. For example, increments of $10–15\,\text{W} \cdot \text{min}^{-1}$ ($61–92\,\text{kg} \cdot \text{m} \cdot \text{min}^{-1}$) can be used on the cycle ergometer for older individuals, deconditioned individuals, and patients with CVD or pulmonary disease. Increases in treadmill grade of $1\%–3\% \cdot \text{min}^{-1}$ with constant belt speeds of 1.5–2.5 mph (2.4–4.0 kph) can also be used for such populations.

Submaximal testing is strongly recommended by the American Heart Association (AHA) in post-MI patients prior to discharge (about 4–6 d postevent) for (a) prognostic assessment; (b) physical activity counseling and Ex R$_x$; and (c) evaluation of medical therapy (25). Moreover, submaximal exercise testing may be preferred in health/fitness settings, particularly during the assessment of individuals deemed to be at greater risk of cardiovascular events. These tests are generally terminated at a predetermined level such as an HR of 120 beats · min^{-1}, 70% of heart rate reserve (HRR), 85% of age predicted HR$_{max}$, or 5 METs, but these termination criteria may vary based on the patient and clinical judgment (10). Established treadmill or ergometry exercise testing protocols that are more conservative in nature (*i.e.*, ramp) are typically appropriate for submaximal testing.

UPPER BODY EXERCISE TESTING

An arm cycle ergometer can be purchased as such or modified from an existing stationary cycle ergometer by replacing the pedals with handles and mounting the unit on a table at shoulder height. Similar to leg cycle ergometers, these can be either mechanically or electrically braked. This mode of testing is appropriate in individuals unable to exercise on a treadmill or lower extremity ergometer (*i.e.*, patients with vascular, orthopedic, and neurologic comorbidities). Peak METs obtained during arm ergometry appear to be predictive of adverse events in patients unable to perform treadmill testing (34). Work rates are adjusted by altering the cranking rates and/or resistance against the flywheel. Work rate increments of 5–10 W (30.6–61.2 kg · m · min^{-1}) every 2–3 min at a cadence of 60–75 revolutions · min^{-1} (rpm) are common recommendations (52). Arm ergometry is best performed in the seated position with the fulcrum of the handle adjusted to shoulder height. SBP taken by the standard cuff method immediately after arm crank ergometry are likely to underestimate "true" SBP responses (33). Brachial SBP during arm ergometry can also be approximated using a Doppler stethoscope at the dorsalis pedis artery.

TESTING FOR RETURN TO WORK

The decision to return to work after a cardiac event is a complex one with ~25% of these patients failing to resume work (29). National and cultural customs, local economic conditions, numerous nonmedical variables, employer stereotypes, and worker attitudes may govern failure to return to work. To counteract these deterrents, job modifications should be explored and implemented to facilitate the resumption of gainful employment.

Work assessment and counseling are useful in optimizing return to work decisions. Early discussion of work-related issues with patients, preferably before hospital discharge, may help establish reasonable return to work expectations. Discussion with the patient could include a job history analysis to (a) ascertain job aerobic requirements and potential cardiac demands; (b) establish tentative time lines for work evaluation and return to work; (c) individualize rehabilitation according to job demands; and (d) determine special work-related needs or job contacts (70). The appropriate time to return to work varies with type of cardiac event or intervention, associated complications, and prognosis.

The GXT provides valuable information regarding a patient's ability to safely return to work (25) because (a) the patient's responses can help assess prognosis; and (b) measured or estimated MET capacity can be compared to the estimated aerobic requirements of the patient's job to assess expected relative work energy demands (2). For most patients, physical demands are considered appropriate if the 8 h energy expenditure work requirement averages ≤50% peak METs achieved on the GXT and peak job demands (*e.g.*, 5–45 min) are within guidelines prescribed for a home exercise program (*e.g.*, ≤80% MET_{peak}). Most contemporary job tasks require only very light to light aerobic requirements (*i.e.*, ≤3 METs) (70).

A GXT is commonly the only functional assessment required to determine return to work status. However, some patients may benefit from further functional testing if job demands differ substantially from those evaluated with the GXT, especially patients with (a) borderline physical work capacity in relationship to the anticipated job demands; (b) concomitant left ventricular dysfunction; and/or (c) concerns about resuming a physically demanding occupation. Job tasks that may evoke disproportionate myocardial demands compared to a GXT include those requiring static muscular contraction work combined with temperature stress and intermittent heavy work (70).

Tests simulating the task(s) in question can be administered when insufficient information is available to determine a patient's ability to resume work within a reasonable degree of safety. For patients at risk for serious arrhythmias or silent or symptomatic myocardial ischemia on the job, ambulatory ECG monitoring may be considered in conjunction with simple, inexpensive tests that can be set up to evaluate types of work not evaluated with a GXT (70). For example, a weight carrying test that simulates occupational tasks can be used to evaluate tolerance for light-to-heavy static work combined with light dynamic work.

MEASUREMENTS DURING EXERCISE TESTING

Common variables assessed during clinical exercise testing include BP, ECG changes, subjective ratings, and signs and symptoms. Ventilatory expired gas analysis responses may be included in the exercise test, particularly in certain groups such as patients with CHF and individuals being assessed for unexplained exertional dyspnea. Lastly, arterial blood gas analysis can also be performed during an advanced exercise test assessment.

HEART RATE AND BLOOD PRESSURE

HR and BP should be measured before, during, and after the GXT. *Table 5.2* indicates the recommended frequency and sequence of these measures. A standardized procedure should be adopted for each laboratory so that baseline measures can be assessed more accurately when repeat testing is performed.

TABLE 5.2. Recommended Monitoring Intervals Associated with Exercise Testing

Variable	Before Exercise Test	During Exercise Test	After Exercise Test
ECG	Monitored continuously; recorded supine position and posture of exercise	Monitored continuously; recorded during the last 15 s of each stage (interval protocol) or the last 15 s of each 2 min period (ramp protocols)	Monitored continuously; recorded immediately postexercise, during the last 15 s of first minute of recovery, and then every 2 min thereafter
HR[a]	Monitored continuously; recorded supine position and posture of exercise	Monitored continuously; recorded during the last 5 s of each minute	Monitored continuously; recorded during the last 5 s of each minute
BP[a,b]	Measured and recorded in supine position and posture of exercise	Measured and recorded during the last 45 s of each stage (interval protocol) or the last 45 s of each 2 min period (ramp protocols)	Measured and recorded immediately postexercise and then every 2 min thereafter
Signs and symptoms	Monitored continuously; recorded as observed	Monitored continuously; recorded as observed	Monitored continuously; recorded as observed
RPE	Explain scale	Recorded during the last 15 s of each exercise stage or every 2 min with ramping protocol	Obtain peak exercise value then not measured in recovery
Gas exchange	Baseline reading to ensure proper operational status	Measured continuously	Generally not needed in recovery

[a]In addition, BP and HR should be assessed and recorded whenever adverse symptoms or abnormal ECG changes occur.

[b]An unchanged or decreasing systolic blood pressure with increasing workloads should be retaken (*i.e.*, verified immediately).

BP, blood pressure; ECG, electrocardiogram; HR, heart rate; RPE, rating of perceived exertion.

Adapted and used by permission from (16).

Several devices have been developed to automate BP measurements during exercise and demonstrate reasonable accuracy (52). These devices also typically allow for auditory confirmation of the automated BP measurement, which may improve confidence in the value obtained. When an automated system is used, calibration and maintenance should be followed according to manufacturer specifications, and calibration checks should periodically be performed by comparing automated to manual BP recordings. Despite advances in automated BP measurements during exercise, manual assessment (standard cuff method) is still commonplace. *Boxes 3.4* and *5.1* contain methods for BP assessment at rest and potential sources of error during exercise, respectively. Abnormal hypertensive and hypotensive responses to the GXT are also possible absolute and relative indications for test termination (see *Box 5.2*) (23).

BOX 5.1	Potential Sources of Error in Blood Pressure Assessment

- Inaccurate sphygmomanometer
- Improper cuff size
- Auditory acuity of technician
- Rate of inflation or deflation of cuff pressure
- Experience of technician
- Reaction time of technician
- Faulty equipment
- Improper stethoscope placement or pressure
- Background noise
- Allowing patient to hold treadmill handrails or flex elbow
- Certain physiologic abnormalities (*e.g.*, damaged brachial artery, subclavian steal syndrome, arteriovenous fistula)

ELECTROCARDIOGRAPHIC MONITORING

A high quality ECG is of paramount importance for an appropriately conducted GXT (see *Appendix C*). Proper skin preparation lowers the resistance at the skin electrode interface, and thereby improves the signal to noise ratio. The general areas for electrode placement should be shaved, if necessary, and cleansed with an alcohol saturated gauze pad. The superficial layer of skin should then be removed using light abrasion with fine grain emery paper or gauze and electrodes placed according to standardized anatomic landmarks (23). Although 12 leads are simultaneously recorded and readily available for assessment, three leads — representing the inferior, anterior, and lateral cardiac distribution — are typically monitored in real time, with 12-lead ECGs printed at the end of each stage and at maximal exercise. The limb electrodes are affixed to the torso for the GXT (23). Because torso leads may give a slightly different ECG configuration when compared with the standard 12-lead resting ECG, use of torso leads should be noted on the ECG.

Signal processing techniques have made it possible to average ECG waveforms and attenuate or eliminate electrical interference or artifact. Although this technology continues to evolve, computer driven ECG interpretation should be considered a compliment rather than a replacement to manual interpretation. Moreover, all reports automatically derived from computer interpretation should be over read by a clinician appropriately trained in ECG interpretation (40).

SUBJECTIVE RATINGS AND SYMPTOMS

The measurement of perceptual responses during exercise testing can provide useful clinical information. Somatic ratings of perceived exertion (RPE) (see *Chapters 4, 7,* and *10*) and/or specific symptoms (*e.g.*, degree of chest pain,

BOX 5.2	Indications for Terminating Exercise Testing

ABSOLUTE INDICATIONS
- Drop in systolic BP of ≥10 mm Hg with an increase in work rate, or if systolic BP decreases below the value obtained in the same position prior to testing when accompanied by other evidence of ischemia
- Moderately severe angina (defined as 3 on standard scale)
- Increasing nervous system symptoms (e.g., ataxia, dizziness, or near syncope)
- Signs of poor perfusion (cyanosis or pallor)
- Technical difficulties monitoring the ECG or SBP
- Subject's desire to stop
- Sustained ventricular tachycardia
- ST elevation (+1.0 mm) in leads without diagnostic Q waves (other than V_1 or aVR)

RELATIVE INDICATIONS
- Drop in systolic BP of ≥10 mm Hg with an increase in work rate, or if systolic BP below the value obtained in the same position prior to testing
- ST or QRS changes such as excessive ST depression (>2 mm horizontal or downsloping ST-segment depression) or marked axis shift
- Arrhythmias other than sustained ventricular tachycardia, including multifocal PVCs, triplets of PVCs, supraventricular tachycardia, heart block, or bradyarrhythmias
- Fatigue, shortness of breath, wheezing, leg cramps, or claudication
- Development of bundle-branch block or intraventricular conduction delay that cannot be distinguished from ventricular tachycardia
- Increasing chest pain
- Hypertensive response (SBP of >250 mm Hg and/or a DBP of >115 mm Hg).

aVR, augmented voltage right; BP, blood pressure; DBP, diastolic blood pressure; ECG, electrocardiogram; PVC, premature ventricular contraction; SBP, systolic blood pressure; V_1, chest lead I.
Reprinted with permission from (25).

burning, discomfort, dyspnea, light-headedness, leg discomfort/pain) should be assessed routinely during clinical exercise tests. Patients are asked to provide subjective estimates during the last 15 s of each exercise stage (or every 2 min during ramp protocols) either verbally or manually. For example, the individual can provide a number verbally or point to a number if a mouthpiece or face mask precludes oral communication. The exercise technician should restate the number to confirm the correct rating. Either the 6–20 category scale (see *Chapter 4*) or the 0–10 category-ratio scale may be used to assess RPE during exercise testing (15). Before the start of the exercise test, the patient should be given clear and concise instructions for use of the selected scale.

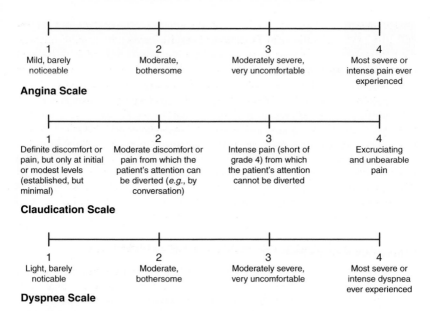

■ FIGURE 5.4. Frequently used scales for assessing the patient's level of angina (*top*), claudication (*middle*), and dyspnea (*bottom*).

Use of alternative rating scales that are specific to subjective symptoms are recommended if subjects become symptomatic during exercise testing. Frequently used scales for assessing the patients' level of angina, claudication, and/or dyspnea can be found in *Figure 5.4*. In general, ratings of ≥3 on the angina scale or a degree of chest discomfort that would cause the patient to stop normal daily activities are reasons to terminate the exercise test (see *Box 5.2*). Interestingly, patients with CVD reporting dyspnea as a primary factor limiting exercise may have a worse prognosis compared to those reporting alternate subjective symptoms (*i.e.*, exercise limited by leg fatigue or angina) (1,18).

GAS EXCHANGE AND VENTILATORY RESPONSES

Currently, the combination of standard GXT procedures and ventilatory expired gas analysis (*i.e.*, cardiopulmonary exercise testing) is the clinical standard for patients with CHF being assessed for transplantation candidacy and individuals with unexplained exertional dyspnea (25). The analysis of ventilatory expired gas overcomes the potential inaccuracies associated with estimating $\dot{V}O_2$ from work rate (*i.e.*, treadmill speed and grade). The direct measurement of $\dot{V}O_2$ is more reliable and reproducible than estimated values from treadmill or cycle ergometer work rates. $\dot{V}O_{2peak}$ is the most accurate measurement of functional capacity and is a useful index of overall cardiopulmonary health (12).

The measurement of $\dot{V}O_2$, $\dot{V}CO_2$, and the subsequent calculation of the respiratory exchange ratio (RER) can also be used to assess the level of physical exertion during the GXT with greater precision than that obtained from age-predicted HR_{max}. The assessment of $\dot{V}E$ also should be made whenever gas exchange responses are obtained. In fact, the combined assessment of $\dot{V}E$ and $\dot{V}CO_2$, commonly expressed as the $\dot{V}E/\dot{V}CO_2$ slope and termed *ventilatory efficiency*, provides robust prognostic information in patients with CHF (12). Because heart and lung diseases frequently lead to ventilatory and/or gas exchange abnormalities during exercise, an integrated analysis of these measures can be useful for differential diagnosis (12). Most currently available ventilatory expired gas analysis systems are also able to perform pulmonary function testing, which is advantageous when performing this type of differential diagnosis. Lastly, collection of gas exchange and ventilatory responses are increasingly being used in clinical trials to objectively assess the response to specific interventions (10).

ARTERIAL BLOOD GAS ASSESSMENT DURING EXERCISE

In patients who present with unexplained exertional dyspnea, pulmonary disease should be considered as a potential underlying cause. It is important to quantify gas partial pressures in these patients because oxygen desaturation may occur during exertion. Although measurement of the partial pressure of oxygen in arterial blood (P_aO_2) and partial pressure of carbon dioxide in arterial blood (P_aCO_2) have been the standard in the past, the availability of pulse oximetry and the estimation of arterial oxygen saturation (SpO_2) has replaced the need to routinely draw arterial blood in most patients. In patients with pulmonary disease, measurements of oxygen saturation in arterial blood (SaO_2) correlate reasonably well with SpO_2 ($\pm 2\%$–3% accuracy rates), provided SpO_2 remains $>85\%$. A decrease of $>5\%$ in SpO_2 during exercise testing is considered an abnormal response suggestive of exercise induced hypoxemia. Invasive assessment of arterial blood gases is still required if a precise measurement is clinically warranted (12).

INDICATIONS FOR EXERCISE TEST TERMINATION

The absolute and relative indications for termination of an exercise test are listed in *Box* 5.2. Absolute indications are unambiguous, whereas relative indications may be superseded by clinical judgment.

POSTEXERCISE PERIOD

Regardless of the postexercise procedures (*i.e.*, active vs. passive recovery), monitoring should continue for at least 6 min after exercise or until ECG changes return to baseline and significant signs and symptoms resolve (23). ST-segment changes that occur only during the postexercise period are currently recognized to be an important diagnostic part of the test (68). HR and BP should also return to near baseline levels before discontinuation of monitoring. In addition, the

HR recovery from exercise is an important prognostic marker that should be recorded (see *Chapter 6*) (25,44).

IMAGING MODALITIES USED IN CONJUNCTION WITH EXERCISE TESTING

Cardiac imaging modalities are being increasingly used in conjunction with GXT to more accurately diagnose myocardial ischemia and assess myocardial function during physical exertion. Commonly used imaging procedures are described in the following sections.

EXERCISE ECHOCARDIOGRAPHY

Exercise echocardiography is an established assessment procedure for patients with suspected myocardial ischemia. Myocardial contractility normally increases with exercise. However, ischemia results in decreased myocardial contractility via hypokinetic (*i.e.*, decreased), dyskinetic (*i.e.*, impaired), or akinetic (*i.e.*, absent) wall motion in the affected segments. Exercise echocardiography is highly indicated in patients with suspected myocardial ischemia with an intermediate pretest probability for CVD and/or an uninterpretable ECG.

Exercise echocardiography is also valuable in the assessment of viable/ischemic myocardium in patients with known CVD that are being considered for a revascularization procedure. Patients with known or suspected CVD and a normal exercise echocardiography response appear to have a low risk for adverse events (49). In patients with valvular disease, exercise echocardiography is highly indicated for the assessment of (a) equivocal aortic stenosis; (b) evidence of low cardiac output; (c) symptomatic patients with mild mitral stenosis; and (d) asymptomatic severe aortic insufficiency or mitral regurgitation where left ventricular size and function are not meeting surgical criteria. In patients with suspected pulmonary hypertension, exercise echocardiography with tissue Doppler imaging may also be advantageous, although the evidence in support of this approach is less robust. A recently published report on the appropriateness of stress echocardiography provides a comprehensive list of indications for this procedure (22).

CARDIAC RADIONUCLIDE IMAGING

Nuclear imaging is now commonly used in conjunction with standard GXT procedures in order to improve the diagnostic accuracy in patients with suspected CVD. There are several different imaging protocols using technetium (Tc)-99m or thallous (thallium) chloride-201. Comparison of the rest and stress images permits the identification of fixed and reversible perfusion abnormalities as well as their differentiation.

Tc-99m permits higher dosing with less radiation exposure than thallium and results in improved images that are sharper and have less artifact and attenuation. Consequently, Tc is the preferred imaging agent when performing tomographic images of the heart using single-photon emission computed tomography (SPECT). SPECT images are obtained with a gamma camera that rotates 180 degrees around the patient stopping at preset angles to record the image. Cardiac images then are displayed in slices from three different axes to allow visualization of the heart in three dimensions. Thus, multiple myocardial segments can be viewed individually without the overlap of segments that occurs with planar imaging. Perfusion defects that are present during exercise but not seen at rest suggest myocardial ischemia. Perfusion defects that are present during exercise and persist at rest suggest previous MI or scar. The extent and distribution of ischemic myocardium can be identified in this manner. Exercise nuclear SPECT imaging has a sensitivity (*i.e.*, percentage of individuals with positive test who have a given disease) of 87% and specificity (*i.e.*, percentage of individuals with negative test who do not have a given disease) of 73% for detecting CVD with ≥50% coronary stenosis (41).

Cardiac radionuclide imaging is highly indicated for patients with an intermediate pretest (see *Table 5.1*) probability for CVD and/or uninterpretable ECG as well as in those patients with a high pretest probability irrespective of ECG interpretability. This procedure is also highly valuable in the assessment of viable/ischemic myocardium in patients with ischemic cardiomyopathy and severe left ventricular dysfunction who are being considered for a revascularization procedure. Patients with known or suspected CVD and a normal cardiac radionuclide imaging study appear to have a low risk for adverse events (49). Conversely, patients with a perfusion defect are at higher risk for adverse events regardless of angiography findings (20). A recently published report on the appropriate criteria for cardiac radionuclide imaging provides a comprehensive list of indications for this procedure (31).

IMAGING MODALITIES NOT USED IN CONJUNCTION WITH EXERCISE TESTING

PHARMACOLOGIC STRESS TESTING

Patients unable to undergo a GXT for reasons such as severe deconditioning, peripheral vascular disease, orthopedic disabilities, neurologic disease, and/or concomitant illness may be evaluated by pharmacologic stress testing. The two most commonly used pharmacologic tests are dobutamine stress echocardiography and dipyridamole or adenosine stress nuclear scintigraphy. Some protocols include light intensity exercise in combination with pharmacologic infusion.

Dobutamine elicits wall motion abnormalities by increasing HR, and therefore myocardial oxygen demand. Dobutamine is infused intravenously with the dose increased gradually until the maximal dose or an endpoint is achieved. Endpoints may include new or worsening wall motion abnormalities, an adequate HR response, serious arrhythmias, angina, significant ST depression, intolerable side effects, and a significant increase or decrease in BP. Atropine may be given if an adequate HR is not achieved or other endpoints have not been reached at peak dobutamine dose. HR, BP, ECG, and echocardiographic images are obtained throughout the infusion of atropine. Echocardiographic images are obtained similar to exercise echocardiography. A new or worsening wall motion abnormality constitutes a positive test for ischemia.

Vasodilators such as dipyridamole and adenosine are commonly used to assess coronary perfusion in conjunction with a nuclear imaging agent. Dipyridamole and adenosine cause maximal coronary vasodilation in normal epicardial arteries, but not in stenotic segments. As a result, a coronary steal phenomenon occurs with a relatively increased flow to normal arteries and a relatively decreased flow to stenotic arteries. Nuclear perfusion imaging under resting conditions is then compared with imaging obtained after coronary vasodilation. Interpretation is similar to that for exercise nuclear testing. Severe side effects are uncommon, but both dipyridamole and adenosine may induce marked bronchospasm, particularly in patients with asthma or reactive airway disease. Thus, administration of these agents is contraindicated in such patients (41). The bronchospasm can be treated with theophylline, although this is rarely needed with adenosine because the half-life is very short. Caffeine and other methylxanthines can block the vasodilator effects of dipyridamole and adenosine, and thus reduce the sensitivity of the test. Therefore, it is recommended that these substances be avoided for at least 24 h before the stress test. The diagnostic accuracy of pharmacologic nuclear stress testing is similar to that of exercise nuclear stress testing (41).

COMPUTED TOMOGRAPHY IN THE ASSESSMENT OF CARDIOVASCULAR DISEASE

Advances in cardiac computed tomography (CT) offer additional methods for the clinical assessment of CVD. Although there are several types of cardiac CT, electron beam computed tomography (EBCT) has been available since 1987 and provides the most robust scientific data. EBCT is a highly sensitive method for the detection of coronary artery calcified plaque (17).

However, it is important to understand the presence of calcified plaque does not in itself indicate the presence of a flow obstructing coronary lesion; conversely, the absence of coronary calcium does not itself indicate the absence of atherosclerotic plaque. A coronary calcium score of zero makes the presence of atherosclerotic plaque including vulnerable plaque highly unlikely. Moreover, a score of zero is associated with a low annual risk (0.1%) of a cardiovascular event over the next 2–5 yr, whereas a high calcium score (>100) is associated with a high annual risk (>2%). Calcium scores correlate poorly with stenosis severity, although a score >400 is frequently associated with perfusion ischemia from obstructive CVD. Measurement of coronary artery calcium appears to improve risk prediction in individuals with an intermediate Framingham risk score (i.e., those with 10%–20% 10 yr likelihood of a cardiovascular event). Thus, in clinically selected intermediate risk patients (see *Table 5.1*), it may be reasonable to use EBCT to further refine risk prediction. However, the measurement of coronary artery calcium is not recommended in individuals with a low (i.e., <10% 10 yr likelihood of a cardiovascular event) or high (i.e., >20% 10 yr likelihood of a cardiovascular event) Framingham risk score. A recently published consensus statement on coronary artery calcium scoring provides a comprehensive discussion on the appropriate indications for this procedure (26).

SUPERVISION OF EXERCISE TESTING

Although clinical exercise tests are generally considered to be safe, the potential for adverse events does exist. The risk of complications requiring hospital admission, acute MI, and sudden cardiac death occurring during or immediately postexercise is ≤0.20%, 0.04%, and 0.01%, respectively (52). Accordingly, individuals who supervise exercise tests must have the necessary cognitive and technical skills to safely administer an exercise test. The American College of Cardiology (ACC), AHA, and ACCP, with broad involvement from other professional organizations involved with exercise testing including the American College of Sports Medicine (ACSM), have outlined the cognitive skills needed to competently supervise exercise tests (68). These skills are presented in *Box 5.3*.

| **BOX 5.3** | **Cognitive Skills Required to Competently Supervise Exercise Tests** |

- Knowledge of appropriate indications for exercise testing
- Knowledge of alternative physiologic cardiovascular tests
- Knowledge of appropriate contraindications, risks, and risk assessment of testing
- Knowledge to promptly recognize and treat complications of exercise testing
- Competence in cardiopulmonary resuscitation and successful completion of an American Heart Association-sponsored course in advance cardiovascular life support and renewal on a regular basis
- Knowledge of various exercise protocols and indications for each
- Knowledge of basic cardiovascular and exercise physiology including hemodynamic response to exercise
- Knowledge of cardiac arrhythmia and the ability to recognize and treat serious arrhythmias (see *Appendix C*)
- Knowledge of cardiovascular drugs and how they can affect exercise performance, hemodynamics, and the electrocardiogram (see *Appendix A*)
- Knowledge of the effects of age and disease on hemodynamic and the electrocardiographic response to exercise
- Knowledge of principles and details of exercise testing including proper lead placement and skin preparation
- Knowledge of endpoints of exercise testing and indications to terminate exercise testing

Adapted from (68).

In most cases, clinical exercise tests can be supervised by properly trained health care professionals such as exercise physiologists, nurses, and physician assistants who are working under the supervision of a physician (*i.e.*, the physician must be in the immediate vicinity and available for emergencies for exercise testing of individuals at high risk) (see *Chapter 2* and *Appendix B*) (68). Several studies have demonstrated that the incidence of cardiovascular complications during GXT is similar with experienced and appropriately trained nonphysician personnel supervising the test and physicians in the immediate vicinity compared to those conducted with direct physician supervision (52). In situations in which the patient is deemed to be at increased risk for an adverse event during the GXT, the physician should be immediately available to manage potential emergency situations. Such cases include, but are not limited to, patients undergoing symptom-limited testing following recent acute events (*i.e.*, acute coronary syndrome or MI), severe left ventricular dysfunction, severe valvular stenosis (*e.g.*, aortic stenosis), or known complex arrhythmias (68) (see *Chapter 2*).

THE BOTTOM LINE

The ACSM Clinical Exercise Testing Key Points are as follows:

- Although a clinical exercise test may not be indicated for most individuals about to begin an exercise program (see *Chapter 2*), the high value of information obtained from this procedure is not debatable.
- Aerobic capacity may be one of the single best prognostic markers in all individuals regardless of health status.
- Standard clinical exercise testing is well accepted for the assessment of individuals with signs and/or symptoms suggestive of CVD.
- The use of cardiopulmonary exercise testing, which combines standard clinical exercise testing with simultaneous ventilatory expired gas analysis, is common practice in patients with CHF as well as those with unexplained exertional dyspnea.
- The recent recognition that appropriately trained nonphysician personnel can safely perform a clinical exercise test may result in the expanded use of this valuable procedure in various clinical settings.

Online Resources

Scientific Statements and Guidelines from the Amercian Heart Association (10,12,23,25,44,52):
http://my.americanheart.org/professional/StatementsGuidelines/Statements-Guidelines_UCM_316885_SubHomePage.jsp

REFERENCES

1. Abidov A, Rozanski A, Hachamovitch R, et al. Prognostic significance of dyspnea in patients referred for cardiac stress testing. *N Engl J Med.* 2005;353(18):1889–98.
2. Ainsworth BE, Haskell WL, Whitt MC, et al. Compendium of physical activities: an update of activity codes and MET intensities. *Med Sci Sports Exerc.* 2000;32(9 Suppl):S498–504.
3. American Thoracic Society, American College of Chest Physicians. ATS/ACCP Statement on cardiopulmonary exercise testing. *Am J Respir Crit Care Med.* 2003;167(2):211–77.
4. Amsterdam EA, Kirk JD, Bluemke DA, et al. Testing of low-risk patients presenting to the emergency department with chest pain: a scientific statement from the American Heart Association. *Circulation.* 2010;122(17):1756–76.
5. Amsterdam EA, Kirk JD, Diercks DB, Lewis WR, Turnipseed SD. Immediate exercise testing to evaluate low-risk patients presenting to the emergency department with chest pain. *J Am Coll Cardiol.* 2002;40(2):251–6.
6. Arena R, Lavie CJ, Milani RV, Myers J, Guazzi M. Cardiopulmonary exercise testing in patients with pulmonary arterial hypertension: an evidence-based review. *J Heart Lung Transplant.* 2010;29(2):159–73.
7. Arena R, Myers J, Abella J, et al. Determining the preferred percent-predicted equation for peak oxygen consumption in patients with heart failure. *Circ Heart Fail.* 2009;2(2):113–20.
8. Arena R, Myers J, Guazzi M. The clinical and research applications of aerobic capacity and ventilatory efficiency in heart failure: an evidence-based review. *Heart Fail Rev.* 2008;13(2):245–69.
9. Arena R, Myers J, Guazzi M. The future of aerobic exercise testing in clinical practice: is it the ultimate vital sign? *Future Cardiol.* 2010;6(3):325–42.
10. Arena R, Myers J, Williams MA, et al. Assessment of functional capacity in clinical and research settings: a scientific statement from the American Heart Association Committee on Exercise, Rehabilitation, and Prevention of the Council on Clinical Cardiology and the Council on Cardiovascular Nursing. *Circulation.* 2007;116(3):329–43.
11. Ashley E, Myers J, Froelicher V. Exercise testing scores as an example of better decisions through science. *Med Sci Sports Exerc.* 2002;34(8):1391–8.
12. Balady GJ, Arena R, Sietsema K, et al. Clinician's guide to cardiopulmonary exercise testing in adults. A scientific statement from the American Heart Association. *Circulation.* 2010;122(2):191–225.
13. Balady GJ, Larson MG, Vasan RS, Leip EP, O'Donnell CJ, Levy D. Usefulness of exercise testing in the prediction of coronary disease risk among asymptomatic persons as a function of the Framingham risk score. *Circulation.* 2004;110(14):1920–5.
14. Balady GJ, Weiner DA, McCabe CH, Ryan TJ. Value of arm exercise testing in detecting coronary artery disease. *Am J Cardiol.* 1985;55(1):37–9.
15. Borg G. *Borg's Perceived Exertion and Pain Scales.* Champaign (IL): Human Kinetics; 1998. 104 p.
16. Brubaker PH, Kaminsky LA, Whaley MH. *Coronary Artery Disease: Essentials of Prevention and Rehabilitation Programs.* Champaign (IL): Human Kinetics; 2002. 364 p.
17. Budoff MJ, Achenbach S, Blumenthal RS, et al. Assessment of coronary artery disease by cardiac computed tomography: a scientific statement from the American Heart Association Committee on Cardiovascular Imaging and Intervention, Council on Cardiovascular Radiology and Intervention, and Committee on Cardiac Imaging, Council on Clinical Cardiology. *Circulation.* 2006;114(16):1761–91.
18. Chase P, Arena R, Myers J, et al. Prognostic usefulness of dyspnea versus fatigue as reason for exercise test termination in patients with heart failure. *Am J Cardiol.* 2008;102(7):879–82.
19. Colice GL, Shafazand S, Griffin JP, Keenan R, Bolliger CT, American College of Chest Physicians. Physiologic evaluation of the patient with lung cancer being considered for resectional surgery: ACCP evidenced-based clinical practice guidelines (2nd edition). *Chest.* 2007;132(3 Suppl):161S–77S.
20. Delcour KS, Khaja A, Chockalingam A, Kuppuswamy S, Dresser T. Outcomes in patients with abnormal myocardial perfusion imaging and normal coronary angiogram. *Angiology.* 2009;60(3):318–21.
21. Dorn J, Naughton J, Imamura D, Trevisan M. Results of a multicenter randomized clinical trial of exercise and long-term survival in myocardial infarction patients: the National Exercise and Heart Disease Project (NEHDP). *Circulation.* 1999;100(17):1764–9.
22. Douglas PS, Khandheria B, Stainback RF, et al. ACCF/ASE/ACEP/AHA/ASNC/SCAI/SCCT/SCMR 2008 appropriateness criteria for stress echocardiography: a report of the American College of Cardiology Foundation Appropriateness Criteria Task Force, American Society of Echocardiography, American College of Emergency Physicians, American Heart Association, American Society of Nuclear Cardiology, Society for Cardiovascular Angiography and Interventions, Society of Cardiovascular Computed Tomography, and Society for Cardiovascular Magnetic Resonance: endorsed by the Heart Rhythm Society and the Society of Critical Care Medicine. *Circulation.* 2008;117(11):1478–97.
23. Fletcher GF, Balady GJ, Amsterdam EA, et al. Exercise standards for testing and training: a statement for healthcare professionals from the American Heart Association. *Circulation.* 2001;104(14):1694–740.
24. Franklin BA. Exercise testing, training and arm ergometry. *Sports Med.* 1985;2(2):100–19.

25. Gibbons RJ, Balady GJ, Bricker JT, et al. Committee to Update the 1997 Exercise Testing Guidelines. ACC/AHA 2002 guideline update for exercise testing: summary article. A report of the American College of Cardiology/American Heart Association Task Force on Practice Guidelines (Committee to Update the 1997 Exercise Testing Guidelines). *J Am Coll Cardiol.* 2002;40(8):1531–40.

26. Greenland P, Bonow RO, Brundage BH, et al. ACCF/AHA 2007 clinical expert consensus document on coronary artery calcium scoring by computed tomography in global cardiovascular risk assessment and in evaluation of patients with chest pain: a report of the American College of Cardiology Foundation Clinical Expert Consensus Task Force (ACCF/AHA Writing Committee to Update the 2000 Expert Consensus Document on Electron Beam Computed Tomography). *Circulation.* 2007;115(3):402–26.

27. Guazzi M, Arena R. The impact of pharmacotherapy on the cardiopulmonary exercise test response in patients with heart failure: a mini review. *Curr Vasc Pharmacol.* 2009;7(4):557–69.

28. Gulati M, Black HR, Shaw LJ, et al. The prognostic value of a nomogram for exercise capacity in women. *N Engl J Med.* 2005;353(5):468–75.

29. Hallberg V, Palomaki A, Kataja M, et al. Return to work after coronary artery bypass surgery. A 10-year follow-up study. *Scand Cardiovasc J.* 2009;43(5):277–84.

30. Hambrecht RP, Schuler GC, Muth T, et al. Greater diagnostic sensitivity of treadmill versus cycle exercise testing of asymptomatic men with coronary artery disease. *Am J Cardiol.* 1992;70(2):141–6.

31. Hendel RC, Berman DS, Di Carli MF, et al. ACCF/ASNC/ACR/AHA/ASE/SCCT/SCMR/SNM 2009 appropriate use criteria for cardiac radionuclide imaging: a report of the American College of Cardiology Foundation Appropriate Use Criteria Task Force, the American Society of Nuclear Cardiology, the American College of Radiology, the American Heart Association, the American Society of Echocardiography, the Society of Cardiovascular Computed Tomography, the Society for Cardiovascular Magnetic Resonance, and the Society of Nuclear Medicine. *Circulation.* 2009;119(22):e561–87.

32. Hiraga T, Maekura R, Okuda Y, et al. Prognostic predictors for survival in patients with COPD using cardiopulmonary exercise testing. *Clin Physiol Funct Imaging.* 2003;23(6):324–31.

33. Hollingsworth V, Bendick P, Franklin B, Gordon S, Timmis GC. Validity of arm ergometer blood pressures immediately after exercise. *Am J Cardiol.* 1990;65(20):1358–60.

34. Ilias NA, Xian H, Inman C, Martin WH,3rd. Arm exercise testing predicts clinical outcome. *Am Heart J.* 2009;157(1):69–76.

35. Kaminsky LA, Whaley MH. Evaluation of a new standardized ramp protocol: the BSU/Bruce Ramp protocol. *J Cardiopulm Rehabil.* 1998;18(6):438–44.

36. Katritsis DG, Pantos J, Efstathopoulos E. Hemodynamic factors and atheromatic plaque rupture in the coronary arteries: from vulnerable plaque to vulnerable coronary segment. *Coron Artery Dis.* 2007;18(3):229–37.

37. Kavanagh T, Mertens DJ, Hamm LF, et al. Peak oxygen intake and cardiac mortality in women referred for cardiac rehabilitation. *J Am Coll Cardiol.* 2003;42(12):2139–43.

38. Kavanagh T, Mertens DJ, Hamm LF, et al. Prediction of long-term prognosis in 12 169 men referred for cardiac rehabilitation. *Circulation.* 2002;106(6):666–71.

39. Kim ES, Ishwaran H, Blackstone E, Lauer MS. External prognostic validations and comparisons of age- and gender-adjusted exercise capacity predictions. *J Am Coll Cardiol.* 2007;50(19):1867–75.

40. Kligfield P, Gettes LS, Bailey JJ, et al. Recommendations for the standardization and interpretation of the electrocardiogram: part I: the electrocardiogram and its technology: a scientific statement from the American Heart Association Electrocardiography and Arrhythmias Committee, Council on Clinical Cardiology; the American College of Cardiology Foundation; and the Heart Rhythm Society: endorsed by the International Society for Computerized Electrocardiology. *Circulation.* 2007;115(10):1306–24.

41. Klocke FJ, Baird MG, Lorell BH, et al. ACC/AHA/ASNC guidelines for the clinical use of cardiac radionuclide imaging—executive summary: a report of the American College of Cardiology/American Heart Association Task Force on Practice Guidelines (ACC/AHA/ASNC Committee to Revise the 1995 Guidelines for the Clinical Use of Cardiac Radionuclide Imaging). *Circulation.* 2003;108(11):1404–18.

42. Kodama S, Saito K, Tanaka S, et al. Cardiorespiratory fitness as a quantitative predictor of all-cause mortality and cardiovascular events in healthy men and women: a meta-analysis. *JAMA.* 2009;301(19):2024–35.

43. Kogan A, Shapira R, Lewis BS, Tamir A, Rennert G. The use of exercise stress testing for the management of low-risk patients with chest pain. *Am J Emerg Med.* 2009;27(7):889–92.

44. Lauer M, Froelicher ES, Williams M, et al. Exercise testing in asymptomatic adults: a statement for professionals from the American Heart Association Council on Clinical Cardiology, Subcommittee on Exercise, Cardiac Rehabilitation, and Prevention. *Circulation.* 2005;112(5):771–6.

45. Loewen GM, Watson D, Kohman L, et al. Preoperative exercise Vo2 measurement for lung resection candidates: results of Cancer and Leukemia Group B Protocol 9238. *J Thorac Oncol.* 2007;2(7):619–25.

46. Madsen T, Mallin M, Bledsoe J, et al. Utility of the emergency department observation unit in ensuring stress testing in low-risk chest pain patients. *Crit Pathw Cardiol.* 2009;8(3):122–4.

47. Mark DB, Shaw L, Harrell FE Jr, et al. Prognostic value of a treadmill exercise score in outpatients with suspected coronary artery disease. *N Engl J Med.* 1991;325(12):849–53.

48. McCullough PA, Gallagher MJ, Dejong AT, et al. Cardiorespiratory fitness and short-term complications after bariatric surgery. *Chest.* 2006;130(2):517–25.

49. Metz LD, Beattie M, Hom R, Redberg RF, Grady D, Fleischmann KE. The prognostic value of normal exercise myocardial perfusion imaging and exercise echocardiography: a meta-analysis. *J Am Coll Cardiol.* 2007;49(2):227–37.

50. Miki K, Maekura R, Hiraga T, et al. Impairments and prognostic factors for survival in patients with idiopathic pulmonary fibrosis. *Respir Med.* 2003;97(5):482–90.

51. Morris CK, Myers J, Froelicher VF, Kawaguchi T, Ueshima K, Hideg A. Nomogram based on metabolic equivalents and age for assessing aerobic exercise capacity in men. *J Am Coll Cardiol.* 1993;22(1):175–82.

52. Myers J, Arena R, Franklin B, et al. Recommendations for clinical exercise laboratories: a scientific statement from the American Heart Association. *Circulation.* 2009;119(24):3144–61.

53. Myers J, Buchanan N, Smith D, et al. Individualized ramp treadmill. Observations on a new protocol. *Chest.* 1992;101(5 Suppl):236S–41S.

54. Myers J, Buchanan N, Walsh D, et al. Comparison of the ramp versus standard exercise protocols. *J Am Coll Cardiol.* 1991;17(6):1334–42.

55. Myers J, Prakash M, Froelicher V, Do D, Partington S, Atwood JE. Exercise capacity and mortality among men referred for exercise testing. *N Engl J Med.* 2002;346(11):793–801.

56. Myers J, Voodi L, Umann T, Froelicher VF. A survey of exercise testing: methods, utilization, interpretation, and safety in the VAHCS. *J Cardiopulm Rehabil.* 2000;20(4):251–8.

57. Noel M, Jobin J, Marcoux A, Poirier P, Dagenais G, Bogaty P. Comparison of myocardial ischemia on the ergocycle versus the treadmill in patients with coronary heart disease. *Am J Cardiol.* 2010;105(5):633–9.

58. Noel M, Jobin J, Poirier P, Dagenais GR, Bogaty P. Different thresholds of myocardial ischemia in ramp and standard bruce protocol exercise tests in patients with positive exercise stress tests and angiographically demonstrated coronary arterial narrowing. *Am J Cardiol.* 2007;99(7):921–4.

59. Normal values. In: Wasserman K, Hansen JE, Sue DY, Stringer W, Whipp BJ, editors. *Principles of Exercise Testing and Interpretation: Including Pathophysiology and Clinical Applications.* 4th ed. Baltimore: Lippincott Williams & Wilkins; 2005. p. 160–182.

60. Oga T, Nishimura K, Tsukino M, Sato S, Hajiro T. Analysis of the factors related to mortality in chronic obstructive pulmonary disease: role of exercise capacity and health status. *Am J Respir Crit Care Med.* 2003;167(4):544–9.

61. Older P, Hall A, Hader R. Cardiopulmonary exercise testing as a screening test for perioperative management of major surgery in the elderly. *Chest.* 1999;116(2):355–62.

62. O'Neill JO, Young JB, Pothier CE, Lauer MS. Peak oxygen consumption as a predictor of death in patients with heart failure receiving beta-blockers. *Circulation.* 2005;111(18):2313–8.

63. Patterson RE, Horowitz SF. Importance of epidemiology and biostatistics in deciding clinical strategies for using diagnostic tests: a simplified approach using examples from coronary artery disease. *J Am Coll Cardiol.* 1989;13(7):1653–65.

64. Peveler WW. Effects of saddle height on economy in cycling. *J Strength Cond Res.* 2008;22(4):1355–9.

65. Peveler WW, Green JM. Effects of saddle height on economy and anaerobic power in well-trained cyclists. *J Strength Cond Res.* 2011;25(3):633.

66. Peveler WW, Pounders JD, Bishop PA. Effects of saddle height on anaerobic power production in cycling. *J Strength Cond Res.* 2007;21(4):1023–7.

67. Pollock ML. *Exercise in Health and Disease: Evaluation and Prescription for Prevention and Rehabilitation.* 2nd ed. Philadelphia (PA): W.B. Saunders; 1990. 741 p.

68. Rodgers GP, Ayanian JZ, Balady G, et al. American College of Cardiology/American Heart Association Clinical Competence Statement on Stress Testing. A Report of the American College of Cardiology/American Heart Association/American College of Physicians-American Society of Internal Medicine Task Force on Clinical Competence. *Circulation.* 2000;102(14):1726–38.

69. Shah SJ, Thenappan T, Rich S, Sur J, Archer SL, Gomberg-Maitland M. Value of exercise treadmill testing in the risk stratification of patients with pulmonary hypertension. *Circ Heart Fail.* 2009;2(4):278–86.

70. Sheldahl LM, Wilke NA, Tristani FE. Evaluation and training for resumption of occupational and leisure-time physical activities in patients after a major cardiac event. *Med Exerc Nutr Health.* 1995;4:273–89.

71. Stein RA, Chaitman BR, Balady GJ, et al. Safety and utility of exercise testing in emergency room chest pain centers: An advisory from the Committee on Exercise, Rehabilitation, and Prevention, Council on Clinical Cardiology, American Heart Association. *Circulation.* 2000;102(12):1463–7.

72. Wilson PW, D'Agostino RB, Levy D, Belanger AM, Silbershatz H, Kannel WB. Prediction of coronary heart disease using risk factor categories. *Circulation.* 1998;97(18):1837–47.

6

Interpretation of Clinical Exercise Test Results

This chapter addresses the interpretation and clinical significance of exercise test results with specific reference to hemodynamic, electrocardiographic (ECG), and ventilatory expired gas responses. The diagnostic and prognostic value of the exercise test will be discussed along with screening for atherosclerotic cardiovascular disease (CVD).

EXERCISE TESTING AS A SCREENING TOOL FOR CORONARY ARTERY DISEASE

The probability of a patient having CVD cannot be estimated accurately from the exercise test result and diagnostic characteristics of the test alone. It also depends on the likelihood of having disease before the test is administered. Bayes' theorem states that the posttest probability of having a disease is determined by the disease probability *before* the test and the probability that the test will provide a true result (50). The probability of a patient having a disease before the test is most importantly related to the presence of symptoms (particularly chest pain characteristics), in addition to the patient's age, sex, and the presence of major CVD risk factors (see *Table 2.2*).

Exercise testing in individuals with known CVD (*i.e.*, prior myocardial infarction [MI], angiographically documented coronary stenoses, and/or prior coronary revascularization) is warranted if there is a reemergence of symptoms postintervention (18). The description of symptoms can be most helpful among individuals in whom the diagnosis is in question. Typical or definite angina (*i.e.*, substernal chest discomfort that may radiate to the back, jaw, or arms, and symptoms provoked by exertion or emotional stress and relieved by rest and/or nitroglycerin) makes the pretest probability so high that the test result does not dramatically change the likelihood of underlying CVD. Atypical angina (*i.e.*, chest discomfort that lacks one of the mentioned characteristics of typical angina) generally indicates an intermediate pretest likelihood of CVD in men >30 yr and women >50 yr (see *Table 5.1* and *Figure 5.1*). In fact, the use of exercise testing to assist in the diagnosis of CVD may be most beneficial in those individuals with an intermediate pretest probability (see *Chapter 5*).

The use of exercise testing in screening asymptomatic individuals, particularly among individuals without diabetes mellitus or major CVD risk factors, is diagnostically problematic in view of the low to very low pretest likelihood of CVD (see *Table 5.1*). An American Heart Association Scientific Statement on exercise testing in asymptomatic adults concluded that there is currently insufficient evidence to support exercise testing as a routine screening modality for atherosclerotic CVD in asymptomatic individuals (35). Given the limited ability of exercise testing to indentify atherosclerotic CVD and predict risk of adverse events during exercise, this assessment is not indicated prior to initiation of an exercise program in asymptomatic individuals (see *Chapter 2*). Even so, the use of exercise testing in asymptomatic individuals may be useful to health/fitness and clinical exercise professionals given its ability to (a) reflect general health; (b) identify normal and abnormal physiologic responses to physical exertion; (c) provide information to more precisely design the exercise prescription (Ex R_x); and (d) provide prognostic insight, especially among those with multiple CVD risk factors (35).

INTERPRETATION OF RESPONSES TO GRADED EXERCISE TESTING

Before interpreting clinical exercise test data, it is important to consider the purpose of the test (*e.g.*, diagnostic, prognostic, therapeutic applications, Ex R_x) and the individual clinical characteristics that may influence the exercise test or its interpretation (*e.g.*, age, sex). Medical conditions influencing test interpretation include orthopedic limitations, pulmonary disease, obesity, neurologic disorders, and deconditioning. Medication effects (see *Appendix A*) and resting ECG abnormalities (see *Appendix C*) also must be considered, especially resting ST-segment changes secondary to conduction defects, left ventricular hypertrophy (LVH), and other factors that may contribute to spurious ST-segment depression.

Although total body and myocardial oxygen consumption ($M\dot{V}O_2$) are directly related, the relationship between these variables can be altered by exercise training, medications, and disease. For example, exercise-induced myocardial ischemia may cause left ventricular dysfunction, exercise intolerance, and a hypotensive blood pressure (BP) response (see *Box 5.2*). The severity of symptomatic ischemia is inversely related to exercise capacity; however, left ventricular ejection fraction does not correlate well with exercise tolerance (39,45).

Responses to exercise tests are useful in evaluating the need for and effectiveness of various types of therapeutic interventions. The following variables are important to quantify accurately when assessing the diagnostic, prognostic, and therapeutic applications of the test. Each is described in the following sections and summarized in *Box 6.1*:

- Hemodynamics: assessed by the heart rate (HR) and systolic BP (SBP)/diastolic BP (DBP) responses.
- ECG waveforms: particularly ST-segment displacement and supraventricular and ventricular dysrhythmias.
- Limiting clinical signs or symptoms.
- Ventilatory gas exchange responses (*e.g.*, $\dot{V}O_2$, minute ventilation [$\dot{V}E$], carbon dioxide production [$\dot{V}CO_2$]).

| BOX 6.1 | **Electrocardiographic, Cardiorespiratory, and Hemodynamic Responses to Exercise Testing and Their Clinical Significance** |

Variable	Clinical Significance
ST-segment depression (ST ↓)	An abnormal ECG response is defined as ≥1 mm of horizontal or downsloping ST ↓ 60–80 ms beyond the J point, suggesting myocardial ischemia.
ST-segment elevation (ST ↑)	ST ↑ in leads displaying a previous Q wave MI almost always reflects an aneurysm or wall motion abnormality. In the absence of significant Q waves, exercise-induced ST ↑ often is associated with a fixed high-grade coronary stenosis.
Supraventricular dysrhythmias	Isolated atrial ectopic beats or short runs of SVT commonly occur during exercise testing and do not appear to have any diagnostic or prognostic significance for CVD.
Ventricular dysrhythmias	The suppression of resting ventricular dysrhythmias during exercise *does not* exclude the presence of underlying CVD; conversely, PVCs that increase in frequency, complexity, or both do not necessarily signify underlying ischemic heart disease. Complex ventricular ectopy, including paired or multiform PVCs, and runs of ventricular tachycardia (≥3 successive beats) are likely to be associated with significant CVD and/or a poor prognosis if they occur in conjunction with signs and/or symptoms of myocardial ischemia in patients with a history of sudden cardiac death, cardiomyopathy, or valvular heart disease. Frequent ventricular ectopy during recovery has been found to be a better predictor of mortality than ventricular ectopy that occurs only during exercise.
Heart rate (HR)	The normal HR response to progressive exercise is a relatively linear increase, corresponding to 10 ± 2 beats $\cdot$ MET^{-1} for physically inactive subjects. Chronotropic incompetence may be signified by the following: 1. A peak exercise HR that is >2 SD ($\approx$20 beats $\cdot$ min^{-1}) below the age-predicted HR$_{max}$ or an inability to achieve ≥85% of the age-predicted HR$_{max}$ for subjects who are limited by volitional fatigue and are not taking β-blockers 2. A chronotropic index (CI) <0.8 (35); where CI is calculated as the percentage of heart rate reserve to percent metabolic reserve achieved at any test stage
Heart rate recovery	An abnormal (slowed) HR recovery is associated with a poor prognosis. HR recovery has frequently been defined as a decrease ≤12 beats $\cdot$ min^{-1} at 1 min (walking in recovery), or ≤22 beats $\cdot$ min^{-1} at 2 min (supine position in recovery).
Systolic blood pressure (SBP)	The normal response to exercise is a progressive increase in SBP, typically 10 ± 2 mm Hg $\cdot$ MET^{-1} with a possible plateau at peak exercise. Exercise testing should be discontinued with SBP values of >250 mm Hg. Exertional hypotension (SBP that fails to rise or falls [>10 mm Hg]) may signify myocardial ischemia and/or LV dysfunction. Maximal exercise SBP of <140 mm Hg suggests a poor prognosis.
Diastolic blood pressure (DBP)	The normal response to exercise is no change or a decrease in DBP. A DBP of >115 mm Hg is considered an endpoint for exercise testing.

(continued)

BOX 6.1	Electrocardiographic, Cardiorespiratory, and Hemodynamic Responses to Exercise Testing and Their Clinical Significance (*Continued*)

Variable	Clinical Significance
Anginal symptoms	Can be graded on a scale of 1–4, corresponding to perceptible but mild, moderate, moderately severe, and severe, respectively. A rating of 3 (moderately severe) generally should be used as an endpoint for exercise testing.
Cardiorespiratory fitness	Average values of $\dot{V}O_{2max}/\dot{V}O_{2peak}$ expressed as METs, expected in healthy sedentary men and women, can be predicted from one of several regression equations (28). Also, see *Table 4.9* for age-specific $\dot{V}O_{2max}$ norms. Recent meta-analysis suggests each 1 MET increase in aerobic capacity equates to 13% and 15% decrease in all-cause mortality and cardiovascular events, respectively (32).
Ventilatory efficiency	Normal $\dot{V}E/\dot{V}CO_2$ slope value <30. Elevated value is strongly prognostic in patients with heart failure and potentially patients with pulmonary hypertension. Values of ~45 or more are indicative of particularly poor prognosis in patients with heart failure. Elevated values are clearly indicative of worsening ventilation perfusion abnormalities in heart failure and pulmonary hypertension populations and thus provide an accurate depiction of disease severity (8).
Partial pressure of end-tidal carbon dioxide ($P_{ET}CO_2$)	$P_{ET}CO_2$ is normally 36–42 mm Hg at rest; increases 3–8 mm Hg during exercise at mild-to-moderate workloads and decreases at maximal exercise. Abnormally low values at rest and during exercise reflective of worsening ventilation perfusion abnormalities and in heart failure and pulmonary hypertension populations, and thus provide an accurate depiction of disease severity and indicate poor prognosis. Also appears to reflect cardiac function in patients with heart failure (4,8).

CVD, cardiovascular disease; ECG, electrocardiographic; LV, left ventricular; MET, metabolic equivalent; MI, myocardial infarction; PVC, premature ventricular contraction; SD, standard deviation; SVT, supraventricular tachycardia; $\dot{V}E$, minute ventilation; $\dot{V}CO_2$, carbon dioxide production; $\dot{V}O_{2max}$, maximal oxygen uptake; $\dot{V}O_{2peak}$, peak oxygen uptake.

HEART RATE RESPONSE

Maximal heart rate (HR_{max}) may be predicted from age using any of several published equations (21,23,56) (see *Chapter 7*). For the most used equation ($220 - age$), the relationship between age and HR_{max} for a large sample of subjects is well established; however, interindividual variability is high (± 12 beats $\cdot$ min^{-1}). As a result, there is a potential for considerable error in the use of methods that extrapolate submaximal test data to an age-predicted HR_{max}.

It has yet to be demonstrated alternate equations that claim higher accuracy and less variability provide clinically superior information compared to use of the $220 - age$ equation (52). Using the $220 - age$ equation, failure to achieve an age-predicted $HR_{max} \geq 85\%$ in the presence of maximal effort (*i.e.*, chronotropic incompetence) is an ominous prognostic marker. In addition, failure to achieve an age-predicted HR_{max} >80% (*i.e.*, chronotropic incompetence), using the equation $\{[HR_{peak} - HR_{rest}]/[(220 - age) - HR_{rest}]\}$, is also an indicator of increased risk for adverse events (35). A delayed decrease in HR early in recovery after a symptom-limited maximal exercise test (*i.e.*, ≤12 beats · min^{-1} decrease after the first minute in recovery) is also a powerful independent predictor of overall mortality and should therefore be included in the exercise test assessment (35).

Achievement of age-predicted HR_{max} should not be used as an absolute test endpoint or as an indication that effort has been maximal because of its high intersubject variability. The clinical indications for stopping an exercise test are presented in *Box 5.2*. Good judgment on the part of the supervising health/fitness, clinical exercise, or health care professional remains the most important criterion for terminating an exercise test.

BLOOD PRESSURE RESPONSE

The normal BP response to dynamic upright exercise consists of a progressive increase in SBP, no change or a slight decrease in DBP, and a widening of the pulse pressure (see *Box 6.1*). The following are key points concerning interpretation of the BP response to progressive dynamic exercise:

- A drop in SBP (≥10 mm Hg decrease in SBP with an increase in workload), or failure of SBP to increase with increased workload, is considered an abnormal test response. Exercise-induced decreases in SBP (*i.e.*, exertional hypotension) may occur in patients with CVD, valvular heart disease, cardiomyopathies, aortic outflow obstruction, and serious dysrhythmias. Occasionally, patients without clinically significant heart disease demonstrate exertional hypotension caused by antihypertensive therapy, prolonged strenuous exercise, and/or vasovagal responses. However, exertional hypotension correlates with myocardial ischemia, left ventricular dysfunction, and an increased risk of subsequent cardiac events (17). In some cases, this response is improved after coronary artery bypass graft surgery (CABG). An SBP >250 mm Hg and/or a DBP >115 mm Hg continue to be used as termination criteria for exercise testing. Moreover, an excessive BP response to exercise is predictive of future hypertension and CVD (55).

- The normal postexercise response is a progressive decline in SBP. During passive recovery in an upright posture, SBP may decrease abruptly because of peripheral pooling (and usually normalizes upon resuming the supine position). SBP remains below pretest resting values for several hours after the test, an expected physiologic response termed *postexercise hypotension*, which occurs in most individuals (51). A failure to decrease or a rise in SBP over the first several minutes of recovery may indicate increased mortality risk (26). DBP also remains below pretest resting values during the postexercise period in most individuals.

- In patients on vasodilators, calcium channel blockers, angiotensin-converting enzyme inhibitors, and α- and β-adrenergic blockers, the BP response to exercise is variably attenuated and cannot be accurately predicted in the absence of clinical test data (see *Appendix A*).

- Although HR_{max} is comparable for men and women, men generally have higher SBPs ($\sim$20 $\pm$5 mm Hg) during maximal treadmill testing. However, the sex difference is no longer apparent after 70 yr. The rate pressure product (RPP), or double product (SBP mm Hg $\times$ HR beats $\cdot$ min^{-1}), is an indicator of myocardial oxygen demand. Maximal double product values during exercise testing are typically between 25,000 (10th percentile) and 40,000 (90th percentile) (17). Signs and symptoms of ischemia generally occur at a reproducible double product.

ELECTROCARDIOGRAPH WAVEFORMS

Appendix C provides information to aid in the interpretation of resting and exercise ECGs. Moreover, a detailed review of ECG analysis is provided in the *ACSM Resource Manual for Guidelines for Exercise Testing and Prescription, Seventh Edition* (54). It should be noted an athlete's resting ECG may present with several benign normal variants including respiratory sinus arrhythmia, sinus bradycardia, incomplete right bundle-branch block, early repolarization, and increased voltage in the precordial leads (24). Additional information is provided here with respect to common exercise-induced changes in ECG variables. The normal ECG response to exercise includes the following:

- Minor and insignificant changes in P wave morphology.
- Superimposition of the P and T waves of successive beats.
- Increases in septal Q wave amplitude.
- Slight decreases in R wave amplitude.
- Increases in T wave amplitude (although wide variability exists among clients/patients).
- Minimal shortening of the QRS duration.
- Depression of the J point.
- Rate-related shortening of the QT interval.

However, some changes in ECG wave morphology may be indicative of underlying pathology. For example, although QRS duration tends to decrease slightly with exercise (and increasing HR) in healthy individuals, it may increase in patients with either angina or left ventricular dysfunction. Exercise-induced P wave changes are rarely seen and are of questionable significance. Many factors affect R wave amplitude; consequently, such changes during exercise have no independent predictive power (44).

ST-Segment Displacement

ST-segment changes are widely accepted criteria for myocardial ischemia and injury. The interpretation of ST-segments may be affected by the resting ECG configuration (*e.g.*, bundle-branch blocks, LVH) and pharmacologic agents (*e.g.*, digitalis therapy). There may be J point depression and tall, peaked T waves at high exercise intensities and during recovery in healthy individuals (49).

Depression of the J point that leads to marked ST-segment upsloping is caused by competition between normal repolarization and delayed terminal depolarization forces rather than by ischemia (41). Exercise-induced myocardial ischemia may be manifested by different types of ST-segment changes on the ECG as shown in *Figure 6.1.*

ST-Segment Elevation

- ST-segment elevation (early repolarization) may be seen in the normal resting ECG in various patterns. Recent data suggest that an early repolarization pattern in the inferior leads may indicate an increased risk of cardiac mortality in middle-aged individuals (53,57). Benign early repolarization can be common in the ECG of athletes and is typically localized to the chest leads V2–V5 (24). Early repolarization exclusively observed in the anterolateral left precordial leads is not thought to be associated with increased risk for sustained ventricular arrhythmias, whereas global early repolarization (*i.e.,* limb and precordial leads) appears to indicate a higher risk (3). Increasing HR usually causes these elevated ST-segments to return to the isoelectric line.
- Exercise-induced ST-segment elevation in leads with Q waves consistent with a prior MI may be indicative of wall motion abnormalities, ischemia, or both (10).

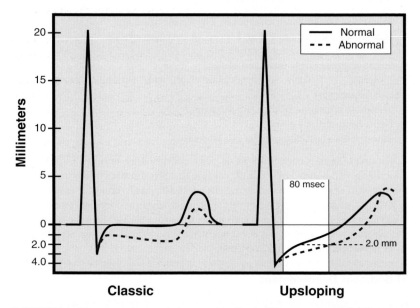

■ **FIGURE 6.1.** ST-segment changes during exercise. Classic ST-segment depression (first complex) is defined as a horizontal or downsloping ST-segment that is ≥1.0 mm below the baseline 60–80 ms past the J point. Slowly upsloping ST-segment depression (second complex) should be considered a borderline response, and added emphasis should be placed on other clinical and exercise variables.

- Exercise-induced ST-segment elevation on an otherwise normal ECG (except in augmented voltage right [aVR] or chest leads V1 and V2) generally indicates significant myocardial ischemia and localizes the ischemia to a specific area of myocardium (48). This response may also be associated with ventricular arrhythmias and myocardial injury.

ST-Segment Depression

- ST-segment depression (*i.e.*, depression of the J point and the slope at 80 ms past the J point) is the most common manifestation of exercise-induced myocardial ischemia.
- Horizontal or downsloping ST-segment depression is more indicative of myocardial ischemia than is upsloping depression.
- The standard criterion for a positive test is ≥ 1.0 mm (0.1 mV) of horizontal or downsloping ST-segment at the J point extending for 60–80 ms.
- Slowly upsloping ST-segment depression should be considered a borderline response, and added emphasis should be placed on other clinical and exercise variables.
- ST-segment depression does not localize ischemia to a specific area of myocardium.
- The more leads with (apparent) ischemic ST-segment shifts, the more severe the disease.
- Significant ST-segment depression occurring only in recovery likely represents a true positive response and should be considered an important diagnostic finding (34).
- Adjustment of the ST-segment relative to the HR may provide additional diagnostic information. The ST/HR index is the ratio of the maximal ST-segment change (μV) to the maximal change in HR from rest to peak exercise (beats $\cdot$ min^{-1}). An ST/HR index of >1.6 μV $\cdot$ beats^{-1} $\cdot$ min^{-1} is defined as abnormal. The ST/HR slope reflects the maximal slope relating the amount of the ST-segment depression (μV) to HR (beats $\cdot$ min^{-1}) during exercise. An ST/HR slope of ≥ 2.4 μV $\cdot$ beats^{-1} $\cdot$ min^{-1} is defined as abnormal (29,30).

ST-Segment Normalization or Absence of Change

- Ischemia may be manifested by normalization of resting ST-segments. ECG abnormalities at rest including T-wave inversion and ST-segment depression may return to normal during anginal symptoms and during exercise in some patients (36).

Dysrhythmias

Exercise-associated dysrhythmias occur in healthy individuals as well as patients with CVD. Increased sympathetic drive and changes in extracellular and intracellular electrolytes, pH, and oxygen tension contribute to disturbances in myocardial and conducting tissue automaticity and reentry, which are major mechanisms of dysrhythmias.

Supraventricular Dysrhythmias

Isolated premature atrial contractions (PACs) are common and require no special precautions. Atrial flutter or atrial fibrillation may occur in organic heart disease or may reflect endocrine, metabolic, or medication effects. Sustained supraventricular tachycardia (SVT) occasionally is induced by exercise and may require pharmacologic treatment or electroconversion if discontinuation of exercise fails to abolish the rhythm. Patients who experience paroxysmal atrial tachycardia may be evaluated by repeating the exercise test after appropriate treatment.

Ventricular Dysrhythmias

Isolated premature ventricular complexes or contractions (PVCs) can occur during exercise in apparently healthy or asymptomatic individuals as well as those diagnosed with CVD. In some individuals, progressive exercise to maximal exertion induces PVCs, whereas in others, it reduces their occurrence. The clinical significance of exercise-induced PVCs remains a matter of debate, although there are data to suggest the occurrence of ventricular ectopy during exercise warrants clinical consideration (9). The suppression of PVCs that are present at rest with exercise testing does not exclude the presence of CVD, and PVCs that increase in frequency, complexity, or both do not necessarily signify underlying ischemic heart disease (9,16). Serious forms of ventricular ectopy include paired or multiform PVCs or runs of ventricular tachycardia (≥3 PVCs in succession). These dysrhythmias are likely to be associated with significant CVD, a poor prognosis, or both, if they occur in conjunction with signs or symptoms of myocardial ischemia, or in patients with a history of resuscitated sudden cardiac death, cardiomyopathy, or valvular heart disease.

Some data indicate that exercise-induced PVCs are associated with a higher mortality in asymptomatic individuals (27). In a cohort referred for clinical exercise testing who were free of heart failure, the occurrence of PVCs during recovery rather than during exercise was prognostically significant (14). Another investigation assessing a large cohort referred for exercise testing ($n > 29,000$) defined frequent ventricular ectopy as, "the presence of >7 PVCs per minute, ventricular bigeminy or trigeminy, ventricular couplets or triplets, ventricular tachycardia, ventricular flutter, torsade de pointes, or ventricular fibrillation" (20). Frequent ventricular ectopy in this study during exercise and recovery was a significant predictor of mortality, although its occurrence in recovery was a significantly stronger prognostic marker.

Criteria for terminating exercise tests based on ventricular ectopy include sustained ventricular tachycardia, multifocal PVCs, and short runs of ventricular tachycardia. The decision to terminate an exercise test should also be influenced by simultaneous evidence of myocardial ischemia and/or adverse signs or symptoms (see *Box 5.2*).

LIMITING SIGNS AND SYMPTOMS

Although patients with exercise-induced ST-segment depression can be asymptomatic, when concomitant angina occurs, the likelihood that the ECG changes result from CVD is significantly increased (59). In addition, angina pectoris *without* ischemic ECG changes may be as predictive of CVD as ST-segment changes alone (12). Angina pectoris and ST-segment changes are currently considered independent variables that identify patients at increased risk for subsequent coronary events. Moderate-to-severe angina (*i.e.*, rating of 3–4 on a 4-point scale) is an absolute indication for exercise test termination (17). Individuals undergoing exercise testing for the assessment of CVD who complain of dyspnea with physical exertion may have a poorer prognosis compared to those who complain of other (*i.e.*, angina) or no exertional symptoms (2). Lastly, termination of exercise testing secondary to dyspnea as opposed to lower extremity fatigue may indicate a worse prognosis in patients with heart disease (11).

In the absence of untoward signs or symptoms, patients generally should be encouraged to give their best effort so that maximal exercise tolerance can be determined. However, the determination of what constitutes "maximal" effort, although important for interpreting test results, can be difficult. Various criteria have been used to confirm that a maximal effort has been elicited during graded exercise testing (GXT). However, all of the following criteria for maximal effort can be subjective and therefore possess limitations to varying degrees:

- Failure of HR to increase with further increases in exercise intensity.
- A plateau in $\dot{V}O_2$ (or failure to increase $\dot{V}O_2$ by 150 mL $\cdot$ min^{-1}) with increased workload (58). This criterion has fallen into disfavor because a plateau is inconsistently seen during GXT and is confused by various definitions and how data are sampled during exercise (46).
- A respiratory exchange ratio (RER) $\geq$1.10 is a minimal threshold that may be obtained in most individuals putting forth a maximal effort, although there may be considerable interindividual variability with an RER $\geq$1.10 (37).
- Various postexercise venous lactic acid concentrations (*e.g.*, 8–10 mmol $\cdot$ L^{-1}) have been used; however, there is also significant interindividual variability in this response.
- A rating of perceived exertion (RPE) >17 on the 6–20 scale or >9 on the 0–10 scale.

Although all of the aforementioned criteria possess limitations, peak RER is perhaps the most accurate and objective noninvasive indicator of subject effort during a GXT (8,52).

VENTILATORY EXPIRED GAS RESPONSES TO EXERCISE

Direct measurement of ventilatory expired gas during exercise provides a more precise assessment of exercise capacity and prognosis and helps to distinguish causes of exercise intolerance. The combination of this technology with standard GXT procedures is typically referred to as *cardiopulmonary exercise testing* (CPX) (8). These responses can be used to assess client/patient effort during an exercise test, particularly when a reduction in maximal exercise capacity is suspected. Submaximal efforts from the client/patient on a maximal GXT can interfere with the interpretation of the test results and subsequent patient management. Moreover, the use of CPX may be advantageous when serial testing is needed for either research or clinical purposes to ensure consistent effort among assessments (6). Maximal oxygen uptake ($\dot{V}O_{2max}$) or peak oxygen uptake ($\dot{V}O_{2peak}$) provides important information about cardiorespiratory fitness and is a powerful marker of prognosis. Population-specific nomograms (see *Figure 5.2*) and/or population norms (see *Table 4.9*) may be used to compare $\dot{V}O_{2peak}$ with the expected value according to age, sex, and physical fitness status (28,47). Additionally, the assessment of ventilatory efficiency (*i.e.*, $\dot{V}E/\dot{V}CO_2$ slope and partial pressure of end-tidal carbon dioxide [$P\text{ET}CO_2$]) provides robust prognostic and/or diagnostic information in patients with congestive heart failure (CHF) and pulmonary hypertension (4,5).

Ventilatory expired gas responses often are used in clinical settings as an estimation of the point at which lactate accumulation in the blood occurs, sometimes referred to as the *lactate* or *anaerobic threshold*. Assessment of this physiologic phenomenon through ventilatory expired gas is typically referred to as *ventilatory threshold* (VT). Several different methods using ventilatory expired gas responses exist for the estimation of this point. These include the ventilatory equivalents and V-slope method (6). Whichever approach is used, it should be remembered VT provides only an estimation, and the concept of anaerobic threshold during exercise is controversial (45). Because exercise beyond the lactate threshold is associated with metabolic acidosis, hyperventilation, and a reduced capacity to perform work, its estimation is a useful physiologic measurement when evaluating interventions in patients with heart and pulmonary disease as well as studying the limits of performance in apparently healthy individuals. However, it should be noted that secondary to abnormal ventilatory responses observed in a significant proportion of patients with CHF (*i.e.*, exercise oscillatory ventilation), determination of VT may not be possible (13).

In addition to estimating when blood lactate values begin to increase, maximal minute ventilation ($\dot{V}E_{max}$) can be used in conjunction with the maximal voluntary ventilation (MVV) to assist in determining if there is a ventilatory limitation to maximal exercise. A comparison between $\dot{V}E_{max}$ and MVV can be used when evaluating responses to a CPX. MVV can be directly measured by a 12–15 s deep and rapid breathing maneuver or estimated from the equation: forced expiratory volume in 1 s [($FEV_{1.0}$) × 40] (8). MVV is preferred to [$FEV_{1.0}$ × 40] to ensure a precise quantification of ventilatory capacity. The relationship between $\dot{V}E_{max}$ and MVV, typically referred to as the *ventilatory reserve*, traditionally is defined as the percentage of the MVV achieved at maximal exercise (*i.e.*, the $\dot{V}E_{max}$/MVV ratio). In most normal healthy individuals, the $\dot{V}E_{max}$/MVV ratio is ≤0.80 (6). Values surpassing this threshold are indicative of a reduced ventilatory reserve and a possible pulmonary limitation to exercise.

Pulse oximetry should also be assessed when CPX is used to assess possible pulmonary limitations to exercise. A decrease in pulse oximeter saturation >5% during exercise also indicates a pulmonary limitation. Lastly, most currently available ventilatory expired gas systems also possess capabilities for pulmonary function testing. Obstructive or restrictive patterns on baseline pulmonary function testing provide insight into the mechanism of limitations to exercise. Moreover, a $\geq$15% decrease in $FEV_{1.0}$ and/or peak expiratory flow following CPX compared to baseline values is indicative of exercise-induced bronchospasm (6).

DIAGNOSTIC VALUE OF EXERCISE TESTING

The diagnostic value of conventional exercise testing for the detection of CVD is influenced by the principles of conditional probability (see *Box 6.2*). The factors that determine the predictive outcomes of exercise testing (and other diagnostic tests) are the sensitivity and specificity of the test procedure and prevalence of CVD in the population tested (50). Sensitivity and specificity determine how effective the test is in making correct diagnoses in individuals with and without disease, respectively. Disease prevalence is an important determinant of the predictive value of the test. Moreover, non-ECG criteria (*e.g.*, duration of exercise or maximal metabolic equivalent [MET] level, hemodynamic responses, symptoms of angina or dyspnea) should be considered in the overall interpretation of exercise test results.

SENSITIVITY

Sensitivity refers to the percentage of patients tested with known CVD who demonstrate significant ST-segment (*i.e.*, positive) changes. Exercise ECG sensitivity

BOX 6.2	Sensitivity, Specificity, and Predictive Value of Diagnostic Graded Exercise Testing

sensitivity = TP/(TP + FN) = the percentage of patients with CVD who have a positive test

specificity = TN/(TN + FP) = the percentage of patients without CVD who have a negative test

predictive value (*positive test*) = TP/(TP + FP) = the percentage of patients with a positive test result who have CVD

predictive value (*negative test*) = TN/(TN + FN) = the percentage of patients with a negative test who do not have CVD

CVD, cardiovascular disease; FN, false negative (negative exercise test and CVD); FP, false positive (positive exercise test and no CVD); TN, true negative (negative exercise test and no CVD); TP, true positive (positive exercise test and CVD).

BOX 6.3	Causes of False Negative Test Results

- Failure to reach an ischemic threshold
- Monitoring an insufficient number of leads to detect ECG changes
- Failure to recognize non-ECG signs and symptoms that may be associated with underlying CVD (*e.g.*, exertional hypotension)
- Angiographically significant CVD compensated by collateral circulation
- Musculoskeletal limitations to exercise preceding cardiac abnormalities
- Technical or observer error

CVD, cardiovascular disease; ECG, electrocardiographic.

for the detection of CVD usually is based on subsequent angiographically determined coronary artery stenosis of ≥70% in at least one vessel. A true positive (TP) exercise test reveals horizontal or downsloping ST-segment depression of ≥1.0 mm and correctly identifies a patient with CVD. False negative (FN) test results show no or nondiagnostic ECG changes and fail to identify patients with underlying CVD.

Common factors that contribute to FN exercise tests are summarized in *Box 6.3*. Test sensitivity is decreased by inadequate myocardial stress, medications that attenuate cardiac demands to exercise or reduce myocardial ischemia (*e.g.*, β-blockers, nitrates, calcium channel blocking agents), and insufficient ECG lead monitoring. Preexisting ECG changes such as LVH, left bundle-branch block (LBBB), or the preexcitation syndrome (Wolff-Parkinson-White syndrome [W-P-W]) limit the ability to interpret exercise-induced ST-segment changes as ischemic ECG responses. The exercise test is most accurate for detecting CVD by applying validated multivariate scores (*i.e.*, pretest risk markers in addition to ST-segment changes and other exercise test responses) (7).

SPECIFICITY

The *specificity* of exercise tests refers to the percentage of patients without CVD who demonstrate nonsignificant (*i.e.*, negative) ST-segment changes. A true negative test correctly identifies an individual without CVD. Many conditions may cause abnormal exercise ECG responses in the absence of significant obstructive CVD (see *Box 6.4*).

Reported values for the specificity and sensitivity of exercise ECG testing vary because of differences in patient selection, test protocols, ECG criteria for a positive test, and the angiographic definition of CVD. In studies that controlled for these variables, the pooled results show a sensitivity of 68% and specificity of 77% (22). Sensitivity, however, is somewhat lower, and specificity is higher when workup bias (*i.e.*, only assessing individuals with a higher likelihood for a given disease) is removed (19,42).

| BOX 6.4 | **Causes of Abnormal ST-Segment Changes in the Absence of Obstructive Cardiovascular Disease[a]** |

- Resting repolarization abnormalities (*e.g.*, left bundle-branch block)
- Cardiac hypertrophy
- Accelerated conduction defects (*e.g.*, Wolff-Parkinson-White syndrome)
- Digitalis
- Nonischemic cardiomyopathy
- Hypokalemia
- Vasoregulatory abnormalities
- Mitral valve prolapsed
- Pericardial disorders
- Technical or observer error
- Coronary spasm in the absence of significant coronary artery disease
- Anemia
- Being a woman

[a]Selected variables simply may be associated with rather than be causes of abnormal test results.

PREDICTIVE VALUE

The predictive value of exercise testing is a measure of how accurately a test result (positive or negative) correctly identifies the presence or absence of CVD in tested patients. For example, the predictive value of a positive test is the percentage of those individuals with an abnormal test who have CVD. Nevertheless, a test should not be classified as "negative" unless the patient has attained an adequate level of myocardial stress, generally defined as having achieved ≥85% of predicted HR_{max} during the test, although this criterion is inherently flawed given the large variability in the HR response at maximal exercise (52). Predictive value cannot be estimated directly from a test's specificity or sensitivity because it depends on the prevalence of disease in the population being tested.

COMPARISON WITH IMAGING STRESS TESTS

Several imaging tests including echocardiography and nuclear techniques are often used in association with exercise testing to diagnose CVD. Guidelines are available that describe these techniques and their accuracy for detecting CVD (15,31). A recent meta-analysis suggests stress echocardiography is superior to nuclear imaging in detecting left main or triple vessel CVD (38). Patients with nuclear imaging studies positive for reversible perfusion defects appear to have a worse prognosis compared to individuals with a normal study (1). An abnormal echocardiography response during exercise (*i.e.*, increased left ventricular filling pressure) also appears to be indicative of an increased risk for future adverse events (25).

PROGNOSTIC APPLICATIONS OF THE EXERCISE TEST

Risk or prognostic evaluation is an important activity in medical practice on which many patient management decisions are based. In patients with CVD, several clinical factors contribute to patient outcome including (a) severity and stability of symptoms; (b) left ventricular function; (c) angiographic extent and severity of CVD; (d) electrical stability of the myocardium; and (e) the presence of other comorbid conditions. Unless cardiac catheterization and immediate coronary revascularization are indicated, an exercise test should be performed in individuals with known or suspected CVD to assess risk of future cardiac events and to assist in subsequent management decisions. As stated in *Chapter 5*, data derived from the exercise test are most useful when considered in the context of other clinical information. Important prognostic variables that can be derived from the exercise test are summarized in *Box 6.1*.

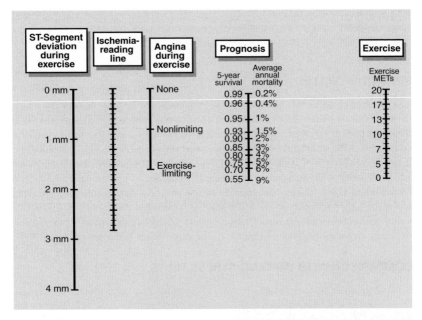

■ **FIGURE 6.2.** Duke nomogram uses five steps to estimate prognosis for a given individual from the parameters of the Duke score. First, the observed amount of ST depression is marked on the ST-segment deviation line. Second, the observed degree of angina is marked on the line for angina, and these two points are connected. Third, the point where this line intersects the ischemia reading line is noted. Fourth, the observed exercise tolerance is marked on the line for exercise capacity. Finally, the mark on the ischemia reading line is connected to the mark on the exercise capacity line, and the estimated 5-yr survival or average annual mortality rate is read from the point at which this line intersects the prognosis scale (40).

Several multivariate prognostic scores such as the Veteran's Administration score (43) (validated for the male veteran population) and the Duke nomogram (39) (validated for the general population including women) (see *Figure 6.2*) can be helpful when applied appropriately. The Duke nomogram does not appear to be valid in patients >75 yr (33). Patients who recently have suffered an acute MI and received thrombolytic therapy and/or have undergone coronary revascularization generally have a low subsequent cardiac event rate. Exercise testing still can provide prognostic information in this population, as well as assist in physical activity counseling and Ex R_x.

THE BOTTOM LINE

- Interpreting the results of a clinical exercise test requires a multivariable approach.
- The HR, hemodynamic, and ECG response to exercise are key objective parameters that require intricate assessment from an experienced clinician. In addition, the subjective symptoms including RPE, angina, and dyspnea are important components of exercise test interpretation.
- When ventilatory expired gas is assessed during the clinical exercise test, a highly accurate determination of aerobic capacity is possible in addition to a potentially more accurate quantification of exercise effort (*i.e.*, peak RER) and assessment of submaximal exercise performance and ventilatory efficiency.
- Clinical exercise testing assists in the diagnosis of CVD as well as the physiologic mechanisms for abnormal functional limitations such as unexplained exertional dyspnea.
- The diagnostic accuracy of clinical exercise testing depends on the characteristics of the patient who is undergoing the assessment and the quality of the test.
- Clinical exercise testing data, and in particular aerobic capacity, provide valuable prognostic information in virtually all individuals undergoing this procedure.

Online Resources

ACSM Position Stands:
http://journals.lww.com/acsm-msse/pages/default.aspx

The American Heart Association:
http://www.americanheart.org/

REFERENCES

1. Abidov A, Hachamovitch R, Hayes SW, et al. Are shades of gray prognostically useful in reporting myocardial perfusion single-photon emission computed tomography? *Circ Cardiovasc Imaging.* 2009; 2(4):290–8.
2. Abidov A, Rozanski A, Hachamovitch R, et al. Prognostic significance of dyspnea in patients referred for cardiac stress testing. *N Engl J Med.* 2005;353(18):1889–98.
3. Antzelevitch C, Yan GX. J wave syndromes. *Heart Rhythm.* 2010;7(4):549–58.
4. Arena R, Lavie CJ, Milani RV, Myers J, Guazzi M. Cardiopulmonary exercise testing in patients with pulmonary arterial hypertension: an evidence-based review. *J Heart Lung Transplant.* 2010;29(2): 159–73.
5. Arena R, Myers J, Guazzi M. The clinical and research applications of aerobic capacity and ventilatory efficiency in heart failure: an evidence-based review. *Heart Fail Rev.* 2008;13(2):245–69.
6. Arena R, Myers J, Williams MA, et al. Assessment of functional capacity in clinical and research settings: a scientific statement from the American Heart Association Committee on Exercise, Rehabilitation, and Prevention of the Council on Clinical Cardiology and the Council on Cardiovascular Nursing. *Circulation.* 2007;116(3):329–43.
7. Ashley E, Myers J, Froelicher V. Exercise testing scores as an example of better decisions through science. *Med Sci Sports Exerc.* 2002;34(8):1391–8.
8. Balady GJ, Arena R, Sietsema K, et al. Clinician's guide to cardiopulmonary exercise testing in adults. A scientific statement from the American Heart Association. *Circulation.* 2010;122(2):191–225.
9. Beckerman J, Wu T, Jones S, Froelicher VF. Exercise test-induced arrhythmias. *Prog Cardiovasc Dis.* 2005;47(4):285–305.
10. Bruce RA, Fisher LD, Pettinger M, Weiner DA, Chaitman BR. ST segment elevation with exercise: a marker for poor ventricular function and poor prognosis. Coronary Artery Surgery Study (CASS) confirmation of Seattle Heart Watch results. *Circulation.* 1988;77(4):897–905.
11. Chase P, Arena R, Myers J, et al. Prognostic usefulness of dyspnea versus fatigue as reason for exercise test termination in patients with heart failure. *Am J Cardiol.* 2008;102(7):879–82.
12. Cole JP, Ellestad MH. Significance of chest pain during treadmill exercise: correlation with coronary events. *Am J Cardiol.* 1978;41(2):227–32.
13. Corra U, Giordano A, Bosimini E, et al. Oscillatory ventilation during exercise in patients with chronic heart failure: clinical correlates and prognostic implications. *Chest.* 2002;121(5):1572–80.
14. Dewey FE, Kapoor JR, Williams RS, et al. Ventricular arrhythmias during clinical treadmill testing and prognosis. *Arch Intern Med.* 2008;168(2):225–34.
15. Douglas PS, Khandheria B, Stainback RF, et al. ACCF/ASE/ACEP/AHA/ASNC/SCAI/SCCT/SCMR 2008 appropriateness criteria for stress echocardiography: a report of the American College of Cardiology Foundation Appropriateness Criteria Task Force, American Society of Echocardiography, American College of Emergency Physicians, American Heart Association, American Society of Nuclear Cardiology, Society for Cardiovascular Angiography and Interventions, Society of Cardiovascular Computed Tomography, and Society for Cardiovascular Magnetic Resonance: endorsed by the Heart Rhythm Society and the Society of Critical Care Medicine. *Circulation.* 2008;117(11):1478–97.
16. Evans CH, Froelicher V. Some common abnormal responses to exercise testing: what to do when you see them. *Prim Care.* 2001;28(1):219–32, ix.
17. Fletcher GF, Balady GJ, Amsterdam EA, et al. Exercise standards for testing and training: a statement for healthcare professionals from the American Heart Association. *Circulation.* 2001;104(14):1694–740.
18. Fletcher GF, Mills WC, Taylor WC. Update on exercise stress testing. *Am Fam Physician.* 2006; 74(10):1749–54.
19. Froelicher VF, Lehmann KG, Thomas R, et al. The electrocardiographic exercise test in a population with reduced workup bias: diagnostic performance, computerized interpretation, and multivariable prediction. Veterans Affairs Cooperative Study in Health Services #016 (QUEXTA) Study Group. Quantitative Exercise Testing and Angiography. *Ann Intern Med.* 1998;128(12 Pt 1):965–74.
20. Frolkis JP, Pothier CE, Blackstone EH, Lauer MS. Frequent ventricular ectopy after exercise as a predictor of death. *N Engl J Med.* 2003;348(9):781–90.
21. Gellish RL, Goslin BR, Olson RE, McDonald A, Russi GD, Moudgil VK. Longitudinal modeling of the relationship between age and maximal heart rate. *Med Sci Sports Exerc.* 2007;39(5):822–9.
22. Gibbons RJ, Balady GJ, Bricker JT, et al. ACC/AHA 2002 guideline update for exercise testing: summary article: a report of the American College of Cardiology/American Heart Association Task Force on Practice Guidelines (Committee to Update the 1997 Exercise Testing Guidelines). *Circulation.* 2002;106(14):1883–92.
23. Gulati M, Shaw LJ, Thisted RA, Black HR, Merz CN, Arnsdorf MF. Heart rate response to exercise stress testing in asymptomatic women. The St. James Women Take Heart project. *Circulation.* 2010; 122(2):130–7.

24. Higgins JP. Normal resting electrocardiographic variants in young athletes. *Phys Sportsmed.* 2008; 36(1):69–75.

25. Holland DJ, Prasad SB, Marwick TH. Prognostic implications of left ventricular filling pressure with exercise. *Circ Cardiovasc Imaging.* 2010;3(2):149–56.

26. Huang CL, Su TC, Chen WJ, et al. Usefulness of paradoxical systolic blood pressure increase after exercise as a predictor of cardiovascular mortality. *Am J Cardiol.* 2008;102(5):518–23.

27. Jouven X, Zureik M, Desnos M, Courbon D, Ducimetiere P. Long-term outcome in asymptomatic men with exercise-induced premature ventricular depolarizations. *N Engl J Med.* 2000;343(12): 826–33.

28. Kim ES, Ishwaran H, Blackstone E, Lauer MS. External prognostic validations and comparisons of age- and gender-adjusted exercise capacity predictions. *J Am Coll Cardiol.* 2007;50(19):1867–75.

29. Kligfield P, Ameisen O, Okin PM. Heart rate adjustment of ST segment depression for improved detection of coronary artery disease. *Circulation.* 1989;79(2):245–55.

30. Kligfield P. Principles of simple heart rate adjustment of ST segment depression during exercise electrocardiography. *Cardiol J.* 2008;15(2):194–200.

31. Klocke FJ, Baird MG, Lorell BH, et al. ACC/AHA/ASNC guidelines for the clinical use of cardiac radio-nuclide imaging—executive summary: a report of the American College of Cardiology/American Heart Association Task Force on Practice Guidelines (ACC/AHA/ASNC Committee to Revise the 1995 Guidelines for the Clinical Use of Cardiac Radionuclide Imaging). *Circulation.* 2003;108(11): 1404–18.

32. Kodama S, Saito K, Tanaka S, et al. Cardiorespiratory fitness as a quantitative predictor of all-cause mortality and cardiovascular events in healthy men and women: a meta-analysis. *JAMA.* 2009; 301(19):2024–35.

33. Kwok JM, Miller TD, Hodge DO, Gibbons RJ. Prognostic value of the Duke treadmill score in the elderly. *J Am Coll Cardiol.* 2002;39(9):1475–81.

34. Lachterman B, Lehmann KG, Abrahamson D, Froelicher VF. "Recovery only" ST-segment depression and the predictive accuracy of the exercise test. *Ann Intern Med.* 1990;112(1):11–6.

35. Lauer M, Froelicher ES, Williams M, et al. Exercise testing in asymptomatic adults: a statement for professionals from the American Heart Association Council on Clinical Cardiology, Subcommittee on Exercise, Cardiac Rehabilitation, and Prevention. *Circulation.* 2005;112(5):771–6.

36. Lavie CJ, Oh JK, Mankin HT, Clements IP, Giuliani ER, Gibbons RJ. Significance of T-wave pseudo-normalization during exercise. A radionuclide angiographic study. *Chest.* 1988;94(3):512–6.

37. Lucia A, Rabadan M, Hoyos J, et al. Frequency of the VO2max plateau phenomenon in world-class cyclists. *Int J Sports Med.* 2006;27(12):984–92.

38. Mahajan N, Polavaram L, Vankayala H, et al. Diagnostic accuracy of myocardial perfusion imaging and stress echocardiography for the diagnosis of left main and triple vessel coronary artery disease: a comparative meta-analysis. *Heart.* 2010;96(12):956–66.

39. Mark DB, Hlatky MA, Harrell FE Jr, Lee KL, Califf RM, Pryor DB. Exercise treadmill score for predicting prognosis in coronary artery disease. *Ann Intern Med.* 1987;106(6):793–800.

40. Mark DB, Shaw L, Harrell FE Jr, et al. Prognostic value of a treadmill exercise score in outpatients with suspected coronary artery disease. *N Engl J Med.* 1991;325(12):849–53.

41. Mirvis DM, Ramanathan KB, Wilson JL. Regional blood flow correlates of ST segment depression in tachycardia-induced myocardial ischemia. *Circulation.* 1986;73(2):365–73.

42. Morise AP. Accuracy of heart rate-adjusted ST segments in populations with and without posttest referral bias. *Am Heart J.* 1997;134(4):647–55.

43. Morrow K, Morris CK, Froelicher VF, et al. Prediction of cardiovascular death in men undergoing noninvasive evaluation for coronary artery disease. *Ann Intern Med.* 1993;118(9):689–95.

44. Myers J, Ahnve S, Froelicher V, Sullivan M. Spatial R wave amplitude changes during exercise: relation with left ventricular ischemia and function. *J Am Coll Cardiol.* 1985;6(3):603–8.

45. Myers J, Froelicher VF. Hemodynamic determinants of exercise capacity in chronic heart failure. *Ann Intern Med.* 1991;115(5):377–86.

46. Noakes TD. Maximal oxygen uptake: "classical" versus "contemporary" viewpoints: a rebuttal. *Med Sci Sports Exerc.* 1998;30(9):1381–98.

47. Normal values. In: Wasserman K, Hansen JE, Sue DY, Stringer W, Whipp BJ, editors. *Principles of Exercise Testing and Interpretation: Including Pathophysiology and Clinical Applications.* 4th ed. Baltimore: Lippincott Williams & Wilkins; 2005. p. 160–82.

48. Nosratian FJ, Froelicher VF. ST elevation during exercise testing. *Am J Cardiol.* 1989;63(13):986–8.

49. Okin PM, Kligfield P. Heart rate adjustment of ST segment depression and performance of the exercise electrocardiogram: a critical evaluation. *J Am Coll Cardiol.* 1995;25(7):1726–35.

50. Patterson RE, Horowitz SF. Importance of epidemiology and biostatistics in deciding clinical strategies for using clinical diagnostic tests: a simplified approach using examples from coronary artery disease. *J Am Coll Cardiol.* 1989;13(7):1653–65.

51. Pescatello LS, Franklin BA, Fagard R, et al. American College of Sports Medicine position stand. Exercise and hypertension. *Med Sci Sports Exerc.* 2004;36(3):533–53.

52. Pinkstaff S, Peberdy MA, Kontos MC, Finucane S, Arena R. Quantifying exertion level during exercise stress testing using percentage of age-predicted maximal heart rate, rate pressure product, and perceived exertion. *Mayo Clin Proc.* 2010;85(12):1095–100.

53. Rosso R, Kogan E, Belhassen B, et al. J-point elevation in survivors of primary ventricular fibrillation and matched control subjects: incidence and clinical significance. *J Am Coll Cardiol.* 2008; 52(15):1231–8.

54. Swain DP, American College of Sports Medicine. *ACSM's Resource Manual for Guidelines for Exercise Testing and Prescription.* 7th ed. Baltimore (MD): Lippincott Williams & Wilkins; 2014.

55. Syme AN, Blanchard BE, Guidry MA, et al. Peak systolic blood pressure on a graded maximal exercise test and the blood pressure response to an acute bout of submaximal exercise. *Am J Cardiol.* 2006;98(7):938–43.

56. Tanaka H, Monahan KD, Seals DR. Age-predicted maximal heart rate revisited. *J Am Coll Cardiol.* 2001;37(1):153–6.

57. Tikkanen JT, Anttonen O, Junttila MJ, et al. Long-term outcome associated with early repolarization on electrocardiography. *N Engl J Med.* 2009;361(26):2529–37.

58. Wasserman K, Whipp BJ, Koyl SN, Beaver WL. Anaerobic threshold and respiratory gas exchange during exercise. *J Appl Physiol.* 1973;35(2):236–43.

59. Whinnery JE, Froelicher VFJr, Longo MR Jr, Triebwasser JH. The electrocardiographic response to maximal treadmill exercise of asymptomatic men with right bundle branch block. *Chest.* 1977;71(3):335–40.

Exercise Prescription

DEBORAH RIEBE, PHD, FACSM, ACSM-HFS, *Associate Editor*

General Principles of Exercise Prescription

AN INTRODUCTION TO THE PRINCIPLES OF EXERCISE PRESCRIPTION

The scientific evidence demonstrating the beneficial effects of exercise is indisputable, and the benefits of exercise far outweigh the risks in most adults (20,38) (see *Chapters 1* and *2*). An exercise training program ideally is designed to meet *individual* health and physical fitness goals. The principles of exercise prescription (Ex R$_x$) presented in this chapter are intended to guide health/fitness, public health, clinical exercise, and health care professionals in the development of an *individually* tailored Ex R$_x$ for the apparently healthy adult whose goal is to improve physical fitness and health and also may apply to adults with certain chronic diseases, disabilities, or health conditions, when appropriately screened (see *Chapters 2, 8–10*). Recreational and competitive athletes will benefit from more advanced training techniques than are presented in this chapter. This edition of the *Guidelines* employs the Frequency (how often), Intensity (how hard), Time (duration or how long), and Type (mode or what kind), with the addition of total Volume (amount) and Progression (advancement) or the *FITT-VP* principle of Ex R$_x$ to be consistent with the American College of Sports Medicine (ACSM) recommendations made in its companion evidence-based position stand (20).

The FITT-VP principles of Ex R$_x$ presented in this chapter are based on the application of the existing scientific evidence on the physiologic, psychological, and health benefits of exercise (20) (see *Chapter 1*). Nonetheless, some individuals may not respond as expected because there is appreciable individual variability in the magnitude of response to a particular exercise regimen (20). Furthermore, the FITT-VP principle of Ex R$_x$ may not apply because of individual characteristics (*e.g.*, health status, physical ability, age) or athletic and performance goals. For individuals with clinical conditions and healthy individuals with special considerations, accommodations should be made to the Ex R$_x$ as indicated in other related chapters of the *Guidelines* (see *Chapters 8–10*).

For most adults, an exercise program including aerobic, resistance, flexibility, and neuromotor exercise training is *indispensable* to improve and maintain physical fitness and health (20). Details of the FITT-VP principle of the Ex R$_x$ are provided later in this chapter. These Ex R$_x$ guidelines present *recommended targets* for exercise derived from the available scientific evidence showing most individuals will realize benefit when following the stated quantity and quality of exercise. However, some individuals will want to or need to include only some of the health-related components of physical fitness in their training regimen or exercise less than suggested by the guidelines presented in this chapter. Even if an individual cannot meet the recommended targets in this chapter, performing *some* exercise is beneficial, especially in inactive or deconditioned individuals, and, for that reason, should be encouraged except where there are safety concerns.

The guidelines presented in *Chapter 7* are consistent with other evidence-based exercise recommendations including relevant ACSM position stands (5,17,20,25,32) and other professional scientific statements (7,38,51,54).

GENERAL CONSIDERATIONS FOR EXERCISE PRESCRIPTION

A program of regular exercise for most adults should include a variety of exercises *beyond* activities performed as part of daily living (20). The optimal Ex R_x should address the health-related physical fitness components of cardiorespiratory (aerobic) fitness (CRF), muscular strength and endurance, flexibility, body composition, and neuromotor fitness. Reduction in the time spent in sedentary activities (*e.g.*, television watching, computer use, sitting in a car or at a desk) *in addition to* regular exercise is important for the health of physically active and inactive individuals. As detailed elsewhere, long periods of sedentary activity are associated with elevated risks of cardiovascular disease (CVD) mortality, worsened cardiometabolic disease biomarkers, and depression (20,34). Even in physically active individuals who meet the recommended targets for exercise, periods of physical inactivity are detrimental to health (20,34). When periods of physical inactivity are broken up by short bouts of standing or physical activity (*e.g.*, a very short walk around the office or home), the adverse effects of physical inactivity are reduced (20,34). Therefore, the Ex R_x should include a plan to decrease periods of physical inactivity in addition to an increase in physical activity (20,31,34).

Overuse injuries (*i.e.*, tissue damage resulting from repetitive demand over time, termed *cumulative trauma disorders*) and other musculoskeletal injuries are of concern to adults. To reduce the potential for overuse disorders and injury, an assortment of exercise modalities may be helpful (20). Common components of the Ex R_x seem to be helpful at least under some circumstances to reduce musculoskeletal injury and complications. These include the warm-up and cool-down, stretching exercises, and gradual progression of volume and intensity (20). The serious risk of CVD complications, which is of particular concern in middle-aged and older adults, can be minimized by (a) following the preparticipation health screening and evaluation procedures outlined in *Chapters 2* and *3*, respectively; (b) beginning a new program of exercise at light-to-moderate intensity; and (c) employing a gradual progression of the quantity and quality of exercise (20). Also important to the Ex R_x are behavioral factors that may enhance the adoption and adherence to exercise participation (see *Chapter 11*).

Bone health is of great importance to younger and older adults (see *Chapters 8* and *10*), especially among women. The ACSM recommends loading exercises

BOX 7.1	Components of the Exercise Training Session

Warm-up: at least 5–10 min of light-to-moderate intensity cardiorespiratory and muscular endurance activities

Conditioning: at least 20–60 min of aerobic, resistance, neuromotor, and/or sports activities (exercise bouts of 10 min are acceptable if the individual accumulates at least 20–60 min · d^{-1} of daily aerobic exercise)

Cool-down: at least 5–10 min of light-to-moderate intensity cardiorespiratory and muscular endurance activities

Stretching: at least 10 min of stretching exercises performed after the warm-up or cool-down phase

Adapted from (20,52).

(*i.e.*, weight bearing and resistance exercise) to maintain bone health (4,5,7,20,32), and these types of exercises should be part of an exercise program, particularly in individuals at risk for low bone density (*i.e.*, osteopenia) and osteoporosis.

An individual's goals, physical ability, physical fitness, health status, schedule, physical and social environment, and available equipment and facilities should be considered when designing the FITT-VP principle of Ex R_x for a client or patient. *Box 7.1* provides general recommendations for the components to be included in an exercise training session for apparently healthy adults. This chapter presents the scientific evidence-based recommendations for aerobic, resistance, flexibility, and neuromotor exercise training based on a combination of the FITT-VP principles of Ex R_x. The following sections present specific recommendations for the Ex R_x to improve health and fitness.

COMPONENTS OF THE EXERCISE TRAINING SESSION

A single exercise session should include the following phases:

- Warm-up.
- Conditioning and/or sports-related exercise.
- Cool-down.
- Stretching.

The warm-up phase consists of a minimum of 5–10 min of light-to-moderate intensity aerobic and muscular endurance activity (see *Table 7.1* for definitions of exercise intensity). The warm-up is a transitional phase that allows the body to adjust to the changing physiologic, biomechanical, and bioenergetic demands placed on it during the conditioning or sports phase of the exercise session. Warming up also improves range of motion (ROM) and may reduce the risk of injury (20). For the purpose of enhancing the *performance* of cardiorespiratory

TABLE 7.1. Methods of Estimating Intensity of Cardiorespiratory and Resistance Exercise

| | Cardiorespiratory Endurance Exercise | | | | | | | | | | | Resistance Exercise |
| | Relative Intensity | | | | Intensity ($\%\dot{V}O_{2max}$) Relative to Maximal Exercise Capacity in MET | | | Absolute Intensity | Absolute Intensity (MET) by Age | | | Relative Intensity |
Intensity	%HRR or %$\dot{V}O_2$R	%HR_{max}	%$\dot{V}O_{2max}$	Perceived Exertion (Rating on 6–20 RPE Scale)	20 METs %$\dot{V}O_{2max}$	10 METs %$\dot{V}O_{2max}$	5 METs %$\dot{V}O_{2max}$	MET	Young (20–39 yr)	Middle Age (40–64 yr)	Older (≥65 yr)	% One Repetition Maximum
Very light	<30	<57	<37	Very light (RPE ≤9)	<34	<37	<44	<2	<2.4	<2.0	<1.6	<30
Light	30–<40	57–<64	37–<45	Very light to fairly light (RPE 9–11)	34–<43	37–<46	44–<52	2.0–<3	<4.8	<4.0	<3.2	30–<50
Moderate	40–<60	64–<76	46–<64	Fairly light to somewhat hard (RPE 12–13)	43–<62	46–<64	52–<68	3.0–<6	4.8–<7.2	4.0–<6.0	3.2–<4.8	50–<70
Vigorous	60–<90	76–<96	64–<91	Somewhat hard to very hard (RPE 14–17)	62–<91	64–<91	68–<92	6.0–<8.8	7.2–<10.2	6.0–<8.5	4.8–<6.8	70–<85
Near maximal to maximal	≥90	≥96	≥91	≥ Very hard (RPE ≥18)	≥91	≥91	≥92	≥8.8	≥10.2	≥8.5	≥6.8	≥85

HR_{max}, maximal heart rate; HRR, heart rate reserve; MET, metabolic equivalent; RPE, rating of perceived exertion; $\dot{V}O_{2max}$, maximum oxygen consumption; $\dot{V}O_2$R, oxygen uptake reserve.

Adapted from (20).

endurance, aerobic exercise, sports, or resistance exercise, especially activities that are of long duration or with many repetitions, a dynamic, cardiorespiratory endurance exercise warm-up is superior to flexibility exercise (20).

The conditioning phase includes aerobic, resistance, flexibility, and neuro-motor exercise, and/or sports activities. Specifics about these modes of exercise are discussed in subsequent sections of this chapter. The conditioning phase is followed by a cool-down period involving aerobic and muscular endurance activity of light-to-moderate intensity lasting at least 5–10 min. The purpose of the cool-down period is to allow for a gradual recovery of heart rate (HR) and blood pressure (BP) and removal of metabolic end products from the muscles used during the more intense exercise conditioning phase.

The stretching phase is distinct from the warm-up and cool-down phases and may be performed following the warm-up or cool-down phase or following the application of heat packs, because warming the muscles improves ROM (20).

AEROBIC (CARDIORESPIRATORY ENDURANCE) EXERCISE

FREQUENCY OF EXERCISE

The frequency of physical activity (*i.e.*, the number of days per week dedicated to an exercise program) is an important contributor to health/fitness benefits that result from exercise. Aerobic exercise is recommended on 3–5 d · wk^{-1} for most adults, with the frequency varying with the intensity of exercise (20,25,32,38,52). Improvements in CRF are attenuated with exercise frequencies >3 d · wk^{-1} and a plateau in improvement with exercise done >5 d · wk^{-1} (20). Vigorous intensity exercise performed >5 d · wk^{-1} might increase the incidence of musculoskeletal injury, so this amount of vigorous intensity, physical activity is not recommended for most adults (20). However, if a variety of exercise modes placing different impact stresses on the body (*e.g.*, running, cycling) or using different muscle groups (*e.g.*, swimming, running) are included in the exercise program, daily vigorous intensity, physical activity may be recommended for some individuals. Alternatively, a weekly combination of 3 to 5 d · wk^{-1} of moderate and vigorous intensity exercise can be performed (20,32,52).

Health/fitness benefits can occur in some individuals who exercise once or twice per week at moderate-to-vigorous intensity, especially with large volumes of exercise as can occur in the "weekend warrior" pattern of exercise (20). In spite of the possible benefits, exercising 1–2 times · wk^{-1} is not recommended for the most adults because the risk of musculoskeletal injury and adverse cardiovascular events is higher in individuals who are not physically active on a regular basis and those who engage in unaccustomed exercise (20).

AEROBIC EXERCISE FREQUENCY RECOMMENDATION

FITT

Moderate intensity, aerobic exercise done at least 5 d · wk^{-1}; or vigorous intensity, aerobic exercise done at least 3 d · wk^{-1}; or a weekly combination of 3–5 d · wk^{-1} of moderate and vigorous intensity exercise is recommended for most adults to achieve and maintain health/fitness benefits.

INTENSITY OF EXERCISE

There is a positive dose response of health/fitness benefits that results from increasing exercise intensity (20). The overload principle of training states exercise below a minimum intensity, or *threshold*, will not challenge the body sufficiently to result in changes in physiologic parameters, including increased maximal oxygen consumption ($\dot{V}O_{2max}$) (20). However, more recent findings demonstrate the minimum threshold of intensity for benefit seems to vary depending on an individual's CRF level and other factors such as age, health status, physiologic differences, genetics, habitual physical activity, and social and psychological factors (20,46,47). Therefore, it may be difficult to precisely define an exact threshold to improve CRF (20,46). For example, individuals with an exercise capacity of 11–14 metabolic equivalents (METs) seemingly require an exercise intensity of at least 45% oxygen uptake reserve ($\dot{V}O_2R$) to increase $\dot{V}O_{2max}$, but no threshold is apparent in individuals with a baseline fitness of <11 METs (20,46). Highly trained athletes may need to exercise at "near maximal" (*i.e.*, 95%–100% $\dot{V}O_{2max}$) training intensities to improve $\dot{V}O_{2max}$, whereas 70%–80% $\dot{V}O_{2max}$ may provide a sufficient stimulus in moderately trained athletes (20,46).

Interval training involves varying the exercise intensity at fixed intervals during a single exercise bout. The duration and intensity of the intervals can be varied depending on the goals of the training session and physical fitness level of the client or patient. Interval training can increase the total volume and/or average exercise intensity performed during an exercise session. Improvements in CRF and cardiometabolic biomarkers with short-term (≤3 mo) interval training are similar to or greater than with single intensity exercise in healthy adults and individuals with metabolic, cardiovascular, or pulmonary disease (20). The use of interval training in adults appears beneficial, but the long-term effects and the safety of interval training remain to be evaluated.

AEROBIC EXERCISE INTENSITY RECOMMENDATION

F I T T

Moderate (*e.g.*, 40%–<60% heart rate reserve [HRR] or $\dot{V}O_2R$) to vigorous (*e.g.*, 60%–<90% HRR or $\dot{V}O_2R$) intensity aerobic exercise is recommended for most adults, and light (*e.g.*, 30%–<40% HRR or $\dot{V}O_2R$) to moderate intensity aerobic exercise can be beneficial in individuals who are deconditioned. Interval training may be an effective way to increase the total volume and/or average exercise intensity performed during an exercise session and may be beneficial for adults.

Methods of Estimating Intensity of Exercise

Several effective methods for prescribing exercise intensity result in improvements in CRF that can be recommended for individualized Ex R$_x$ (20). *Table 7.1* shows the approximate classification of exercise intensity commonly used in practice. One method of determining exercise intensity is not necessarily equivalent to the intensity derived using another method, because no studies have compared all of the methods of measurement of exercise intensity simultaneously. In addition, the relationships among measures of actual energy expenditure (EE) and the absolute (*i.e.*, $\dot{V}O_2$ and METs) and relative methods to prescribe exercise intensity (*i.e.*, %HRR, %HR$_{max}$ [maximal heart rate], and %$\dot{V}O_{2max}$) can vary considerably depending on exercise test protocol, exercise mode, exercise intensity, and characteristics of the client or patient (*i.e.*, resting HR, physical fitness level, age, and body composition) as well as other factors (20).

The HRR or $\dot{V}O_2$R methods may be preferable for Ex R$_x$ because exercise intensity can be underestimated or overestimated when using the HR (*i.e.*, %HR$_{max}$) or $\dot{V}O_2$ (*i.e.*, %$\dot{V}O_{2max}$) methods (20,44). However, the advantage of the HRR or $\dot{V}O_2$R methods is not universally accepted (20,44). Furthermore, the accuracy of any of these methods may be influenced by the method of measurement or estimation used (20).

The formula "220 − age" is commonly used to predict HR$_{max}$ (19). This formula is simple to use, but it can underestimate or overestimate measured HR$_{max}$ (21,23,48,58). Specialized regression equations for estimating HR$_{max}$ may be superior to the equation of 220 − age, at least in some individuals (21,26,48,58). Although these equations are promising, they cannot yet be recommended for universal application, although they may be applied to populations similar to those in which they were derived (20). *Table 7.2* shows some of the more commonly used equations to estimate HR$_{max}$. For greater accuracy in determining exercise intensity for the Ex R$_x$, using the directly measured HR$_{max}$ is preferred to estimated methods; but when not feasible, estimation of exercise intensity is acceptable.

Measured or estimated measures of absolute exercise intensity include caloric expenditure (kcal $\cdot$ min^{-1}), absolute oxygen uptake (mL $\cdot$ min^{-1} or L $\cdot$ min^{-1}), and METs. These absolute measures can result in misclassification

TABLE 7.2. Commonly Used Equations for Estimating Maximal Heart Rate

Author	Equation	Population
Fox (19)	HR$_{max}$ = 220 − age.	Small group of men and women
Astrand (9)	HR$_{max}$ = 216.6 − (0.84 × age)	Men and women ages 4−34 yr
Tanaka (48)	HR$_{max}$ = 208 − (0.7 × age)	Healthy men and women
Gellish (21)	HR$_{max}$ = 207 − (0.7 × age)	Men and women participants in an adult fitness program with broad range of age and fitness levels
Gulati (23)	HR$_{max}$ = 206 − (0.88 × age)	Asymptomatic middle-aged women referred for stress testing

HR$_{max}$, maximum heart rate.

of exercise intensity (*e.g.*, moderate and vigorous intensity) because they do not take into consideration individual factors such as body weight, sex, and fitness level (1,2,27). Measurement error, and consequently misclassification, is greater when using estimated rather than directly measured absolute EE and under free living compared to laboratory conditions (1,2,27). For example, an older individual working at 6 METs may be exercising at a vigorous-to-maximal intensity, whereas a younger individual working at the same absolute intensity will be exercising moderately (27). Therefore, for individual Ex R_x, a *relative* measure of intensity (*i.e.*, the energy cost of the activity relative to the individual's maximal capacity such as % $\dot{V}O_2$ [*i.e.*, $\dot{V}O_2$ mL $\cdot$ kg^{-1} $\cdot$ min^{-1}], HRR, and $\dot{V}O_2R$) is more appropriate, especially for older and deconditioned individuals (27,32).

A summary of methods for calculating exercise intensity using HR, $\dot{V}O_2$, and METs are presented in *Box 7.2*. Intensity of exercise training is usually determined as a range so the calculation using the formulae presented in *Box 7.2* need to be repeated twice (*i.e.*, once for the lower limit of the desired intensity range and once for the upper limit of the desired intensity range). The prescribed exercise intensity range for an individual should be determined by taking various factors into consideration, including age, habitual physical activity level, physical fitness level, and health status. Examples illustrating the use of several methods for prescribing exercise intensity are found in *Figure 7.1*. The reader is directed to other ACSM publications (*e.g.*, [20,45] for further explanation and examples using these additional methods of prescribing exercise intensity).

BOX 7.2	**Summary of Methods for Prescribing Exercise Intensity Using Heart Rate (HR), Oxygen Uptake ($\dot{V}O_2$), and Metabolic Equivalents (METs)**

- HRR method: Target HR (THR) = $[(\text{HR}_{max/peak}{}^a - \text{HR}_{rest}) \times \%$ intensity desired] + HR_{rest}
- $\dot{V}O_2R$ method: Target $\dot{V}O_2R^c$ = $[(\dot{V}O_{2max/peak}{}^b - \dot{V}O_{2rest}) \times \%$ intensity desired] + $\dot{V}O_{2rest}$
- HR method: Target HR = $\text{HR}_{max/peak}{}^a \times \%$ intensity desired
- $\dot{V}O_2$ method: Target $\dot{V}O_2{}^c$ = $\dot{V}O_{2max/peak}{}^b \times \%$ intensity desired
- MET method: Target MET^c = $[(\dot{V}O_{2max/peak}{}^b)/3.5$ mL $\cdot$ kg^{-1} $\cdot$ min$^{-1}] \times \%$ intensity desired

[a]$\text{HR}_{max/peak}$ is the highest value obtained during maximal/peak exercise or it can be estimated by 220 − age or some other prediction equation (see *Table 7.2*).
[b]$\dot{V}O_{2max/peak}$ is the highest value obtained during maximal/peak exercise or it can be estimated from a submaximal exercise test. Please see The Concept of Maximal Oxygen Uptake in *Chapter 4* for the distinction between $\dot{V}O_{2max}$ and $\dot{V}O_{2peak}$.
[c]Activities at the target $\dot{V}O_2$ and MET can be determined using a compendium of physical activity (1, 2) or metabolic calculations (22) (*Table 7.3*).
$\text{HR}_{max/peak}$, maximal or peak heart rate; HR_{rest}, resting heart rate; HRR, heart rate reserve; $\dot{V}O_2R$, oxygen uptake reserve.

Heart Rate Reserve (HRR) Method
    Available test data:
        HR_{rest}: 70 beats $\cdot$ min^{-1}
        HR_{max}: 180 beats $\cdot$ min^{-1}
    Desired exercise intensity range: 50%–60%
    Formula: Target Heart Rate (THR) = $[(HR_{max} - HR_{rest}) \times \%$ intensity$] + HR_{rest}$
        1)   Calculation of HRR:
                $HRR = (HR_{max} - HR_{rest})$
                $HRR = (180$ beats $\cdot$ $min^{-1} - 70$ beats $\cdot$ $min^{-1}) = 110$ beats $\cdot$ min^{-1}
        2)   Determination of exercise intensity as %HRR:
                Convert desired %HRR into a decimal by dividing by 100
                %HRR = desired intensity $\times$ HRR
                %HRR = 0.5×110 beats $\cdot$ $min^{-1} = 55$ beats $\cdot$ min^{-1}
                %HRR = 0.6×110 beats $\cdot$ $min^{-1} = 66$ beats $\cdot$ min^{-1}
        3)   Determine THR range:
                THR = $(\%HRR) + HR_{rest}$
                To determine lower limit of THR range:
                    THR = 55 beats $\cdot$ $min^{-1} + 70$ beats $\cdot$ $min^{-1} = 125$ beats $\cdot$ min^{-1}
                To determine upper limit of THR range:
                    THR = 66 beats $\cdot$ $min^{-1} + 70$ beats $\cdot$ $min^{-1} = 136$ beats $\cdot$ min^{-1}
                THR range: 125 beats $\cdot$ min^{-1} to 136 beats $\cdot$ min^{-1}

$\dot{V}O_2$ *Reserve ($\dot{V}O_2R$) Method*
    Available test data:
        $\dot{V}O_{2max}$: 30 mL $\cdot$ kg^{-1} $\cdot$ min^{-1}
        $\dot{V}O_{2rest}$: 3.5 mL $\cdot$ kg^{-1} $\cdot$ min^{-1}
    Desired exercise intensity range: 50%–60%
    Formula: Target $\dot{V}O_2$ = $[(\dot{V}O_{2max} - \dot{V}O_{2rest}) \times \%$ intensity$] + \dot{V}O_{2rest}$
        1)   Calculation of $\dot{V}O_2R$:
                $\dot{V}O_2R = \dot{V}O_{2max} - \dot{V}O_{2rest}$
                $\dot{V}O_2R = 30$ mL $\cdot$ kg^{-1} $\cdot$ $min^{-1} - 3.5$ mL $\cdot$ kg^{-1} $\cdot$ min^{-1}
                $\dot{V}O_2R = 26.5$ mL $\cdot$ kg^{-1} $\cdot$ min^{-1}
        2)   Determination of exercise intensity as $\%\dot{V}O_2R$:
                Convert desired intensity ($\%\dot{V}O_2R$) into a decimal by dividing by 100
                $\%\dot{V}O_2R$ = desired intensity $\times$ $\%\dot{V}O_2R$
                Calculate $\%\dot{V}O_2R$:
                $\%\dot{V}O_2R = 0.5 \times 26.5$ mL $\cdot$ kg^{-1} $\cdot$ $min^{-1} = 13.3$ mL $\cdot$ kg^{-1} $\cdot$ min^{-1}
                $\%\dot{V}O_2R = 0.6 \times 26.5$ mL $\cdot$ kg^{-1} $\cdot$ $min^{-1} = 15.9$ mL $\cdot$ kg^{-1} $\cdot$ min^{-1}
        3)   Determine target $\dot{V}O_2R$ range:
                $(\%\dot{V}O_2R) + \dot{V}O_{2rest}$
                To determine the lower target $\dot{V}O_2$ range:
                    Target $\dot{V}O_2 = 13.3$ mL $\cdot$ kg^{-1} $\cdot$ $min^{-1} + 3.5$ mL $\cdot$ kg^{-1} $\cdot$ $min^{-1} =$
                    16.8 mL $\cdot$ kg^{-1} $\cdot$ min^{-1}
                To determine upper target $\dot{V}O_2$ range:
                      Target $\dot{V}O_2 = 15.9$ mL $\cdot$ kg^{-1} $\cdot$ $min^{-1} + 3.5$ mL $\cdot$ kg^1 $\cdot$ $min^{-1} =$
                    19.4 mL $\cdot$ kg^{-1} $\cdot$ min^{-1}
                Target $\dot{V}O_2$ range: 16.8 mL $\cdot$ kg^{-1} $\cdot$ min^{-1} to 19.4 mL $\cdot$ kg^{-1} $\cdot$ min^{-1}

■ **FIGURE 7.1.** Examples of the application of various methods for prescribing exercise intensity. HR_{max}, maximal heart rate; HR_{rest}, resting heart rate; MET, metabolic equivalent; $\dot{V}O_2$, volume of oxygen consumed per unit of time; $\dot{V}O_{2max}$, maximal volume of oxygen consumed per unit of time. Adapted from (49).

4) Determine MET target range (optional):

$1 \text{ MET} = 3.5 \text{ mL} \cdot \text{kg}^{-1} \cdot \text{min}^{-1}$

Calculate lower MET target:

$1 \text{ MET}/3.5 \text{ mL} \cdot \text{kg}^{-1} \cdot \text{min}^{-1} = \times \text{ MET}/16.8 \text{ mL} \cdot \text{kg}^{-1} \cdot \text{min}^{-1}$

$\times \text{ MET} = 16.8 \text{ mL} \cdot \text{kg}^{-1} \cdot \text{min}^{-1}/3.5 \text{ mL} \cdot \text{kg}^{-1} \cdot \text{min}^{-1} = 4.8 \text{ METs}$

Calculate upper MET target:

$1 \text{ MET}/3.5 \text{ mL} \cdot \text{kg}^{-1} \cdot \text{min}^{-1} = \times \text{ MET}/19.4 \text{ mL} \cdot \text{kg}^{-1} \cdot \text{min}^{-1}$

$\times \text{ MET} = 19.4 \text{ mL} \cdot \text{kg}^{-1} \cdot \text{min}^{-1}/3.5 \text{ mL} \cdot \text{kg}^{-1} \cdot \text{min}^{-1} = 5.5 \text{ METs}$

5) Identify physical activities requiring EE within the target range from compendium of physical activities (1,2) or by using metabolic calculations shown in *Table 7.3* or reference (22). Also see the following examples of use of metabolic equations.

%HR$_{max}$ (Measured Or Estimated) Method:

Available data:

A man 45 yr of age

Desired exercise intensity: 70%–80%

Formula: $\text{THR} = \text{HR}_{max} \times$ desired %

Calculate estimated HR$_{max}$ (if measured HR$_{max}$ not available):

$\text{HR}_{max} = 220 - \text{age}$

$\text{HR}_{max} = 220 - 45 = 175 \text{ beats} \cdot \text{min}^{-1}$

1) Determine THR range:

$\text{THR} = \text{Desired \%} \times \text{HR}_{max}$

Convert desired % HR$_{max}$ into a decimal by dividing by 100

Determine lower limit of THR range:

$\text{THR} = 175 \text{ beats} \cdot \text{min}^{-1} \times 0.70 = 123 \text{ beats} \cdot \text{min}^{-1}$

Determine upper limit of THR range:

$\text{THR} = 175 \text{ beats} \cdot \text{min}^{-1} \times 0.80 = 140 \text{ beats} \cdot \text{min}^{-1}$

THR range: $123 \text{ beats} \cdot \text{min}^{-1}$ to $140 \text{ beats} \cdot \text{min}^{-1}$

%$\dot{V}O_2$ (Measured or Estimated) Method

Available data:

A woman 45 yr of age

Estimated $\dot{V}O_{2max}$: $30 \text{ mL} \cdot \text{kg}^{-1} \cdot \text{min}^{-1}$

Desired $\dot{V}O_2$ range: 50%–60%

Formula: $\dot{V}O_{2max} \times$ desired %

Determine target $\dot{V}O_2$ range:

$\text{Target } \dot{V}O_2 = \text{Desired \%} \times \dot{V}O_{2max}$

Convert desired intensity (%$\dot{V}O_2$) into a decimal by dividing by 100

Determine lower limit of target $\dot{V}O_2$ range:

$\text{Target } \dot{V}O_2 = 0.50 \times 30 \text{ mL} \cdot \text{kg}^{-1} \cdot \text{min}^{-1} = 15 \text{ mL} \cdot \text{kg}^{-1} \cdot \text{min}^{-1}$

Determine upper limit of target $\dot{V}O_{2max}$ range:

$\text{Target } \dot{V}O_2 = 0.60 \times 30 \text{ mL} \cdot \text{kg}^{-1} \cdot \text{min}^{-1} = 18 \text{ mL} \cdot \text{kg}^{-1} \cdot \text{min}^{-1}$

Target $\dot{V}O_2$ range: $15 \text{ mL} \cdot \text{kg}^{-1} \cdot \text{min}^{-1}$ to $18 \text{ mL} \cdot \text{kg}^{-1} \cdot \text{min}^{-1}$

1) Determine MET target range (optional):

$1 \text{ MET} = 3.5 \text{ mL} \cdot \text{kg}^{-1} \cdot \text{min}^{-1}$

Calculate lower MET target:

$1 \text{ MET}/3.5 \text{ mL} \cdot \text{kg}^{-1} \cdot \text{min}^{-1} = \times \text{ MET}/15.0 \text{ mL} \cdot \text{kg}^{-1} \cdot \text{min}^{-1}$

$\times \text{ MET} = 15.0 \text{ mL} \cdot \text{kg}^{-1} \cdot \text{min}^{-1}/3.5 \text{ mL} \cdot \text{kg}^{-1} \cdot \text{min}^{-1} = 4.3 \text{ METs}$

Calculate upper MET target:

$1 \text{ MET}/3.5 \text{ mL} \cdot \text{kg}^{-1} \cdot \text{min}^{-1} = \times \text{ MET}/18.0 \text{ mL} \cdot \text{kg}^{-1} \cdot \text{min}^{-1}$

$\times \text{ MET} = 18.0 \text{ mL} \cdot \text{kg}^{-1} \cdot \text{min}^{-1}/3.5 \text{ mL} \cdot \text{kg}^{-1} \cdot \text{min}^{-1} = 5.1 \text{ METs}$

■ **Figure 7.1.** (*Continued*)

2) Identify physical activities requiring EE within the target range from compendium of physical activities (1,2) or by using metabolic calculations shown in *Table 7.3* and reference (22). See the following examples of use of metabolic equations.

Using metabolic calculations (22) *or (Table 7.3) to determine running speed on a treadmill*
Available data:

A man 32 yr of age
Weight: 130 lb (59 kg)
Height: 70 in (177.8 cm)
$\dot{V}O_{2max}$: 54 mL $\cdot$ kg^{-1} $\cdot$ min^{-1}

Desired treadmill grade: 2.5%
Desired exercise intensity: 80%
Formula: $\dot{V}O_2 = 3.5 + (0.2 \times speed) + (0.9 \times speed \times \% \ grade)$

1. Determine target $\dot{V}O_2$:
   Target $\dot{V}O_2$ = desired % $\times$ $\dot{V}O_{2max}$
   Target $\dot{V}O_2$ = 0.80 $\times$ 54 mL $\cdot$ kg^{-1} $\cdot$ min^{-1} = 43.2 mL $\cdot$ kg^{-1} $\cdot$ min^{-1}
2. Determine treadmill speed:
   $\dot{V}O_2 = 3.5 + (0.2 \times speed) + (0.9 \times speed \times \% \ grade)$
   43.2 mL $\cdot$ kg^{-1} $\cdot$ min^{-1} = 3.5 + (0.2 $\times$ speed) + (0.9 $\times$ speed $\times$ 0.025)
   39.7 = (0.2 $\times$ speed) + (0.9 $\times$ speed $\times$ 0.025)
   39.7 = (0.2 $\times$ speed) + (0.0225 $\times$ speed)
   39.7 = 0.2225 $\times$ speed
   178.4 m $\cdot$ min^{-1} = speed
   Speed on treadmill: 10.7 km $\cdot$ h^{-1} (6.7 mi $\cdot$ h^1)

Using metabolic calculations (22) *(Table 7.2) to determine % grade during walking on a treadmill*
Available data:

A man 54 yr of age who is moderately physically active
Weight: 190 lb (86.4 kg)
Height: 70 in (177.8 cm)

Desired walking speed: 2.5 mi $\cdot$ h^{-1} (4 km $\cdot$ h^{-1}; 67 m $\cdot$ min^{-1})
Desired MET: 5 METs
Formula: $\dot{V}O_2 = 3.5 + (0.1 \times speed) + (1.8 \times speed \times \% \ grade)$

1. Determine target $\dot{V}O_2$:
   Target $\dot{V}O_2$ = MET $\times$ 3.5 mL $\cdot$ kg^{-1} $\cdot$ min^{-1}
   Target $\dot{V}O_2$ = 5 $\times$ 3.5 mL $\cdot$ kg^{-1} $\cdot$ min^{-1} = 17.5 mL $\cdot$ kg^{-1} $\cdot$ min^{-1}
2. Determine treadmill grade:
   $\dot{V}O_2 = 3.5 + (0.1 \times speed) + (1.8 \times speed \times \% \ grade)$
   17.5 mL $\cdot$ kg^{-1} $\cdot$ min^{-1} = 3.5 + (0.1 $\times$ 67 m $\cdot$ s^{-1}) + (1.8 $\times$ 67 m $\cdot$ s^{-1} $\times$ % grade)
   14 = (0.1 $\times$ 67 m $\cdot$ s^{-1}) + (1.8 $\times$ 67 m $\cdot$ s^{-1} $\times$ % grade)
   14 = 6.7 + (120.6 $\times$ % grade)
   7.3 = 120.6 $\times$ % grade
   0.06 = % grade
   % grade = 6%

■ **Figure 7.1.** (*Continued*)

Using metabolic calculations (22) (Table 7.3) to determine target work rate (kg · m · min^{-1}) on a Monarch leg cycle ergometer

Available data:

A woman 42 yr of age
Weight: 190 lb (86.4 kg)
Height: 70 in (177.8 cm)
Desired $\dot{V}O_2$: 18 kg · m · min^{-1}
Formula: $\dot{V}O_2 = 7.0 + (1.8 \times$ work rate)/body mass

1. Calculate work rate on cycle ergometer:
$\dot{V}O_2 = 7.0 + (1.8 \times$ work rate)/body mass)
18 mL · kg^{-1} · min^{-1} = 7.0 + (1.8 × work rate)/86.4 kg
11 = (1.8 × work rate)/86.4
950.4 = 1.8 × work rate
528 = work rate
Work rate = 528 kg · m · min^{-1} = 86.6 W

■ **Figure 7.1.** (*Continued*)

TABLE 7.3. Metabolic Calculations for the Estimation of Energy Expenditure ($\dot{V}O_{2max}$ [mL · kg^{-1} · min^{-1}]) During Common Physical Activities

| Activity | Resting Component | Sum of Resting + Horizontal + Vertical/Resistance Components | | Limitations |
		Horizontal Component	Vertical Component/ Resistance Component	
Walking	3.5	0.1 × speed[a]	1.8 × speed[a] × grade[b]	Most accurate for speeds of 1.9–3.7 mi · h^{-1} (50–100 m · min^{-1})
Running	3.5	0.2 × speed [a]	0.9 × speed [a] × grade[b]	Most accurate for speeds >5 mi · h^{-1} (134 m · min^{-1})
Stepping	3.5	0.2 × steps · min^{-1}	1.33 × (1.8 × step height[c] × steps · min^{-1})	Most accurate for stepping rates of 12–30 steps · min^{-1}
Leg cycling	3.5	3.5	(1.8 × work rate[d])/body mass[e]	Most accurate for work rates of 300–1,200 kg · m · min^{-1} (50–200 W)
Arm cycling	3.5		(3 × work rate[d])/body mass[e]	Most accurate for work rates between 150–750 kg · m · min^{-1} (25–125 W)

[a]Speed in m · min^{-1}.

[b]Grade is percent grade expressed in decimal format (*e.g.,* 10% = 0.10).

[c]Step height in m.

Multiply by the following conversion factors:

lb to kg: 0.454; in to cm: 2.54; ft to m: 0.3048; mi to km: 1.609; mi · h^{-1} to m · min^{-1}: 26.8; kg · m · min^{-1} to W: 0.164; W to kg · m · min^{-1}: 6.12; $\dot{V}O_{2max}$ L · min^{-1} to kcal · min^{-1}: 4.9; $\dot{V}O_2$ MET to mL · kg^{-1} · min^{-1}: 3.5.

[d]Work rate in kilogram meters per minute (kg · m · min^{-1}) is calculated as resistance (kg) × distance per revolution of flywheel × pedal frequency per minute. Note: Distance per revolution is 6 m for Monark leg ergometer, 3 m for the Tunturi and BodyGuard ergometers, and 2.4 m for Monark arm ergometer.

[e]Body mass in kg

$\dot{V}O_{2max}$, maximal volume of oxygen consumed per unit of time.

Adapted from (8).

When using $\dot{V}O_2$ or METs to prescribe exercise, health/fitness, public health, clinical exercise, and health care professionals can identify activities within the desired $\dot{V}O_2$ or MET range by using a compendium of physical activities (1,2) or metabolic calculations (22) (see *Table 7.3* and *Figure 7.1*). There are metabolic equations for estimation of EE during walking, running, cycling, and stepping. Although there are preliminary equations for other modes of exercise such as the elliptical trainer, there is insufficient data to recommend these for universal use at this time. A direct method of Ex R_x by plotting the relationship between HR and $\dot{V}O_2$ may be used when HR and $\dot{V}O_2$ are measured during an exercise test (see *Figure 7.2*). This method may be particularly useful when prescribing exercise in individuals taking medications such as β-blockers or who have a chronic disease or health conditions such as diabetes mellitus or atherosclerotic CVD that alters the HR response to exercise (see *Appendix A* and *Chapters 9* and *10*).

Measures of perceived effort and affective valence (*i.e.*, the pleasantness of exercise) can be used to modulate or refine the prescribed exercise intensity (see *Chapter 11*). These include the Borg Rating of Perceived Exertion (RPE) Scales (12–14,33), OMNI Scales (40,41,55), Talk Test (35), and Feeling Scale (24). These methods have been validated against several physiologic markers, but the evidence is insufficient to support using these methods as a *primary* method of prescribing exercise intensity (20).

METHODS OF ESTIMATING INTENSITY   FITT

Several methods can be used to estimate intensity during exercise. There are no studies available comparing all exercise intensity prescription methods simultaneously. Thus, the various methods described in this chapter to quantify exercise intensity may not necessarily be equivalent to each other (see *Box 7.2*).

EXERCISE TIME (DURATION)

Exercise time/duration is prescribed as a measure of the amount of time physical activity is performed (*i.e.*, time · session^{-1}, d^{-1}, and wk^{-1}). It is recommended that most adults accumulate 30–60 min · d^{-1} (≥150 min · wk^{-1}) of moderate intensity exercise, 20–60 min · d^{-1} (≥75 min · wk^{-1}) of vigorous intensity exercise, or a combination of moderate and vigorous intensity exercise per day to attain the volumes of exercise recommended in the following discussion (20,52). However, less than 20 min of exercise per day can be beneficial, especially in previously sedentary individuals (20,52). For weight management, longer durations of exercise (≥60–90 min · d^{-1}) may be needed, especially in individuals who spend large amounts of time in sedentary behaviors (17). (See *Chapter 10* and the ACSM position stand on overweight and obesity (17) for additional information regarding the Ex R_x recommendations for promoting and maintaining weight loss.)

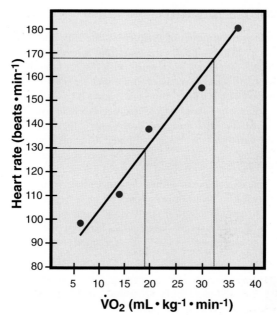

■ **FIGURE 7.2.** Prescribing exercise heart rate using the relationship between heart rate and $\dot{V}O_2$. A line of best fit has been drawn through the data points on this plot of HR and $\dot{V}O_2$ during a hypothetical exercise test in which $\dot{V}O_{2max}$ was observed to be 38 mL · kg^{-1} · min^{-1} and HR$_{max}$ was 184 beats · min^{-1}. A THR range was determined by finding the HR that corresponds to 50% and 85% $\dot{V}O_{2max}$. For this individual, 50% $\dot{V}O_{2max}$ was ~19 mL · kg^{-1} · min^{-1}, and 85% $\dot{V}O_{2max}$ was ~32 mL · kg^{-1} · min^{-1}. The corresponding THR range is 130–168 beats · min^{-1} [8].

The recommended time/duration of physical activity may be performed continuously (*i.e.*, one session) or intermittently and can be accumulated over the course of a day in one or more sessions of physical activity that total at least 10 min · session^{-1}. Exercise bouts of <10 min may yield favorable adaptations in very deconditioned individuals, but further study is needed to confirm the effectiveness of these shorter bouts of exercise [20].

AEROBIC EXERCISE TIME (DURATION) RECOMMENDATION

FITT

Most adults should accumulate 30–60 min · d^{-1} (≥150 min · wk^{-1}) of moderate intensity exercise, 20–60 min · d^{-1} (≥75 min · wk^{-1}) of vigorous intensity exercise, or a combination of moderate and vigorous intensity exercise daily to attain the recommended targeted volumes of exercise. This recommended amount of exercise may be accumulated in one continuous exercise session or in bouts of ≥10 min over the course of a day. Durations of exercise less than recommended can be beneficial in some individuals.

EXERCISE VOLUME (QUANTITY)

Exercise volume is the product of Frequency, Intensity, and Time (duration) or *FIT* of exercise. Evidence supports the important role of exercise volume in realizing health/fitness outcomes, particularly with respect to body composition and weight management. Thus, exercise volume may be used to estimate the gross EE of an individual's Ex R_x. MET-min $\cdot$ wk^{-1} and kcal $\cdot$ wk^{-1} can be used to estimate exercise volume in a standardized manner. *Box 7.3* shows the definition and calculations for METs, MET-min, and kcal $\cdot$ min^{-1} for a wide array of physical activities. These variables can also be estimated using previously published tables (1, 2). MET-min and kcal $\cdot$ min^{-1} can then be used to calculate MET-min $\cdot$ wk^{-1} and kcal $\cdot$ wk^{-1} that is accumulated as part of an exercise program to evaluate whether the exercise volume is within the ranges described later in this chapter that will likely result in health/fitness benefits.

The results of epidemiological studies and randomized clinical trials have shown there is a dose-response *association* between the volume of exercise and health/fitness outcomes (*i.e.*, with greater amounts of physical activity, the

---

BOX 7.3   Calculation of METs, MET-Min^{-1}, and Kcal $\cdot$ Min^{-1}

Metabolic Equivalents (METs): An index of EE. "[A MET is the ratio of the rate of energy expended during an activity to the rate of energy expended at rest. . . . (One) MET is the rate of EE while sitting at rest . . . by convention, [1 MET is equal to] an oxygen uptake of 3.5 [mL $\cdot$ kg^{-1} $\cdot$ min^{-1}]" (38).

MET-min: An index of EE that quantifies the total amount of physical activity performed in a standardized manner across individuals and types of activities (38). Calculated as the product of the number of METs associated with one or more physical activities and the number of minutes the activities were performed (*i.e.*, METs × min); usually standardized per week or per day as a measure of exercise volume.

Kilocalorie (kcal): The energy needed to increase the temperature of 1 kg of water by 1° C. To convert METs to kcal $\cdot$ min^{-1}, it is necessary to know an individual's body weight, kcal $\cdot$ min^{-1} = [(METs × 3.5 mL $\cdot$ kg^{-1} $\cdot$ min^{-1} × body wt in kg) ÷ 1000)] × 5. Usually standardized as kilocalorie per week or per day as a measure of exercise volume.

Example:

Jogging (at ~7 METs) for 30 min on 3 d $\cdot$ wk^{-1} for a 70 kg male:
7 METs × 30 min × 3 times per week = 630 MET-min $\cdot$ wk^{-1}
[(7 METs × 3.5 mL $\cdot$ kg^{-1} $\cdot$ min^{-1} × 70 kg) ÷ 1000)] × 5 = 8.575 kcal $\cdot$ min^{-1}
8.575 kcal $\cdot$ min^{-1} × 30 min × 3 times per week = 771.75 kcal $\cdot$ wk^{-1}

Adapted from (20).

health/fitness benefits also increase) (16,20,52). It is not clear whether or not there is a minimum or maximum amount of exercise that is needed to attain health/fitness benefits. However, a total EE of $\geq$500–1,000 MET-min $\cdot$ wk^{-1} is consistently associated with lower rates of CVD and premature mortality. Thus, $\geq$500–1,000 MET-min $\cdot$ wk^{-1} is a reasonable target volume for an exercise program for most adults (20,52). This volume is approximately equal to (a) 1,000 kcal $\cdot$ wk^{-1} of moderate intensity, physical activity (or about 150 min wk^{-1}); (b) an exercise intensity of 3–5.9 METs (for individuals weighing ~68–91 kg [~150–200 lb]); and (c) 10 MET-h $\cdot$ wk^{-1} (20,52). It should be noted that lower volumes of exercise (i.e., 4 kcal $\cdot$ kg^{-1} $\cdot$ wk^{-1} or 330 kcal $\cdot$ wk^{-1}) can result in health/fitness benefits in some individuals, especially in individuals who are deconditioned (16,20,52). Even lower volumes of exercise may also have benefit, but evidence is lacking to make definitive recommendations (20).

Pedometers are effective tools for promoting physical activity and can be used to approximate exercise volume in steps per day (50). The goal of 10,000 steps $\cdot$ d^{-1} is often cited, but it appears that achieving a pedometer step count of at least 5,400–7,900 steps $\cdot$ d^{-1} can meet recommended exercise targets (20,50). To achieve step counts of 5,400–7,900 steps $\cdot$ d^{-1}, one can estimate total exercise volume by considering the following: (a) walking 100 steps $\cdot$ min^{-1} provides a very rough approximation of moderate intensity exercise; (b) walking 1 mile $\cdot$ d^{-1} yields about 2,000 steps $\cdot$ d^{-1}; and (c) walking at a moderate intensity for 30 min $\cdot$ d^{-1} yields about 3,000–4,000 steps $\cdot$ d^{-1} (10,20,28,50). For weight management, higher step counts may be necessary, and a population-based study estimated men may require 11,000–12,000 steps $\cdot$ d^{-1}, and women 8,000–12,000 steps $\cdot$ d^{-1}, respectively, to maintain a normal weight (20,50). Because of the substantial errors of prediction when using pedometer step counts, using steps $\cdot$ min^{-1} *combined with* currently recommended time/durations of exercise (e.g., 100 steps $\cdot$ min^{-1} for 30 min $\cdot$ session^{-1} and 150 min $\cdot$ wk^{-1}) is judicious (20).

AEROBIC EXERCISE VOLUME RECOMMENDATION   FITT

A target volume of $\geq$500–1,000 MET-min $\cdot$ wk^{-1} is recommended for most adults. This volume is approximately equal to 1,000 kcal $\cdot$ wk^{-1} of moderate intensity, physical activity, ~150 min $\cdot$ wk^{-1} of moderate intensity exercise, or pedometer counts of $\geq$5,400–7,900 steps $\cdot$ d^{-1}. Because of the substantial errors in prediction when using pedometer step counts, use steps $\cdot$ d^{-1} *combined with* currently recommended time/durations of exercise. Lower exercise volumes can have health/fitness benefits for deconditioned individuals, and greater volumes may be needed for weight management.

TYPE (MODE)

Rhythmic, aerobic type exercises involving large muscle groups are recommended for improving CRF (20). The modes of physical activity that result in improvement and maintenance of CRF are found in *Table 7.4*. The principle of

TABLE 7.4. Modes Of Aerobic (Cardiorespiratory Endurance) Exercises to Improve Physical Fitness

Exercise Group	Exercise Description	Recommended for	Examples
A	Endurance activities requiring minimal skill or physical fitness to perform	All adults	Walking, leisurely cycling, aqua-aerobics, slow dancing
B	Vigorous intensity endurance activities requiring minimal skill	Adults (as per the preparticipation screening guidelines in *Chapter 2*) who are habitually physically active and/or at least average physical fitness	Jogging, running, rowing, aerobics, spinning, elliptical exercise, stepping exercise, fast dancing
C	Endurance activities requiring skill to perform	Adults with acquired skill and/or at least average physical fitness levels	Swimming, cross-country skiing, skating
D	Recreational sports	Adults with a regular exercise program and at least average physical fitness	Racquet sports, basketball, soccer, down-hill skiing, hiking

Adapted from (8).

specificity of training should be kept in mind when selecting the exercise modalities to be included in the Ex R$_x$. The specificity principle states that the physiologic adaptations to exercise are specific to the type of exercise performed (20).

Table 7.4 shows aerobic or cardiorespiratory endurance exercises categorized by the intensity and skill demands. Type A exercises, recommended for all adults, require little skill to perform, and the intensity can easily be modified to accommodate a wide range of physical fitness levels. Type B exercises are typically performed at a vigorous intensity and are recommended for individuals who are at least of average physical fitness and who have been doing some exercise on a regular basis. Type C exercises require skill to perform, and therefore are best for individuals who have reasonably developed motor skills and physical fitness to perform the exercises safely. Type D exercises are recreational sports that can improve physical fitness but which are generally recommended as ancillary physical activities performed in addition to recommended conditioning physical activities. Type D physical activities are recommended only for individuals who possess adequate motor skills and physical fitness to perform the sport; however, many of these sports may be modified to accommodate individuals of lower skill and physical fitness levels.

AEROBIC EXERCISE TYPE RECOMMENDATION   F I T T

Rhythmic, aerobic exercise of at least moderate intensity that involves large muscle groups and requires little skill to perform is recommended for all adults to improve health and CRF. Other exercise and sports requiring skill to perform or higher levels of fitness are recommended only for individuals possessing adequate skill and fitness to perform the activity.

RATE OF PROGRESSION

The recommended rate of progression in an exercise program depends on the individual's health status, physical fitness, training responses, and exercise program goals. Progression may consist of increasing any of the components of the FITT principle of Ex R$_x$ as tolerated by the individual. During the initial phase of the exercise program, increasing exercise time/duration (*i.e.*, min · session^{-1}) is recommended. An increase in exercise time/duration per session of 5–10 min every 1–2 wk over the first 4–6 wk of an exercise training program is reasonable for the average adult (20). After the individual has been exercising regularly for ≥1 mo, the FIT of exercise is gradually adjusted upward over the next 4–8 mo — or longer for older adults and very deconditioned individuals — to meet the recommended quantity and quality of exercise presented in the *Guidelines*. Any progression in the FITT-VP principle of Ex R$_x$ should be made gradually avoiding large increases in any of the FITT-VP components to minimize risks of muscular soreness, injury, undue fatigue, and the long-term risk of overtraining. Following any adjustments in the Ex R$_x$, the individual should be monitored for any adverse effects of the increased volume, such as excessive shortness of breath, fatigue, and muscle soreness, and downward adjustments should be made if the exercise is not well tolerated (20).

THE FITT-VP PRINCIPLE OF EX R$_x$ SUMMARY   F I T T

The FITT-VP principle of Ex R$_x$ features an individu-
ally tailored exercise program that includes specification of the Frequency (F), Intensity (I), Time or duration (T), Type or mode (T), Volume (V), and Progression (P) of exercise to be performed. The exact composition of FITT-VP will vary depending on the characteristics and goals of the individual. The FITT-VP principle of Ex R$_x$ will need to be revised according to the individual response, need, limitation, and adaptations to exercise as well as evolution of the goals and objectives of the exercise program. *Table* 7.5 summarizes the FITT-VP principle of Ex R$_x$ recommendations for aerobic exercise.

MUSCULAR FITNESS

The health benefits of enhancing muscular fitness (*i.e.*, the functional parameters of muscle strength, endurance, and power) are well established (5,20,52). Higher levels of muscular strength are associated with a significantly better cardiometabolic risk factor profile, lower risk of all cause mortality, fewer CVD events, lower risk of developing physical function limitations, and lower risk for nonfatal disease (20). In addition to greater strength, there is an impressive array of changes in health-related biomarkers that can be derived from regular participation in resistance training, including improvements in body composition, blood glucose levels, insulin sensitivity, and BP in individuals

TABLE 7.5. Aerobic (Cardiovascular Endurance) Exercise Evidence-Based Recommendations

FITT-VP	Evidence-Based Recommendation
Frequency	• ≥5 d · wk^{-1} of moderate exercise, or ≥3 d · wk^{-1} of vigorous exercise, or a combination of moderate and vigorous exercise on ≥3–5 d · wk^{-1} is recommended.
Intensity	• Moderate and/or vigorous intensity is recommended for most adults. • Light-to-moderate intensity exercise may be beneficial in deconditioned individuals.
Time	• 30–60 min · d^{-1} of purposeful moderate exercise, or 20–60 min · d^{-1} of vigorous exercise, or a combination of moderate and vigorous exercise per day is recommended for most adults. • <20 min of exercise per day can be beneficial, especially in previously sedentary individuals.
Type	• Regular, purposeful exercise that involves major muscle groups and is continuous and rhythmic in nature is recommended.
Volume	• A target volume of ≥500–1,000 MET-min · wk^{-1} is recommended. • Increasing pedometer step counts by ≥2,000 steps · d^{-1} to reach a daily step count ≥7,000 steps · d^{-1} is beneficial. • Exercising below these volumes may still be beneficial for individuals unable or unwilling to reach this amount of exercise.
Pattern	• Exercise may be performed in one (continuous) session per day or in multiple sessions of ≥10 min to accumulate the desired duration and volume of exercise per day. • Exercise bouts of <10 min may yield favorable adaptations in very deconditioned individuals.
Progression	• A gradual progression of exercise volume by adjusting exercise duration, frequency, and/or intensity is reasonable until the desired exercise goal (maintenance) is attained. • This approach may enhance adherence and reduce risks of musculoskeletal injury and adverse cardiac events.

Adapted from (20).

with pre-hypertension to Stage 1 hypertension (6,17,20,36) (see *Chapter 10*). Accordingly, resistance training may be effective for preventing and treating the "metabolic syndrome" (20) (see *Chapter 10*). Importantly, exercise that promotes muscle strength and mass also effectively increases bone mass (*i.e.*, bone mineral density and content) and bone strength of the specific bones stressed and may serve as a valuable measure to prevent, slow, or even reverse the loss of bone mass in individuals with osteoporosis (3,4,20,52) (see *Chapter 10*). Because muscle weakness has been identified as a risk factor for the development of osteoarthritis, resistance training may reduce the chance of developing this musculoskeletal disorder (20,43) (see *Chapter 10*). In individuals with osteoarthritis, resistance training can reduce pain and disability (20,31). Preliminary work suggests that resistance training may prevent and improve depression and anxiety, increase vigor, and reduce fatigue (20).

Each component of muscular fitness improves consequent to an appropriately designed resistance training regimen and correctly performed resistance exercises. As the trained muscles strengthen and enlarge (*i.e.*, hypertrophy), the resistance must be progressively increased if additional gains are to be accrued.

To optimize the efficacy of resistance training, the FITT-VP principle of Ex R$_x$ should be tailored to the individual's goals (5, 20).

Although muscular power is important for athletic events such as the shot put or javelin throw, muscular strength and endurance are of greater importance in a general training regimen focusing on health/fitness outcomes for young and middle-aged adults. In addition to focusing on muscular strength and endurance, older adults (≥65 yr) may benefit from power training because this element of muscle fitness declines most rapidly with aging and insufficient power has been associated with a greater risk of accidental falls (11,15).

GOALS FOR A HEALTH-RELATED RESISTANCE TRAINING PROGRAM F I T T

For adults of all ages, the goals of a health-related resistance training program should be to (a) make activities of daily living (ADL) (*e.g.*, stair climbing, carrying bags of groceries) less stressful physiologically; and (b) effectively manage, attenuate, and even prevent chronic diseases and health conditions such as osteoporosis, Type 2 diabetes mellitus, and obesity. *For these reasons, although resistance training is important across the age span, its importance becomes even greater with age* (7,20,32).

The guidelines described in this chapter for resistance training are dedicated to improving health and most appropriate for an overall or general physical fitness program that includes but does not necessarily emphasize muscle development (5,20).

FREQUENCY OF RESISTANCE EXERCISE

For general muscular fitness, particularly among those who are untrained or recreationally trained (*i.e.*, not engaged in a formal training program), an individual should resistance train each major muscle group (*i.e.*, the muscle groups of the chest, shoulders, upper and lower back, abdomen, hips, and legs) 2–3 d · wk^{-1} with at least 48 h separating the exercise training sessions for the same muscle group (5,20). Depending on the individual's daily schedule, all muscle groups to be trained may be done so in the same session (*i.e.*, whole body), or each session may "split" the body into selected muscle groups so that only a few of groups are trained in any one session (5,20). For example, muscles of the lower body may be trained on Mondays and Thursdays, and upper body muscles may be trained on Tuesdays and Fridays. This split weight training routine entails 4 d · wk^{-1} to train each muscle group 2 times · wk^{-1}; however, each session is of shorter duration than a whole body session used to train all muscle groups. The split and whole body methods are effective as long as each muscle group is trained 2–3 d · wk^{-1}. Having these different resistance training options provides the individual with more flexibility in scheduling, which may help to improve the likelihood of adherence to a resistance training regimen.

RESISTANCE TRAINING FREQUENCY RECOMMENDATION

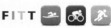

Resistance training of each major muscle group 2–3 d · wk^{-1} with at least 48 h separating the exercise training sessions for the same muscle group is recommended for all adults.

TYPES OF RESISTANCE EXERCISES

Many types of resistance training equipment can effectively be used to improve muscular fitness including free weights, machines with stacked weights or pneumatic resistance, and even resistance bands. Resistance training regimens should include multijoint or compound exercises that affect more than one muscle group (*e.g.*, chest press, shoulder press, pull-down, dips, lower back extension, abdominal crunch/curl-up, leg press, squats). Single joint exercises targeting major muscle groups such as biceps curls, triceps extensions, quadriceps extensions, leg curls, and calf raises can also be included in a resistance training program (5,20).

To avoid creating muscle imbalances that may lead to injury, opposing muscle groups (*i.e.*, agonists and antagonists), such as the lower back and abdomen or the quadriceps and hamstring muscles, should be included in the resistance training routine (5,20). Examples of these types of resistance exercises are low back extensions and abdominal crunches to target the muscles in the lower back and abdomen, and leg presses and leg curls to exercise the quadriceps and hamstring muscles.

TYPES OF RESISTANCE EXERCISES

Many types of resistance training equipment can effectively be used to improve muscular fitness. Multijoint exercises affecting more than one muscle group and targeting agonist and antagonist muscle groups are recommended for all adults. Single joint exercises targeting major muscle groups may also be included in a resistance training program.

VOLUME OF RESISTANCE EXERCISE (SETS AND REPETITIONS)

Each muscle group should be trained for a total of two to four sets. These sets may be derived from the same exercise or from a combination of exercises affecting the same muscle group (5,20). For example, the pectoral muscles of the chest region may be trained either with four sets of bench presses or with two sets of bench presses and two sets of dips (37). A reasonable rest interval between sets is 2–3 min. Using different exercises to train the same muscle group adds variety, may prevent long-term mental "staleness," and may improve adherence to the training program, although evidence that these factors improve adherence is lacking (20).

Four sets per muscle group is more effective than two sets; however, even a single set per exercise will significantly improve muscular strength, particularly among novices (5,20,37). By completing one set of two different exercises that affect the same muscle group, the muscle has executed two sets. For example, bench presses and dips affect the pectoralis muscles of the chest so that by completing one set of each the muscle group has performed a total of two sets. Moreover, compound exercises such as the bench press and dips also train the triceps muscle group. From a practical standpoint of program adherence, each individual should carefully assess her/his daily schedule, time demands, and level of commitment to determine how many sets per muscle should be performed during resistance training sessions. Of paramount importance is the adoption of a resistance training program that will be realistically maintained over the long term.

The resistance training intensity and number of repetitions performed with each set are inversely related. That is, the greater the intensity or resistance, the fewer the number of repetitions that will need to be completed. To improve muscular strength, mass, and — to some extent — endurance, a resistance exercise that allows an individual to complete 8–12 repetitions per set should be selected. This translates to a resistance that is ~60%–80% of the individual's one repetition maximum (1-RM) or the greatest amount of weight lifted for a single repetition. For example, if an individual's 1-RM in the shoulder press is 100 lb (45.5 kg), then, when performing that exercise during the training sessions, he/she should choose a resistance between 60 and 80 lb (27–36 kg). If an individual performs multiple sets per exercise, the number of repetitions completed before fatigue occurs will be at or close to 12 repetitions with the first set and will decline to about 8 repetitions during the last set for that exercise. Each set should be performed to the point of muscle fatigue but not failure because exerting muscles to the point of failure increases the likelihood of injury or debilitating residual muscle soreness, particularly among novices (5,20,37).

If the objective of the resistance training program is mainly to improve muscular endurance rather than strength and mass, a higher number of repetitions, perhaps 15–25, should be performed per set along with shorter rest intervals and fewer sets (i.e., 1 or 2 sets per muscle group) (5,20). This regimen necessitates a lower intensity of resistance typically of no more than 50% 1-RM. Similarly, older and very deconditioned individuals who are more susceptible to musculotendinous injury should begin a resistance training program conducting more repetitions (i.e., 10–15) at a moderate intensity of 60%–70% of 1-RM, or an RPE of 5–6 on a 10-point scale (5,20,32) assuming the individual has the capacity to use this intensity while maintaining proper lifting technique. Subsequent to a period of adaptation to resistance training and improved musculotendinous conditioning, older individuals may choose to follow guidelines for younger adults (i.e., higher intensity with 8–12 repetitions per set) (20) (see *Chapter 8*).

VOLUME OF RESISTANCE EXERCISE (SETS AND REPETITIONS) RECOMMENDATION

F I T T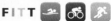

Adults should train each muscle group for a total of 2–4 sets with 8–12 repetitions per set with a rest interval of 2–3 min between sets to improve muscular fitness. For older adults and very deconditioned individuals, ≥1 set of 10–15 repetitions of moderate intensity (*i.e.*, 60%–70% 1-RM), resistance exercise is recommended.

RESISTANCE EXERCISE TECHNIQUE

To ensure optimal health/fitness gains and minimize the chance of injury, each resistance exercise should be performed with proper technique regardless of training status or age. The exercises should be executed using correct form and technique, including performing the repetitions deliberately and in a controlled manner, moving through the full ROM of the joint, and employing proper breathing techniques (*i.e.*, exhalation during the concentric phase and inhalation during the eccentric phase and avoid the Valsalva maneuver) (5,20). However, it is not recommended resistance training be composed exclusively of eccentric or lengthening contractions conducted at very high intensities (*e.g.*, >100% 1-RM) because of the significant chance of injury and severe muscle soreness as well as serious complications such as rhabdomyolysis (*i.e.*, muscle damage resulting in excretion of myoglobin into the urine that may harm kidney function) that can ensue (5,20). Individuals who are naïve to resistance training should receive instruction on proper technique from a qualified health/fitness professional (*e.g.*, ACSM Certified Health Fitness Specialist[SM], ACSM Certified Personal Trainer®) on each exercise used during resistance training sessions (5,20).

RESISTANCE EXERCISE TECHNIQUE RECOMMENDATIONS

F I T T

All individuals should perform resistance training using correct technique. Proper resistance exercise techniques employ controlled movements through the full ROM and involve concentric and eccentric muscle actions.

PROGRESSION/MAINTENANCE

As muscles adapt to a resistance exercise training program, the participant should continue to subject them to overload or greater stimuli to continue to increase muscular strength and mass. This "progressive overload" principle may be performed in several ways. The most common approach is to increase the amount of resistance lifted during training. For example, if an individual is using 100 lb (45.5 kg) of resistance for a given exercise, and her/his muscles have adapted to the point to which 12 repetitions are easily performed, then the resistance should be increased so that no more than 12 repetitions are completed without significant muscle fatigue and difficulty in completing the last repetition of that set. Other ways to progressively overload muscles include performing more sets per muscle group and increasing the number of $d \cdot wk^{-1}$ the muscle groups are trained (5,20).

On the other hand, if the individual has attained the desired levels of muscular strength and mass, and he/she seeks to simply maintain that level of muscular fitness, it is not necessary to progressively increase the training stimulus. That is, increasing the overload by adding resistance, sets, or training sessions per week is not required during a maintenance resistance training program. Muscular strength may be maintained by training muscle groups as little as $1 \ d \cdot wk^{-1}$ as long as the training intensity or the resistance lifted is held constant (5,20).

The FITT-VP principle of Ex R_x for resistance training is summarized in *Table 7.6*. Because these guidelines are most appropriate for a general fitness program, a more rigorous training program must be employed if one's goal is to maximally increase muscular strength and mass, particularly among competitive athletes in sports such as football and bodybuilding. If the reader is interested in more than health/fitness

TABLE 7.6 Resistance Exercise Evidence-Based Recommendations

FITT-VP	Evidence-Based Recommendation
Frequency	• Each major muscle group should be trained on 2–3 $d \cdot wk^{-1}$.
Intensity	• 60%–70% 1-RM (moderate-to-vigorous intensity) for novice to intermediate exercisers to improve strength • ≥80% 1-RM (vigorous-to-very vigorous intensity) for experienced strength trainers to improve strength • 40%–50% RM (very light-to-light intensity) for older individuals beginning exercise to improve strength • 40%–50% 1-RM (very light-to-light intensity) may be beneficial for improving strength in sedentary individuals beginning a resistance training program • <50% 1-RM (light-to-moderate intensity) to improve muscular endurance • 20%–50% 1-RM in older adults to improve power
Time	• No specific duration of training has been identified for effectiveness.
Type	• Resistance exercises involving each major muscle group are recommended. • Multijoint exercises affecting more than one muscle group and targeting agonist and antagonist muscle groups are recommended for all adults. • Single joint exercises targeting major muscle groups may also be included in a resistance training program, typically after performing multijoint exercise(s) for that particular muscle group. • A variety of exercise equipment and/or body weight can be used to perform these exercises.
Repetitions	• 8–12 repetitions is recommended to improve strength and power in most adults. • 10–15 repetitions is effective in improving strength in middle-aged and older individuals starting exercise. • 15–20 repetitions are recommended to improve muscular endurance.
Sets	• 2–4 sets are recommended for most adults to improve strength and power. • A single set of resistance exercise can be effective especially among older and novice exercisers. • ≤2 sets are effective in improving muscular endurance.
Pattern	• Rest intervals of 2–3 min between each set of repetitions are effective. • A rest of ≥48 h between sessions for any single muscle group is recommended.
Progression	• A gradual progression of greater resistance, and/or more repetitions per set, and/or increasing frequency is recommended.

1-RM, one repetition maximum.

Adapted from (20).

and general outcomes or instead desires to maximally develop muscular strength and mass, he/she is referred to the ACSM position stand on progression models in resistance training for healthy adults for additional information (5,20).

PROGRESSION/MAINTENANCE OF RESISTANCE TRAINING RECOMMENDATION   FITT

As muscles adapt to a resistance exercise training program, the participant should continue to subject them to overload to continue to increase muscular strength and mass by gradually increasing resistance, number of sets, or frequency of training.

FLEXIBILITY EXERCISE (STRETCHING)

Joint ROM or flexibility can be improved across all age groups by engaging in flexibility exercises (20,32). The ROM around a joint is improved immediately after performing flexibility exercise and shows chronic improvement after about 3–4 wk of regular stretching at a frequency of at least 2–3 times · wk^{-1} (20). Postural stability and balance can also be improved by engaging in flexibility exercises, especially when combined with resistance exercise (20). It is possible that regular flexibility exercise may result in a reduction of musculotendinous injuries, prevention of low back pain, or delayed onset of muscle soreness, but the evidence is far from being definitive (20).

The goal of a flexibility program is to develop ROM in the major muscle/ tendon groups in accordance with individualized goals. Certain performance standards discussed later in this chapter enhance the effectiveness of flexibility exercises. It is most effective to perform flexibility exercise when the muscle temperature is increased through warm-up exercises or passively through methods such as moist heat packs or hot baths, although this benefit may vary across muscle tendon units (20).

Stretching exercises may result in an immediate, short-term decrease in muscle strength, power, and sports performance performed after stretching, with the negative effect particularly apparent when strength and power is important to performance (20, 29). Before specific recommendations can be made, more research is needed on the immediate effects of flexibility exercises on the performance of fitness-related activities. Nevertheless, it is reasonable based on the available evidence to recommend when feasible, individuals engaging in a general fitness program perform flexibility exercise *following* cardiorespiratory or resistance exercise — or alternatively — as a stand alone program (20).

FLEXIBILITY EXERCISE RECOMMENDATION   FITT

ROM is improved acutely and chronically following flexibility exercises. Flexibility exercises are most effective when the muscles are warm. Flexibility exercises may acutely reduce power and strength so it is recommended that flexibility exercises be performed after exercise and sports where strength and power are important for performance.

TYPES OF FLEXIBILITY EXERCISES

Flexibility exercise should target the major muscle tendon units of the shoulder girdle, chest, neck, trunk, lower back, hips, posterior and anterior legs, and ankles (20). *Box 7.4* shows the several types of flexibility exercises that can improve ROM. Although often considered "contraindicated," properly performed ballistic stretching may be considered for adults, particularly for individuals engaging in activities that involve ballistic movements such as basketball and is equally effective as static stretching in increasing joint ROM (20). Proprioceptive neuromuscular facilitation (PNF) techniques that require a partner to perform and static stretching are superior to dynamic or slow movement stretching in increasing ROM around a joint (20). PNF techniques typically involve an isometric contraction followed by a static stretch in the same muscle/tendon group (*i.e.*, contract-relax).

BOX 7.4   **Flexibility Exercise Definitions**

Ballistic methods or "bouncing" stretches use the momentum of the moving body segment to produce the stretch (57).

Dynamic or slow movement stretching involves a gradual transition from one body position to another, and a progressive increase in reach and range of motion as the movement is repeated several times (30).

Static stretching involves slowly stretching a muscle/tendon group and holding the position for a period of time (*i.e.*, 10–30 s). Static stretches can be active or passive (56).

Active static stretching involves holding the stretched position using the strength of the agonist muscle as is common in many forms of yoga (20).

Passive static stretching involves assuming a position while holding a limb or other part of the body with or without the assistance of a partner or device (such as elastic bands or a ballet barre) (20).

Proprioceptive neuromuscular facilitation (PNF) methods take several forms but typically involve an isometric contraction of the selected muscle/tendon group followed by a static stretching of the same group (*i.e.*, contract-relax) (39,42).

Adapted from (20).

FLEXIBILITY TYPE RECOMMENDATION   FITT

A series of flexibility exercises targeting the major muscle tendon units should be performed. A variety of static, dynamic, and PNF flexibility exercises can improve ROM around a joint.

VOLUME OF FLEXIBILITY EXERCISE (TIME, REPETITIONS, AND FREQUENCY)

Holding a stretch for 10–30 s to the point of tightness or slight discomfort enhances joint ROM, and there seems to be little additional benefit resulting from holding the strength for a longer duration, except for older individuals (20). In older adults, stretching for 30–60 s may result in greater flexibility gains than shorter duration stretches (20) (see *Chapter 8*). For PNF stretches, it is recommended that the individuals of all ages hold a light-to-moderate contraction (*i.e.*, 20%–75% of maximum voluntary contraction) for 3–6 s, followed by an assisted stretch for 10–30 s (20). Flexibility exercises should be repeated 2–4 times to accumulate a total of 60 s of stretching for each flexibility exercise by adjusting time/duration and repetitions according to individual needs (20). The goal of 60 s of stretch time can be attained by, for example, two, 30 s stretches or four, 15 s stretches (20). Performing flexibility exercises $\geq$2–3 d $\cdot$ wk^{-1} will improve ROM but stretching exercises are most effective when performed daily (20). A stretching routine following these guidelines can be completed by most individuals in $\leq$10 min (20). A summary of the FITT-VP principle of Ex R$_x$ for flexibility exercise is found in *Table 7.7*.

TABLE 7.7. Flexibility Exercise Evidence-Based Recommendations	
FITT-VP	**Evidence-Based Recommendation**
*F*requency	• $\geq$2–3 d $\cdot$ wk^{-1} with daily being most effective
*I*ntensity	• Stretch to the point of feeling tightness or slight discomfort
*T*ime	• Holding a static stretch for 10–30 s is recommended for most adults.
	• In older individuals, holding a stretch for 30–60 s may confer greater benefit.
	• For proprioceptive neuromuscular facilitation (PNF) stretching, a 3–6 s light-to-moderate contraction (*e.g.*, 20%–75% of maximum voluntary contraction) followed by a 10–30 s assisted stretch is desirable.
*T*ype	• A series of flexibility exercises for each of the major muscle-tendon units is recommended.
	• Static flexibility (*i.e.*, active or passive), dynamic flexibility, ballistic flexibility, and PNF are each effective.
*V*olume	• A reasonable target is to perform 60 s of total stretching time for each flexibility exercise.
*P*attern	• Repetition of each flexibility exercise 2–4 times is recommended.
	• Flexibility exercise is most effective when the muscle is warmed through light-to-moderate aerobic activity or passively through external methods such as moist heat packs or hot baths.
*P*rogression	• Methods for optimal progression are unknown.

PNF, proprioceptive neuromuscular facilitation.

FLEXIBILITY VOLUME RECOMMENDATION   F I T T

A total of 60 s of flexibility exercise per joint is recommended. Holding a single flexibility exercise for 10–30 s to the point
of tightness or slight discomfort is effective. Older adults can benefit from
holding the stretch for 30–60 s. A 20%–75% maximum voluntary contraction held for 3–6 s followed by a 10–30 s assisted stretch is recommended
for PNF techniques. Performing flexibility exercises $\geq$2–3 d $\cdot$ wk^{-1} is
recommended with daily flexibility exercise being most effective.

NEUROMOTOR EXERCISE

Neuromotor exercise training involves motor skills such as balance, coordination,
gait, and agility, and proprioceptive training and is sometimes called *functional
fitness training*. Other multifaceted physical activities sometimes considered to
be neuromotor exercise involve varying combinations of neuromotor exercise,
resistance exercise, and flexibility exercise and include physical activities such as
tai ji (tai chi), qigong, and yoga. For older individuals, the benefits of neuromotor
exercise training are clear. Neuromotor exercise training results in improvements
in balance, agility, and muscle strength, and reduces the risk of falls and the fear
of falling (7,20,32) among older adults (see *Chapter 8*). There are few studies of
the benefits of neuromotor training in younger adults, although limited study
suggests that balance and agility training may result in reduced injury in athletes
(20). Because of a lack of research on middle age and younger adults, definitive
recommendations for benefit of neuromotor exercise training cannot be made;
nonetheless, there *may* be benefit especially for individuals participating in physical activities requiring agility, balance, and other motor skills (20).

The optimal effectiveness of the various types of neuromotor exercise, doses
(*i.e.*, FIT), and training regimens are not known for adults of any age (20,32).
Studies that have resulted in improvements have mostly employed training frequencies of $\geq$2–3 d wk^{-1} with exercise sessions of $\geq$20–30 min duration for a
total of $\geq$60 min of neuromotor exercise per week (20,32). There is no available
evidence concerning the number of repetitions of exercises needed, the intensity
of the exercise, or optimal methods for progression. A summary of the FITT-VP
principle of Ex R$_x$ for neuromotor exercise is found in *Table 7.8*.

NEUROMOTOR EXERCISE RECOMMENDATIONS F I T T

Neuromotor exercises involving balance, agility, coor-
dination, and gait are recommended on $\geq$2–3 d $\cdot$ wk^{-1} for older individuals and are likely beneficial for younger adults as well. The optimal duration or number of repetitions of these exercises is not known, but neuromotor exercise routines of $\geq$20–30 min in duration for a total of $\geq$60 min
of neuromotor exercise per week are effective.

TABLE 7.8. Neuromotor Exercise Evidence-Based Recommendations

FITT-VP	Evidence-Based Recommendation
Frequency	• ≥2–3 d · wk^{-1} is recommended
Intensity	• An effective intensity of neuromotor exercise has not been determined.
Time	• ≥20–30 min · d^{-1} may be needed
Type	• Exercises involving motor skills (*e.g.*, balance, agility, coordination, gait), proprioceptive exercise training, and multifaceted activities (*e.g.*, tai ji, yoga) are recommended for older individuals to improve and maintain physical function and reduce falls in those at risk for falling. • The effectiveness of neuromotor exercise training in younger and middle-aged individuals has not been established but there is probable benefit.
Volume	• The optimal volume (*e.g.*, number of repetitions, intensity) is not known.
Pattern	• The optimal pattern of performing neuromotor exercise is not known.
Progression	• Methods for optimal progression are not known.

Adapted from (20).

EXERCISE PROGRAM SUPERVISION

The health/fitness and clinical exercise professional may determine the level of supervision that is optimal for an individual by evaluating information derived from the preparticiption health screening (see *Chapter 2*) and the preexercise evaluation (see *Chapter 3*) that may include health screening, medical evaluation, and/or exercise testing as indicated by the individual's exercise goals and health status. Supervision by an experienced exercise leader can enhance adherence to exercise and may improve safety for individuals with chronic diseases and health conditions (20,32) (see *Chapter 11*). Individualized exercise instruction may be helpful for sedentary adults initiating a new exercise program (20,32).

THE BOTTOM LINE

- An exercise program that includes aerobic, resistance, flexibility, and neuromotor exercise training beyond ADL to improve and maintain physical fitness and health is essential for health/fitness benefits among most adults.
- This edition of the *Guidelines* employs the FITT-VP principle of Ex R$_x$, that is, Frequency (how often), Intensity (how hard), Time (duration or how long), and Type (mode or what kind), with the addition of total Volume (amount) and Progression (advancement).
- The ACSM recommends that most adults engage in moderate intensity, aerobic exercise training ≥30 min · d^{-1}, ≥5 d · wk^{-1} to total ≥150 min · wk^{-1}; vigorous intensity cardiorespiratory exercise training ≥20 min · d^{-1}, ≥3 d · wk^{-1} to total ≥75 min · wk^{-1}; or a combination of moderate and vigorous intensity exercise to total an EE of ≥500–1,000 MET-min · wk^{-1}.

- On 2–3 d · wk^{-1}, adults should also perform resistance exercises for each of the major muscle groups and neuromotor exercise involving balance, agility, gait, and coordination (*e.g.*, such as standing on one leg, walking or running through cones, dance steps).
- A series of flexibility exercises for each of the major muscle tendon groups ≥2–3 d · wk^{-1} is recommended to maintain joint ROM.
- The exercise program should be modified according to an individual's habitual physical activity, physical function, physical fitness level, health status, exercise responses, and stated goals.
- Adults, including physically active adults, should concurrently reduce total time engaged in sedentary behaviors and intersperse frequent, short bouts of standing and physical activity between periods of sedentary activity throughout the day.

Online Resources

2008 Physical Activity Guidelines for All Americans (52):
http://www.health.gov/PAguidelines/

ACSM/AMA ExeRxcise is Medicine:
http://www.exerciseismedicine.org

American College of Sports Medicine position stand on progression models in resistance training (18):
http://www.acsm.org

American College of Sports Medicine position stand on the quantity and quality of Exercise (20):
http://www.acsm.org

American Heart Association:
http://www.heart.org

National Institutes on Aging Exercise and Physical Activity Guide (53):
http://www.nia.nih.gov/HealthInformation/Publications/

National Strength and Conditioning Association:
http://www.nsca-lift.org

Shape Up America:
http://www.shapeup.org

REFERENCES

1. Ainsworth BE, Haskell WL, Leon AS, et al. Compendium of physical activities: classification of energy costs of human physical activities. *Med Sci Sports Exerc.* 1993;25(1):71–80.
2. Ainsworth BE, Haskell WL, Whitt MC, et al. Compendium of physical activities: an update of activity codes and MET intensities. *Med Sci Sports Exerc.* 2000;32(9 Suppl):S498–504.
3. American College of Sports Medicine. American College of Sports Medicine Position Stand. Exercise and physical activity for older adults. *Med Sci Sports Exerc.* 1998;30(6):992–1008.
4. American College of Sports Medicine. American College of Sports Medicine position stand. Osteoporosis and exercise. *Med Sci Sports Exerc.* 1995;27(4):i–vii.
5. American College of Sports Medicine. American College of Sports Medicine position stand. Progression models in resistance training for healthy adults. *Med Sci Sports Exerc.* 2009;41(3):687–708.
6. American College of Sports Medicine, American Diabetes Association. Exercise and type 2 diabetes: American College of Sports Medicine and the American Diabetes Association: joint position statement. Exercise and type 2 diabetes. *Med Sci Sports Exerc.* 2010;42(12):2282–303.

7. American College of Sports Medicine, Chodzko-Zajko WJ, Proctor DN, et al. American College of Sports Medicine position stand. Exercise and physical activity for older adults. *Med Sci Sports Exerc.* 2009;41(7):1510–30.

8. Armstrong LE, Brubaker PH, Whaley MH, Otto RM, American College of Sports Medicine. *ACSM's Guidelines for Exercise Testing and Prescription.* 7th ed. Baltimore (MD): Lippincott Williams & Wilkins; 2005. 366 p.

9. Astrand PO. *Experimental Studies of Physical Working Capacity in Relation to Sex and Age.* Copenhagen (Denmark): Musksgaard; 1952. 171 p.

10. Bassett DR Jr, Wyatt HR, Thompson H, Peters JC, Hill JO. Pedometer-measured physical activity and health behaviors in U.S. adults. *Med Sci Sports Exerc.* 2010;42(10):1819–25.

11. Bonnefoy M, Jauffret M, Jusot JF. Muscle power of lower extremities in relation to functional ability and nutritional status in very elderly people. *J Nutr Health Aging.* 2007;11(3):223–8.

12. Borg GA. Perceived exertion. *Exerc Sport Sci Rev.* 1974;2:131–53.

13. Borg G, Hassmen P, Lagerstrom M. Perceived exertion related to heart rate and blood lactate during arm and leg exercise. *Eur J Appl Physiol Occup Physiol.* 1987;56(6):679–85.

14. Borg G, Ljunggren G, Ceci R. The increase of perceived exertion, aches and pain in the legs, heart rate and blood lactate during exercise on a bicycle ergometer. *Eur J Appl Physiol Occup Physiol.* 1985;54(4):343–9.

15. Chan BK, Marshall LM, Winters KM, Faulkner KA, Schwartz AV, Orwoll ES. Incident fall risk and physical activity and physical performance among older men: the Osteoporotic Fractures in Men Study. *Am J Epidemiol.* 2007;165(6):696–703.

16. Church TS, Earnest CP, Skinner JS, Blair SN. Effects of different doses of physical activity on cardiorespiratory fitness among sedentary, overweight or obese postmenopausal women with elevated blood pressure: a randomized controlled trial. *JAMA.* 2007;297(19):2081–91.

17. Donnelly JE, Blair SN, Jakicic JM, et al. American College of Sports Medicine Position Stand. Appropriate physical activity intervention strategies for weight loss and prevention of weight regain for adults. *Med Sci Sports Exerc.* 2009;41(2):459–71.

18. Ehrman JK, American College of Sports Medicine. *ACSM's Resource Manual for Guidelines for Exercise Testing and Prescription.* 6th ed. Baltimore (MD): Lippincott Williams & Wilkins; 2009. 868 p.

19. Fox SM 3rd, Naughton JP, Haskell WL. Physical activity and the prevention of coronary heart disease. *Ann Clin Res.* 1971;3(6):404–32.

20. Garber CE, Blissmer B, Deschenes MR, et al. American College of Sports Medicine Position Stand. The quantity and quality of exercise for developing and maintaining cardiorespiratory, musculoskeletal, and neuromotor fitness in apparently healthy adults: guidance for prescribing exercise. *Med Sci Sports Exerc.* 2011;43(7):1334–59.

21. Gellish RL, Goslin BR, Olson RE, McDonald A, Russi GD, Moudgil VK. Longitudinal modeling of the relationship between age and maximal heart rate. *Med Sci Sports Exerc.* 2007;39(5):822–9.

22. Glass S, Dwyer GB, American College of Sports Medicine. *ACSM's Metabolic Calculations Handbook.* Baltimore (MD): Lippincott Williams & Wilkins; 2007. 128 p.

23. Gulati M, Shaw LJ, Thisted RA, Black HR, Merz CN, Arnsdorf MF. Heart rate response to exercise stress testing in asymptomatic women. The St. James Women Take Heart Project. *Circulation.* 2010; 122(2):130–7.

24. Hardy CJ, Rejeski WJ. Not what, but how one feels: the measurement of affect during exercise. *J Sport Exer Psych.* 1989;11:304–17.

25. Haskell WL, Lee IM, Pate RR, et al. Physical activity and public health: updated recommendation for adults from the American College of Sports Medicine and the American Heart Association. *Med Sci Sports Exerc.* 2007;39(8):1423–34.

26. Hawkins S, Wiswell R. Rate and mechanism of maximal oxygen consumption decline with aging: implications for exercise training. *Sports Med.* 2003;33(12):877–88.

27. Howley ET. Type of activity: resistance, aerobic and leisure versus occupational physical activity. *Med Sci Sports Exerc.* 2001;33(6 Suppl):S364,9; discussion S419–20.

28. Kang M, Marshall SJ, Barreira TV, Lee JO. Effect of pedometer-based physical activity interventions: a meta-analysis. *Res Q Exerc Sport.* 2009;80(3):648–55.

29. McHugh MP, Cosgrave CH. To stretch or not to stretch: the role of stretching in injury prevention and performance. *Scand J Med Sci Sports.* 2010;20(2):169–81.

30. McMillian DJ, Moore JH, Hatler BS, Taylor DC. Dynamic vs. static-stretching warm up: the effect on power and agility performance. *J Strength Cond Res.* 2006;20(3):492–9.

31. Messier SP. Obesity and osteoarthritis: disease genesis and nonpharmacologic weight management. *Med Clin North Am.* 2009;93(1):145,59, xi–xii.

32. Nelson ME, Rejeski WJ, Blair SN, et al. Physical activity and public health in older adults: recommendation from the American College of Sports Medicine and the American Heart Association. *Med Sci Sports Exerc.* 2007;39(8):1435–45.

33. Noble BJ, Borg GA, Jacobs I, Ceci R, Kaiser P. A category-ratio perceived exertion scale: relationship to blood and muscle lactates and heart rate. *Med Sci Sports Exerc.* 1983;15(6):523–8.

34. Owen N, Healy GN, Matthews CE, Dunstan DW. Too much sitting: the population health science of sedentary behavior. *Exerc Sport Sci Rev.* 2010;38(3):105–13.

35. Persinger R, Foster C, Gibson M, Fater DC, Porcari JP. Consistency of the talk test for exercise prescription. *Med Sci Sports Exerc.* 2004;36(9):1632–6.

36. Pescatello LS, Franklin BA, Fagard R, et al. American College of Sports Medicine position stand. Exercise and hypertension. *Med Sci Sports Exerc.* 2004;36(3):533–53.

37. Peterson MD, Rhea MR, Alvar BA. Applications of the dose-response for muscular strength development: a review of meta-analytic efficacy and reliability for designing training prescription. *J Strength Cond Res.* 2005;19(4):950–8.

38. *Physical Activity Guidelines Advisory Committee Report, 2008* [Internet]. Washington (DC): U.S. Department of Health and Human Services; 2008. 78 p. [cited 2011 Jan 6]. Available from: http://www.health.gov/paguidelines/Report/pdf/CommitteeReport.pdf

39. Rees SS, Murphy AJ, Watsford ML, McLachlan KA, Coutts AJ. Effects of proprioceptive neuromuscular facilitation stretching on stiffness and force-producing characteristics of the ankle in active women. *J Strength Cond Res.* 2007;21(2):572–7.

40. Robertson RJ, Goss FL, Dube J, et al. Validation of the adult OMNI scale of perceived exertion for cycle ergometer exercise. *Med Sci Sports Exerc.* 2004;36(1):102–8.

41. Robertson RJ, Goss FL, Rutkowski J, et al. Concurrent validation of the OMNI perceived exertion scale for resistance exercise. *Med Sci Sports Exerc.* 2003;35(2):333–41.

42. Sharman MJ, Cresswell AG, Riek S. Proprioceptive neuromuscular facilitation stretching: mechanisms and clinical implications. *Sports Med.* 2006;36(11):929–39.

43. Slemenda C, Heilman DK, Brandt KD, et al. Reduced quadriceps strength relative to body weight: a risk factor for knee osteoarthritis in women? *Arthritis Rheum.* 1998;41(11):1951–9.

44. Swain DP. Energy cost calculations for exercise prescription: an update. *Sports Med.* 2000;30(1):17–22.

45. Swain DP, American College of Sports Medicine. *ACSM's Resource Manual for Guidelines for Exercise Testing and Prescription.* 7th ed. Baltimore (MD): Lippincott Williams & Wilkins; 2014.

46. Swain DP, Franklin BA. VO(2) reserve and the minimal intensity for improving cardiorespiratory fitness. *Med Sci Sports Exerc.* 2002;34(1):152–7.

47. Swain DP, Leutholtz BC. Heart rate reserve is equivalent to %VO2 reserve, not to %VO2max. *Med Sci Sports Exerc.* 1997;29(3):410–4.

48. Tanaka H, Monahan KD, Seals DR. Age-predicted maximal heart rate revisited. *J Am Coll Cardiol.* 2001;37(1):153–6.

49. Thompson WR, Gordon NF, Pescatello LS, American College of Sports Medicine. *ACSM's Guidelines for Exercise Testing and Prescription.* 8th ed. Baltimore (MD): Lippincott Williams & Wilkins; 2010. 400 p.

50. Tudor-Locke C, Hatano Y, Pangrazi RP, Kang M. Revisiting "how many steps are enough?" *Med Sci Sports Exerc.* 2008;40(7 Suppl):S537–43.

51. U.S. Department of Agriculture. *Report of the Dietary Guidelines Advisory Committee on the Dietary Guidelines for Americans, 2010* [Internet]. Washington (DC): U.S. Goverment Printing Office; 2010. 453 p. [cited 2011 Jan 6]. Available from: http://www.cnpp.usda.gov/DGAs2010-DGACReport.htm

52. U.S. Department of Health and Human Services. *2008 Physical Activity Guidelines for Americans* [Internet]. Washington (DC): U.S. Department of Health and Human Services; 2008. 78 p. [cited 2011 Jan 6]. Available from: http://www.health.gov/paguidelines/pdf/paguide.pdf

53. U.S. Department of Health and Human Services. *Exercise & Physical Activity: Your Everyday Guide from the National Institute on Aging* [Internet]. Bethesda (MD): National Institute on Aging, U.S. National Institutes of Health; 2011. 126 p. [cited 2011 Apr 15]. Available from: http://www.nia.nih.gov/HealthInformation/Publications/ExerciseGuide/

54. U.S. Department of Health and Human Services, United States Department of Agriculture, United States Dietary Guidelines Advisory Committee. *Dietary Guidelines for Americans, 2005.* 6th ed. Washington (DC): G.P.O; 2005. 71 p.

55. Utter AC, Robertson RJ, Green JM, Suminski RR, McAnulty SR, Nieman DC. Validation of the Adult OMNI Scale of perceived exertion for walking/running exercise. *Med Sci Sports Exerc.* 2004;36(10):1776–80.

56. Winters MV, Blake CG, Trost JS, et al. Passive versus active stretching of hip flexor muscles in subjects with limited hip extension: a randomized clinical trial. *Phys Ther.* 2004;84(9):800–7.

57. Woolstenhulme MT, Griffiths CM, Woolstenhulme EM, Parcell AC. Ballistic stretching increases flexibility and acute vertical jump height when combined with basketball activity. *J Strength Cond Res.* 2006;20(4):799–803.

58. Zhu N, Suarez-Lopez JR, Sidney S, et al. Longitudinal examination of age-predicted symptom-limited exercise maximum HR. *Med Sci Sports Exerc.* 2010;42(8):1519–27.

8

Exercise Prescription for Healthy Populations with Special Considerations and Environmental Considerations

PREGNANCY

The acute physiologic responses to exercise are generally increased during pregnancy compared with nonpregnancy (121) (see *Table 8.1*). Healthy, pregnant women without exercise contraindications (2) (see *Box 8.1*) are encouraged to exercise throughout pregnancy. Regular exercise during pregnancy provides health/fitness benefits to the mother and child (2,34). Exercise may also reduce the risk of developing conditions associated with pregnancy such as pregnancy-induced hypertension and gestational diabetes mellitus (34,60). The American College of Sports Medicine (ACSM) endorses guidelines (76) regarding exercise in pregnancy and the postpartum period set forth by the American College of Obstetricians and Gynecologists (2,11), the Joint Committee of the Society of Obstetricians and Gynecologists of Canada (32), and the Canadian Society for Exercise Physiology (CSEP) (32). Collectively, these guidelines outline the importance of exercise during pregnancy and also provide guidance on exercise prescription (Ex R_x) and contraindications to beginning and continuing exercise during pregnancy. The CSEP Physical Activity Readiness Medical Examination, termed the *PARmed-X for Pregnancy*, should be used for the health screening of pregnant women before their participation in exercise programs (88) (see *Figure 8.1*).

EXERCISE TESTING

Maximal exercise testing should not be performed on women who are pregnant unless medically necessary (2,11,32). If a maximal exercise test is warranted, the test should be performed with physician supervision after the woman has been medically evaluated for contraindications to exercise (see *Figure 8.1*). A woman who was sedentary before pregnancy or who has a medical condition (see *Box 8.1*) should receive clearance from her physician or midwife before beginning an exercise program.

EXERCISE PRESCRIPTION

The recommended Ex R_x for women who are pregnant should be modified according to the woman's symptoms, discomforts, and abilities during pregnancy. It is important to be aware of contraindications for exercising during pregnancy (see *Box 8.1*).

TABLE 8.1. Physiologic Responses to Acute Exercise during Pregnancy Compared to Nonpregnancy (121)

Oxygen uptake (during weight-dependent exercise)	Increase
Heart rate	Increase
Stroke volume	Increase
Cardiac output	Increase
Tidal volume	Increase
Minute ventilation	Increase
Ventilatory equivalent for oxygen ($\dot{V}E/\dot{V}O_2$)	Increase
Ventilatory equivalent for carbon dioxide ($\dot{V}O_{2max}/\dot{V}CO_2$)	Increase
Systolic blood pressure	No change/decrease
Diastolic blood pressure	No change/decrease

BOX 8.1   Contraindications for Exercising during Pregnancy

RELATIVE
- Severe anemia
- Unevaluated maternal cardiac dysrhythmia
- Chronic bronchitis
- Poorly controlled Type 1 diabetes mellitus
- Extreme morbid obesity
- Extreme underweight
- History of extremely sedentary lifestyle
- Intrauterine growth restriction in current pregnancy
- Poorly controlled hypertension
- Orthopedic limitations
- Poorly controlled seizure disorder
- Poorly controlled hyperthyroidism
- Heavy smoker

ABSOLUTE
- Hemodynamically significant heart disease
- Restrictive lung disease
- Incompetent cervix/cerclage
- Multiple gestation at risk for premature labor
- Persistent second or third trimester bleeding
- Placenta previa after 26 wk of gestation
- Premature labor during the current pregnancy
- Ruptured membranes
- Preeclampsia/pregnancy-induced hypertension

Reprinted with permission from (2).

Physical Activity Readiness
Medical Examination for
Pregnancy (2002)

PARmed-X for PREGNANCY PHYSICAL ACTIVITY READINESS
MEDICAL EXAMINATION

PARmed-X for PREGNANCY is a guideline for health screening prior to participation in a prenatal fitness class or other exercise.

Healthy women with uncomplicated pregnancies can integrate physical activity into their daily living and can participate without significant risks either to themselves or to their unborn child. Postulated benefits of such programs include improved aerobic and muscular fitness, promotion of appropriate weight gain, and facilitation of labour. Regular exercise may also help to prevent gestational glucose intolerance and pregnancy-induced hypertension.

The safety of prenatal exercise programs depends on an adequate level of maternal-fetal physiological reserve. PARmed-X for PREGNANCY is a convenient checklist and prescription for use by health care providers to evaluate pregnant patients who want to enter a prenatal fitness program and for ongoing medical surveillance of exercising pregnant patients.

Instructions for use of the 4-page PARmed-X for PREGNANCY are the following:

1. The patient should fill out the section on PATIENT INFORMATION and the PRE-EXERCISE HEALTH CHECKLIST (PART 1, 2, 3, and 4 on p. 1) and give the form to the health care provider monitoring her pregnancy.
2. The health care provider should check the information provided by the patient for accuracy and fill out SECTION C on CONTRAINDICATIONS (p. 2) based on current medical information.
3. If no exercise contraindications exist, the HEALTH EVALUATION FORM (p. 3) should be completed, signed by the health care provider, and given by the patient to her prenatal fitness professional.

In addition to prudent medical care, participation in appropriate types, intensities and amounts of exercise is recommended to increase the likelihood of a beneficial pregnancy outcome. PARmed-X for PREGNANCY provides recommendations for individualized exercise prescription (p. 3) and program safety (p. 4).

NOTE: Sections A and B should be completed by the patient before the appointment with the health care provider.

A PATIENT INFORMATION

NAME _____
ADDRESS _____
TELEPHONE _____ BIRTHDATE _____ HEALTH INSURANCE No. _____
NAME OF PRENATAL FITNESS PROFESSIONAL _____
PRENATAL FITNESS PROFESSIONAL?S PHONE NUMBER _____

B PRE-EXERCISE HEALTH CHECKLIST

PART 1: GENERAL HEALTH STATUS

In the past, have you experienced (check YES or NO):

	YES	NO
1. Miscarriage in an earlier pregnacy?	❑	❑
2. Other pregnancy complications?	❑	❑
3. I have completed a PAR-Q within the last 30 days.	❑	❑

If you answered YES to question 1 or 2, please explain:

Number of previous pregnancies? _____

PART 2: STATUS OF CURRENT PREGNANCY

Due Date: _____

During this pregnancy, have you experienced:

	YES	NO
1. Marked fatigue?	❑	❑
2. Bleeding from the vagina ("spotting")?	❑	❑
3. Unexplained faintness or dizziness?	❑	❑
4. Unexplained abdominal pain?	❑	❑
5. Sudden swelling of ankles, hands or face?	❑	❑
6. Persistent headaches or problems with headaches?	❑	❑
7. Swelling, pain or redness in the calf of one leg?	❑	❑
8. Absence of fetal movement after 6th month?	❑	❑
9. Failure to gain weight after 5th month?	❑	❑

If you answered YES to any of the above questions, please explain:

PART 3: ACTIVITY HABITS DURING THE PAST MONTH

1. List only regular fitness/recreational activities:

INTENSITY	FREQUENCY (times/week)			TIME (minutes/day)		
	1-2	2-4	4+	<20	20-40	40+
Heavy	___	___	___	___	___	___
Medium	___	___	___	___	___	___
Light	___	___	___	___	___	___

2. Does your regular occupation (job/home) activity involve:

	YES	NO
Heavy Lifting?	❑	❑
Frequent walking/stair climbing?	❑	❑
Occasional walking (>once/hr)?	❑	❑
Prolonged standing?	❑	❑
Mainly sitting?	❑	❑
Normal daily activity?	❑	❑
3. Do you currently smoke tobacco?*	❑	❑
4. Do you consume alcohol?*	❑	❑

PART 4: PHYSICAL ACTIVITY INTENTIONS

What physical activity do you intend to do?

Is this a change from what you currently do? ❑ YES ❑ NO

*NOTE: PREGNANT WOMEN ARE STRONGLY ADVISED NOT TO SMOKE OR CONSUME ALCOHOL DURING PREGNANCY AND DURING LACTATION.

CSEP © Canadian Society for Exercise Physiology
SCPE Société canadienne de physiologie de l'exercice

Supported by: Health Santé Canada Canada

■ **FIGURE 8.1.** Physical Activity Readiness (PARmed-X) for Pregnancy. Reprinted with permission from (88).

Physical Activity Readiness
Medical Examination for
Pregnancy (2002)

PARmed-X for PREGNANCY PHYSICAL ACTIVITY READINESS MEDICAL EXAMINATION

C CONTRAINDICATIONS TO EXERCISE: to be completed by your health care provider

Absolute Contraindications			Relative Contraindications		
Does the patient have:			*Does the patient have:*		
	YES	NO		YES	NO
1. Ruptured membranes, premature labour?	❑	❑	1. History of spontaneous abortion or premature labour in previous pregnancies?	❑	❑
2. Persistent second or third trimester bleeding/placenta previa?	❑	❑	2. Mild/moderate cardiovascular or respiratory disease (e.g., chronic hypertension, asthma)?	❑	❑
3. Pregnancy-induced hypertension or pre-eclampsia?	❑	❑	3. Anemia or iron deficiency? (Hb < 100 g/L)?	❑	❑
4. Incompetent cervix?	❑	❑	4. Malnutrition or eating disorder (anorexia, bulimia)?	❑	❑
5. Evidence of intrauterine growth restriction?	❑	❑	5. Twin pregnancy after 28th week?	❑	❑
6. High-order pregnancy (e.g., triplets)?	❑	❑	6. Other significant medical condition?	❑	❑
7. Uncontrolled Type I diabetes, hypertension or thyroid disease, other serious cardiovascular, respiratory or systemic disorder?	❑	❑	Please specify: _____		
			NOTE: Risk may exceed benefits of regular physical activity. The decision to be physically active or not should be made with qualified medical advice.		
PHYSICAL ACTIVITY RECOMMENDATION: ❑ Recommended/Approved ❑ Contraindicated					

■ **FIGURE 8.1.** (*Continued*)

FITT RECOMMENDATIONS FOR WOMEN WHO ARE PREGNANT

FITT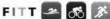

Aerobic Exercise

Frequency: 3–4 d · wk^{-1}. Research suggests an ideal frequency of 3–4 d · wk^{-1} because frequency has been shown to be a determinant of birth weight. Women who do not exercise within the recommended frequency (*i.e.*, ≥5 d · wk^{-1} or ≤2 d · wk^{-1}) increase their risk of having a low-birth-weight baby (19). Infants with a low birth weight for gestational age are at risk for perinatal complications and developmental problems (19), thus prevention of low birth weight is an important health goal.

Intensity: Because maximal exercise testing is rarely performed with women who are pregnant, heart rate (HR) ranges that correspond to moderate intensity exercise have been developed and validated for low-risk pregnant women based on age while taking fitness levels into account (see *Box 8.2*) (32,76). Moderate intensity exercise is recommended for women with a prepregnancy body mass index (BMI) <25 kg · m^2. Light intensity exercise is recommended for women with a prepregnancy BMI ≥25 kg · m^2 (31,32,76).

Time: ≥15 min · d^{-1} gradually increasing to a maximum of 30 min · d^{-1} of accumulated moderate intensity exercise to total 120 min · wk^{-1}. A 10–15 min warm-up and a 10–15 min cool-down of light intensity, physical activity is suggested before and after the exercise session, respectively (32), resulting in approximately 150 min · wk^{-1} of accumulated exercise. Women with a prepregnancy BMI of ≥ 25 kg $\cdot$ m^2 who have been medically prescreened can exercise at a light intensity start- ing at 25 min $\cdot$ d^{-1}, adding 2 min $\cdot$ wk^{-1} until 40 min 3–4 d $\cdot$ wk^{-1} is achieved (77).

Type: Dynamic, rhythmic physical activities that use large muscle groups such as walking and cycling.

Progression: The optimal time to progress is after the first trimester (13 wk) because the discomforts and risks of pregnancy are lowest at that time. Gradual progression from a minimum of 15 min $\cdot$ d^{-1}, 3 d $\cdot$ wk^{-1} (at the appropriate target HR or RPE) to a maximum of approximately 30 min $\cdot$ d^{-1}, 4 d $\cdot$ wk^{-1} (at the appropriate target HR or RPE) (32).

BOX 8.2	Heart Rate Ranges That Correspond to Moderate Intensity Exercise for Low-Risk Normal Weight Women Who Are Pregnant and to Light Intensity Exercise for Low-Risk Women Who Are Pregnant and Overweight or Obese (32,76)

BMI <25 kg $\cdot$ m^2

Age (yr)	Fitness Level	Heart Rate Range (beats $\cdot$ min^{-1})[a]
<20	—	140–155
20–29	Low	129–144
	Active	135–150
	Fit	145–160
30–39	Low	128–144
	Active	130–145
	Fit	140–156

BMI ≥ 25 kg $\cdot$ m^2

Age (yr)	Heart Rate Range (beats $\cdot$ min^{-1})[a]
20–29	102–124
30–39	101–120

BMI, body mass index.
[a]Target HR ranges were derived from peak exercise tests in medically prescreened low-risk women who were pregnant (76).

SPECIAL CONSIDERATIONS

- Women who are pregnant and sedentary or have a medical condition should gradually increase physical activity levels to meet the recommended levels earlier as per preparticipation completion of the PARmed-X for Pregnancy (88) (see *Figure 8.1*).
- Women who are pregnant and severely obese and/or have gestational diabetes mellitus or hypertension should consult their physician before beginning an exercise program and have their Ex R_x adjusted to their medical condition, symptoms, and physical fitness level.
- Women who are pregnant should avoid contact sports and sports/activities that may cause loss of balance or trauma to the mother or fetus. Examples of sports/activities to avoid include soccer, basketball, ice hockey, roller blading, horseback riding, skiing/snow boarding, scuba diving, and vigorous intensity, racquet sports.
- Exercise should be terminated immediately with medical follow-up should any of these signs or symptoms occur: vaginal bleeding, dyspnea before exertion, dizziness, headache, chest pain, muscle weakness, calf pain or swelling, preterm labor, decreased fetal movement (once detected), and amniotic fluid leakage (2). In the case of calf pain and swelling, thrombophlebitis should be ruled out.
- Women who are pregnant should avoid exercising in the supine position after 16 wk of pregnancy to ensure that venous obstruction does not occur (32).
- Women who are pregnant should avoid performing the Valsalva maneuver during exercise.
- Women who are pregnant should avoid exercising in a hot humid environment, be well hydrated, and dressed appropriately to avoid heat stress. See this chapter and the ACSM position stands on exercising in the heat (6) and fluid replacement (8) for additional information.
- During pregnancy, the metabolic demand increases by $\sim$300 kcal $\cdot$ d^{-1}. Women should increase caloric intake to meet the caloric costs of pregnancy and exercise. To avoid excessive weight gain during pregnancy, consult appropriate weight gain guidelines based on prepregnancy BMI available from the Institute of Medicine and the National Research Council (118).
- Women who are pregnant may participate in a strength training program that incorporates all major muscle groups with a resistance that permits multiple submaximal repetitions (*i.e.*, 12–15 repetitions) to be performed to a point of moderate fatigue. Isometric muscle actions and the Valsalva maneuver should be avoided as should the supine position after 16 wk of pregnancy (32). Kegel exercises and those that strengthen the pelvic floor are recommended to decrease the risk of incontinence (75).
- Generally, gradual exercise in the postpartum period may begin $\sim$4–6 wk after a normal vaginal delivery or about 8–10 wk (with medical clearance) after a cesarean section delivery (75). Deconditioning typically occurs during the initial postpartum period so women should gradually increase physical activity levels until prepregnancy physical fitness levels are achieved. Light-to-moderate intensity exercise does not interfere with breastfeeding (75).

THE BOTTOM LINE

• Women who are pregnant and healthy are encouraged to exercise throughout pregnancy with the Ex R_x modified according to symptoms, discomforts, and abilities. Women who are pregnant should exercise 3–4 d · wk^{-1} for ≥15 min · d^{-1} gradually increasing to a maximum of 30 min · d^{-1} for each exercise session, accumulating a total of 150 min · wk^{-1} of physical activity that includes the warm up and cool down. Moderate intensity exercise is recommended for women with a prepregnancy BMI <25 kg · m^2. Light intensity exercise is recommended for women with a prepregnancy BMI of ≥25 kg · m^2.

Online Resources

The American Congress of Obstetricians and Gynecologists:
http://www.acog.org

The Canadian Society for Exercise Physiology (PARmed-X for Pregnancy):
http://www.csep.ca/english/view.asp?x=698

The Society of Obstetricians and Gynecologists of Canada:
http://www.sogc.org

CHILDREN AND ADOLESCENTS

Children and adolescents (defined as individuals 6–17 yr) are more physically active than their adult counterparts. However, only our youngest children are as physically active as recommended by experts (114), and most young individuals above the age of 10 yr do not meet prevailing physical activity guidelines. The *2008 Physical Activity Guidelines* call for children and adolescents to engage in at least 60 min · day^{-1} of moderate-to-vigorous intensity, physical activity and to include vigorous intensity, physical activity, resistance exercise, and bone loading activity on at least 3 d · wk^{-1} (114). In the United States, the prevalence of meeting this guideline was 42% in children aged 6–11 yr, and in adolescents aged 12–19 yr the prevalence was only 8% (113).

Children and adolescents are physiologically adaptive to endurance exercise training (52,85), resistance training (14,69), and bone loading exercise (66,68). Further, exercise training produces improvements in cardiometabolic risk factors (63,80). Thus, the benefits of exercise are much greater than the risks. However, because prepubescent children have immature skeletons, younger children should not participate in excessive amounts of vigorous intensity exercise.

Most young individuals are healthy, and it is safe for them to start moderate intensity exercise training without medical screening. Clinical exercise testing should be reserved for children in whom there is a specific clinical indication. Physiologic responses to acute, graded exercise are qualitatively similar to those seen in adults. However, there are important quantitative differences, many of which are related to the effects of body mass, muscle mass, and height. In addition, it is notable children have a much lower anaerobic capacity than adults limiting their ability to perform sustained vigorous intensity exercise (14).

EXERCISE TESTING

Generally, the adult guidelines for standard exercise testing apply to children and adolescents (see *Chapter 5*). However, the physiologic responses during exercise differ from those of adults (see *Table 8.2*) so that the following issues should be considered (87,121):

- Exercise testing for clinical or health/fitness purposes is generally not indicated for children or adolescents unless there is a health concern.
- The exercise testing protocol should be based on the reason the test is being performed and the functional capability of the child or adolescent.
- Children and adolescents should be familiarized with the test protocol and procedure before testing to minimize stress and maximize the potential for a successful test.
- Treadmill and cycle ergometers should be available for testing. Treadmills tend to elicit a higher peak oxygen uptake ($\dot{V}O_{2peak}$) and maximum HR (HR_{max}). Cycle ergometers provide less risk for injury but need to be correctly sized for the child or adolescent.
- Compared to adults, children and adolescents are mentally and psychologically immature and may require extra motivation and support during the exercise test.

In addition, health/fitness testing may be performed outside of the clinical setting. In these types of settings, the Fitnessgram test battery may be used to

TABLE 8.2. Physiologic Responses to Acute Exercise in Children Compared to Adults (56,111)

Variable	
Absolute oxygen uptake	Lower
Relative oxygen uptake	Higher
Heart rate	Higher
Cardiac output	Lower
Stroke volume	Lower
Systolic blood pressure	Lower
Diastolic blood pressure	Lower
Respiratory rate	Higher
Tidal volume	Lower
Minute ventilation	Lower
Respiratory exchange ratio	Lower

assess the components of health-related fitness in youth (39). The components of the Fitnessgram test battery include body composition (*i.e.*, BMI or skinfold thicknesses), cardiorespiratory fitness (CRF) (*i.e.*, 1-min walk/run and PACER), muscular fitness (*i.e.*, curl-up test and pull-up/push-up tests), and flexibility (*i.e.*, sit-and-reach test).

EXERCISE PRESCRIPTION

The Ex R$_x$ guidelines outlined in this chapter for children and adolescents establish the minimal amount of physical activity needed to achieve the health/fitness benefits associated with regular physical activity (114). Children and adolescents should be encouraged to participate in various physical activities that are enjoyable and age appropriate.

FITT RECOMMENDATIONS FOR CHILDREN AND ADOLESCENTS

FITT

Aerobic Exercise

Frequency: Daily.

Intensity: Most should be moderate-to-vigorous intensity aerobic exercise and should include vigorous intensity at least 3 d · wk^{-1}. Moderate intensity corresponds to noticeable increases in HR and breathing. Vigorous intensity corresponds to substantial increases in HR and breathing.

Time: ≥60 min · d^{-1}.

Type: Enjoyable and developmentally appropriate aerobic physical activities, including running, brisk walking, swimming, dancing, and bicycling.

Muscle Strengthening Exercise

Frequency: ≥3 d · wk^{-1}.

Time: As part of their 60 min · d^{-1} or more of exercise.

Type: Muscle strengthening physical activities can be unstructured (*e.g.*, playing on playground equipment, climbing trees, tug-of-war) or structured (*e.g.*, lifting weights, working with resistance bands).

Bone Strengthening Exercise

Frequency: ≥3 d · wk^{-1}.

Time: As part of 60 min · d^{-1} or more of exercise.

Type: Bone strengthening activities include running, jumping rope, basketball, tennis, resistance training, and hopscotch.

SPECIAL CONSIDERATIONS

- Children and adolescents may safely participate in strength training activities provided they receive proper instruction and supervision. Generally, adult guidelines for resistance training may be applied (see *Chapter 7*). Eight to 15 submaximal repetitions of an exercise should be performed to the point of moderate fatigue with good mechanical form before the resistance is increased.

- Because of immature thermoregulatory systems, youth should avoid exercise in hot humid environments and be properly hydrated. See this chapter and the ACSM position stands on exercising in the heat (6) and fluid replacement (8) for additional information.

- Children and adolescents who are overweight or physically inactive may not be able to achieve 60 min $\cdot$ d^{-1} of moderate-to-vigorous intensity, physical activity. These individuals should start out with moderate intensity, physical activity as tolerated and gradually increase the frequency and time of physical activity to achieve the 60 min $\cdot$ d^{-1} goal. Vigorous intensity, physical activity can then be gradually added at least 3 d $\cdot$ wk^{-1}.

- Children and adolescents with diseases or disabilities such as asthma, diabetes mellitus, obesity, cystic fibrosis, and cerebral palsy should have their Ex R$_x$ tailored to their condition, symptoms, and physical fitness level (see *Chapter 10*).

- Efforts should be made to decrease sedentary activities (*i.e.*, television watching, surfing the Internet, and playing video games) and increase activities that promote lifelong activity and fitness (*i.e.*, walking and cycling).

THE BOTTOM LINE

- Most children >10 yr do not meet the recommended physical activity guidelines. Children and adolescents should participate in a variety of age appropriate physical activities to develop CRF and muscular and bone strength. Exercise supervisors and leaders should be mindful of the external temperature and hydration levels of children who exercise because of their immature thermoregulatory systems.

Online Resources

U.S. Department of Health and Human Services. *2008 Physical Activity Guidelines for Americans* (2008). U.S. Department of Health and Human Services [Internet]:
http://www.health.gov/paguidelines/default/aspx

U.S. Department of Health and Human Services (2008). *Physical Activity Guidelines Advisory Committee Report, 2008.* Washington (DC): USDHHS (91):
http://www.health.gov/paguidelines/committeereport.aspx

OLDER ADULTS

The term *older adult* (defined as individuals ≥65 yr and individuals 50–64 yr with clinically significant conditions or physical limitations that affect movement, physical fitness, or physical activity) represents a diverse spectrum of ages and physiologic capabilities (107). Because physiologic aging does not occur uniformly across the population, individuals of similar chronological age may differ dramatically in their response to exercise. In addition, it is difficult to distinguish the effects of aging on physiologic function from the effects of deconditioning or disease. Health status is often a better indicator of ability to engage in physical activity than chronological age. Individuals with chronic disease should be in consultation with a health care provider who can guide them with their exercise program.

Overwhelming evidence exists that supports the benefits of physical activity in (a) slowing physiologic changes of aging that impair exercise capacity; (b) optimizing age-related changes in body composition; (c) promoting psychological and cognitive well-being; (d) managing chronic diseases; (e) reducing the risks of physical disability; and (f) increasing longevity (7,106). Despite these benefits, older adults are the least physically active of all age groups. Although recent trends indicate a slight improvement in reported physical activity, only about 22% of individuals ≥65 yr engage in regular physical activity. The percentage of reported physical activity decreases with advancing age with fewer than 11% of individuals >85 yr engaging in regular physical activity (38).

To safely administer an exercise test and develop a sound Ex R$_x$ requires knowledge of the effects of aging on physiologic function at rest and during exercise. *Table 8.3* provides a list of age-related changes in key physiologic variables. Underlying disease and medication use may alter the expected response to acute exercise.

TABLE 8.3. Effects of Aging on Selected Physiologic and Health-Related Variables (107)

Variable	Change
Resting heart rate	Unchanged
Maximum heart rate	Lower
Maximum cardiac output	Lower
Resting and exercise blood pressure	Higher
Absolute and relative maximum oxygen uptake reserve ($\dot{V}O_2R_{max}$ L · min^{-1} and mL · kg^{-1} · min^{-1})	Lower
Residual volume	Higher
Vital capacity	Lower
Reaction time	Slower
Muscular strength	Lower
Flexibility	Lower
Bone mass	Lower
Fat-free body mass	Lower
% Body fat	Higher
Glucose tolerance	Lower
Recovery time	Longer

EXERCISE TESTING

Most older adults do not require an exercise test prior to initiating a moderate intensity, physical activity program. For older adults with multiple risk factors as defined in *Table 2.2*, an individual is considered at moderate risk for adverse responses to exercise and is advised to undergo medical examination and exercise testing before initiating vigorous intensity exercise (see *Figure 2.4*). Exercise testing may require subtle differences in protocol, methodology, and dosage. The following list details the special considerations for testing older adults (107):

- The initial workload should be light (*i.e.*, <3 metabolic equivalents [METs]) and workload increments should be small (*i.e.*, 0.5–1.0 MET) for those with low work capacities. The Naughton treadmill protocol is a good example of such a protocol (see *Figure 5.3*).
- A cycle ergometer may be preferable to a treadmill for those with poor balance, poor neuromotor coordination, impaired vision, impaired gait patterns, weight-bearing limitations, and/or foot problems. However, local muscle fatigue may be a factor for premature test termination when using a cycle ergometer.
- Adding a treadmill handrail support may be required because of reduced balance, decreased muscular strength, poor neuromotor coordination, and fear. However, handrail support for gait abnormalities will reduce the accuracy of estimating peak MET capacity based on the exercise duration or peak workload achieved.
- Treadmill workload may need to be adapted according to walking ability by increasing grade rather than speed.
- For those who have difficulty adjusting to the exercise protocol, the initial stage may need to be extended, the test restarted, or the test repeated. In these situations, also consider an intermittent protocol (see *Chapter 5*).
- Exercise-induced dysrhythmias are more frequent in older adults than in individuals in other age groups.
- Prescribed medications are common and may influence the electrocardiographic (ECG) and hemodynamic responses to exercise (see *Appendix A*).
- The exercise ECG has higher sensitivity (*i.e.*, ~84%) and lower specificity (*i.e.*, ~70%) than in younger age groups (*i.e.*, <50% sensitivity and >80% specificity). The higher rate of false positive outcomes may be related to the greater frequency of left ventricular hypertrophy (LVH) and the presence of conduction disturbances among older rather than younger adults (45).

There are no specific exercise test termination criteria for older adults beyond those presented for all adults in *Chapter 5*. The increased prevalence of cardiovascular, metabolic, and orthopedic problems among older adults increases the likelihood of an early test termination. In addition, many older adults exceed the age-predicted HR_{max} during a maximal exercise test.

Exercise Testing for the Oldest Segment of the Population

The oldest segment of the population ($\geq$75 yr and individuals with mobility limitations) most likely has one or more chronic medical conditions. The likelihood of physical limitations also increases with age. The approach described earlier is not applicable for the oldest segment of the population and for individuals with mobility limitations because (a) a prerequisite exercise test may be perceived as a barrier to physical activity promotion; (b) exercise testing is advocated before initiation of vigorous intensity exercise, but relatively few individuals in the oldest segment of the population are capable or likely to participate in vigorous intensity exercise, especially upon initiation of an exercise program; (c) the distinction between moderate and vigorous intensity exercise among older adults is difficult (*e.g.*, a moderate walking pace for one individual may be near the upper limit of capacity for an older, unfit adult with multiple chronic conditions); and (d) there is a paucity of evidence of increased mortality or cardiovascular event risk during exercise or exercise testing in this segment of the population. Therefore, the following recommendations are made for the aging population:

- In lieu of an exercise test, a thorough medical history and physical examination should serve to determine cardiac contraindications to exercise.
- Individuals with cardiovascular disease (CVD) symptoms or diagnosed disease can be risk classified and treated according to standard guidelines (see *Chapter 2*).
- Individuals free from CVD symptoms and disease should be able to initiate a light intensity (<3 METs) exercise program without undue risk (46).

Physical Performance Testing

Physical performance testing has largely replaced exercise stress testing for the assessment of functional status of older adults (50). Some test batteries have been developed and validated as correlates of underlying fitness domains, whereas others have been developed and validated as predictors of subsequent disability, institutionalization, and death. Physical performance testing is appealing in that most performance tests require little space, equipment, and cost; can be administered by lay or health/fitness personnel with minimal training; and are considered extremely safe in healthy and clinical populations (24,96). The most widely used physical performance tests have identified cut points indicative of functional limitations associated with poorer health status that can be targeted for an exercise intervention. Some of the most commonly used physical performance tests are described in *Table 8.4*. Before performing these assessments, (a) carefully consider the specific population for which each test was developed; (b) be aware of known floor or ceiling effects; and (c) understand the context (*i.e.*, the sample, age, health status, and intervention) in which change scores or predictive capabilities are attributed.

TABLE 8.4. Commonly Used Physical Performance Tests

Measure and Description	Administration Time	Cut-point Indicative of Lower Function
Senior Fitness Test (96)	30 min total	≤25th percentile of age-based norms
Seven items: 30 s chair stand, 30 s arm curls, 8 ft up and go, 6-min walk, 2-min step test, sit and reach, and back scratch with normative scales for each test.	Individual items range from 2 to 10 min each	
Short Physical Performance Battery (51)	10 min	10 points
A test of lower extremity functioning that combines scores from usual gait speed and timed tests of balance and chair stands. Scores range from 0 to 12 with higher score indicating better functioning.		
Usual Gait Speed	<2 min	1 m · s^{-1}
Usually assessed as the better of two trials of time to walk a short distance (3–10 m) at a usual pace.		
6-Min Walk Test	<10 min	≤25th percentile of age-based norms (97)
Widely used as an indicator of cardiorespiratory endurance. Assessed as the most distance an individual can walk in 6 min. A change of 50 m is considered a substantial change (49).		
Continuous Scale Physical Performance Test (29)	60 min	57 points
Two versions — long and short — are available. Each consists of serial performance of daily living tasks such as carrying a weighted pot of water, donning and removing a jacket, getting down and up from the floor, climbing stairs, carrying groceries, and others, performed within an environmental context that represent underlying physical domains. Scores range from 0 to 100 with higher scores representing better functioning.		

The *Senior Fitness Test* was developed using a large, healthy community dwelling sample and has published normative data for men and women 60–94 yr for items representing upper and lower body strength, upper and lower body flexibility, cardiorespiratory endurance, agility, and dynamic balance (96). The Short Physical Performance Battery (SPPB) (51), a test of lower extremity functioning, is best known for its predictive capabilities for disability, institutionalization, and death but also has known ceiling effects that limit its use as an outcome for exercise interventions in generally healthy older adults. A change of 0.5 points in the SPPB is considered a small meaningful change, whereas a change of 1.0 points is considered a substantial change (49). Usual gait speed, widely considered the simplest test of walking ability, has comparable predictive validity to the SPPB (90), but its sensitivity to change with exercise interventions has not been consistent. A change in usual gait speed of 0.05 m · s^{-1} is considered a small meaningful change and a change of 0.10 m · s^{-1} is considered a substantial change (49).

EXERCISE PRESCRIPTION

The general principles of Ex R$_x$ apply to adults of all ages (see *Chapter* 7). The relative adaptations to exercise and the percentage of improvement in the components of physical fitness among older adults are comparable with those reported in younger adults and are important for maintaining health and functional ability and attenuating many of the physiologic changes that are associated with aging (see *Table* 8.3). Low functional capacity, muscle weakness, and deconditioning are more common in older adults than in any other age group and contribute to loss of independence (7). An Ex R$_x$ should include aerobic, muscle strengthening/ endurance, and flexibility exercises. Individuals who are frequent fallers or have mobility limitations may also benefit from specific neuromotor exercises to improve balance, agility, and proprioceptive training in addition to the other components of health-related physical fitness. However, age should not be a barrier to physical activity promotion because positive improvements are attainable at any age.

For Ex R$_x$, an important distinction between older adults and their younger counterparts should be made relative to intensity. For apparently healthy adults, moderate and vigorous intensity, physical activities are defined relative to METs, with moderate intensity activities defined as 3–<6 METs and vigorous intensity activities as ≥6 METs. In contrast for older adults, activities should be defined relative to an individual's physical fitness within the context of perceived physical exertion using a 10-point scale, on which 0 is considered an effort equivalent to sitting and 10 is considered an all out effort, a moderate intensity, physical activity is defined as 5 or 6, and a vigorous intensity, physical activity as 7 or 8. A moderate intensity, physical activity should produce a noticeable increase in HR and breathing, whereas a vigorous intensity, physical activity should produce a substantial increase in HR or breathing (82).

FITT RECOMMENDATIONS FOR OLDER ADULTS

Aerobic Exercise

To promote and maintain health, older adults should adhere to the following Ex R$_x$ for aerobic (cardiorespiratory) physical activities. When older adults cannot do these recommended amounts of physical activity because of chronic conditions, they should be as physically active as their abilities and conditions allow.

Frequency: ≥5 d · wk^{-1} for moderate intensity, physical activities or ≥3 d · wk^{-1} for vigorous intensity, physical activities or some combination of moderate and vigorous intensity exercise 3–5 d · wk^{-1}.

Intensity: On a scale of 0–10 for level of physical exertion, 5–6 for moderate intensity and 7–8 for vigorous intensity (82).

Time: For moderate intensity, physical activities, accumulate at least 30 or up to 60 (for greater benefit) min · d^{-1} in bouts of at least 10 min each to total 150–300 min · wk^{-1}, or at least 20–30 min · d^{-1} of more vigorous intensity, physical activities to total 75–100 min · wk^{-1} or an equivalent combination of moderate and vigorous intensity, physical activity.

Type: Any modality that does not impose excessive orthopedic stress — walking is the most common type of activity. Aquatic exercise and stationary cycle exercise may be advantageous for those with limited tolerance for weight-bearing activity.

Muscle Strengthening/Endurance Exercise

Frequency: ≥2 d · wk^{-1}.

Intensity: Moderate intensity (*i.e.*, 60%–70% one repetition maximum [1-RM]). Light intensity (*i.e.*, 40%–50% 1-RM) for older adults beginning a resistance training program. When 1-RM is not measured, intensity can be prescribed between moderate (5–6) and vigorous (7–8) intensity on a scale of 0–10 (82).

Type: Progressive weight-training program or weight-bearing calisthenics (8–10 exercises involving the major muscle groups; ≥1 set of 10–15 repetitions each), stair climbing, and other strengthening activities that use the major muscle groups.

Flexibility Exercise

Frequency: ≥2 d · wk^{-1}.

Intensity: Stretch to the point of feeling tightness or slight discomfort.

Time: Hold stretch for 30–60 s.

Type: Any physical activities that maintain or increase flexibility using slow movements that terminate in sustained stretches for each major muscle group using static stretches rather than rapid ballistic movements.

Neuromotor (Balance) Exercises for Frequent Fallers or Individuals with Mobility Limitations

There are no specific recommendations for exercises that incorporate neuromotor (balance) training into an Ex R$_x$. However, neuromotor exercise training, which combines balance, agility, and proprioceptive training, is effective in reducing and preventing falls if performed 2–3 d · wk^{-1} (7,44). General recommendations include using the following: (a) progressively difficult postures that gradually reduce the base of support (*e.g.*, two-legged stand, semitandem stand, tandem stand, one-legged stand); (b) dynamic movements that perturb the center of gravity (*e.g.*, tandem walk, circle turns); (c) stressing postural muscle groups (*e.g.*, heel, toe stands); (d) reducing sensory input (*e.g.*, standing with eyes closed); and (e) tai chi. Supervision of these activities may be warranted (5).

SPECIAL CONSIDERATIONS

There are numerous considerations that should be taken into account to maximize the effective development of an exercise program including the following:

- Intensity and duration of physical activity should be light at the beginning in particular for older adults who are highly deconditioned, functionally limited, or have chronic conditions that affect their ability to perform physical tasks.
- Progression of physical activities should be individualized and tailored to tolerance and preference; a conservative approach may be necessary for the most deconditioned and physically limited older adults.
- Muscular strength decreases rapidly with age, especially for those >50 yr. Although resistance training is important across the lifespan, it becomes more rather than less important with increasing age (7,44,82).
- For strength training involving use of weightlifting machines, initial training sessions should be supervised and monitored by personnel who are sensitive to the special needs of older adults (see *Chapter 7*).
- In the early stages of an exercise program, muscle strengthening/endurance physical activities may need to precede aerobic training activities among very frail individuals. Individuals with sarcopenia, a marker of frailty, need to increase muscular strength before they are physiologically capable of engaging in aerobic training.
- Older adults should gradually exceed the recommended minimum amounts of physical activity and attempt continued progression if they desire to improve and/or maintain their physical fitness.
- If chronic conditions preclude activity at the recommended minimum amount, older adults should perform physical activities as tolerated to avoid being sedentary.
- Older adults should consider exceeding the recommended minimum amounts of physical activity to improve management of chronic diseases and health conditions for which a higher level of physical activity is known to confer a therapeutic benefit.
- Moderate intensity, physical activity should be encouraged for individuals with cognitive decline given the known benefits of physical activity on cognition. Individuals with significant cognitive impairment can engage in physical activity but may require individualized assistance.
- Structured physical activity sessions should end with an appropriate cool-down, particularly among individuals with CVD. The cool-down should include a gradual reduction of effort and intensity and optimally, flexibility exercises.
- Incorporation of behavioral strategies such as social support, self-efficacy, the ability to make healthy choices, and perceived safety all may enhance participation in a regular exercise program (see *Chapter 11*).

- The health/fitness and clinical exercise professional should also provide regular feedback, positive reinforcement, and other behavioral/programmatic strategies to enhance adherence.

THE BOTTOM LINE

All older adults should be guided in the development of a personalized Ex R$_x$ or physical activity plan that meets their needs and personal preferences. The Ex R$_x$ should include aerobic, muscle strengthening and endurance, flexibility, and neuromotor exercises, and focus on maintaining and improving functional ability. In addition to standard physical fitness assessments, physical performance tests can be used. These tests identify functional limitations associated with poorer heath status that can be targeted for exercise intervention.

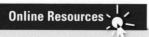

Online Resources

Continuous Scale Physical Functional Performance Battery (28):
http://www.coe.uga.edu/cs-pfp/index.html

Short Physical Performance Battery (12):
http://www.grc.nia.nih.gov/branches/ledb/sppb/index.htm

LOW BACK PAIN

Low back pain (LBP) is traditionally described as pain that is primarily localized to the lumbar and lumbosacral area that may or may not be associated with leg pain. However, LBP is actually a complex multidimensional phenomenon. For some individuals, LBP is a recurrent and uncomfortable inconvenience, whereas for others, chronic LBP is a major cause of chronic disability and distress. The mere description of the problem of LBP based on spatial characteristics of pain belies the complexity of the problem and its impact. Best evidence clinical guidelines now recommend physical activity as a key component of management across the spectrum of the condition (4,27,115).

Most cases of LBP show rapid improvement in pain and symptoms within the first month of symptom occurrence (89). Roughly one-half to three-quarters of individuals, however, will experience some level of persistent or recurrent symptoms, with the prevalence of LBP being twice as high for individuals with a prior history of LBP (57). Furthermore, recurrent episodes tend toward increased severity and duration, and higher levels of disability including work disability and higher medical and indemnity costs (117).

Individuals with LBP can be subgrouped into one of three general categories: (a) LBP associated with a potentially serious pathology (*e.g.*, cancer or fracture);

(b) LBP with specific neurological signs and symptoms (*e.g.*, radiculopathy or spinal stenosis); and (c) nonspecific LBP (17), the latter of which accounts for up to 90% of cases (57). For the purposes of management, LBP may be further subgrouped according to the duration of symptoms: (a) acute (the initial 4–6 wk); (b) subacute (<3 mo); and (c) chronic (≥3 mo) (27,115). It should be noted, however, that LBP is often characterized by remission and exacerbation of symptoms that may or may not be attributable to known physical or psychological stressors.

When LBP is a symptom of another serious pathology (*e.g.*, cancer), exercise testing and Ex R_x should be guided by considerations related to the primary condition. For all other causes, and in the absence of a comorbid condition (*e.g.*, CVD with its associated risk factors), recommendations for exercise testing and Ex R_x are similar as for healthy individuals (see *Chapters* 2 and 7). Some considerations, however, must be given to individuals with LBP who are fearful of pain and/or reinjury, and thus avoid physical activity, as well as to those individuals who persist in physical activity despite worsening symptoms (54). Individuals with LBP who are fearful of pain and/or reinjury often misinterpret any aggravation of symptoms as a worsening of their spinal condition, and hold the mistaken belief that pain equates with tissue damage (103). In contrast, those with LBP who persist in physical activity may not allow injured tissues the time that is needed to heal. Both behaviors are associated with chronic pain.

EXERCISE TESTING

Exercise and physical fitness testing is common in individuals with chronic LBP with little to no evidence of contraindication based on LBP alone. If LBP is acute, guidelines generally recommend a gradual return to physical activity. As such, exercise testing should be symptom limited in the first weeks following symptom onset (1).

Cardiorespiratory Fitness

Many clients/patients with chronic LBP have reduced CRF levels compared to the normal population. Current evidence, however, has failed to find a clear relationship between CRF and pain (116). What is clear, however, is that chronic LBP cannot be fully explained by deconditioning or avoidance of physical activity for fear of pain. Despite this, the advice to stay physically active is nearly universal in current clinical practice guidelines for LBP (4,27,115).

The guidelines for standard CRF testing apply to individuals with LBP (see *Chapter* 4) with the following considerations:

- Compared to cycle and upper extremity ergometry, treadmill testing produces the highest $\dot{V}O_{2peak}$ in individuals with LBP. Actual or anticipated pain may limit performance (120).
- Actual or anticipated pain may limit submaximal testing as often as maximal testing (36,59,109,110). Therefore, the choice of maximal versus submaximal

testing in individuals with LBP should be guided by the same considerations as for the general population.

Muscular Strength and Endurance

Reduced muscle strength and endurance in the trunk has been associated with LBP (1), as have changes in strength and endurance ratios (*e.g.*, flexors vs. extensors) (15). There has also been the suggestion neuromotor imbalances may exist between paired muscles such as the erector spinae in individuals with LBP (94). How these muscular and neuromotor changes relate to the development, progression, and potential treatment of LBP symptoms remains unclear and may be multifactorial.

General testing of muscular strength and endurance in individuals with LBP should be guided by the same considerations as for the general population (see *Chapter 4*). In addition, tests of the strength and endurance of the trunk musculature are common in individuals with LBP (48). When interpreting these results, however, several factors must be kept in mind:

- Assessments using isokinetic dynamometers with back attachments, selectorized machines, and back hyperextension benches specifically test the trunk muscles in individuals with LBP. The reliability of these tests is questionable because of considerable learning effect in particular between the first and second sessions (33,64,92).
- For individuals with LBP, performance is often limited by actual or anticipated fear of reinjury (65).

Flexibility

There is no clear relationship between gross spinal flexibility and LBP or associated disability (4). A range of studies have shown associations between measures of spine flexibility, hip flexibility, and LBP (72). The nature of these associations, however, is likely complex, and requires further study. Assessing spine flexibility is still recommended as part of a standard clinical evaluation in LBP (13) and may provide insight into the condition of the individual. Furthermore, there appears to be some justification, although based on relatively weak evidence, for flexibility testing in the lower limbs, and in particular the hips of individuals with LBP.

In general, flexibility testing in individuals with LBP should be guided by the same considerations as for the general population (see *Chapter 4*). It is essential, however, to identify whether the assessment is limited by stretch tolerance of the target structures or exacerbation of LBP symptoms.

Physical Performance

Physical performance tests afford another indicator of the functional impact of LBP when added to the traditional impairment-based measures such as muscle strength and flexibility (105) for they assess the impact of LBP and its associated

BOX 8.3	Physical Performance Measures for Low Back Pain (9,104,105)

Test	Reliable	Valid	Responsive
Repeated Trunk Flexion — from standing, the participant flexes the lumbar spine to end-range and returns to the upright position 10 times as fast as possible, self-selecting a speed that does not aggravate symptoms. Time to completion is recorded (s). Averaging two trials improves reliability.	✓	✓	
Repeated Sit-to-Stand — the participant stands up five times from a chair without the use of the arms as fast as possible. Time to completion is recorded (s). Averaging two trials improves reliability.	✓	✓	✓
50-Foot Walk — the participant walks 50 ft as fast as possible without a walking aid. Time to completion is recorded (s).	✓	✓	
5-Min Walk — the participant walks as far as possible in 5 min without a walking aid. Distance is recorded (ft or m).	✓	✓	
1-Min Stair Climbing—the participant walks up and down 5 stairs for 1 min as fast as possible using the rail for support if required. The total amount of steps climbed is recorded.	✓	✓	✓

psychomotor slowing. Such testing is complementary to self-reports of function. Examples of such tests mostly include a timed component and are presented in *Box 8.3*.

EXERCISE PRESCRIPTION

Clinical practice guidelines for the management of LBP consistently recommend staying physically active and avoiding bed rest (17). Although it may be best to avoid exercise in the very immediate aftermath of an acute and severe episode of LBP so as not to exacerbate symptoms (1,27), individuals with subacute and chronic LBP as well as recurrent LBP are encouraged to be physically active (1).

Current evidence does not provide any consensus on the type of exercise that should be promoted in individuals with LBP or on how to best manage the program variables for these individuals (17). When recommendations are provided, they should follow very closely the recommendations for the general population (see *Chapter 7*) combining resistance, aerobic, and flexibility exercise (1). In chronic LBP, exercise programs that incorporate individual tailoring, supervision, stretching, and strengthening are associated with the best outcomes (27,55). A complete exercise program based on the exercise preferences of the individual and health/fitness, clinical exercise, and/or health care professional may be most appropriate (4). Minimum levels for intensity and volume should be the same as for a healthy population (see *Chapter 7*).

SPECIAL CONSIDERATIONS

- Exercises to promote spinal stabilization (71,95) are often recommended based on the suggestion that intervertebral instability may be a cause of certain cases of LBP (86).
  - This approach provides no clear additional benefit over other approaches to the management of nonspecific LBP (67).
  - This approach may be beneficial when LBP is related to a mechanical instability (58), however, further research is required.
  - There does not appear to be any detrimental effect of including spinal stabilization exercises within a general exercise program for individuals with LBP based on the preference of the individual and the health/fitness, clinical exercise, and/or health care professional.
- Certain exercises or positions may aggravate symptoms of LBP.
  - Walking, especially walking downhill, may aggravate symptoms in individuals with spinal stenosis (62).
  - Certain individuals with LBP may experience a "peripheralization" of symptoms, that is, a distal spread of pain into the lower limb with certain sustained or repeated movements of the lumbar spine (3). In such a situation, exercise or activities that aggravate peripheralization should temporarily be avoided.
- Exercises or movements that result in a "centralization" of symptoms (*i.e.*, a reduction of pain in the lower limb from distal to proximal) should be encouraged (3,108,119).
- Flexibility exercises are generally encouraged as part of an overall exercise program.
  - Hip and lower limb flexibility should be promoted, although no stretching intervention studies have shown efficacy in treating or preventing LBP (35).
  - It is generally not recommended to use trunk flexibility as a treatment goal in LBP (112).

THE BOTTOM LINE

LBP is a complex multidimensional phenomenon. Recommendations for exercise testing and Ex R$_x$ are similar to those for healthy individuals when LBP is not associated with another serious pathology (*e.g.*, cancer). It may be best to avoid exercise in the very immediate aftermath of an acute and severe episode of LBP so as not to exacerbate symptoms. However, individuals with subacute and chronic LBP as well as recurrent LBP should participate in physical activity. Performance is often limited by actual or anticipated fear of reinjury and/or pain.

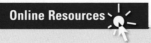

ENVIRONMENTAL CONSIDERATIONS

EXERCISE IN HOT ENVIRONMENTS

Muscular contractions produce metabolic heat that is transferred from the active muscles to the blood and then to the body's core. Subsequent body temperature elevations elicit heat loss responses of increased skin blood flow and increased sweat secretion so that heat can be dissipated to the environment via evaporation (100). Thus, the cardiovascular system plays an essential role in temperature regulation. Heat exchange between skin and environment via sweating and dry heat exchange is governed by biophysical properties dictated by surrounding temperature, humidity and air motion, sky and ground radiation, and clothing (43). However, when the amount of metabolic heat exceeds heat loss, hyperthermia (*i.e.*, elevated internal body temperature) may develop. Sweat that drips from the body or clothing provides no cooling benefit. If secreted sweat drips from the body and is not evaporated, a higher sweating rate will be needed to achieve the evaporative cooling requirements (100). Sweat losses vary widely and depend on the amount and intensity of physical activity and environmental conditions (46). Other factors can alter sweat rates and ultimately fluid needs. For example, heat acclimatization results in higher and more sustained sweating rates, whereas aerobic exercise training has a modest effect on enhancing sweating rate responses (100).

Dehydration increases physiologic strain as measured by core temperature, HR, and perceived exertion responses during exercise-induced heat stress (98). The greater the body water deficit, the greater the increase in physiologic strain for a given exercise task (74). Dehydration can augment core temperature elevations during exercise in temperate (83) as well as in hot environments (102). The typical reported core temperature augmentation with dehydration is an increase of 0.1° to 0.2° C (0.2° to 0.4° F) with each 1% of dehydration (99). The greater heat storage with dehydration is associated with a proportionate decrease in heat loss. Thus, decreased sweating rate (*i.e.*, evaporative heat loss) and decreased cutaneous blood flow (*i.e.*, dry heat loss) are responsible for greater heat storage observed during exercise when hypohydrated (79).

Counteracting Dehydration

Dehydration (*i.e.*, 3%–5% body mass loss) likely does not degrade muscular strength (37) or anaerobic performance (25). Dehydration >2% of body mass decreases aerobic exercise performance in temperate, warm, and hot environments;

and as the level of dehydration increases, aerobic exercise performance is reduced proportionally (61). The critical water deficit (*i.e.*, >2% body mass for most individuals) and magnitude of performance decrement are likely related to environmental temperature, exercise task, and the individuals' unique biological characteristics (*e.g.*, tolerance to dehydration). Acute dehydration impairs endurance performance regardless of whole body hyperthermia or environmental temperature; and endurance capacity (*i.e.*, time to exhaustion) is reduced more in a hot environment than in a temperate or cold one.

Individuals have varying sweat rates, and as such, fluid needs for individuals performing similar tasks under identical conditions can be different. Determining sweat rate ($L \cdot h^{-1}$ or $q \cdot h^{-1}$) by measuring body weight before and after exercise provides a fluid replacement guide. Active individuals should drink at least 1 pt of fluid for each pound of body weight lost. Meals can help stimulate thirst resulting in restoration of fluid balance. Snack breaks during longer training sessions can help replenish fluids and be important in replacing sodium and other electrolytes. In a field setting, the additive use of first morning body mass measurements in combination with some measure of first morning urine concentration and gross thirst perception can provide a simple and inexpensive way to dichotomize euhydration from gross dehydration (see *Figure 8.2*) (26). Paler color urine indicates adequate hydration; the darker yellow/brown the urine color, the greater the degree of dehydration. Urine color can provide a simple and inexpensive way to dichotomize euhydration from gross dehydration (26). *Box 8.4* provides recommendations for hydration prior to, during, and following exercise or physical activity (8).

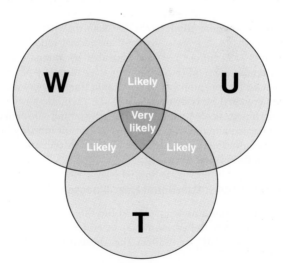

■ **FIGURE 8.2. W** stands for "weight." **U** stands for "urine." **T** stands for "thirst." When two or more simple markers are present, dehydration is likely. If all three markers are present, dehydration is very likely. Reprinted with permission from (26).

| BOX 8.4 | Fluid Replacement Recommendations before, during, and after Exercise |

	Fluid	Comments
Before exercise	• Drink 5–7 mL · kg^{-1} (0.08–0.11 oz · lb^{-1}) at least 4 h before exercise (12–17 oz for 154-lb individual).	• If urine is not produced or very dark, drink another 3–5 mL · kg^{-1} (0.05–0.08 oz · lb^{-1}) 2 h before exercise. • Sodium-containing beverages or slated snacks will help retain fluid.
During exercise	• Monitor individual body weight changes during exercise to estimate sweat loss. • Composition of fluid should include 20–30 mEq · L^{-1} of sodium, 2–5 mEq · L^{-1} of potassium, and 5%–10% of carbohydrate.	• Prevent a >2% loss in body weight. • Amount and rate of fluid replacement depends on individual sweating rate, environment, and exercise duration.
After exercise	• Consumption of normal meals and beverages will restore euhydration. • If rapid recovery is needed, drink 1.5 L · kg^{-1} (23 oz · lb^{-1}) of body weight lost.	• Goal is to fully replace fluid and electrolyte deficits. • Consuming sodium will help recovery by stimulating thirst and fluid retention.

Adapted from (6,8).

Overdrinking hypotonic fluid is the mechanism that leads to exercise-associated hyponatremia, a state of lower than normal blood sodium concentration (typically <135 mEq · L^{-1}) accompanied by altered cognitive status. Hyponatremia tends to be more common in long duration physical activities and is precipitated by consumption of hypotonic fluid (water) alone in excess of sweat losses (typified by body mass gains). The syndrome can be prevented by not drinking in excess of sweat rate and by consuming salt-containing fluids or foods when participating in exercise events that result in many hours of continuous or near continuous sweating. For additional information, see the ACSM position stand on fluid replacement (8).

Medical Considerations: Exertional Heat Illnesses

Heat illnesses range from muscle cramps to life-threatening hyperthermia and are described in *Table 8.5*. Dehydration may be either a direct (*i.e.*, heat cramps and heat exhaustion) (101) or indirect (*i.e.*, heatstroke) (22) factor in heat illness.

Heat cramps are muscle pains or spasms most often in the abdomen, arms, or legs that may occur in association with strenuous activity. Muscle fatigue, water loss, and significant sweat sodium are contributing factors. Heat cramps respond

TABLE 8.5. A Comparison of the Signs and Symptoms of Illnesses that Occur in Hot Environments (6)

Disorder	Prominent Signs and Symptoms	Mental Status Changes	Core Temperature Elevation
Exertional heatstroke	Disorientation, dizziness, irrational behavior, apathy, headache, nausea, vomiting, hyperventilation, wet skin	Marked (disoriented, unresponsive)	Marked (>40° C)
Exertional heat exhaustion	Low blood pressure, elevated heart rate and respiratory rates, skin is wet and pale, headache, weakness, dizziness, decreased muscle coordination, chills, nausea, vomiting, diarrhea	Little or none, agitated	None to moderate (37° to 40° C)
Heat syncope	Heart rate and breathing rates are slow; skin is pale; patient may experience sensations of weakness, tunnel vision, vertigo, or nausea before syncope	Brief fainting episode	Little or none
Exertional heat cramps	Begins as feeble, localized, wandering spasms that may progress to debilitating cramps	None	Moderate (37° to 40° C)

well to rest, prolonged stretching, dietary sodium chloride (*i.e.*, ⅛–¼ tsp of table salt or one to two salt tablets added to 300–500 mL of fluid, bullion broth, or salty snacks), or intravenous normal saline fluid.

Heat syncope is a temporary circulatory failure caused by the pooling of blood in the peripheral veins, particularly of the lower extremities. Heat syncope tends to occur more often among physically unfit, sedentary, and nonacclimatized individuals. It is caused by standing erect for a long period; or at the cessation of strenuous, prolonged, upright exercise because maximal cutaneous vessel dilation results in a decline of blood pressure (BP) and insufficient oxygen delivery to the brain. Symptoms range from light-headedness to loss of consciousness; however, recovery is rapid once individuals sit or lay supine. Complete recovery of stable BP and HR may take a few hours. See the ACSM position stand on heat illness during exercise for additional information (6).

Heat exhaustion is the most common form of serious heat illness. It occurs during exercise/physical activity in the heat when the body cannot sustain the level of cardiac output ($\dot{Q}$) needed to support skin blood flow for thermoregulation and blood flow for metabolic requirements of exercise. It is characterized by prominent fatigue and progressive weakness without severe hyperthermia. Oral fluids are preferred for rehydration in individuals who are conscious, able to swallow, and not losing fluid (*i.e.*, vomiting and diarrhea). Intravenous fluid administration facilitates recovery in those unable to ingest oral fluids or who have severe dehydration.

Exertional heatstroke is caused by hyperthermia and is characterized by elevated body temperature (>40° C or 104° F), profound central nervous system dysfunction, and multiple organ system failure that can result in delirium, convulsions, or coma. The greatest risk for heatstroke exists during high intensity prolonged exercise when the ambient wet-bulb globe temperature (WBGT) exceeds 28° C (82° F). It is a life-threatening medical emergency that requires immediate and effective whole body cooling with cold water and ice water immersion therapy. Inadequate physical fitness, excess adiposity, improper clothing, protective pads, incomplete heat acclimatization, illness, or medications also increase risk.

Exercise Prescription

Health/fitness and clinical exercise professionals may use standards established by the National Institute for Occupational Safety and Health to define WBGT levels at which the risk of heat injury is increased, but exercise may be performed if preventive steps are taken (81). These steps include required rest breaks between exercise periods.

Individuals whose Ex R_x specifies a target heart rate (THR) will achieve this THR at a lower absolute workload when exercising in a warm/hot versus a cooler environment. For example, in hot or humid weather, an individual will achieve their THR with a reduced running speed. Reducing one's workload to maintain the same THR in the heat will help to reduce the risk of heat illness during acclimatization. As heat acclimatization develops, a progressively higher exercise intensity will be required to elicit the THR. The first exercise session in the heat may last as little as 5–10 min for safety reasons but can be increased gradually.

Developing a Personalized Plan

Adults and children who are adequately rested, nourished, hydrated, and acclimatized to heat are at less risk for exertional heat illnesses. The following factors should be considered when developing an individualized plan to minimize the effects of hyperthermia and dehydration along with the questions in Box 8.5 (26):

- Monitor the environment: Use the WBGT index to determine appropriate action.
- Modify activity in extreme environments: Enable access to ample fluid, provide longer and/or more rest breaks to facilitate heat dissipation, and shorten or delay playing times. Perform exercise at times of the day when conditions will be cooler compared to midday (early morning, later evening). Children and older adults should modify activities in conditions of high-ambient temperatures accompanied by high humidity (see Box 8.6).
- Consider heat acclimatization status, physical fitness, nutrition, sleep deprivation, and age of participants; intensity, time/duration, and time of day for exercise; availability of fluids; and playing surface heat reflection (i.e., grass vs. asphalt). Allow at least 3 h, and preferably 6 h, of recovery and rehydration time between exercise sessions.
- Heat acclimatization: These adaptations include decreased rectal temperature, HR, and RPE; increased exercise tolerance time; increased sweating rate; and a reduction in sweat salt. Acclimatization results in the following: (a) improved

BOX 8.5	Questions to Evaluate Readiness to Exercise in a Hot Environment (10)

Adults should ask the following questions to evaluate readiness to exercise in a hot environment. Corrective action should be taken if any question is answered "no."

- Have I developed a plan to avoid dehydration and hyperthermia?
- Have I acclimatized by gradually increasing exercise duration and intensity for 10–14 d?
- Do I limit intense exercise to the cooler hours of the day (early morning)?
- Do I avoid lengthy warm-up periods on hot, humid days?
- When training outdoors, do I know where fluids are available, or do I carry water bottles in a belt or a backpack?
- Do I know my sweat rate and the amount of fluid that I should drink to replace body weight loss?
- Was my body weight this morning within 1% of my average body weight?
- Is my 24 h urine volume plentiful?
- Is my urine color "pale yellow" or "straw colored"?
- When heat and humidity are high, do I reduce my expectations, my exercise pace, the distance, and/or duration of my workout or race?
- Do I wear loose-fitting, porous, lightweight clothing?
- Do I know the signs and symptoms of heat exhaustion, exertional heatstroke, heat syncope, and heat cramps (see *Table 8.4*)?
- Do I exercise with a partner and provide feedback about his/her physical appearance?
- Do I consume adequate salt in my diet?
- Do I avoid or reduce exercise in the heat if I experience sleep loss, infectious illness, fever, diarrhea, vomiting, carbohydrate depletion, some medications, alcohol, or drug abuse?

BOX 8.6	Modifications to Activities for Children

WBGT °F MODIFICATION

<75.0	All activities allowed, be alert for signs or symptoms of heat-related illness in prolonged events.
75.0–78.6	Longer rest periods in the shade; enforce drinking every 15 min
79.0–84.0	Stop activity of unacclimatized individuals and those in high-risk categories; limit activities of all others (disallow long-distance races, cut duration of other activities)
>85.0	Cancel all athletic activities

Adapted from (8).

heat transfer from the body's core to the external environment; (b) improved cardiovascular function; (c) more effective sweating; and (d) improved exercise performance and heat tolerance. Seasonal acclimatization will occur gradually during late spring and early summer months with sedentary exposure to the heat. However, this process can be facilitated with a structured program of moderate exercise in the heat across 10–14 d to stimulate adaptations to warmer ambient temperatures.

- Clothing: Clothes that have a high wicking capacity may assist in evaporative heat loss. Athletes should remove as much clothing and equipment (especially headgear) as possible to permit heat loss and reduce the risks of hyperthermia, especially during the initial days of acclimatization.
- Education: The training of participants, personal trainers, coaches, and community emergency response teams enhances the reduction, recognition (see *Table 8.5*), and treatment of heat-related illness. Such programs should emphasize the importance of recognizing signs/symptoms of heat intolerance, being hydrated, fed, rested, and acclimatized to heat. Educating individuals about dehydration, assessing hydration state, and using a fluid replacement program can help maintain hydration.

Organizational Planning

When clients exercise in hot/humid conditions, personnel in fitness facilities and organizations should formulate a standardized heat stress management plan that incorporates the following considerations:

- Screening and surveillance of at-risk participants.
- Environmental assessment (*i.e.*, WBGT index) and criteria for modifying or canceling exercise.
- Heat acclimatization procedures.
- Easy access to fluids and bathroom facilities.
- *Optimized but not maximized* fluid intake that (a) matches the volume of fluid consumed to the volume of sweat lost; and (b) limits body weight change to <2% of body weight.
- Awareness of the signs and symptoms of heatstroke, heat exhaustion, heat cramps, and heat syncope (see *Table 8.5*).
- Implementation of specific emergency procedures.

THE BOTTOM LINE

Metabolic heat produced by muscular contractions increases body temperature during exercise. Heat illness ranges from muscle cramps to life-threatening hyperthermia. In addition, dehydration has been associated with an increased risk for heat exhaustion and is a risk factor for heatstroke. Sweat losses vary widely among individuals and depend on exercise intensity and environmental conditions. Thus, fluid needs will be highly variable among individuals. The risk of dehydration and hyperthermia can be minimized by monitoring the environment; modifying activities in hot, humid environments; wearing appropriate clothing; and knowing the signs and symptoms of heat illness.

EXERCISE IN COLD ENVIRONMENTS

Individuals exercise and work in many cold weather environments (*i.e.*, low temperature, high winds, low solar radiation, and rain/water exposure). For the most part, cold temperatures are not a barrier to performing physical activity, although some individuals may perceive them to be. Many factors including the environment, clothing, body composition, health status, nutrition, age, and exercise intensity interact to determine if exercising in the cold elicits additional physiologic strain and injury risk beyond that associated with the same exercise done under temperate conditions. In most cases, exercise in the cold does not increase cold injury risk. However, there are scenarios (*i.e.*, immersion, rain, and low-ambient temperature with wind) where whole body or local thermal balance cannot be maintained during exercise-related cold stress that contributes to hypothermia, frostbite, and diminished exercise capability and performance. Furthermore, exercise-related cold stress may increase the risk of morbidity and mortality in at-risk populations such as those with CVD and asthmatic conditions. Inhalation of cold air may also exacerbate these conditions.

Hypothermia develops when heat loss exceeds heat production causing the body heat content to decrease (93). The environment, individual characteristics, and clothing all impact the development of hypothermia. Some specific factors that increase the risk of developing hypothermia include immersion, rain, wet clothing, low body fat, older age (*i.e.*, ≥60 yr), and hypoglycemia (23).

Medical Considerations: Cold Injuries

Frostbite occurs when tissue temperatures fall lower than 0° C (32° F) (30,73). Frostbite is most common in exposed skin (*i.e.*, nose, ears, cheeks, and exposed wrists) but also occurs in the hands and feet. Contact frostbite may occur by touching cold objects with bare skin, particularly highly conductive metal or stone that causes rapid heat loss.

Wind Speed (mph)

Air Temperature (°F)

	40	35	30	25	20	15	10	5	0	-5	-10	-15	-20	-25	-30	-35	-40	-45
5	36	31	25	19	13	7	1	-5	-11	-16	-22	-28	-34	-40	-46	-52	-57	-63
10	34	27	21	15	9	3	-4	-10	-16	-22	-28	-35	-41	-47	-53	-59	-66	-72
15	32	25	19	13	6	0	-7	-13	-19	-26	-32	-39	-45	-51	-58	-64	-71	-77
20	30	24	17	11	4	-2	-9	-15	-22	-29	-35	-42	-48	-55	-61	-68	-74	-81
25	29	23	16	9	3	-4	-11	-17	-24	-31	-37	-44	-51	-58	-64	-71	-78	-84
30	28	22	15	8	1	-5	-12	-19	-26	-33	-39	-46	-53	-60	-67	-73	-80	-87
35	28	21	14	7	0	-7	-14	-21	-27	-34	-41	-48	-55	-62	-69	-76	-82	-89
40	27	20	13	6	-1	-8	-15	-22	-29	-36	-43	-50	-57	-64	-71	-78	-84	-91
45	26	19	12	5	-2	-9	-16	-23	-30	-37	-44	-51	-58	-65	-72	-79	-86	-93
50	26	19	12	4	-3	-10	-17	-24	-31	-38	-45	-52	-60	-67	-74	-81	-88	-95
55	25	18	11	4	-3	-11	-18	-25	-32	-39	-46	-54	-61	-68	-75	-82	-89	-97
60	25	17	10	3	-4	-11	-19	-26	-33	-40	-48	-55	-62	-69	-76	-84	-91	-98

Frostbite times: ☐ Frostbite could occur in 30 min
▨ Frostbite could occur in 10 min
▩ Frostbite could occur in 5 min

■ **FIGURE 8.3.** Wind Chill Temperature Index in Fahrenheit and Celsius and frostbite times for exposed facial skin (20,84).

The principal cold stress determinants for frostbite are air temperature, wind speed, and wetness. Wind exacerbates heat loss by facilitating convective heat loss and reduces the insulative value of clothing. The Wind Chill Temperature Index (WCT) (see *Figure 8.3*) integrates wind speed and air temperature to provide an estimate of the cooling power of the environment. WCT is specific in that its correct application only estimates the danger of cooling for the exposed skin of individuals walking at $1.3 \text{ m} \cdot \text{s}^{-1}$ ($3 \text{ mi} \cdot \text{h}^{-1}$). Important information about wind and the WCT incorporates the following considerations:

- Wind does not cause an exposed object to become cooler than the ambient temperature.
- Wind speeds obtained from weather reports do not take into account man-made wind (*e.g.*, running, skiing).
- The WCT presents the relative risk of frostbite and predicted times to freezing (see *Figure 8.3*) of exposed facial skin. Facial skin was chosen because this area of the body is typically not protected.
- Frostbite cannot occur if the air temperature is >0° C (32° F).
- Wet skin exposed to the wind cools faster. If the skin is wet and exposed to wind, the ambient temperature used for the WCT table should be 10° C lower than the actual ambient temperature (18).
- The risk of frostbite is <5% when the ambient temperature is greater than −15° C (5° F), but increased safety surveillance of exercisers is warranted when the WCT falls lower than −27° C (−8° F). In those conditions, frostbite can occur in 30 min or less in exposed skin (23).

Clothing Considerations

Cold weather clothing protects against hypothermia and frostbite by reducing heat loss through the insulation provided by the clothing and trapped air within and between clothing layers (23). Typical cold weather clothing consists of three layers: (a) an inner layer (*i.e.*, lightweight polyester or polypropylene); (b) a middle layer (*i.e.*, polyester fleece or wool) that provides the primary insulation; and (c) an outer layer designed to allow moisture transfer to the air while repelling wind and rain. Recommendations for clothing wear include the following considerations (23):

- Adjust clothing insulation to minimize sweating.
- Use clothing vents to reduce sweat accumulation.
- Do not wear an outer layer unless rainy or very windy.
- Reduce clothing insulation as exercise intensity increases.
- Do not impose a single clothing standard on an entire group of exercisers.
- Wear appropriate footwear to minimize the risks of slipping and falling in snowy or icy conditions.

Exercise Prescription

Whole body and facial cooling theoretically lower the threshold for the onset of angina during aerobic exercise. The type and intensity of exercise-related cold stress also modifies the risk for an individual with CVD. Activities that involve the upper body or increase metabolism potentially increase risk:

- Shoveling snow raises the HR to 97% HR_{max} and systolic BP increases to 200 mm Hg (40).
- Walking in snow that is either packed or soft significantly increases energy requirements and myocardial oxygen demands so that individuals with atherosclerotic CVD may have to slow their walking pace.
- Swimming in water <25° C (77° F) may be a threat to individuals with CVD because they may not be able to recognize angina symptoms; and therefore may place themselves at greater risk (23).

THE BOTTOM LINE

In general, cold temperatures are not a barrier to performing physical activity. However, exercise-related cold stress may increase the risk of morbidity and mortality in individuals with CVD and asthmatic conditions. The risk of frostbite is <5% when the ambient temperature is greater than −15° C (5° F). Frostbite can occur when the WCT is lower than −27° C (−8° F). Dressing appropriately for the type of weather expected and understanding the risks most likely to be encountered during exercise will reduce the risk of cold injuries substantially.

EXERCISE IN HIGH ALTITUDE ENVIRONMENTS

The progressive decrease in atmospheric pressure associated with ascent to higher altitudes reduces the partial pressure of oxygen in the inspired air, resulting in decreased arterial oxygen levels. Immediate compensatory responses include increased ventilation and $\dot{Q}$, the latter usually through elevated HR (70). For most individuals, the effects of altitude appear at and above 3,950 ft (1,200 m). In this section, *low altitude* refers to locations <3,950 ft (1,200 m), *moderate altitude* to locations between 3,950 and 7,900 ft (1,200–2,400 m), *high altitude* between 7,901 and 13,125 ft (2,400–4,000 m), and *very high altitude* >13,125 ft (4,000 m) (78).

Physical performance decreases with increasing altitude >3,950 ft (1,200 m). In general, the physical performance decrement will be greater as elevation, physical activity duration, and muscle mass increases, but is lessened with altitude acclimatization. The most common altitude effect on physical task performance is an increased time for task completion or more frequent rest breaks. With altitude exposure of ≥1 wk, significant altitude acclimatization occurs. The time to complete a task is reduced but the time remains longer relative to sea level. The estimated percentage increases in performance time to complete tasks of various durations during initial altitude exposure and after 1 wk of altitude acclimatization are given in *Table 8.6* (42).

Medical Considerations: Altitude Illnesses

Rapid ascent to high and very high altitude increases individual susceptibility to altitude illness. The primary altitude illnesses are acute mountain sickness

TABLE 8.6. Estimated Impact of Increasing Altitude on Time to Complete Physical Tasks at Various Altitudes (42)

	Percentage Increase in Time To Complete Physical Tasks Relative to Sea Level							
	Tasks Lasting <2 min		Tasks Lasting 2–5 min		Tasks Lasting 10–30 min		Tasks Lasting >3 h	
Altitude	Initial	>1 wk	Initial	>1 wk	Initial	>1 wk	Initial	>1 wk
Moderate	0	0	2–7	0–2	4–11	1–3	7–18	3–10
High	0–2	0	12–18	5–9	20–45	9–20	40–65	20–45
Very high	2	0	50	25	90	60	200	90

(AMS), high altitude cerebral edema (HACE), and high altitude pulmonary edema (HAPE). Additionally, many individuals develop a sore throat and bronchitis that may produce disabling, severe coughing spasms at high altitudes. Susceptibility to altitude sickness is increased in individuals with a prior history and by prolonged physical exertion and dehydration early in the altitude exposure.

AMS is the most common form of altitude sickness. Symptoms include headache, nausea, fatigue, decreased appetite, and poor sleep, and in severe cases, poor balance and mild swelling in the hands, feet, or face. AMS develops within the first 24 h of altitude exposure. Its incidence and severity increases in direct proportion to ascent rate and altitude. The estimated incidence of AMS in unacclimatized individuals rapidly ascending directly to moderate altitudes is 0%–20%; to high altitudes, 20%–60%; and to very high altitudes, 50%–80% (97). In most individuals, if ascent is stopped and physical exertion is limited, recovery from AMS occurs over 24–48 h after symptoms have peaked.

HACE is a potentially fatal, although not common, illness that occurs in <2% of individuals ascending >12,000 ft (3,658 m). HACE is an exacerbation of unresolved, severe AMS. HACE most often occurs in individuals who have AMS symptoms and continue to ascend.

HAPE is a potentially fatal, although not common, illness that occurs in <10% of individuals ascending >12,000 ft (3,658 m). Individuals making repeated ascents and descents >12,000 ft (3,658 m) and who exercise strenuously early in the exposure have an increased susceptibility to HAPE. The presence of crackles and rales in the lungs may indicate increased susceptibility to developing HAPE. Blue lips and nail beds may be present with HAPE.

Prevention and Treatment of Altitude Sickness

Altitude acclimatization is the best countermeasure to all altitude sickness. Minimizing sustained exercise/physical activity and maintaining adequate hydration and food intake will reduce susceptibility to altitude sickness and facilitate recovery. When moderate to severe symptoms and signs of an altitude-related sickness develop, the preferred treatment is to descend to a lower altitude. Descents of 1,000–3,000 ft (305–914 m) with an overnight stay are effective in prevention and recovery of all altitude sickness.

AMS may be significantly diminished or prevented with prophylactic or therapeutic use of acetazolamide (i.e., acetazolamide [Diamox]). Headaches may be treated with aspirin, acetaminophen, ibuprofen, indomethacin, or naproxen (see *Appendix A*). Oxygen or hyperbaric chamber therapy will usually relieve some symptoms such as headache, fatigue, and poor sleep. Prochlorperazine (Compazine) may be used to help relieve nausea and vomiting. Dexamethasone (Decadron, Hexadrol) may be used if other treatments are not available or effective (53). Acetazolamide (Diamox) may be helpful (53). Treatment of individuals diagnosed with HACE or HAPE includes descent, oxygen therapy, and/ or hyperbaric bag therapy. Dexamethasone (Decadron, Hexadrol) and acetazolamide (Diamox) are also helpful.

Rapid Ascent

Many unacclimatized individuals travel directly to high mountainous areas for skiing or trekking vacations. Beginning within hours after rapid ascent to a given altitude up to about 14,000 ft (4,300 m), and lasting for the first couple of days, AMS may be present and physical and cognitive performances will be at their nadir for these individuals. During this time, voluntary physical activity should not be excessive, whereas endurance exercise training should be stopped or its intensity greatly reduced to minimize the possibility that AMS will be exacerbated. After this time when AMS subsides because of partial altitude acclimatization, individuals may resume all normal activities and exercise training, if desired. Monitoring exercise HR provides a safe, easy, and objective means to quantify exercise intensity at altitude, as it does at sea level. For example, using an age-predicted maximal HR equation such as "220 − age" and multiplying the result by the same percentage intensity desired at altitude as at sea level provides a similar training stimulus as long as the weekly number and durations of the training sessions are also maintained. Be mindful that for the same perceived effort, jogging or running pace will be reduced at altitude relative to sea level, independent of altitude acclimatization status.

Altitude Acclimatization

With altitude acclimatization, individuals can achieve optimal physical and cognitive performance for the altitude to which they are acclimatized. Altitude acclimatization consists of physiologic adaptations that develop in a time-dependent manner during repeated or continuous exposures to moderate or high altitudes and decreases susceptibility to altitude sickness. In addition to achieving acclimatization by residing continuously at a given target altitude, at least partial altitude acclimatization can develop by living at a moderate elevation, termed *staging*, before ascending to a higher target elevation. The goal of staged ascents is to gradually promote development of altitude acclimatization while averting the adverse consequences (*e.g.*, altitude sickness) of rapid ascent to high altitudes. Breathing low concentrations of oxygen using masks, hoods, or rooms (*i.e.*, normobaric hypoxia) is not as effective as being exposed to the natural altitude environment (*i.e.*, hypobaric hypoxia) for inducing functionally useful altitude acclimatization (41).

For individuals ascending from low altitude, the first stage of all staged ascent protocols should be ≥3 d of residence at moderate altitude. At this altitude, individuals will experience small decrements in physical performance and a low incidence of altitude sickness. At any given altitude, almost all of the acclimatization response is attained between 7 and 12 d of residence at that altitude. Short stays of 3–7 d at moderate altitudes will decrease susceptibility to altitude sickness at higher altitudes. Stays of 6–12 d are required to improve physical work performance. The magnitude of the acclimatization response is increased with additional higher staging elevations or a longer duration at a given staging elevation. The final staging elevation should be as close as

BOX 8.7	Staging Guideline for Exercise at High Altitudes

The general staging guideline is as follows: For every day spent >3,950 ft (1,200 m), an individual is prepared for a subsequent rapid ascent to a higher altitude equal to the number of days at that altitude times 1,000 ft (305 m). For example, if an individual stages at 6,000 ft (1,829 m) for 6 d, physical performance will be improved and altitude sickness will be reduced at altitudes to 12,000 ft (3,637 m). This guideline applies to altitudes up to 14,000 ft (4,267 m).

possible to the target elevation. See *Box 8.7* for the staging guideline for exercise at high altitudes.

Assessing Individual Altitude Acclimatization Status

The best indices of altitude acclimatization over time at a given elevation is a decline (or absence) of altitude sickness, improved physical performance, decreased HR, and an increase in arterial oxygen saturation (SaO_2). The presence and severity of AMS may be evaluated by the extent of its symptoms (*i.e.*, headache, nausea, fatigue, decreased appetite, and poor sleep) and signs (*i.e.*, poor balance, and mild swelling in the hands, feet, or face). The uncomplicated resolution of AMS or its absence in the first 3–4 d following ascent indicates a normal acclimatization response. After about 1–2 wk of acclimatization, physical performance improves such that most tasks can be performed for longer periods of time and with less perceived effort relative to the initial exposure to the same elevation. Another early sign of appropriate adaptation to altitude is increased urine volume, which generally occurs during the first several days at a given elevation. Urine volume will continue to increase with additional ascent and decrease with subsequent adaptation.

Measurement of SaO_2 by noninvasive pulse oximetry is a very good indicator of acclimatization. Pulse oximetry should be performed under quiet, resting conditions. From its nadir on the first day at a given altitude, SaO_2 should progressively increase over the first 3–7 d before stabilizing. For example, with initial exposure to an altitude of 14,000 ft (4,300 m), resting SaO_2 is 81%; after a week of continuous residence at the same elevations, resting SaO_2 progressively rises to ~88%.

Exercise Prescription

During the first few days at high altitudes, individuals should minimize their exercise/physical activity to reduce susceptibility to altitude illness. After this period, individuals whose Ex R_x specifies a THR should maintain the same exercise HR at higher altitudes. The personalized number of weekly training sessions and the duration of each session at altitude can remain similar to those used at sea level for a given individual. This approach reduces the risk of altitude illness and excessive physiologic strain. For example, at high altitudes, reduced speed, distance, or resistance will achieve the same THR as at lower altitudes. Because altitude acclimatization develops, the THR will be achieved at progressively higher exercise intensity.

Developing a Personalized Plan

Adults and children who are acclimatized to altitude, adequately rested, nourished, and hydrated minimize their risk for developing altitude sickness and maximize their physical performance capabilities for the altitude to which they are acclimatized. The following factors should be considered to further minimize the effects of high altitude:

- Monitor the environment: High altitude regions usually are associated with more daily extremes of temperature, humidity, wind, and solar radiation. Follow appropriate guidelines for hot (8) and cold (23) environments.
- Modify activity at high altitudes: Consider altitude acclimatization status, physical fitness, nutrition, sleep quality and quantity, age, exercise time and intensity, and availability of fluids. Provide longer and/or more rest breaks to facilitate rest and recovery and shorten activity times. Longer duration activities are affected more by high altitude than shorter duration activities.
- Develop an altitude acclimatization plan: Monitor progress.
- Clothing: Individual clothing and equipment need to provide protection over a greater range of temperature and wind conditions.
- Education: The training of participants, personal trainers, coaches, and community emergency response teams enhances the reduction, recognition, and treatment of altitude-related illnesses.

Organizational Planning

When clients exercise in high altitude locations, physical fitness facilities and organizations should formulate a standardized management plan that includes the following procedures:

- Screening and surveillance of at-risk participants.
- Using altitude acclimatization procedures to minimize the risk of altitude sickness and enhance physical performance.
- Consideration of the hazards of mountainous terrain when designing exercise programs and activities.
- Awareness of the signs and symptoms of altitude illness.
- Develop organizational procedures for emergency medical care of altitude illnesses.
- Team physicians should consider maintaining a supply of oxygen and pharmaceuticals for preventing and treating altitude sickness.

THE BOTTOM LINE

Physical performance decreases with increasing altitude >3,950 ft (1,200 m), with greater decrements associated with higher elevation, longer activity duration, and larger muscle mass. During the first few days at high altitudes, individuals should minimize their physical activity to reduce susceptibility to altitude illness. After this period, individuals whose Ex R$_x$ specifies a THR should maintain the same exercise HR at higher altitudes.

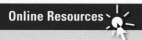

Online Resources

United States Army Institute of Environmental Medicine (USARIEM):
http://www.usariem.army.mil

REFERENCES

1. Abenhaim L, Rossignol M, Valat J, et al. The role of activity in the therapeutic management of back pain. Report of the International Paris Task Force on Back Pain. *Spine.* 2000;25(4):1S–33S.
2. ACOG Committee Obstetric Practice. ACOG Committee opinion. Number 267, January 2002: exercise during pregnancy and the postpartum period. *Obstet Gynecol.* 2002;99(1):171–3.
3. Aina A, May S, Clare H. The centralization phenomenon of spinal symptoms—a systematic review. *Man Ther.* 2004;9:134–43.
4. Airaksinen O, Brox J, Cedraschi C, et al. Chapter 4 European guidelines for the management of chronic nonspecific low back pain. *Eur Spine J.* 2006;15:s192–300.
5. American College of Sports Medicine. Position stand. Exercise and physical activity for older adults. *Med Sci Sports Exerc.* 1998;30(6):992–1008.
6. American College of Sports Medicine, Armstrong LE, Casa DJ, et al. American College of Sports Medicine position stand. Exertional heat illness during training and competition. *Med Sci Sports Exerc.* 2007;39(3):556–72.
7. American College of Sports Medicine, Chodzko-Zajko WJ, Proctor DN, et al. American College of Sports Medicine position stand. Exercise and physical activity for older adults. *Med Sci Sports Exerc.* 2009;41(7):1510–30.
8. American College of Sports Medicine, Sawka MN, Burke LM, et al. American College of Sports Medicine position stand. Exercise and fluid replacement. *Med Sci Sports Exerc.* 2007;39(2):377–90.
9. Andersson EI, Lin CC, Smeets RJ. Performance tests in people with chronic low back pain: responsiveness and minimal clinically important change. *Spine (Phila Pa 1976).* 2010;35(26):E1559–63.
10. Armstrong LE. Heat and humidity. In: Armstrong LE, editor. *Performing in Extreme Environments.* Champaign: Human Kinetics; 2000. p. 15–70.
11. Artal R, O'Toole M. Guidelines of the American College of Obstetricians and Gynecologists for exercise during pregnancy and the postpartum period. *Br J Sports Med.* 2003;37(1):6–12; discussion 12.
12. *Assessing Physical Performance in the Older Patient* [Internet]. Bethesda (MD): National Institute on Aging, U.S. National Institutes of Health; [cited 2011 Feb 4]. Available from: http://www.grc.nia.nih.gov/branches/ledb/sppb/index.htm
13. Atlas S, Deyo R. Evaluating and managing acute low back pain in the primary care setting. *J Gen Intern Med.* 2001;16(2):120–31.
14. Bar-Or O, Rowland TW. *Pediatric Exercise Medicine: From Physiological Principles to Health Care Application.* Champaign (IL): Human Kinetics; 2004. 501 p.
15. Beimborn D, Morrissey M. A review of the literature related to trunk muscle performance. *Spine.* 1988;13(6):655–60.
16. Binkley HM, Beckett J, Casa DJ, Kleiner DM, Plummer PE. National Athletic Trainers' Association Position Statement: exertional heat illnesses. *J Athl Train.* 2002;37(3):329–43.
17. Bouwmeester W, van Enst A, van Tulder M. Quality of low back pain guidelines improved. *Spine.* 2009;34(23):2563–7.

18. Brajkovic D, Ducharme MB. Facial cold-induced vasodilation and skin temperature during exposure to cold wind. *Eur J Appl Physiol.* 2006;96(6):711–21.

19. Campbell MK, Mottola MF. Recreational exercise and occupational activity during pregnancy and birth weight: a case-control study. *Am J Obstet Gynecol.* 2001;184(3):403–8.

20. *Canada's Windchill Index: Windchill Hazards and What To Do* [Internet]. Gatineau (Quebec): Environment Canada; [cited 2011 Feb 4]. Available from: http://www.ec.gc.ca/meteo-weather/default.asp?lang=En&n=5FBF816A-1

21. Cappaert TA, Stone JA, Castellani JW, et al. National Athletic Trainers' Association position statement: environmental cold injuries. *J Athl Train.* 2008;43(6):640–58.

22. Carter R,3rd, Cheuvront SN, Williams JO, et al. Epidemiology of hospitalizations and deaths from heat illness in soldiers. *Med Sci Sports Exerc.* 2005;37(8):1338–44.

23. Castellani JW, Young AJ, Ducharme MB, et al. American College of Sports Medicine position stand: prevention of cold injuries during exercise. *Med Sci Sports Exerc.* 2006;38(11):2012–29.

24. Cesari M, Kritchevsky SB, Newman AB, et al. Added value of physical performance measures in predicting adverse health-related events: results from the health, aging and body composition study. *J Am Geriatr Soc.* 2009;57(2):251–9.

25. Cheuvront SN, Carter R,3rd, Haymes EM, Sawka MN. No effect of moderate hypohydration or hyperthermia on anaerobic exercise performance. *Med Sci Sports Exerc.* 2006;38(6):1093–7.

26. Cheuvront SN, Sawka MN. Hydration assessment of athletes. *Gatorade Sports Sci Exch.* 2005;18(2):1–5.

27. Chou R, Qaseem A, Snow V, et al. Diagnosis and treatment of low back pain: a joint clinical practice guideline from the American College of Physicians and the American Pain Society. *Ann Intern Med.* 2007;147:478–91.

28. *Continuous Scale Physical Functional Performance: Evaluation of Functional Performance in Older Adults* [Internet]. Athens (GA): University of Georgia; [cited 2011 Feb 4]. Available from: http://www.coe.uga.edu/cs-pfp/index.html

29. Cress ME, Buchner DM, Questad KA, Esselman PC, deLateur BJ, Schwartz RS. Continuous-scale physical functional performance in healthy older adults: a validation study. *Arch Phys Med Rehabil.* 1996;77(12):1243–50.

30. Danielsson U. Windchill and the risk of tissue freezing. *J Appl Physiol.* 1996;81(6):2666–73.

31. Davenport MH, Charlesworth S, Vanderspank D, Sopper MM, Mottola MF. Development and validation of exercise target heart rate zones for overweight and obese pregnant women. *Appl Physiol Nutr Metab.* 2008;33(5):984–9.

32. Davies GA, Wolfe LA, Mottola MF, et al. Joint SOGC/CSEP clinical practice guideline: exercise in pregnancy and the postpartum period. *Can J Appl Physiol.* 2003;28(3):330–41.

33. Demoulin C, Vanderthommen M, Duysens C, Crielaard J. Spinal muscle evaluation using the Sorensen test: a critical appraisal of the literature. *Joint Bone Spine.* 2004;73(1):43–50.

34. Dempsey JC, Butler CL, Williams MA. No need for a pregnant pause: physical activity may reduce the occurrence of gestational diabetes mellitus and preeclampsia. *Exerc Sport Sci Rev.* 2005;33(3):141–9.

35. Dugan S. The role of exercise in the prevention and management of acute low back pain. *Clin Occup Environ Med.* 2006;5(3):615–32.

36. Duque I, Parra J, Duvallet A. Aerobic fitness and limiting factors of maximal performance in chronic low back pain patients. *J Back Musculoskelet Rehabil.* 2009;22(2):113–9.

37. Evetovich TK, Boyd JC, Drake SM, et al. Effect of moderate dehydration on torque, electromyography, and mechanomyography. *Muscle Nerve.* 2002;26(2):225–31.

38. Federal Interagency Forum on Aging-Related Statistics (U.S.). *Older Americans 2004: Key Indicators of Well-Being.* Washington (DC): Federal Interagency Forum on Aging-Related Statistics; 2004. 141 p.

39. *Fitnessgram/Activitygram Reference Guide* [Internet]. Dallas (TX): The Cooper Institute; 2008 [cited 2011 Jan 26]. 206 p. Available from: http://www.cooperinstitute.org/ourkidshealth/fitnessgram/documents/FITNESSGRAM_ReferenceGuide.pdf

40. Franklin BA, Hogan P, Bonzheim K, et al. Cardiac demands of heavy snow shoveling. *JAMA.* 1995;273(11):880–2.

41. Fulco CS, Muza SR, Beidleman BA, et al. Effect of repeated normobaric hypoxia exposures during sleep on acute mountain sickness, exercise performance, and sleep during exposure to terrestrial altitude. *Am J Physiol Regul Integr Comp Physiol.* 2011;300(2):R428–36.

42. Fulco CS, Rock PB, Cymerman A. Maximal and submaximal exercise performance at altitude. *Aviat Space Environ Med.* 1998;69(8):793–801.

43. Gagge AP, Gonzalez RR. Mechanisms of heat exchange: biophysics and physiology. In: Fregly MJ, editor. *Handbook of Physiology/Section 4, Environmental Physiology.* Bethesda: American Physiological Society; 1996. p. 45–84.

44. Garber CE, Blissmer B, Deschenes MR, et al. American College of Sports Medicine position stand. Quantity and quality of exercise for developing and maintaining cardiorespiratory, musculoskeletal,

and neuromotor fitness in apparently healthy adults: guidance for prescribing exercise. *Med Sci Sports Exerc*. 2011;43(7):1334–559.

45. Gibbons RJ, Balady GJ, Bricker JT, et al. ACC/AHA 2002 guideline update for exercise testing: summary article: a report of the American College of Cardiology/American Heart Association Task Force on Practice Guidelines (Committee to Update the 1997 Exercise Testing Guidelines). *Circulation*. 2002;106(14):1883–92.

46. Gill TM, DiPietro L, Krumholz HM. Role of exercise stress testing and safety monitoring for older persons starting an exercise program. *JAMA*. 2000;284(3):342–9.

47. Gonzalez RR, Cheuvront SN, Montain SJ, et al. Expanded prediction equations of human sweat loss and water needs. *J Appl Physiol*. 2009;107(2):379–88.

48. Gruther W, Wick F, Paul B, et al. Diagnostic accuracy and reliability of muscle strength and endurance measurements in patients with chronic low back pain. *J Rehabil Med*. 2009;41(8):613–9.

49. Guralnik JM, Ferrucci L, Pieper CF, et al. Lower extremity function and subsequent disability: consistency across studies, predictive models, and value of gait speed alone compared with the short physical performance battery. *J Gerontol A Biol Sci Med Sci*. 2000;55(4):M221–31.

50. Guralnik JM, Leveille S, Volpato S, Marx MS, Cohen-Mansfield J. Targeting high-risk older adults into exercise programs for disability prevention. *J Aging Phys Activ*. 2003;11(2):219–28.

51. Guralnik JM, Simonsick EM, Ferrucci L, et al. A short physical performance battery assessing lower extremity function: association with self-reported disability and prediction of mortality and nursing home admission. *J Gerontol*. 1994;49(2):M85–94.

52. Gutin B, Barbeau P, Owens S, et al. Effects of exercise intensity on cardiovascular fitness, total body composition, and visceral adiposity of obese adolescents. *Am J Clin Nutr*. 2002;75(5):818–26.

53. Hackett PH, Roach RC. High-altitude illness. *N Engl J Med*. 2001;345(2):107–14.

54. Hasenbring M, Hallner D, Rusu A. Fear-avoidance- and endurance-related responses to pain: development and validation of the Avoidance-Endurance Questionnaire (AEQ). *European Journal of Pain* [Internet]. 2008 [cited 2012 Jan 7]. doi:10.1016/j.ejpain.2008.11.001

55. Hayden J, van Tulder M, Tomlinson G. Systematic review: strategies for using exercise therapy to improve outcomes in chronic low back pain. *Ann Intern Med*. 2005;142:776–85.

56. Hebestreit HU, Bar-Or O. Differences between children and adults for exercise testing and prescription. In: Skinner JS, editor. *Exercise Testing and Exercise Prescription for Special Cases: Theoretical Basis and Clinical Application*. 3rd ed. Baltimore: Lippincott Williams & Wilkins; 2005. p. 68–84.

57. Hestbaek L, Leboeuf-Yde C, Manniche C. Low back pain: what is the long-term course? A review of studies of general patient populations. *Eur Spine J*. 2003;12(2):149–65.

58. Hicks G, Fritz J, Delitto A, McGill S. Preliminary development of a clinical prediction rule for determining which patients with low back pain will respond to a stabilization exercise program. *Arch Phys Med Rehabil*. 2005;86:1753–62.

59. Hodselmans A, Dijkstra P, Geertzen J, van der Schans C. Exercise capacity in non-specific chronic low back pain patients: a lean body mass-based Astrand bicycle test; reliability, validity and feasibility. *J Occup Rehabil*. 2008;18(3):282–9.

60. Impact of physical activity during pregnancy and postpartum on chronic disease risk. *Med Sci Sports Exerc*. 2006;38(5):989–1006.

61. Institute of Medicine (É.U.). Panel on Dietary Reference Intakes for Electrolytes and Water. *Dietary Reference Intakes for Water, Potassium, Sodium, Chloride, and Sulfate*. Washington (DC): National Academies Press; 2005. 617 p.

62. Jensen O, Schmidt-Olsen S. A new functional test in the diagnostic evaluation of neurogenic intermittent claudication. *Clin Rheumatol*. 1989;8(3):363–7.

63. Kang HS, Gutin B, Barbeau P, et al. Physical training improves insulin resistance syndrome markers in obese adolescents. *Med Sci Sports Exerc*. 2002;34(12):1920–7.

64. Larivière C, Da Silva R, Arsenault B, Nadeau S, Plamondon A, Vadeboncoeur R. Specificity of a back muscle exercise machine in healthy and low back pain subjects. *Med Sci Sports Exerc*. 2010;42(3):592–9.

65. Lee C, Simmonds M, Novy D, Jones S. Functional self-efficacy, perceived gait ability and perceived exertion in walking performance of individuals with low back pain. *Physiother Theory Pract*. 2002;18(4):193–203.

66. Macdonald HM, Kontulainen SA, Khan KM, McKay HA. Is a school-based physical activity intervention effective for increasing tibial bone strength in boys and girls? *J Bone Miner Res*. 2007; 22(3):434–46.

67. Macedo LG, Maher CG, Latimer J, McAuley JH. Motor control exercise for persistent, nonspecific low back pain: a systematic review. *Phys Ther*. 2009;89(1):9–25.

68. MacKelvie KJ, Petit MA, Khan KM, Beck TJ, McKay HA. Bone mass and structure are enhanced following a 2-year randomized controlled trial of exercise in prepubertal boys. *Bone*. 2004;34(4):755–64.

69. Malina RM. Weight training in youth-growth, maturation, and safety: an evidence-based review. *Clin J Sport Med*. 2006;16(6):478–87.

70. Mazzeo RS, Fulco CS. Physiological systems and their responses to conditions to hypoxia. In: Tipton CM, editor. *ACSM's Advanced Exercise Physiology*. Baltimore: Lippincott Williams & Wilkins; 2006. p. 564–580.

71. McGill S, Karpowicz A. Exercises for spine stabilization: motion/motor patterns, stability progressions, and clinical technique. *Arch Phys Med Rehabil*. 2009;90(1):118–26.

72. McGregor AH, Hukins DW. Lower limb involvement in spinal function and low back pain. *J Back Musculoskelet Rehabil*. 2009;22(4):219–22.

73. Molnar GW, Hughes AL, Wilson O, Goldman RF. Effect of skin wetting on finger cooling and freezing. *J Appl Physiol*. 1973;35(2):205–7.

74. Montain SJ, Latzka WA, Sawka MN. Control of thermoregulatory sweating is altered by hydration level and exercise intensity. *J Appl Physiol*. 1995;79(5):1434–9.

75. Mottola MF. Exercise in the postpartum period: practical applications. *Curr Sports Med Rep*. 2002; 1(6):362–8.

76. Mottola MF, Davenport MH, Brun CR, Inglis SD, Charlesworth S, Sopper MM. VO2peak prediction and exercise prescription for pregnant women. *Med Sci Sports Exerc*. 2006;38(8):1389–95.

77. Mottola MF, Giroux I, Gratton R, et al. Nutrition and exercise prevent excess weight gain in overweight pregnant women. *Med Sci Sports Exerc*. 2010;42(2):265–72.

78. Muza SR, Fulco C, Beidleman BA, Cymerman A. *Altitude Acclimatization and Illness Management*. Washington (DC): Department of the Army Technical Bulletin: TB MED 505; 2010. 120 p.

79. Nadel ER, Fortney SM, Wenger CB. Circulatory adjustments during heat stress. In: Cerretelli P, Whipp BJ, editors. *Exercise Bioenergetics and Gas Exchange: Proceedings of the International Symposium on Exercise Bioenergetics and Gas Exchange, Held in Milan, Italy, July 7–9, 1980, a Satellite of the XXVIII International Congress of Physiological Sciences*. Amsterdam (NY): Elsevier/North-Holland Biomedical Press; sole distributors for the USA and Canada, Elsevier North Holland; 1980. p. 303–313.

80. Nassis GP, Papantakou K, Skenderi K, et al. Aerobic exercise training improves insulin sensitivity without changes in body weight, body fat, adiponectin, and inflammatory markers in overweight and obese girls. *Metabolism*. 2005;54(11):1472–9.

81. National Institute for Occupational Safety and Health, Division of Standards Development and Technology Transfer. *Working in Hot Environments*. Cincinnati (OH): NIOSH; 1992. 12 p.

82. Nelson ME, Rejeski WJ, Blair SN, et al. Physical activity and public health in older adults: recommendation from the American College of Sports Medicine and the American Heart Association. *Med Sci Sports Exerc*. 2007;39(8):1435–45.

83. Neufer PD, Young AJ, Sawka MN. Gastric emptying during exercise: effects of heat stress and hypohydration. *Eur J Appl Physiol Occup Physiol*. 1989;58(4):433–9.

84. *NWS Windchill Chart* [Internet]. Silver Spring (MD): NOAA, National Weather Service; 2009 [cited 2011 Feb 4]. Available from: http://www.nws.noaa.gov/om/windchill/index.shtml

85. Obert P, Mandigouts S, Nottin S, Vinet A, N'Guyen LD, Lecoq AM. Cardiovascular responses to endurance training in children: effect of gender. *Eur J Clin Invest*. 2003;33(3):199–208.

86. Panjabi M, Lydon C, Vasavada A, Grob D, Crisco J, Dvorak J. On the understanding of clinical instability. *Spine*. 1994;19(23):2642–50.

87. Paridon SM, Alpert BS, Boas SR, et al. Clinical stress testing in the pediatric age group: a statement from the American Heart Association Council on Cardiovascular Disease in the Young, Committee on Atherosclerosis, Hypertension, and Obesity in Youth. *Circulation*. 2006;113(15):1905–20.

88. *PARmed-X for Pregnancy* [Internet]. Ottawa (Ontario): Canadian Society for Exercise Physiology; 2002 [cited 2011 Feb 4]. 4 p. Available from: http://www.csep.ca/english/view.asp?x=698

89. Pengel L, Herbert R, Maher C, Refshauge K. Acute low back pain: systematic review of its prognosis. *BMJ*. 2003;327:323.

90. Perera S, Mody SH, Woodman RC, Studenski SA. Meaningful change and responsiveness in common physical performance measures in older adults. *J Am Geriatr Soc*. 2006;54(5):743–9.

91. *Physical Activity Guidelines Advisory Committee Report, 2008* [Internet]. Washington (DC): U.S. Department of Health and Human Services; 2008 [cited 2011 Jan 6]. 683 p. Available from: http://www.health.gov/paguidelines/Report/pdf/CommitteeReport.pdf

92. Pincus T, Burton A, Vogel S, Field A. A systematic review of psychological factors as predictors of chronicity/disability in prospective cohorts of low back pain. *Spine*. 2002;27(5):E109–20.

93. Pozos RS, Danzl DF. Human physiological responses to cold stress and hypothermia. In: Pandolf KB, editor. *Textbooks of Military Medicine: Medical Aspects of Harsh Environments*. Falls Church: Office of the Surgeon General, United States Army; 2002. p. 351–382.

94. Renkawitz T, Boluki D, Grifka J. The association of low back pain, neuromuscular imbalance, and trunk extension strength in athletes. *Spine J*. 2006;6(6):673–783.

95. Richardson C, Jull G, Hodges P, Hides J. *Therapeutic Exercise for Spinal Segmental Stabilization in Low Back Pain*. Toronto (Ontario): Churchill Livingstone; 1999.

96. Rikli RE, Jones CJ. *Senior Fitness Test Manual*. Champaign (IL): Human Kinetics; 2001. 161 p.
97. Roach R, Stepanek J, Hackett P. Acute mountain sickness and high-altitude cerebral edema. In: Pandolf KB, Burr RE, editors. *Textbooks of Military Medicine: Medical Aspects of Harsh Environments*. Falls Church: Office of the Surgeon General, United States Army; 2002. p. 760–88.
98. Sawka MN, Coyle EF. Influence of body water and blood volume on thermoregulation and exercise performance in the heat. *Exerc Sport Sci Rev*. 1999;27:167–218.
99. Sawka MN, Francesconi RP, Young AJ, Pandolf KB. Influence of hydration level and body fluids on exercise performance in the heat. *JAMA*. 1984;252(9):1165–9.
100. Sawka MN, Young AJ. Physiological systems and their responses to conditions of heat and cold. In: Tipton CM, American College of Sports Medicine, editors. *ACSM's Advanced Exercise Physiology*. Baltimore: Lippincott Williams & Wilkins; 2006. p. 535–63.
101. Sawka MN, Young AJ, Latzka WA, Neufer PD, Quigley MD, Pandolf KB. Human tolerance to heat strain during exercise: influence of hydration. *J Appl Physiol*. 1992;73(1):368–75.
102. Senay LC,Jr. Relationship of evaporative rates to serum [Na+], [K+], and osmolarity in acute heat stress. *J Appl Physiol*. 1968;25(2):149–52.
103. Simmonds MJ, Goubert L, Moseley GL, Verbunt JA. Moving with pain. In: Flor H, Kalso E, Dostrovsky JO, editors. *Proceedings of the 11th World Congress on Pain, Sydney, Australia, August 21–26, 2005*. Seattle: IASP Press; 2006. p. 799–811.
104. Simmonds MJ, Lee CE. Physical performance tests: an expanded model of assessment and outcome. In: Liebenson C, Czech School of Manual Medicine, editors. *Rehabilitation of the Spine: A Practitioner's Manual*. Baltimore: Lippincott, Williams & Wilkins; 2006. p. 260–275.
105. Simmonds MJ, Olson S, Jones S, et al. Psychometric characteristics and clinical usefulness of physical performance tests in patients with low back pain. *Spine*. 1998;23(22):2412–21.
106. Singh MA. Exercise comes of age: rationale and recommendations for a geriatric exercise prescription. *J Gerontol A Biol Sci Med Sci*. 2002;57(5):M262–82.
107. Skinner JS. Aging for exercise testing and exercise prescription. In: Skinner JS, editor. *Exercise Testing and Exercise Prescription for Special Cases: Theoretical Basis and Clinical Application*. 3rd ed. Baltimore: Lippincott Williams & Wilkins; 2005. p. 85–99.
108. Skytte L, May S, Petersen P. Centralization: its prognostic value in patients with referred symptoms and sciatica. *Spine*. 2005;30(11):E293–9.
109. Smeets R, van Geel K, Verbunt J. Is the fear avoidance model associated with the reduced level of aerobic fitness in patients with chronic low back pain? *Arch Phys Med Rehabil*. 2009;90(1): 109–17.
110. Smeets R, Wittink H, Hidding A, Knottnerus J. Do patients with chronic low back pain have a lower level of aerobic fitness than healthy controls?: are pain, disability, fear of injury, working status, or level of leisure time activity associated with the difference in aerobic fitness level? *Spine*. 2006;31(1):90–7.
111. Strong WB, Malina RM, Blimkie CJ, et al. Evidence based physical activity for school-age youth. *J Pediatr*. 2005;146(6):732–7.
112. Sullivan M, Shoaf L, Riddle D. The relationship of lumbar flexion to disability in patients with low back pain. *Phys Ther*. 2000;80(3):240–50.
113. Troiano RP, Berrigan D, Dodd KW, Masse LC, Tilert T, McDowell M. Physical activity in the United States measured by accelerometer. *Med Sci Sports Exerc*. 2008;40(1):181–8.
114. U.S. Department of Health and Human Services. *2008 Physical Activity Guidelines for Americans* [Internet]. Washington (DC): U.S. Department of Health and Human Services; 2008 [cited 2011 Jan 6]. 76 p. Available from: http://www.health.gov/paguidelines/pdf/paguide.pdf
115. van Tulder M, Becker A, Bekkering T, et al. Chapter 3 European guidelines for the management of acute nonspecific low back pain in primary care. *Eur Spine J*. 2006;15:s169–91.
116. Verbunt JA, Smeets RJ, Wittink HM. Cause or effect? Deconditioning and chronic low back pain. *Pain*. 2010;149(3):428–30.
117. Wasiak R, Kim J, Pransky G. Work disability and costs caused by recurrence of low back pain: longer and more costly than in first episodes. *Spine*. 2006;31(2):219–25.
118. *Weight Gain During Pregnancy: Reexamining the Guideline. Report Brief* [Internet]. Washington (DC): National Academy of Sciences; 2009 [cited 2011 Jan 13]. 4 p. Available from: http://www.iom.edu/Reports/2009/Weight-Gain-During-Pregnancy-Reexamining-the-Guidelines.aspx
119. Werneke M, Hart D, Cook D. A descriptive study of the centralization phenomenon: a prospective analysis. *Spine*. 1999;24(7):676–83.
120. Wittink H, Michel T, Kulich R, et al. Aerobic fitness testing in patients with chronic low back pain: which test is best? *Spine*. 2000;25(13):1704–10.
121. Wolfe LA. Pregnancy. In: Skinner JS, editor. *Exercise Testing and Exercise Prescription for Special Cases: Theoretical Basis and Clinical Application*. 3rd ed. Baltimore: Lippincott Williams & Wilkins; 2005. p. 377–391.

9

Exercise Prescription for Patients with Cardiovascular and Cerebrovascular Disease

The intent of this chapter is to describe the guidelines for developing an exercise prescription (Ex R$_x$) among individuals with cardiovascular (CVD) and cerebrovascular disease (see *Box 9.1*). Specifically, this chapter will focus on (a) exercise training procedures for inpatient and outpatient cardiac rehabilitation programs; (b) resistance training guidelines; and (c) procedures for preparing patients to return to work.

INPATIENT REHABILITATION PROGRAMS

Following a documented physician referral, patients hospitalized after a cardiac event or procedure associated with coronary artery disease (CAD), cardiac valve replacement, or myocardial infarction (MI) should be provided with a program consisting of early assessment and mobilization, identification of and education regarding CVD risk factors, assessment of the patient's level of readiness for physical activity, and comprehensive discharge planning.

The goals for inpatient rehabilitation programs are as follows:

- Identify patients with significant cardiovascular, physical, or cognitive impairments that may influence the performance of physical activity.
- Offset the deleterious physiologic and psychological effects of bed rest.
- Provide additional medical surveillance of patients and their responses to physical activity.
- Evaluate and begin to enable patients to safely return to activities of daily living (ADL) within the limits imposed by their CVD.
- Prepare the patient and support system at home or in a transitional setting to optimize recovery following acute care hospital discharge.
- Facilitate physician referral and patient entry into an outpatient cardiac rehabilitation program.

Before beginning formal physical activity in the inpatient setting, a baseline assessment should be conducted by a health care provider who possesses the skills and competencies necessary to assess and document vital signs, heart and lung sounds, and musculoskeletal strength and flexibility. Initiation and progression of physical activity depends on the findings of the initial assessment and

BOX 9.1	Manifestations of Cardiovascular Disease

Acute coronary syndromes: the manifestation of coronary artery disease (CAD) as increasing symptoms of angina pectoris, myocardial infarction (MI), or sudden death

Cardiovascular disease (CVD): diseases that involve the heart and/or blood vessels; includes hypertension, CAD, peripheral arterial disease; includes but not limited to atherosclerotic arterial disease

Cerebrovascular disease (stroke): diseases of the blood vessels that supply the brain

CAD: disease of the arteries of the heart (usually atherosclerotic)

Myocardial ischemia: temporary lack of adequate coronary blood flow relative to myocardial oxygen demands; it is often manifested as angina pectoris

MI: injury/death of the muscular tissue of the heart

Peripheral arterial disease (PAD): diseases of arterial blood vessels outside the heart and brain

varies with level of risk. Thus, inpatients should be risk stratified as early as possible following their acute cardiac event or procedure. The American College of Sports Medicine (ACSM) has adopted the risk stratification system established by the American Association of Cardiovascular and Pulmonary Rehabilitation (AACVPR) for patients with known CVD because it considers the overall prognosis of the patient and their potential for rehabilitation (31) (see *Box 2.4*).

The indications and contraindications for inpatient and outpatient cardiac rehabilitation are listed in *Box 9.2*. Exceptions should be considered based on the clinical judgment of the physician and the rehabilitation team. Shortened length of hospital stay after the acute event or intervention limits the time available for patient assessment and the rehabilitation intervention. Patients who undergo elective percutaneous coronary intervention are usually discharged within 24 h from admission, and patients with uncomplicated MI or coronary artery bypass graft (CABG) surgery are often discharged within 5 d. Activities and programs during the early recovery period will depend on the size of the MI and the occurrence of any complications and include self-care activities, arm and leg range of motion (ROM), and postural changes. Simple exposure to orthostatic or gravitational stress, such as intermittent sitting or standing during hospital convalescence, reduces much of the deterioration in exercise performance that often follows an acute cardiac event (12). Patients may progress from self-care activities to walking short to moderate distances of 50–500 ft (15–152 m) with minimal or no assistance three to four times per day to independent ambulation on the hospital unit. The optimal dose of exercise for inpatients remains to be better defined. Nevertheless, it depends in part on the patient's medical history,

BOX 9.2	Indications and Contraindications for Inpatient and Outpatient Cardiac Rehabilitation

INDICATIONS
- Medically stable post–myocardial infarction (MI)
- Stable angina
- Coronary artery bypass graft (CABG) surgery
- Percutaneous transluminal coronary angioplasty (PTCA)
- Stable heart failure caused by either systolic or diastolic dysfunction (cardiomyopathy)
- Heart transplantation
- Valvular heart surgery
- Peripheral arterial disease (PAD)
- At risk for coronary artery disease (CAD) with diagnoses of diabetes mellitus, dyslipidemia, hypertension, or obesity
- Other patients who may benefit from structured exercise and/or patient education based on physician referral and consensus of the rehabilitation team

CONTRAINDICATIONS
- Unstable angina
- Uncontrolled hypertension — that is, resting systolic blood pressure (SBP) >180 mm Hg and/or resting diastolic BP (DBP) >110 mm Hg
- Orthostatic BP drop of >20 mm Hg with symptoms
- Significant aortic stenosis (aortic valve area <1.0 cm^2)
- Uncontrolled atrial or ventricular arrhythmias
- Uncontrolled sinus tachycardia (>120 beats · min^{-1})
- Uncompensated heart failure
- Third-degree atrioventricular (AV) block without pacemaker
- Active pericarditis or myocarditis
- Recent embolism
- Acute thrombophlebitis
- Acute systemic illness or fever
- Uncontrolled diabetes mellitus (see *Chapter 10*)
- Severe orthopedic conditions that would prohibit exercise
- Other metabolic conditions, such as acute thyroiditis, hypokalemia, hyperkalemia, or hypovolemia (until adequately treated)

clinical status, and symptoms. The rating of perceived exertion (RPE) provides a useful and complementary guide to heart rate (HR) in gauging exercise intensity (see *Chapter 7*). In general, the criteria for terminating an inpatient exercise session are similar to or slightly more conservative than those for terminating a low-level exercise test (see *Box 9.3*) (2). Although not all patients may be suitable candidates for inpatient exercise, virtually all benefit from some level of inpatient

BOX 9.3	Adverse Responses to Inpatient Exercise Leading to Exercise Discontinuation

- Diastolic blood pressure (DBP) ≥110 mm Hg
- Decrease in systolic blood pressure (SBP) >10 mm Hg during exercise with increasing workload
- Significant ventricular or atrial arrhythmias with or without associated signs/symptoms
- Second- or third-degree heart block
- Signs/symptoms of exercise intolerance including angina, marked dyspnea, and electrocardiogram (ECG) changes suggestive of ischemia

Used with permission from (2).

intervention including the assessment of CVD risk factors (see *Table 2.2*), physical activity counseling, and patient and family education.

Recommendations for inpatient exercise programming include the Frequency, Intensity, Time, and Type of Exercise or the *FITT* principle of Ex R$_x$ as well as progression. Activity goals should be built into the overall plan of care. The exercise program components for patients with CVD are essentially the same as for individuals who are apparently healthy (see *Chapter 7*) or for individuals in the low-risk category (see *Box 2.4*).

FITT RECOMMENDATIONS FOR INPATIENT PROGRAMS

Frequency: Mobilization: two to four times per day for the first 3 d of the hospital stay.

Intensity: Seated or standing resting heart rate (HR$_{rest}$) +20 beats · min^{-1} for patients with an MI and +30 beats · min^{-1} for patients recovering from heart surgery; with an upper limit ≤120 beats · min^{-1} that corresponds to an RPE ≤13 on a scale of 6–20 (6).

Time: Begin with intermittent walking bouts lasting 3–5 min as tolerated with exercise bouts of progressively increasing duration. The rest period may be a slower walk (or complete rest at the patient's discretion) that is shorter than the duration of the exercise bout. Attempt to achieve a 2:1 exercise/rest ratio.

Type: Walking.

Progression: When continuous exercise duration reaches 10–15 min, increase intensity as tolerated within the recommended RPE and HR limits.

By hospital discharge, the patient should demonstrate an understanding of physical activities that may be inappropriate or excessive. Moreover, a safe, progressive plan of exercise should be formulated before leaving the hospital. A predischarge low-level submaximal exercise test is useful for prognostic assessment (see *Chapter 5*), evaluation of medical therapy or coronary interventions, Ex R$_x$, and physical activity counseling (16). Until evaluated with an exercise test or entry into a clinically supervised outpatient cardiac rehabilitation program, the upper limit of exercise should not exceed those levels observed during the inpatient program while closely monitoring for signs and symptoms of exercise intolerance. Patients should be counseled to identify abnormal signs and symptoms suggesting exercise intolerance and the need for medical evaluation. All patients also should be educated and encouraged to investigate outpatient exercise program options with appropriately qualified staff and be provided with information regarding the use of home exercise equipment. All patients, especially moderate- to high-risk patients (see *Box 2.4*), should be strongly encouraged to participate in a clinically supervised outpatient cardiac rehabilitation program.

OUTPATIENT EXERCISE PROGRAMS

Outpatient cardiac rehabilitation programs may begin as soon as possible after hospital discharge (32). The goals for outpatient rehabilitation are listed in *Box 9.4*.

At program entry, the following assessments should be performed:

- Medical and surgical history including the most recent cardiovascular event, comorbidities, and other pertinent medical history.
- Physical examination with an emphasis on the cardiopulmonary and musculoskeletal systems.
- Review of recent cardiovascular tests and procedures including 12-lead electrocardiogram (ECG), coronary angiogram, echocardiogram, stress test

---

| BOX 9.4 | Goals for Outpatient Cardiac Rehabilitation |

- Develop and assist the patient to implement a safe and effective formal exercise and lifestyle physical activity program.
- Provide appropriate supervision and monitoring to detect change in clinical status.
- Provide ongoing surveillance data to the patient's health care providers in order to enhance medical management.
- Return the patient to vocational and recreational activities or modify these activities based on the patient's clinical status.
- Provide patient and spouse/partner/family education to optimize secondary prevention (*e.g.*, risk factor modification) through aggressive lifestyle management and judicious use of cardioprotective medications.

(exercise or imaging studies), revascularization, and pacemaker/implantable defibrillator implantation.

- Current medications including dose, route of administration, and frequency
- CVD risk factors (see *Table* 2.2).

Exercise training is safe and effective for most patients with CVD; however, all patients should be stratified based on their risk for occurrence of a cardiac-related event during exercise training (see *Box* 2.4). Routine preexercise assessment of risk for exercise (see *Chapters* 3 and 5) should be performed before, during, and after each rehabilitation session, as deemed appropriate by the qualified staff and include the following:

- HR.
- Blood pressure (BP).
- Body weight (weekly).
- Symptoms or evidence of change in clinical status not necessarily related to activity (*e.g.*, dyspnea at rest, light-headedness or dizziness, palpitations or irregular pulse, chest discomfort).
- Symptoms and evidence of exercise intolerance.
- Change in medications and adherence to the prescribed medication regimen.
- Consideration of ECG surveillance that may consist of telemetry or hardwire monitoring, "quick-look" monitoring using defibrillator paddles, or periodic rhythm strips depending on the risk status of the patient and the need for accurate rhythm detection.

EXERCISE PRESCRIPTION

The "American College of Cardiology (ACC)/American Heart Association (AHA) 2002 Guideline Update for Exercise Testing" (16) states exercise testing at baseline is essential for the development of an Ex R_x in patients who suffered from MI with (Class I recommendation) or without (Class IIa recommendation) revascularization, as well as those patients who have undergone coronary revascularization alone (Class IIa recommendation). The test should be completed while the patient is stable on guideline-based medications.

Prescriptive techniques for determining exercise dosage or the FITT principle of Ex R_x for the general apparently healthy population are detailed in *Chapter* 7. The Ex R_x techniques used for the apparently healthy adult population classified as low-to-moderate risk for occurrence of a cardiac-related event during exercise training (see *Figure* 2.3) may be applied to many low- and moderate-risk patients with CVD. This chapter provides specific considerations and modifications of the Ex R_x for patients with known CVD.

Key variables to be considered in the development of an Ex R_x for patients with CVD include the following:

- Safety factors including clinical status, risk stratification category (see *Box* 2.4), exercise capacity, ischemic/anginal threshold, musculoskeletal limitations,

and cognitive/psychological impairment that might result in nonadherence and/or inability to meet exercise guidelines.
- Associated factors including premorbid activity level, vocational and avocational requirements, and personal health/fitness goals.

FITT RECOMMENDATIONS FOR OUTPATIENT PROGRAMS

FITT

Frequency: Exercise should be performed at least 3 d but preferably on most days of the week. Frequency of exercise depends on several factors including baseline exercise tolerance, exercise intensity, fitness and other health goals, and types of exercise that are incorporated into the overall program. For patients with very limited exercise capacities, multiple short (1–10 min) daily sessions may be prescribed. Patients should be encouraged to perform some of these exercise sessions independently (*i.e.*, without direct supervision) following the recommendations outlined in this chapter.

Intensity: Exercise intensity may be prescribed using one or more of the following methods:

- Based on results from the baseline exercise test, 40%–80% of exercise capacity using the HR reserve (HRR), oxygen uptake reserve ($\dot{V}O_2R$), or peak oxygen uptake ($\dot{V}O_{2peak}$) methods
- RPE of 11–16 on a scale of 6–20 (6)
- Exercise intensity should be prescribed at a HR below the ischemic threshold; for example, <10 beats, if such a threshold has been determined for the patient. The presence of classic angina pectoris that is induced with exercise and relieved with rest or nitroglycerin is sufficient evidence for the presence of myocardial ischemia

For the purposes of the Ex R_x, it is preferable for individuals to take their prescribed medications at their usual time as recommended by their health care providers. Individuals on a β-adrenergic blocking agent (*i.e.*, β-blocker) may have an attenuated HR response to exercise and an increased or decreased maximal exercise capacity. For patients whose β-blocker dose was altered after an exercise test or during the course of rehabilitation, a new graded exercise test may be helpful, particularly in patients who have not undergone a coronary revascularization procedure or who have been incompletely revascularized (*i.e.*, residual obstructive coronary lesions are present) or who have rhythm disturbances. However, another exercise test may not be medically necessary in patients who have undergone complete coronary revascularization, or when it is logistically impractical.

When patients whose β-blocker dose has been altered exercise without a new exercise test, signs and symptoms should be monitored, and RPE and HR responses should be recorded at previously performed workloads. These new HRs may serve as the patient's new exercise target HR (THR) range. Patients on diuretic therapy may become volume depleted, have hypokalemia, or demonstrate orthostatic hypotension particularly after bouts of exercise. For these patients, the BP response to exercise, symptoms of dizziness or light-headedness, and arrhythmias should be monitored while providing education regarding proper hydration (3). See *Appendix A* for other medications that may influence the hemodynamic response during and after exercise.

Time: Warm-up and cool-down activities of 5–10 min, including static stretching, ROM, and light intensity (*i.e.*, <40% $\dot{V}O_2R$, <64% peak heart rate [HR_{peak}], or <11 RPE) aerobic activities, should be a component of each exercise session and precede and follow the conditioning phase. The goal for the duration of the aerobic conditioning phase is generally 20–60 min per session. After a cardiac-related event, patients may begin with as little as 5–10 min of aerobic conditioning with a gradual increase in aerobic exercise time of 1–5 min per session or an increase in time per session of 10%–20% per week.

Type: The aerobic exercise portion of the session should include rhythmic, large muscle group activities with an emphasis on increased caloric expenditure for maintenance of a healthy body weight and its many other associated health benefits (see *Chapters 1, 7,* and *10*). To promote whole body physical fitness, conditioning that includes the upper and lower extremities and multiple forms of aerobic activities and exercise equipment should be incorporated into the exercise program. The different types of exercise equipment may include the following:

- Arm ergometer
- Combination of upper or lower (dual action) extremity cycle ergometer
- Upright and recumbent cycle ergometer
- Recumbent stepper
- Rower
- Elliptical
- Stair climber
- Treadmill for walking

Aerobic interval training (AIT) involves alternating 3–4 min periods of exercise at high intensity (90%–95% HR_{peak}) with exercise at moderate intensity (60%–70% HR_{peak}). Such training for approximately 40 min, three times per week has been shown to yield a greater improvement in $\dot{V}O_{2peak}$ in patients with heart failure (44) and greater long-term improvements in $\dot{V}O_{2peak}$ in patients after CABG (27) compared to standard continuous, moderate intensity exercise. Although AIT has routinely been used in athletes, its use in patients with CVD appears to have potential but cannot yet be universally recommended until further data regarding safety and efficacy are available.

Progression: There is no standard format for the rate of progression in exercise session duration. Thus, progression should be individualized to patient tolerance. Factors to consider in this regard include initial physical fitness level, patient motivation and goals, symptoms, and musculoskeletal limitations. Exercise sessions may include continuous or intermittent exercise depending on the capability of the patient. *Table 9.1* provides a sample progression using intermittent exercise.

Continuous Electrocardiographic Monitoring

ECG monitoring during supervised exercise sessions may be helpful during the first several weeks. The following recommendations for ECG monitoring are related to patient-associated risks of exercise training (see *Chapter 1*) and are in agreement with those of the AACVPR (2):

- Low-risk cardiac patients may begin with continuous ECG monitoring and decrease to intermittent ECG monitoring after six sessions or sooner as deemed appropriate by the rehabilitation staff.
- Moderate-risk patients may begin with continuous ECG monitoring and decrease to intermittent ECG monitoring after 12 sessions or sooner as deemed appropriate by the rehabilitation staff.
- High-risk patients may begin with continuous ECG monitoring and decrease to intermittent ECG monitoring after 18 sessions or sooner as deemed appropriate by the rehabilitation staff.

TABLE 9.1. Sample Exercise Progression Using Intermittent Exercise (5)

Week	% FC	Total Exercise Time (min) at % FC	Exercise Bout (min)	Rest Bout (min)	Number of Exercise/ Rest Bouts
Functional Capacity ≥4 METs					
1–2	50–60	15–20	3–10	2–5	3–4
3–4	60–70	20–40	10–20	Optional	2
Functional Capacity ≥4 METs					
1–2	40–50	10–20	3–7	3–5	3–4
3–4	50–60	15–30	7–15	2–5	2–3
5	60–70	25–40	12–20	2	2

Continue with two repetitions of continuous exercise with one rest period or progress to a single continuous bout.

FC, functional capacity; MET, metabolic equivalent.

BOX 9.5	Reasons for No Available Preparticipation Exercise Test

- Extreme deconditioning
- Orthopedic limitations
- Recent successful percutaneous intervention or revascularization surgery without residual obstructive coronary artery disease

Exercise Prescription without a Preparticipation Exercise Test

Exercise testing at baseline is important for the development of an Ex R_x in patients experiencing an MI or undergoing a coronary revascularization (16). However, with shorter hospital stays, more aggressive interventions, and greater sophistication of diagnostic procedures, it is not unusual for patients to begin cardiac rehabilitation before having an exercise test (see *Box 9.5*). Until an exercise test is performed, Ex R_x procedures can be based on the recommendations of these *Guidelines* and what was accomplished during the inpatient phase, home exercise activities, and RPE. The rehabilitation staff should closely monitor for signs and symptoms of exercise intolerance such as excessive fatigue, dizziness or light-headedness, chronotropic incompetence, and signs or symptoms of ischemia.

Lifestyle Physical Activity

In addition to formal exercise sessions, patients should be encouraged to gradually return to general ADL such as household chores, yard work, shopping, and hobbies as evaluated and appropriately modified by the rehabilitation staff. Participation in competitive sports should be guided by the recommendations of the ACC Bethesda Conference (42). Relatively inexpensive pedometers can be useful to monitor physical activity and may enhance adherence with walking programs (8). Walking for 30 min $\cdot$ d^{-1} equates to 3,000–4,000 steps, whereas a 1-mi (1.6 km) walk equates to ~2,000 steps. To meet current recommendations for physical activity, adding ~2,000 steps $\cdot$ d^{-1} to reach a daily step count of 5,400–7,000 steps $\cdot$ d^{-1} is beneficial. Pedometers are most effective in increasing physical activity when accompanied by a goal for achieving specific daily step count, such as a goal of 10,000 steps $\cdot$ d^{-1} (8) (see *Chapter 7*).

TYPES OF OUTPATIENT EXERCISE PROGRAMS

Participation in cardiac rehabilitation after suffering or undergoing an indexed cardiac-related event represents guideline-based care to reduce the risk for experiencing a second event, improving exercise tolerance, managing symptoms, and facilitating healthier lifestyle changes. However, cardiac rehabilitation is underused. For example, among Medicare beneficiaries, in 1997, only 14% of patients experiencing an MI and 31% who had undergone CABG received cardiac rehabilitation (41). However, many patients may be unable to participate for various reasons including program location and accessibility, transportation, and work or personal schedules. Accordingly, creative programming that incorporates a mix of supervised and unsupervised sessions (*i.e.*, hybrid design) and/or regular telephone, Internet, or mail contact should be considered as alternatives. In some cases, an independent program with follow-up by the patient's health care providers may be the only option.

It is important that patients eventually transition from a medically supervised program to an independent one (*i.e.*, self-monitored and unsupervised home exercise program). The optimal number of weeks of attendance at a supervised program before entering an independent program is unknown and is likely patient specific. Insurance reimbursement is often a factor that determines the length of time of participation in a supervised program. In any case, the rehabilitation team should develop a program that appropriately prepares the patient for eventual transfer to unsupervised exercise. Some centers offer extended short-term transition programs or long-term maintenance programs. The following issues should be considered in the determination of appropriateness for independent exercise:

- Cardiac symptoms that are stable or absent.
- Appropriate HR, BP, and rhythm responses to exercise (see *Chapters* 4 and 5).
- Demonstrated knowledge of proper exercise principles and awareness of abnormal symptoms.
- Motivation to continue to exercise regularly without close supervision.

SPECIAL CONSIDERATIONS

Patients with Peripheral Artery Disease

Peripheral artery disease (PAD) affects approximately 8 million adults in the United States (34) and increases in prevalence with advancing age (40). Major risk factors for PAD include diabetes mellitus, hypertension, smoking, dyslipidemia, hyperhomocysteinemia, non-Caucasian race, high levels of C-reactive protein, and renal insufficiency (28). Patients with PAD have a 6.6 times greater risk of dying from CVD compared with individuals without PAD (40).

Intermittent claudication, the major symptom of PAD, is characterized by a reproducible aching or cramping sensation in one or both legs that typically is triggered by weight-bearing exercise (38). Intermittent claudication is reported in 5% of the population in the United States older than 55 yr. On initial clinical presentation, up to 35% of individuals with PAD have typical claudication and up to 50% have atypical leg pain (20,28). Because those with either typical or atypical claudication have similar changes in ankle systolic BP (SBP) during treadmill exercise (13), patients with any description of leg pain should be considered to have intermittent claudication until proven otherwise. As the

TABLE 9.2. Fontaine Classification of Peripheral Artery Disease (38)

Stage	Symptoms
1	Asymptomatic
2	Intermittent claudication
2a	Distance to pain onset >200 m
2b	Distance to pain onset <200 m
3	Pain at rest
4	Gangrene, tissue loss

symptoms worsen, they may become severe enough to limit the individual from performing ADL (14).

PAD is caused by the development of atherosclerotic plaque in systemic arteries that leads to significant stenosis, resulting in the reduction of blood flow to regions distal to the area of occlusion. This reduction in blood flow creates a mismatch between oxygen supply and demand causing ischemia to develop in the affected areas that typically are the calf, thigh, or buttocks (18). PAD is staged based on the presence of symptoms as described in *Table 9.2* and by the ankle-brachial index (ABI), with values ranging from >1.0 to <0.5 (see *Table 9.3*) (38). If arterial lesions in the lower extremities progress to severe PAD, resulting in severe claudication or pain at rest, peripheral intervention may be indicated (18,40). In the most severe cases in which critical limb ischemia develops resulting in gangrene or tissue loss, amputation of the lower extremity may be indicated. The recommended treatments for PAD include an initially conservative approach using medications (*e.g.*, cilostazol) (see *Appendix A*) and exercise followed by peripheral revascularization if conservative therapy is not successful (18).

Exercise Testing

Exercise testing is performed in patients with PAD to determine the time of onset of claudication pain pretherapeutic and posttherapeutic intervention, to measure the postexercise ABI, and to diagnose the presence of CVD (45):

- Patients with PAD are classified as high risk (see *Table 2.3*); therefore, exercise testing under medical supervision is indicated (see *Figure 2.4*).
- Medication dose should be noted and repeated in an identical manner in subsequent exercise tests.

TABLE 9.3. Ankle-Brachial Index Scale for Peripheral Arterial Disease (38)

Supine Resting Ankle-Brachial Index	Postexercise Ankle-Brachial Index
>1.0	No change or increase
0.8–0.9	>0.5
0.5–0.8	>0.2
<0.5	<0.2

- Ankle and brachial artery SBP should be measured bilaterally after 5–10 min of rest in the supine position. The ABI should be calculated by dividing the higher ankle SBP reading by the higher brachial artery SBP reading.
- A treadmill protocol beginning with a slow speed with gradual increments in grade is recommended (45) (see *Chapter 5*).
- Claudication pain perception may be monitored using the following scale: 0 = *no pain*, 1 = *onset of pain*, 2 = *moderate pain*, 3 = *intense pain*, and 4 = *maximal pain* (45), or the Borg CR10 Scale (7) (see *Figure 9.1*). The time and distance to the onset of pain and the time and distance to maximal pain should be recorded.
- Following the completion of the exercise test, patients should recover in the supine position for up to 15 min, and ABI should be calculated during this time. The time taken for the pain to resolve after exercise should also be recorded (45).
- In addition to the symptom-limited graded exercise test, the 6-min walking test may be used to assess ambulatory function in patients with PAD (45).

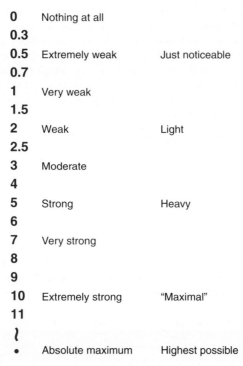

■ **FIGURE 9.1.** The Borg CR10 Scale. The scale with correct instructions can be obtained from Borg Perception, Radisvagen 124, 16573 Hasselby, Sweden. See also the home page: www.borgperception.se/index.html. © Gunnar Borg. Reprinted with permission from (7). Note: This scale is a pain scale that can be adapted to determine dyspnea and most other symptoms.

FITT Recommendations for Individuals with Peripheral Artery Disease

Exercise training is effective in the treatment of individuals with PAD. Training using an interval approach leads to increases in the times and distances to onset of pain and to maximal pain (14). The exercise program should also be designed to target the CVD risk factors that are often associated with PAD (45). The following FITT principle of Ex R$_x$ is recommended for individuals with PAD.

FITT RECOMMENDATIONS FOR PATIENTS WITH PAD   FITT

Frequency: Weight-bearing aerobic exercise 3–5 d · wk^{-1}; resistance exercise at least 2 d · wk^{-1}

Intensity: Moderate intensity (*i.e.*, 40%–<60% $\dot{V}O_2R$) that allows the patient to walk until he or she reaches a pain score of 3 (*i.e.*, intense pain) on the 4-point pain scale (45). Between bouts of activity, individuals should be given time to allow ischemic pain to subside before resuming exercise (19,45).

Time: 30–60 min · d^{-1}, but initially, some patients may need to start with 10 min bouts and exercise intermittently to accumulate a total of 30–60 min · d^{-1}. Many patients may need to begin the program by accumulating only 15 min · d^{-1}, gradually increasing time by 5 min · d^{-1} biweekly.

Type: Weight-bearing aerobic exercise, such as walking, and non–weight-bearing exercise, such as arm and leg ergometry. Cycling may be used as a warm-up but should not be the primary type of activity. Resistance training is recommended to enhance and maintain muscular strength and endurance (see *Chapter 7*).

Other Considerations

- The optimal work to rest ratio has not been determined for individuals with PAD. Nonetheless, the work to rest ratio may need to be adjusted for each patient.
- A cold environment may aggravate the symptoms of intermittent claudication; therefore, a longer warm-up may be necessary (10).
- Encourage patients to stop smoking if they are current smokers.
- For optimal benefit, patients should participate in a supervised exercise program for a minimum of 6 mo (15). Following exercise training programs of this length, improvements in pain-free walking of 106%–177% and 64%–85% in absolute walking ability may occur (9).

Patients with a Sternotomy

Median sternotomy is usually performed as part of CABG and valve replacement surgery in order to gain access to the heart. Although there are various surgical techniques that are used to close the sternum upon completion of the operation, the figure-of-eight interlocking closures with sternal wires, is commonly performed to secure the sternum during the early postoperative period (24). Sternal bone healing to attain adequate sternal stability is usually achieved by 8 wk (35). Healing-related complications that include infection, nonunion, and instability occur in about 2%–5% of cases (24). Several clinical factors such as diabetes mellitus, obesity, immunosuppressive therapy, advanced age, and osteoporosis predispose patients to such complications (24).

In any case, caution must be used in developing an exercise program in patients with a sternotomy, particularly within the first 8–12 wk following the procedure. There are no clinical studies that have adequately evaluated the effect of specific activities and exercise programming on sternal healing and stability. Hence, clinical judgment on the part of the rehabilitation team must be used. The patient's surgeon, health care provider, or appropriately trained rehabilitation staff should routinely evaluate the sternal wound for infection, healing, and stability during the first 8–12 wk following surgery and longer if any unusual symptoms of sternal pain or other complications occur. Upper body movements that exert tension on the sternal wound should be avoided during this early period. Because each patient differs in muscular strength and other factors that may affect healing, no standard weight limits can be recommended during this early period. Subsequently, after appropriate evaluation, ROM exercises and other activities that involve sternal muscles can be gradually introduced and progressed as long as there is no evidence of sternal instability as detected by movement in the sternum, pain, cracking, or popping.

Recent Pacemaker or Implantable Cardioverter Defibrillator Implantation

Cardiac pacemakers are used to restore an optimal HR and to synchronize atrial and ventricular filling and contraction in the setting of abnormal rhythms. Specific indications for pacemakers include sick sinus syndrome with symptomatic bradycardia, acquired atrioventricular (AV) block, and persistent advanced AV block after MI. Cardiac resynchronization pacemakers, sometimes called *biventricular pacemakers*, are used in patients with left ventricular systolic dysfunction who demonstrate ventricular dyssynchrony during contraction of the left and right ventricles. The different types of pacemakers are the following:

- Rate-responsive pacemakers that are programmed to increase or decrease HR to match the level of physical activity (*e.g.*, sitting rest or walking).
- Single-chambered pacemakers that have only one lead placed into the right atrium or the right ventricle.

- Dual-chambered pacemakers that have two leads; one placed in the right atrium and one in the right ventricle.
- Cardiac resynchronization therapy pacemakers that have three leads; one in right atrium, one in right ventricle, and one in coronary sinus or, less commonly, the left ventricular myocardium via an external surgical approach.

The type of pacemaker is identified by a four-letter code as indicated in the following section:

- The first letter of the code describes the chamber paced (*e.g.*, atria [A], ventricle [V], dual [D]).
- The second letter of the code describes the chamber sensed.
- The third letter of the code describes the pacemaker's response to a sensed event.
- The fourth letter of the code describes the rate response capabilities of the pacemaker, (*e.g.*, inhibited [I], rate responsive [R]).

For example, a VVIR code pacemaker means (a) the ventricle is paced (V) and sensed (V); (b) when the pacemaker senses a normal ventricular contraction, it is inhibited (I); and (c) the pulse generator is rate responsive (R).

Implantable cardiac defibrillators (ICDs) are devices that monitor heart rhythms and deliver shocks if life-threatening rhythms are detected. ICDs are used for high-rate ventricular tachycardia or ventricular fibrillation in patients who are at risk for these conditions as a result of previous cardiac arrest, cardiomyopathy, heart failure, or ineffective drug therapy for abnormal heart rhythms. When ICDs detect a too rapid or irregular heartbeat, they may first try to pace the heart into a normal rate and rhythm (*i.e.*, antitachycardia pacing). If unsuccessful, they can then deliver a shock that resets the heart to a more normal HR and electrical pattern (*i.e.*, cardioversion). Thus, ICDs aim to protect against sudden cardiac death from ventricular tachycardia and ventricular fibrillation.

Ex R_x considerations for those with pacemakers are as follows:

- Programmed pacemaker modes, HR limits, and ICD rhythm detection algorithms should be obtained from the patient's cardiologist prior to exercise testing or training.
- Exercise testing should be used to evaluate HR and rhythm responses prior to beginning an exercise program.
- When an ICD is present, the HR_{peak} during the exercise test and exercise training program should be maintained at least 10 beats $\cdot$ min^{-1} below the programmed HR threshold for antitachycardia pacing and defibrillation.
- After the first 24 h following the device implantation, mild upper extremity ROM activities can be performed and may be useful to avoid subsequent joint complications.
- To maintain device and incision integrity, for 3–4 wk after implant, rigorous upper extremity activities such as swimming, bowling, lifting weights, elliptical machines, and golfing should be avoided. However, lower extremity activities are allowable.

Patients with Heart Failure

Exercise training in patients with heart failure has consistently been shown to improve functional capacity, symptoms, and quality of life (21). Furthermore, recent data suggest a modest reduction of rehospitalization rates and mortality (29). Most studies include only patients with left ventricular systolic dysfunction. Data on patients with heart failure and normal ejection fraction (diastolic heart failure) are limited to a few small observational studies. The standard recommendations for exercise training in patients with heart failure are similar to those for patients with known CVD, as defined earlier in this chapter (see *Box 9.1*). Although aerobic exercise remains the mainstay of clinical training programs, resistance training has been shown to increase muscle strength and endurance, reduce symptoms, and improve quality of life (17,30,33,36). Exercise training in patients with heart failure is generally well tolerated and safe (29). A recent large randomized trial has demonstrated that among 490 patients with an ICD in the exercise group, only one experienced ICD firing during an exercise session. Overall, the adverse event rates during the entire study period did not differ between the exercise and control groups (29).

Patients after Cardiac Transplantation

The Ex R_x for patients with cardiac transplantation offers a unique set of challenges. For the first several months after surgery, the transplanted heart does not respond normally to sympathetic nervous stimulation. The cardiac rehabilitation team should be aware of the following hemodynamic alterations that are commonly present during this time: (a) HR_{rest} is elevated; and (b) the HR response to exercise is abnormal such that the increase in HR during exercise is delayed and HR_{peak} is below normal.

Ex R_x for these patients does not include use of a THR but rather should include (a) an extended warm-up and cool-down to patient tolerance if the patient is limited by muscular deconditioning; (b) using RPE to monitor exercise intensity aiming for an RPE of 11–16; and (c) incorporation of stretching and ROM exercises (see *Chapter 7*). However, at 1 yr after surgery, approximately one-third of patients exhibit a partially normalized HR response to exercise and may be given a THR based on results from an exercise test (39). Medical management of the patient with cardiac transplant is aimed at preventing immune system rejection of the transplanted heart while avoiding the many possible adverse side effects of immunosuppressive therapy such as infections, dyslipidemia, hypertension, obesity, osteoporosis, renal dysfunction, and diabetes mellitus.

RESISTANCE TRAINING FOR CARDIAC PATIENTS

Resistance training is now a standard part of the overall exercise training program for most, if not all, patients with CVD (43). Such training yields many benefits, which are outlined in *Box 9.6*. The development of muscular strength

BOX 9.6	**Purposes of Resistance Training for Patients with Cardiac Disease (43)**

- Improve muscular strength and endurance
- Decrease cardiac demands of muscular work (*i.e.*, reduced rate pressure product) during daily activities
- Prevent and treat other diseases and conditions, such as osteoporosis, Type 2 diabetes mellitus, and obesity
- Increase ability to perform activities of daily living
- Improve self-confidence
- Maintain independence
- Slow age and disease-related declines in muscle strength and mass

and endurance facilitates resumption of work and efficient performance of ADL. Patient criteria for participation in resistance training are provided in *Box 9.7* with guidelines for resistance training in *Box 9.8*. See *Chapter 7* for additional information on resistance training.

EXERCISE TRAINING FOR RETURN TO WORK

For those planning to return to work, exercise training should consider the muscle groups and energy systems required to perform occupational tasks, particularly for those patients whose jobs involve manual labor. Exercise training leads to an improved ability to perform physical work, a better perception of job demands, an enhanced self-efficacy, and a greater willingness to resume work and to remain employed following a cardiac event (23,37). *Box 9.9* presents the Ex R$_x$ regarding preparation for return to work.

BOX 9.7	**Patient Criteria for a Resistance Training Program (43)**

- All patients entering cardiac rehabilitation should be considered for resistance training exercise (see *Box 9.8*); particularly those who require strength improvements to perform activities of daily living, work, or recreational activities; and those with controlled heart failure, obesity, or diabetes.
- No evidence of congestive heart failure (CHF), uncontrolled arrhythmias, severe valvular disease, uncontrolled hypertension, and unstable symptoms.

BOX 9.8   Resistance Training Guidelines[a] (43)

- Equipment (Type)
  - Elastic bands
  - Cuff and hand weights
  - Free weights
  - Wall pulleys
  - Machines (dependent on weight of lever arms and range of motion)
- Proper techniques
  - Raise and lower weights with slow, controlled movements to full extension.
  - Maintain regular breathing pattern and avoid breath holding.
  - Avoid straining.
  - Avoid sustained, tight gripping, which may evoke an excessive blood pressure (BP) response.
  - A rating of perceived exertion (RPE) of 11–14 ("light" to "somewhat hard") on a scale of 6–20 may be used as a subjective guide to effort.
  - Terminate exercise if warning signs or symptoms occur including dizziness, arrhythmias, unusual shortness of breath, or anginal discomfort.
- Initial load should allow 10–15 repetitions that can be lifted without straining (~30%–40% one repetition maximum [1-RM] for the upper body; ~50%–60% for the lower body). 1-RM is the maximum load that can be lifted one time. When determination of 1-RM is deemed inappropriately, multiple trials using progressively higher loads can be performed until the patient can perform no more than 10 repetitions without straining. That load can then be used for training.
  - Exercise dosage can be progressed by increasing the resistance, increasing the number of repetitions, or decreasing the rest period between sets or exercises.
  - Increase loads by 5% increments when the patient can comfortably achieve the upper limit of the prescribed repetition range (e.g., 12–15 repetitions).
  - Low-risk patients may progress to 8–12 repetitions with a resistance of ~60%–80% 1-RM.
  - Because of the potential for an elevated BP response, the rate pressure product (RPP) should not exceed that during prescribed endurance exercise as determined from the exercise test.
- Each major muscle group (i.e., chest, shoulders, arms, abdomen, back, hips, and legs) should be trained initially with one set; multiple set regimens may be introduced later as tolerated.
  - Sets may be of the same exercise or from different exercises affecting the same muscle group.

| BOX 9.8 | Resistance Training Guidelines[a] (43) (*Continued*) |

- Perform 8–10 exercises of the major muscle groups.
- Exercise large muscle groups before small muscle groups.
- Include multijoint exercises or "compound" exercises that affect more than one muscle group.
- Frequency: 2–3 d · wk^{-1} with at least 48 h separating training sessions for the same muscle group. All muscle groups to be trained may be done in the same session, that is, whole body or each session may "split" the body into selected muscle groups so that only a few are trained in any one session. Resistance training should be performed after the aerobic component of the exercise session to allow for adequate warm-up.
- Progression: Increase slowly as the patient adapts to the program (~2–5 lb · wk^{-1} [0.91–2.27 kg] for upper body and 5–10 lb · wk^{-1} for lower body [0.91–4.5 kg]).

[a]For additional information on resistance training, see *Chapter 7*.

| BOX 9.9 | Exercise Prescription for Return to Work |

- Assessment of patient's work demands and environment
  - Nature of work
  - Muscle groups used at work
  - Work demands that primarily involve muscular strength and endurance
  - Primary movements performed during work
  - Periods of high metabolic demands vs. periods of low metabolic demands
  - Environmental factors including temperature, humidity, and altitude
- Exercise prescription
  - Emphasize exercise modalities that use muscle groups involved in work tasks.
  - If possible, use exercises that mimic movement patterns used during work tasks.
  - Balance resistance vs. aerobic training relative to work tasks.
  - If environmental stress occurs at work, educate the patient about appropriate precautions including avoidance if need be, and, if possible, expose them to similar environmental conditions while performing activities similar to work tasks (see the American College of Sports Medicine Position Stands [1,2,10] and *Chapter 8* for additional information on environmental precautions).
  - If possible, monitor the physiologic responses to a simulated work environment.

EXERCISE PRESCRIPTION FOR PATIENTS WITH CEREBROVASCULAR DISEASE (STROKE)

Stroke is a brain injury that is caused by either vascular ischemia or intracerebral hemorrhage and is a leading cause of disability in the United States (34). Stroke leads to the adverse combination of reduced functional capacity and increased energy demands to perform routine activities (*i.e.*, diminished physiologic fitness reserve) (34). Among patients suffering from a hemiparetic stroke, the $\dot{V}O_{2peak}$ is approximately half that of age-matched individuals (22), a level that is near the minimum range required for ADL. Standard stroke care during the initial 3–6 mo postevent period focuses on basic mobility function and recovery of ADL. Many patients are discharged from standard physical therapy care without having achieved full recovery and suffer further decline in mobility within a year (22). Hence, exercise interventions that go beyond the early subacute period are needed to optimize functional capacity for the long term.

Randomized exercise training studies using a wide variety of modalities and protocols have demonstrated an 8%–23% improvement in $\dot{V}O_{2peak}$ after 2–6 mo of training (22). However, most research has focused on patients with hemiparesis who have mild-to-moderate gait impairment. Among such patients, treadmill training using progressive intensity and duration appears to offer promising results (25,26). However, at this time, no specific training protocol has been adequately studied or can be recommended for these patients or those with more limiting neuromuscular deficits.

THE BOTTOM LINE

- Following a documented physician referral, patients hospitalized after a cardiac-related event or procedure associated with CAD, cardiac valve replacement, or MI should be provided with a program consisting of early assessment and mobilization, identification of and education regarding CVD risk factors, assessment of the patient's level of readiness for physical activity, and comprehensive discharge planning.
- Inpatients should be educated and encouraged to investigate outpatient exercise program options and be provided with information regarding the use of home exercise equipment. All patients, especially moderate- to high-risk patients with CVD, should be strongly encouraged to participate in a clinically supervised outpatient cardiac rehabilitation program.
- Exercise training is safe and effective for most patients with CVD; however, all patients should be classified according to future risk for occurrence of cardiac-related events during exercise training.
- In addition to formal outpatient exercise sessions, patients should be encouraged to gradually return to general ADL such as household chores, yard work, shopping, and hobbies as evaluated and appropriately modified by the rehabilitation staff.

- It is important that outpatients eventually transition from a medically supervised program to an independent (*i.e.*, self-monitored and unsupervised) home exercise program. The optimal number of weeks of attendance at a supervised program before entering an independent program is unknown and is likely patient specific.
- PAD is a common disorder with increasing prevalence in older adults. Conservative management of patients with asymptomatic PAD and patients with intermittent claudication is recommended to modify risk factors and improve ambulatory ability, whereas patients with more severe PAD typically require revascularization of the lower extremities. Exercise rehabilitation is a highly effective, conservative treatment to improve ambulation in patients with intermittent claudication.
- Resistance training is now a standard part of the overall exercise training program for most, if not all, patients with CVD (see *Chapter 7*).
- Standard stroke care during the initial 3–6 mo postevent period focuses on basic mobility function and recovery of ADL. Exercise interventions that go beyond the early subacute period are needed to optimize functional capacity for the long term.

Online Resources

American Association for Cardiovascular and Pulmonary Rehabilitation (1):
http://www.aacvpr.org

American Heart Association (4):
http://www.americanheart.org

Clinical Exercise Physiology Association (11):
http://www.acsm-cepa.org

Society for Vascular Medicine:
http://www.svmb.org

VascularWeb:
http://www.vascularweb.org

REFERENCES

1. American Association for Cardiovascular and Pulmonary Rehabilitation Web site [Internet]. Chicago (IL): American Association for Cardiovascular and Pulmonary Rehabilitation; [cited 2011 Jan 6]. Available from: http://www.aacvpr.org/
2. American Association of Cardiovascular and Pulmonary Rehabilitation. Cardiac rehabilitation in the inpatient and transitional setting. In: *Guidelines for Cardiac Rehabilitation and Secondary Prevention Programs*. 4th ed. Champaign: Human Kinetics; 2004. p. 31–52.
3. American College of Sports Medicine, Sawka MN, Burke LM, et al. American College of Sports Medicine Position Stand. Exercise and fluid replacement. *Med Sci Sports Exerc.* 2007;39(2):377–90.
4. American Heart Association Web site [Internet]. Dallas (TX): American Heart Association; [cited 2011 Jan 6]. Available from: http://www.americanheart.org/
5. Armstrong LE, Brubaker PH, Whaley MH, Otto RM, American College of Sports Medicine. *ACSM's Guidelines for Exercise Testing and Prescription.* 7th ed. Baltimore (MD): Lippincott Williams & Wilkins; 2005. 366 p.

6. Borg GA. Psychophysical bases of perceived exertion. *Med Sci Sports Exerc*. 1982;14(5):377–81.

7. Borg G. Scaling pain and related subjective somatic symptoms. In: *Borg's Perceived Exertion and Pain Scales*. Champaign: Human Kinetics; 1998. p. 63–67.

8. Bravata DM, Smith-Spangler C, Sundaram V, et al. Using pedometers to increase physical activity and improve health: a systematic review. *JAMA*. 2007;298(19):2296–304.

9. Bulmer AC, Coombes JS. Optimising exercise training in peripheral arterial disease. *Sports Med*. 2004;34(14):983–1003.

10. Castellani JW, Young AJ, Ducharme MB, et al. American College of Sports Medicine Position Stand: prevention of cold injuries during exercise. *Med Sci Sports Exerc*. 2006;38(11):2012–29.

11. Clinical Exercise Physiology Association Web site [Internet]. Indianapolis (IN): Clinical Exercise Physiology Association; [cited 2011 Jun 7]. Available from: http://www.acsm-cepa.org/

12. Convertino VA. Blood volume response to physical activity and inactivity. *Am J Med Sci*. 2007; 334(1):72–9.

13. Gardner AW, Montgomery PS, Afaq A. Exercise performance in patients with peripheral arterial disease who have different types of exertional leg pain. *J Vasc Surg*. 2007;46(1):79–86.

14. Gardner AW, Montgomery PS, Flinn WR, Katzel LI. The effect of exercise intensity on the response to exercise rehabilitation in patients with intermittent claudication. *J Vasc Surg*. 2005; 42(4):702–9.

15. Gardner AW, Poehlman ET. Exercise rehabilitation programs for the treatment of claudication pain. A meta-analysis. *JAMA*. 1995;274(12):975–80.

16. Gibbons RJ, Balady GJ, Bricker JT, et al. ACC/AHA 2002 guideline update for exercise testing: summary article. A report of the American College of Cardiology/American Heart Association Task Force on Practice Guidelines (Committee to Update the 1997 Exercise Testing Guidelines). *J Am Coll Cardiol*. 2002;40(8):1531–40.

17. Hare DL, Ryan TM, Selig SE, Pellizzer AM, Wrigley TV, Krum H. Resistance exercise training increases muscle strength, endurance, and blood flow in patients with chronic heart failure. *Am J Cardiol*. 1999;83(12):1674–7, A7.

18. Hiatt WR, Cox L, Greenwalt M, Griffin A, Schechter C. Quality of the assessment of primary and secondary endpoints in claudication and critical leg ischemia trials. *Vasc Med*. 2005;10(3):207–13.

19. Hirsch AT, Criqui MH, Treat-Jacobson D, et al. Peripheral arterial disease detection, awareness, and treatment in primary care. *JAMA*. 2001;286(11):1317–24.

20. Hirsch AT, Haskal ZJ, Hertzer NR, et al. ACC/AHA 2005 Practice Guidelines for the management of patients with peripheral arterial disease (lower extremity, renal, mesenteric, and abdominal aortic): a collaborative report from the American Association for Vascular Surgery/Society for Vascular Surgery, Society for Cardiovascular Angiography and Interventions, Society for Vascular Medicine and Biology, Society of Interventional Radiology, and the ACC/AHA Task Force on Practice Guidelines (Writing Committee to Develop Guidelines for the Management of Patients with Peripheral Arterial Disease): endorsed by the American Association of Cardiovascular and Pulmonary Rehabilitation; National Heart, Lung, and Blood Institute; Society for Vascular Nursing; TransAtlantic Inter-Society Consensus; and Vascular Disease Foundation. *Circulation*. 2006;113(11):e463–654.

21. Hunt SA, American College of Cardiology, American Heart Association Task Force on Practice Guidelines (Writing Committee to Update the 2001 Guidelines for the Evaluation and Management of Heart Failure). ACC/AHA 2005 guideline update for the diagnosis and management of chronic heart failure in the adult: a report of the American College of Cardiology/American Heart Association Task Force on Practice Guidelines (Writing Committee to Update the 2001 Guidelines for the Evaluation and Management of Heart Failure). *J Am Coll Cardiol*. 2005;46(6):e1–82.

22. Ivey FM, Hafer-Macko CE, Macko RF. Exercise rehabilitation after stroke. *NeuroRx*. 2006;3(4): 439–50.

23. Leon AS, Franklin BA, Costa F, et al. Cardiac rehabilitation and secondary prevention of coronary heart disease: an American Heart Association scientific statement from the Council on Clinical Cardiology (Subcommittee on Exercise, Cardiac Rehabilitation, and Prevention) and the Council on Nutrition, Physical Activity, and Metabolism (Subcommittee on Physical Activity), in collaboration with the American Association of Cardiovascular and Pulmonary Rehabilitation. *Circulation*. 2005;111(3):369–76.

24. Losanoff JE, Jones JW, Richman BW. Primary closure of median sternotomy: techniques and principles. *Cardiovasc Surg*. 2002;10(2):102–10.

25. Luft AR, Macko RF, Forrester LW, et al. Treadmill exercise activates subcortical neural networks and improves walking after stroke: a randomized controlled trial. *Stroke*. 2008;39(12):3341–50.

26. Macko RF, Ivey FM, Forrester LW, et al. Treadmill exercise rehabilitation improves ambulatory function and cardiovascular fitness in patients with chronic stroke: a randomized, controlled trial. *Stroke*. 2005;36(10):2206–11.

27. Moholdt TT, Amundsen BH, Rustad LA, et al. Aerobic interval training versus continuous moderate exercise after coronary artery bypass surgery: a randomized study of cardiovascular effects and quality of life. *Am Heart J.* 2009;158(6):1031–7.

28. Norgren L, Hiatt WR, Dormandy JA, et al. Inter-Society Consensus for the Management of Peripheral Arterial Disease (TASC II). *J Vasc Surg.* 2007;(45 Suppl S):S5–67.

29. O'Connor CM, Whellan DJ, Lee KL, et al. Efficacy and safety of exercise training in patients with chronic heart failure: HF-ACTION randomized controlled trial. *JAMA.* 2009;301(14):1439–50.

30. Oka RK, De Marco T, Haskell WL, et al. Impact of a home-based walking and resistance training program on quality of life in patients with heart failure. *Am J Cardiol.* 2000;85(3):365–9.

31. Outpatient cardiac rehabilitation and secondary prevention. In: American Association of Cardiovascular and Pulmonary Rehabilitation, editor. *Guidelines for Cardiac Rehabilitation and Secondary Prevention Programs.* 4th ed. Champaign: Human Kinetics; 2004. p. 53–68.

32. Paker K. An early cardiac access clinic significantly improves cardiac rehabilitation participation and completion rates in low risk STEMI patients. *Can J Cardiol.* 2011;27(5):619–27.

33. Pu CT, Johnson MT, Forman DE, et al. Randomized trial of progressive resistance training to counteract the myopathy of chronic heart failure. *J Appl Physiol.* 2001;90(6):2341–50.

34. Roger VL, Go AS, Lloyd-Jones DM, et al. Heart disease and stroke statistics—2012 update: A report from the American Heart Association. *Circulation.* 2012;125(1):e2–e220.

35. Sargent LA, Seyfer AE, Hollinger J, Hinson RM, Graeber GM. The healing sternum: a comparison of osseous healing with wire versus rigid fixation. *Ann Thorac Surg.* 1991;52(3):490–4.

36. Selig SE, Carey MF, Menzies DG, et al. Moderate-intensity resistance exercise training in patients with chronic heart failure improves strength, endurance, heart rate variability, and forearm blood flow. *J Card Fail.* 2004;10(1):21–30.

37. Sheldahl LM, Wilke NA, Tristani FE. Evaluation and training for resumption of occupational and leisure-time physical activities in patients after a major cardiac event. *Med Exerc Nutr Health.* 1995;4:273–89.

38. Squires RW. Pathophysiology and clinical features of cardiovascular diseases. In: Kaminsky LA, editor. *ACSM's Resource Manual for Guidelines for Exercise Testing and Prescription.* 5th ed. Baltimore: Lippincott Williams & Wilkins; 2006. p. 411–438.

39. Squires RW, Leung TC, Cyr NS, et al. Partial normalization of the heart rate response to exercise after cardiac transplantation: frequency and relationship to exercise capacity. *Mayo Clin Proc.* 2002; 77(12):1295–300.

40. Stein R, Hriljac I, Halperin JL, Gustavson SM, Teodorescu V, Olin JW. Limitation of the resting ankle-brachial index in symptomatic patients with peripheral arterial disease. *Vasc Med.* 2006; 11(1):29–33.

41. Suaya JA, Shepard DS, Normand SL, Ades PA, Prottas J, Stason WB. Use of cardiac rehabilitation by Medicare beneficiaries after myocardial infarction or coronary bypass surgery. *Circulation.* 2007;116(15):1653–62.

42. Thompson PD, Balady GJ, Chaitman BR, Clark LT, Levine BD, Myerburg RJ. Task Force 6: coronary artery disease. *J Am Coll Cardiol.* 2005;45(8):1348–53.

43. Williams MA, Haskell WL, Ades PA, et al. Resistance exercise in individuals with and without cardiovascular disease: 2007 update: a scientific statement from the American Heart Association Council on Clinical Cardiology and Council on Nutrition, Physical Activity, and Metabolism. *Circulation.* 2007;116(5):572–84.

44. Wisloff U, Stoylen A, Loennechen JP, et al. Superior cardiovascular effect of aerobic interval training versus moderate continuous training in heart failure patients: a randomized study. *Circulation.* 2007;115(24):3086–94.

45. Womack CJ, Gardner AW. Peripheral arterial disease. In: Durstine JL, editor. *ACSM's Exercise Management for Persons with Chronic Diseases and Disabilities.* 2nd ed. Champaign: Human Kinetics; 2003. p. 81–5.

10

Exercise Prescription for Populations with Other Chronic Diseases and Health Conditions

This chapter contains the exercise prescription (Ex R_x) guidelines and recommendations for individuals with chronic diseases and other health conditions. The Ex R_x guidelines and recommendations are presented using the Frequency, Intensity, Time, and Type (FITT) principle of Ex R_x based on the available literature. For information relating to volume and progression, health/fitness, public health, clinical exercise, and health care professionals are referred to *Chapter 7*. Information is often lacking regarding volume and progression for the chronic diseases and health conditions presented in this chapter. In these instances, the guidelines and recommendations provided in *Chapter 7* for apparently healthy populations should be adapted with good clinical judgment for the chronic disease(s) and health condition(s) being targeted.

ARTHRITIS

Arthritis and rheumatic diseases are leading causes of pain and disability. Among adults in the United States ≥18 yr, 22.2% (49.9 million) reported having a doctor's diagnosis of arthritis and 9.4% (21.1 million) reported having an arthritis-related activity limitation (32). The prevalence of arthritis is expected to increase substantially by 2030 because of the aging population and rising prevalence of obesity (14,77,109). There are over 100 rheumatic diseases — the two most common being osteoarthritis and rheumatoid arthritis. *Osteoarthritis* is a local degenerative joint disease that can affect one or multiple joints (*i.e.*, most commonly the hands, hips, spine, and knees). *Rheumatoid arthritis* is a chronic, systemic inflammatory disease in which there is pathological activity of the immune system against joint tissues (130). Other common rheumatic diseases include fibromyalgia (discussed later in this chapter), systemic lupus erythematosus, gout, and bursitis.

Medications are core components of the treatment of arthritis that includes analgesics, nonsteroidal anti-inflammatory drugs, and disease-modifying antirheumatic drugs for rheumatoid arthritis. However, optimal treatment of arthritis involves a multidisciplinary approach including patient education in self-management, physical therapy, and occupational therapy (200,274). In the later stages of disease when pain is refractory to conservative management, total joint replacement and other surgeries can provide substantial relief. Although pain and functional limitations can present challenges to physical activity among individuals with arthritis, regular exercise is essential for managing these conditions. Specifically, exercise reduces pain, maintains muscle strength around affected joints, reduces joint stiffness, prevents functional decline, and improves mental health and quality of life (208,274).

EXERCISE TESTING

Most individuals with arthritis tolerate symptom-limited exercise testing consistent with recommendations for apparently healthy adults (see *Chapters 4* and *5*). The following are special considerations for individuals with arthritis:

- High intensity exercise is contraindicated when there is acute inflammation (*i.e.*, hot, swollen, and painful joints). If individuals are experiencing acute inflammation, exercise testing should be postponed until the flare has subsided.
- Although some individuals with arthritis tolerate treadmill walking, use of cycle leg ergometry alone or combined with arm ergometry may be less painful for some and allow better assessment of cardiorespiratory function. The mode of exercise chosen should be the least painful for the individual being tested.
- Allow ample time for individuals to warm up at a light intensity level prior to beginning the graded exercise test.
- Monitor pain levels during testing. There are many validated scales available including the Borg CR10 Scale (see *Figure 9.1*) (27) and visual numeric scale (see *Figure 10.1*) (205). Testing should be stopped if the patient indicates pain is too severe to continue.
- Muscle strength and endurance can be measured using typical protocols (see *Chapter 4*). However, pain may limit maximum muscle contraction in affected joints.

EXERCISE PRESCRIPTION

Pain can be a major barrier to beginning and maintaining a regular exercise program. Therefore, when prescribing exercise for individuals with arthritis, a key guiding principle should be identifying a program that minimizes pain while gradually progressing toward levels that provide greater health benefits (155). In general, recommendations for Ex R$_x$ are consistent with those for apparently

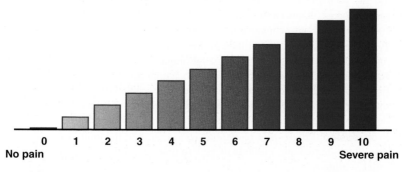

FIGURE 10.1. Visual numeric pain scale. (Reprinted with permission from [205].)

healthy adults (see *Chapter 7*), but FITT recommendations should take into account an individual's' pain, stability, and functional limitations.

FITT RECOMMENDATIONS FOR INDIVIDUALS WITH ARTHRITIS   F I T T

Aerobic, Resistance, and Flexibility Exercise

Frequency: Aerobic exercise 3–5 d · wk^{-1}; resistance exercise 2–3 d · wk^{-1}; flexibility/range of motion (ROM) exercises are essential and should be performed daily if possible.

Intensity: Although an optimal intensity of aerobic exercise has not been determined, light-to-moderate intensity, physical activities are recommended because they are associated with lower risk of injury or pain exacerbation compared to higher intensity activities. A 40%–<60% oxygen consumption reserve ($\dot{V}O_2R$) or heart rate reserve (HRR) is appropriate for most individuals with arthritis. Very light intensity, aerobic exercise (*e.g.*, 30%–<40% $\dot{V}O_2R$ or HRR) is appropriate for individuals with arthritis who are deconditioned.

The appropriate intensity for resistance exercise for patients with arthritis has not been determined, and both light and higher intensity resistance training have shown improvements in function, pain, and strength among patients with rheumatoid arthritis and osteoarthritis (60,104,112,117,255). However, most studies have focused on light or moderate intensity resistance training; that is, a higher number of repetitions (10–15) at a lower percentage of one repetition maximum (1-RM) (40%–60% 1-RM). For patients with rheumatoid arthritis and considerable damage in weight-bearing joints, there is some evidence that more intense physical activity may result in greater progression of joint damage (48). Therefore, lower intensity resistance exercise or physical activity is recommended for these patients (75).

Time: A goal of ≥150 min · wk^{-1} of aerobic exercise is appropriate for many individuals with arthritis, but long continuous bouts of exercise may be difficult for some of these individuals. Therefore, it is appropriate to start with short bouts of 10 min (or less if needed), according to an individual's pain levels. The optimal number of sets and repetitions of resistance exercise is not known. Guidelines for healthy adults typically apply (see *Chapter 7*) with consideration of pain levels.

Type: Aerobic exercise activities with low joint stress are appropriate including walking, cycling, or swimming. High-impact activities such as running, stair climbing, and those with stop and go actions are not recommended if limited by lower body arthritis. Resistance exercise should include all major muscle groups as recommended for healthy adults (see *Chapter 7*). Include flexibility exercise with ROM exercises of all major muscle groups.

Progression: Progression of aerobic, resistance, and flexibility exercises should be gradual and individualized based on an individual's pain and other symptoms.

SPECIAL CONSIDERATIONS

Additional considerations when prescribing exercise for individuals with arthritis are the following (155,157):

- Avoid strenuous exercises during acute flare ups and periods of inflammation. However, it is appropriate to gently move joints through their full ROM during these periods.
- Adequate warm-up and cool-down periods (5–10 min) are critical for minimizing pain. Warm-up and cool-down activities can involve slow movement of joints through their ROM.
- Individuals with significant pain and functional limitation may need interim goals of lower than the recommended ≥150 min · wk^{-1} of aerobic exercise and should be encouraged to undertake and maintain any amount of physical activity that they are able to perform.
- Inform individuals with arthritis that a small amount of discomfort in the muscles or joints during or immediately after exercise is common, and this does not necessarily mean joints are being further damaged. However, if the patient's pain rating 2 h after exercising is higher than it was prior to exercise, the duration and/or intensity of exercise should be reduced in future sessions.
- Encourage individuals with arthritis to exercise during the time of day when pain is typically least severe and/or in conjunction with peak activity of pain medications.
- Appropriate shoes that provide shock absorption and stability are particularly important for individuals with arthritis. Shoe specialists can provide recommendations for appropriate shoes to meet individual biomechanical profiles.
- Incorporate functional exercises such as the sit-to-stand and step-ups as tolerated to improve neuromotor control, balance, and maintenance of activities of daily living (ADL).
- For water exercise, the temperature should be 83° to 88° F (28° to 31° C) because warm water helps to relax muscles and reduce pain.

THE BOTTOM LINE

- Exercise is an essential tool for managing osteoarthritis pain and other symptoms. Moderate aerobic activities with low joint stress are appropriate. Adequate warm-up, cool-down, and stretching are important for minimizing pain. The FITT principle of Ex R$_x$ should accommodate individuals' pain levels.

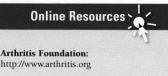

Online Resources

Arthritis Foundation:
http://www.arthritis.org

CANCER

....

Cancer is a group of nearly 200 diseases characterized by the uncontrolled growth and spread of abnormal cells resulting from damage to deoxyribonucleic acid (DNA) by internal factors (*e.g.*, inherited mutations) and environmental exposures (*e.g.*, tobacco smoke). Most cancers are classified according to the cell type from which they originate. Carcinomas develop from the epithelial cells of organs and compose at least 80% of all cancers. Other cancers arise from the cells of the blood (leukemias), immune system (lymphomas), and connective tissues (sarcomas). The lifetime prevalence of cancer is one in two for men and one in three for women (5). Cancer affects all ages but is most common in older adults. About 76% of all cancers are diagnosed in individuals ≥55 yr (5); hence, there is a strong likelihood that individuals diagnosed with cancer will have other chronic diseases (*e.g.*, cardiopulmonary disease, diabetes mellitus, osteoporosis, arthritis).

Treatment for cancer may involve surgery, radiation, chemotherapy, hormones, and immunotherapy. In the process of destroying cancer cells, some treatments also damage healthy tissue. Patients may experience side effects that limit their ability to exercise during treatment and afterward. These long-term and late effects of cancer treatment are described elsewhere (152). Furthermore, overall physical function is generally diminished because of losses of aerobic capacity, muscle tissue, and ROM. Even among cancer survivors who are 5 yr or more posttreatment, more than half report physical performance limitations including crouching/kneeling, standing for 2 h, lifting/carrying 10 lb (4.5 kg), and walking 0.25 mi (0.4 km) (170). In the following sections, the National Coalition for Cancer Survivorship definition of cancer survivor is used; that is, from the time of diagnosis to the balance of life including the time period during treatment (165).

EXERCISE TESTING

A diagnosis of cancer and curative cancer treatments pose challenges for multiple body systems involved in performing exercise and/or affected by exercise. For example, survivors of breast cancer who have had lymph nodes removed may respond differently to inflammation and injury on the side of the body that underwent surgery, having implications for exercise testing and Ex R$_x$. Cancer and cancer therapy have the potential to affect the health-related components of physical fitness (*i.e.*, cardiorespiratory fitness [CRF], muscular strength and endurance, body composition, and flexibility) as well as neuromotor function.

Understanding how an individual has been affected by his or her cancer experience is important prior to exercise testing and designing the Ex R$_x$ for survivors of cancer during and after treatment (121). Every individual with cancer can have a unique experience and response. Because of the diversity in this patient population, the safety guidance for preexercise evaluations of cancer survivors focuses on general as well as cancer site–specific recommendations of the medical assessments (see *Table 10.1*) (221).

TABLE 10.1. Preexercise Medical Assessments for Individuals with Cancer

Cancer Site	Breast	Prostate	Colon	Adult Hematologic (No HSCT)	Adult HSCT	Gynecologic
General medical assessments recommended prior to exercise	Recommend evaluation for peripheral neuropathies and musculoskeletal morbidities secondary to treatment regardless of time since treatment. If there has been hormonal therapy, recommend evaluation of fracture risk. Individuals with known metastatic disease to the bone will require evaluation to discern what is safe prior to starting exercise. Individuals with known cardiac conditions (secondary to cancer or not) require medical assessment of the safety of exercise prior to starting. There is always a risk that metastasis to the bone or cardiac toxicity secondary to cancer treatments will be undetected. This risk will vary widely across the population of survivors. Fitness professionals may want to consult with the patient's medical team to discern this likelihood. However, requiring medical assessment for metastatic disease and cardiotoxicity for all survivors prior to exercise is not recommended, as this would create an unnecessary barrier to obtaining the well-established health benefits of exercise for the majority of survivors, for whom metastasis and cardiotoxicity are unlikely to occur.					
Cancer site specific medical assessments recommended prior to starting an exercise program	Recommend evaluation for arm/shoulder morbidity prior to upper body exercise.	Evaluation of muscle strength & wasting.	Patient should be evaluated as having established consistent and proactive infection prevention behaviors for an existing ostomy prior to engaging in exercise training more vigorous than a walking program.	None	None	Patients with morbid obesity may require additional medical assessment for the safety of activity beyond cancer-specific risk. Recommend evaluation for lower extremity lymphedema prior to vigorous aerobic exercise or resistance training.

HSCT, hematopoietic stem cell transplantation.
Reprinted with permission from (221).

Standard exercise testing methods are generally appropriate for patients with cancer who have been medically cleared for exercise with the following considerations:

- Ideally, patients with cancer should receive a comprehensive assessment of all components of health-related physical fitness (see *Chapter 4*). However, requiring a comprehensive physical fitness assessment prior to starting exercise may create an unnecessary barrier to starting activity. For this reason, no assessments are required to start a light intensity walking, progressive strength training, or flexibility program in survivors.
- Be aware of a survivor's health history, comorbid chronic diseases and health conditions, and any exercise contraindications before commencing health-related fitness assessments or designing the Ex R_x.
- Health-related fitness assessments may be valuable for evaluating the degree to which musculoskeletal strength and endurance or CRF may be affected by cancer-related fatigue or other commonly experienced symptoms that impact function (150).
- There is no evidence the level of medical supervision required for symptom-limited or maximal exercise testing needs to be different for patients with cancer than for other populations (see *Chapter 2*).
- Understanding the most common toxicities associated with cancer treatments including increased risk for fractures, cardiovascular events, and neuropathies related to specific types of treatment and musculoskeletal morbidities secondary to treatment is important (152).
- The evidence-based literature indicates 1-RM testing is safe among survivors of breast cancer (221).

EXERCISE PRESCRIPTION

Survivors of cancer should avoid inactivity during and after treatment; however, there is insufficient evidence to provide precise recommendations regarding the FITT principle of Ex R_x. The recent American College of Sports Medicine (ACSM) expert panel on guidelines for exercise in adult survivors of cancer concluded there is ample evidence exercise is safe both during and after treatment for all types of cancer reviewed (*i.e.*, breast, prostate, colon, hematologic, and gynecologic cancers) (221). Overall recommendations for survivors of cancer are consistent with the guidelines provided in *Chapter 7* and with the American Cancer Society's recommendation of 30–60 min of moderate-to-vigorous intensity, physical activity at least 5 d · wk^{-1} (56). It is important to note, however, that the FITT principle of Ex R_x recommendations for individuals with cancer that follow are based on limited literature. Special considerations needed to ensure the safety of this potentially vulnerable population are in *Table 10.2* (221). To date, there are no recommendations regarding the supervision of exercise across the continuum of survivorship and/or in various exercise settings (*e.g.*, home, health/fitness, clinical). Health/fitness, clinical exercise, and health care professionals should use good judgment in deciding the level of exercise supervision needed on an individual basis.

FITT RECOMMENDATIONS FOR INDIVIDUALS WITH CANCER

FITT

Aerobic, Resistance, and Flexibility Exercise

The appropriate FITT recommendations will vary across the cancer experience and requires individualization of the Ex R_x.

Frequency: For those who have completed treatment, the goal for aerobic exercise should be to increase gradually from the current physical activity level to 3–5 d · wk^{-1} with resistance training 2–3 d · wk^{-1}. Flexibility activities can occur daily, even during treatment. Evidence indicates even those currently undergoing systemic cancer treatments can increase daily physical activity sessions over the course of 1 mo (221).

Intensity: Exercise tolerance may be highly variable during active treatment. Survivors who have completed treatment may increase intensity slowly for all physical activities. Heart rate (HR) may be less reliable for monitoring intensity for cancer survivors currently undergoing treatment. Therefore, educating survivors to use perceived exertion to monitor intensity may be advisable (see *Chapter 7*). If tolerated without adverse effects of symptoms or side effects, exercise intensity need not differ from healthy populations. Aerobic exercise should be moderate (*i.e.*, 40%–<60% $\dot{V}O_2R$ or HRR; rating of perceived exertion [RPE] of 12–13 on a scale of 6–20 [27]) to vigorous (60%–85% $\dot{V}O_2R$ or HRR or RPE of 12–16 on a scale of 6–20 [27]) intensity. Moderate intensity resistance exercise should be 60%–70% 1-RM. Flexibility intensity should be mindful of ROM restrictions resultant to surgery and/or radiation therapy (151).

Time: Several short bouts per day rather than a single bout may be useful, particularly during active treatment. Survivors who have completed treatment can increase duration as tolerated for all activities. When tolerated without exacerbation of symptoms or side effects, exercise session duration should be no different than that for healthy populations. Aerobic exercise should be 75 min · wk^{-1} of vigorous intensity or 150 min · wk^{-1} of moderate intensity activity or an equivalent combination of the two. Resistance training should be at least 1 set of 8–12 repetitions.

Type: Aerobic exercise should be prolonged, rhythmic activities using large muscle groups (*e.g.*, walking, cycling, swimming). Resistance exercise should be weights, resistance machines, or weight-bearing functional tasks (*e.g.*, sit-to-stand) targeting all major muscle groups. Flexibility exercise should be stretching or ROM exercises of all major muscle groups also addressing specific areas of joint or muscle restriction that may have resulted from treatment with steroids, radiation, or surgery.

Progression: Slower progression may be needed among survivors of cancer compared to healthy adults. Awareness of the highly variable impact of exercise on symptoms in survivors of cancer undergoing treatment is needed (222). If exercise progression leads to an increase in fatigue or other common adverse symptoms as a result of prescribed exercise, the FITT principle of Ex R_x should be reduced to a level that is better tolerated.

TABLE 10.2. Review of U.S. DHHS Physical Activity Guidelines (PAGs) for Americans and Alterations Needed for Cancer Survivors

	Breast	Prostate	Colon	Adult Hematologic (No HSCT)	Adult HSCT	Gynecologic
General Statement	Avoid inactivity, return to normal daily activities as quickly as possible after surgery. Continue normal daily activities and exercise as much as possible during and after non-surgical treatments. Individuals with known metastatic bone disease will require modifications to avoid fractures. Individuals with cardiac conditions (secondary to cancer or not) may require modifications and may require greater supervision for safety.					
Aerobic exercise training (volume, intensity, progression)	Recommendations are the same as age appropriate guidelines from the PAGs for Americans.				Ok to exercise every day, lighter intensity and lower progression of intensity recommended.	Recommendations are the same as age appropriate guidelines from the PAGs for Americans. Women with morbid obesity may require additional supervision and altered programming.
Cancer site specific comments on aerobic exercise training prescriptions	Be aware of fracture risk.	Be aware of increased potential for fracture.	Physician permission recommended for patients with an ostomy prior to participation in contact sports (risk of blow).	None	Care should be taken to avoiding over-training given immune effects of vigorous exercise.	If peripheral neuropathy is present, a stationary bike might be preferable over weight bearing exercise.
Resistance training (volume, intensity, progression)	Altered recommendations. See below.	Recommendations same as age appropriate PAGs.	Altered recommendations. See below.	Recommendations same as age appropriate PAGs.	same as age	Altered recommendations. See below.
Cancer site specific comments on resistance training prescription	Start with a supervised program of at least 16 sessions and very low resistance, progress resistance at small increments. No upper limit on the amount of weight to which survivors can progress. Watch for arm/shoulder symptoms, including	Add pelvic floor exercises for those who undergo radical prostatectomy. Be aware of risk for fracture.	Recommendations same as age-appropriate PAGs. For patients with a stoma, start with low resistance and progress	None	Resistance training might be more important than aerobic exercise in BMT patients. See	There is no data on the safety of resistance training in women with lower limb lymphedema secondary to gynecologic cancer. This

	lymphedema, and reduce resistance or stop specific exercises according to symptom response. If a break is taken, lower the level of resistance by 2 wk worth for every wk of no exercise (e.g., a 2 wk exercise vacation = lower to the resistance used 4 wk ago). Be aware of risk for fracture in this population.		resistance slowly to avoid herniation at the stoma.	text for further discussion on this point.	condition is very complex to manage. It may not be possible to extrapolate from the findings on upper limb lymphedema. Proceed with caution if the patient has had lymph node removal and/or radiation to lymph nodes in the groin.
Flexibility training (volume, intensity, progression)	Recommendations are the same as age appropriate PAGs for Americans.		Recommendations same as age appropriate PAGs, with care to avoid excessive intraabdominal pressure for patients with ostomies.	Recommendations are the same as age appropriate PAGs for Americans.	
Exercises with special considerations (e.g., yoga, organized sports, and Pilates)	Yoga appears safe as long as arm and shoulder morbidities are taken into consideration. Dragon boat racing not empirically tested, but the volume of participants provides face validity of safety for this activity. No evidence on organized sport or Pilates.	Research gap.	If an ostomy is present, modifications will be needed for swimming or contact sports. Research gap.	Research gap.	Research gap.

BMT, bone marrow transplantation; HSCT, hematopoietic stem cell transplantation; PAGS, physical activities guidelines; U.S. DHHS, U.S. Department of Health and Human Services.
Reprinted with permission from (221).

SPECIAL CONSIDERATIONS

- Up to 90% of all survivors of cancer will experience cancer-related fatigue at some point (238). Cancer-related fatigue is prevalent in patients receiving chemotherapy and radiation and may prevent or restrict the ability to exercise. In some cases, fatigue may persist for months or years after treatment completion. However, survivors are advised to avoid physical inactivity, even during treatment.
- Bone is a common site of metastases in many cancers, particularly breast, prostate, and lung cancer. Survivors with metastatic disease to the bone will require modification of their exercise program (e.g., reduced impact, intensity, volume) given the increased risk of bone fragility and fractures.
- Cachexia or muscle wasting is prevalent in individuals with advanced gastrointestinal cancers and may limit exercise capacity, depending on the extent of muscle wasting.
- Identify when a patient/client is in an immune suppressed state (e.g., taking immunosuppressive medications after a bone marrow transplant or those undergoing chemotherapy or radiation therapy). There may be times when exercising at home or a medical setting would be more advisable than exercising in a public fitness facility.
- Swimming should not be prescribed for patients with indwelling catheters or central lines and feeding tubes, those with ostomies, those in an immune suppressed state, or those receiving radiation.
- Patients receiving chemotherapy may experience fluctuating periods of sickness and fatigue during treatment cycles that require frequent modifications to the Ex R$_x$ such as periodically reducing the intensity and/or time (duration) of the exercise session during symptomatic periods.
- Safety considerations for exercise training for patients with cancer are presented in *Table 10.3*. As with other populations, the risks associated with physical activity must be balanced against the risks of physical inactivity for survivors of cancer. As with other populations, exercise should be stopped if unusual symptoms are experienced (e.g., dizziness, nausea, chest pain).

THE BOTTOM LINE

- Individuals who have had a diagnosis of cancer should avoid physical inactivity as long as physical activity does not worsen symptoms/side effects. Daily exercise is generally safe, even during intensive active therapies such as bone marrow transplant. The appropriate exercise testing, prescription, and supervision recommendations will vary across the cancer experience, with the greatest need for caution during periods of active treatment, as exercise tolerance will vary during periods of adjuvant curative therapy (e.g., chemotherapy, radiotherapy). Symptom response should be the primary guide to the Ex R$_x$ during active treatment. Even after treatment is over, starting at light

TABLE 10.3. Contraindications for Starting Exercise, Stopping Exercise, and Injury Risk for Cancer Survivors

	Breast	Prostate	Colon	Adult Hematologic (No HSCT)	Adult HSCT	Gynecologic
General contraindications for starting an exercise program common across all cancer sites	Allow adequate time to heal after surgery. The number of weeks required for surgical recovery may be as high as 8. Do not exercise individuals who are experiencing fever, extreme fatigue, significant anemia, or ataxia. Follow *ACSM Guidelines* for exercise prescription with regard to cardiovascular and pulmonary contraindications for starting an exercise program. However, the potential for an adverse cardiopulmonary event might be higher among cancer survivors than age matched comparisons given the toxicity of radiotherapy and chemotherapy and long term/late effects of cancer surgery.					
Cancer specific contraindications for starting an exercise program	Women with acute arm or shoulder problems secondary to breast cancer treatment should seek medical care to resolve those issues prior to exercise training with the upper body.	None	Physician permission recommended for patients with an ostomy prior to participation in contact sports (risk of blow), weight training (risk of hernia).	None	None	Women with swelling or inflammation in the abdomen, groin, or lower extremity should seek medical care to resolve these issues prior to exercise training with the lower body.
Cancer specific reasons for stopping an exercise program. (Note: General *ACSM Guidelines* for stopping exercise remain in place for this population.)	Changes in arm/shoulder symptoms or swelling should result in reductions or avoidance of upper body exercise until after appropriate medical evaluation and treatment resolves the issue.	None	Hernia, ostomy related systemic infection.	None	None	Changes in swelling or inflammation of the abdomen, groin, or lower extremities should result in reductions or avoidance of lower body exercise until after appropriate medical evaluation and treatment resolves the issue.

(continued)

TABLE 10.3. Contraindications for Starting Exercise, Stopping Exercise, and Injury Risk for Cancer Survivors (*Continued*)

	Breast	Prostate	Colon	Adult Hematologic (No HSCT)	Adult HSCT	Gynecologic
General injury risk issues in common across cancer sites	Patients with bone metastases may need to alter their exercise program with regard to intensity, duration, and mode given increased risk for skeletal fractures. Infection risk is higher for patients that are currently undergoing chemotherapy or radiation treatment or have compromised immune function after treatment. Care should be taken to reduce infection risk in fitness centers frequented by cancer survivors. Patients currently in treatment and immediately following treatment may vary from exercise session to exercise session with regard to exercise tolerance, depending on their treatment schedule. Individuals with known metastatic disease to the bone will require modifications and increased supervision to avoid fractures. Individuals with cardiac conditions (secondary to cancer or not) will require modifications and may require increased supervision for safety.					
Cancer specific risk of injury, emergency procedures	The arms/shoulders should be exercised, but proactive injury prevention approaches are encouraged, given the high incidence of arm/shoulder morbidity in breast cancer survivors. Women with lymphedema should wear a well-fitting compression garment during exercise. Be aware of risk for fracture among those treated with hormonal therapy, a diagnosis of osteoporosis, or bony metastases.	Be aware of risk for fracture among patients treated with ADT, a diagnosis of osteoporosis or bony metastases	Advisable to avoid excessive intra-abdominal pressures for patients with an ostomy.	Multiple myeloma patients should be treated as if they are osteoporotic.	None	The lower body should be exercised, but proactive injury prevention approaches are encouraged, given the potential for lower extremity swelling or inflammation in this population. Women with lymphedema should wear a well-fitting compression garment during exercise. Be aware of risk for fractures among those treated with hormonal therapies, with diagnosed osteoporosis, or with bony metastases.

ADT, androgen deprivation therapy; HSCT, hematopoietic stem cell transplantation.
Reprinted with permission from (221).

intensity for a short period of time (duration) and progressing slowly will assist with avoiding the onset or exacerbation of, and may assist with treatment or prevention of, persistent adverse treatment effects such as fatigue or lymphedema.

> **Online Resources**
>
> **American Cancer Society:**
> http://www.cancer.org
>
> **American College of Sports Medicine:**
> http://www.acsm.org to access the expert panel report on exercise and cancer
>
> **National Academies Press (85):**
> http://www.nap.edu/catalog.php?record_id=11468#toc From Cancer Patient to Survivor: Lost in Transition

CEREBRAL PALSY

Cerebral palsy (CP) is a nonprogressive lesion of the brain occurring before, at, or soon after birth that interferes with normal brain development. CP is caused by damage to areas of the brain that control and coordinate muscle tone, reflexes, posture, and movement. The resulting impact on muscle tone and reflexes depends on the location and extent of the injury within the brain. Consequently, the type and severity of dysfunction varies considerably among individuals with CP. In developed countries, the incidence of CP is reported to be between 1.5 and 5 live births per 1,000.

Despite its diverse manifestations, CP predominantly exists in two forms: spastic (70% of those with CP) (142) and athetoid (248). *Spastic CP* is characterized by an increased muscle tone typically involving the flexor muscle groups of the upper extremity (*e.g.*, biceps brachii, brachialis, pronator teres) and extensor muscle groups of the lower extremities (*e.g.*, quadriceps, triceps surae). The antagonistic muscles of the hypertonic muscles are usually weak. *Spasticity* is a dynamic condition decreasing with slow stretching, warm external temperature, and good positioning. However, quick movements, cold external temperature, fatigue, or emotional stress increases hypertonicity. *Athetoid CP* is characterized by involuntary and/or uncontrolled movement that occurs primarily in the extremities. These extraneous movements may increase with effort and emotional stress.

CP can further be categorized topographically (*e.g.*, quadriplegia, diplegia, hemiplegia); however, in the context of Ex R_x, a functional classification as developed by the Cerebral Palsy International Sport and Recreation Association (CP-ISRA) is more relevant (33). CP-ISRA has developed an eight-part comprehensive functional classification scheme for sports participation based on the degree of neuromotor function (see *Table 10.4*). Athletes are classified in

TABLE 10.4. Cerebral Palsy International Sports and Recreation Association (CP-ISRA) Functional Classification System (33)

Class	Functional Ability
1	Severe involvement in all four limbs; limited trunk control; unable to grasp; poor functional strength in upper extremities, often necessitating the use of an electric wheelchair for independence.
2	Severe-to-moderate quadriplegic, normally able to propel a wheelchair very slowly with arms or by pushing with feet; poor functional strength and severe control problems in the upper extremities.
3	Moderate quadriplegia, fair functional strength and moderate control problems in upper extremities and torso; uses wheelchair.
4	Lower limbs have moderate-to-severe involvement; good functional strength and minimal control problem in upper extremities and torso; uses wheelchair.
5	Good functional strength and minimal control problems in upper extremities; may walk with or without assistive devices for ambulatory support.
6	Moderate-to-severe quadriplegia; ambulates without walking aids; less coordination; balance problems when running or throwing; has greater upper extremity involvement.
7	Moderate-to-minimal hemiplegia; good functional ability in nonaffected side; walks/runs with noted limp.
8	Minimally affected; may have minimal coordination problems; able to run and jump freely; has good balance.

eight classes, with Class 1 representing an athlete with severe spasticity and/or athetosis resulting in poor functional ROM and poor functional strength in all extremities and the trunk. The athlete will be dependent on a power wheelchair or assistance for mobility. An athlete classified in Class 8 will demonstrate minimal neuromotor involvement and may appear to have near normal function (33).

The variability in motor control pattern in CP is large and becomes even more complex because of the persistence of primitive reflexes. In normal motor development, reflexes appear, mature, and disappear; whereas other reflexes become controlled or mediated at a higher level (*i.e.*, the cortex). In CP, primitive reflexes (*e.g.*, the palmar and tonic labyrinthine reflexes) may persist and higher level reflex activity (*i.e.*, postural reflexes) may be delayed or absent. Severely involved individuals with CP may primarily move in reflex patterns, whereas those with mild involvement may be only hindered by reflexes during extreme effort or emotional stress (142).

EXERCISE TESTING

The hallmark of CP is disordered motor control; however, CP is often associated with other sensory (*e.g.*, vision, hearing impairment) or cognitive (*e.g.*, intellectual disability, perceptual motor disorder) disabilities that may limit participation as much as or perhaps more than the motor limitations (45). Associated conditions such as convulsive seizures (*i.e.*, epilepsy), which occur in about 25% of those with CP, may significantly interfere with exercise testing and programming. Exercise testing may be done in individuals with CP to uncover challenges or barriers to regular physical activity, to identify risk factors for secondary health conditions, to determine the functional capacity of the individual, and/or to prescribe the appropriate exercise intensity for aerobic and strengthening exercises.

Individuals with CP have decreased physical fitness levels compared with their able-bodied peers. However, investigation in this area is limited focusing almost entirely on children and adolescents and involving primarily individuals with minimal or moderate involvement (i.e., those who are ambulatory) (46,53,187,248). As they age, adolescents with CP may show a decline in gross motor capacity related to loss of ROM, postural changes, or pain as well as reduced aerobic capacity. The decline in aerobic capacity with age appears to be greater in girls than boys (19,258). There are several documented disability-related changes in older adults with CP such as greater physical fatigue, impaired motion/problematic joint contractures, and loss of mobility, which would impact the overall fitness level of the older adult with CP (239).

When exercise testing individuals with CP, consider the following issues:

- Initially, a functional assessment should be taken of the trunk and upper and lower extremity involvement that includes measures of functional ROM, strength, flexibility, and balance. This assessment will facilitate the choice of exercise testing equipment, protocols, and adaptations. Medical clearance should be sought before any physical fitness testing.
- All testing should be conducted using appropriate, and if necessary, adaptive equipment such as straps and holding gloves, and guarantee safety and optimal testing conditions for mechanical efficiency.
- The testing mode used to assess CRF is dependent on the functional capacity of the individual and — if an athlete with CP — the desired sport. In general,
  - Arm and leg ergometry are preferred for individuals with athetoid CP because of the benefit of moving in a closed chain.
  - In individuals with significant involvement (Classes 1 and 2), minimal efforts may result in work levels that are above the anaerobic threshold and in some instances may be maximal efforts.
  - Wheelchair ergometry is recommended for individuals with moderate involvement (Classes 3 and 4) with good functional strength and minimal coordination problems in the upper extremities and trunk.
  - In highly functioning individuals (Classes 5 through 8) who are ambulatory, treadmill testing may be recommended, but care should be taken at the final stages of the protocol when fatigue occurs and the individual's walking or running skill may deteriorate.
- Because of the heterogeneity of the CP population, a maximal exercise test protocol cannot be generalized. It is recommended to test new participants at two or three submaximal levels, starting with a minimal power output before determining the maximal exercise protocol.
- Because of poor economy of movement in this population, true maximal CRF testing may not be appropriate or accurate. Therefore, maximal CRF testing should involve submaximal steady state workloads at levels comparable with sporting conditions. Movement during these submaximal workloads should be controlled to optimize economy of movement (i.e., mechanical efficiency).

For example, with cycle leg ergometry, the choice of resistance or gearing is extremely important in individuals with CP. Some individuals will benefit from a combination of low resistance and high segmental velocity, whereas others will have optimal economy of movement with a high resistance, low segmental velocity combination.

- In individuals with moderate and severe CP, motion is considered a series of discrete bursts of activity. Hence, the assessment of anaerobic power derived from the Wingate anaerobic test gives a good indication of the performance potential of the individual.
- In individuals with athetoid CP, strength tests should be performed through movement in a closed chain (*e.g.*, exercise machines that control the path of the movement). Before initiating open kinetic chain strengthening exercises (*e.g.*, dumbbells, barbells, other free weights), always check the impact of primitive reflexes on performance (*i.e.*, position of head, trunk, and proximal joints of the extremities) and whether the individual has adequate neuromotor control to exercise with free weights.
- In children with CP, eccentric strength training increases eccentric torque production throughout the ROM while decreasing electromyographic (EMG) activity in the exercising muscle. Eccentric training may decrease cocontraction and improve net torque development in muscles exhibiting increased tone (197).
- Results from any exercise test in the same individual with CP may vary considerably from day to day because of fluctuations in muscle tone.

EXERCISE PRESCRIPTION/SPECIAL CONSIDERATIONS

Generally, the FITT principle of Ex R_x recommendations for the general population should be applied to individuals with CP (see *Chapter* 7) (87,102). It is important to note, however, that the FITT principle of Ex R_x recommendations for individuals with CP that follow are based on a very limited literature. For this reason and because of the impact of CP on the neuromotor function, the following FITT principle of Ex R_x recommendations and special considerations are combined in this section:

- The FITT principle of Ex R_x needed to elicit health/fitness benefits in individuals with CP is unclear. Even though the design of exercise training programs to enhance health/fitness benefits should be based on the same principles as the general population, modifications to the training protocol may have to be made based on the individual's functional mobility level, number and type of associated conditions, and degree of involvement of each limb (204).
- Because of lack of movement control, energy expenditure (EE) is high even at low power output levels. In individuals with severe involvement (Classes 1 and 2), aerobic exercise programs should start with frequent but short bouts of moderate intensity (*i.e.*, 40%–50% $\dot{V}O_2R$ or HRR or RPE of 12–13 on a

scale of 6–20). Recovery periods should begin each time this intensity level is exceeded. Exercise bouts should be progressively increased to reach an intensity of 50%–85% $\dot{V}O_2R$ for 20 min. Because of poor economy of movement, some severely involved individuals will not be able to work at these intensity levels for 20 min, so shorter durations that can be accumulated should be considered.

- In moderately to minimally involved individuals, aerobic exercise training should follow the FITT principle of Ex R_x including progression for the general population (see *Chapter 7*). If balance deficits during exercise are an issue, leg ergometry with a tricycle or recumbent stationary bicycle (82) for the lower extremities and hand cycling for the upper extremities are recommended because (a) they allow for a wide range of power output; (b) movements occur in a closed chain; (c) muscle contraction velocity can be changed without changing the power output through the use of resistance or gears; and (d) there is minimal risk for injuries caused by lack of movement or balance control.

- Individuals with CP fatigue easily because of poor economy of movement. Fatigue has a disastrous effect on hypertonic muscles and will further deteriorate the voluntary movement patterns. Training sessions will be more effective, particularly for individuals with high muscle tone, if (a) several short training sessions are conducted rather than one longer session; (b) relaxation and stretching routines are included throughout the session; and (c) new skills are introduced early in the session (30,209).

- Resistance training increases strength in individuals with CP without an adverse effect on muscle tone (53,179). However, the effects of resistance training on functional outcome measures and mobility in this population are inconclusive (158,223). Emphasize the role of flexibility training in conjunction with any resistance training program designed for individuals with CP.

- Resistance exercises designed to target weak muscle groups that oppose hypertonic muscle groups improve the strength of the weak muscle group and normalize the tone in the opposing hypertonic muscle group through reciprocal inhibition. For example, slow concentric elbow extensor activity will normalize the tone in a hypertonic elbow flexor. Other techniques, such as neuromuscular electrical stimulation (179) and whole body vibration (1), increase muscle strength without negative effects on spasticity. Dynamic strengthening exercises over the full ROM that are executed at slow contraction speeds to avoid stretch reflex activity in the opposing muscles are recommended.

- Hypertonic muscles should be stretched slowly to their limits throughout the workout program to maintain length. Stretching for 30 s improves muscle activation of the antagonistic muscle group, whereas sustained stretching for 30 min is effective in temporarily reducing spasticity in the muscle being stretched (269). Ballistic stretching should be avoided.

- Generally, the focus for children with CP is on inhibiting abnormal reflex activity, normalizing muscle tone, and developing reactions to increase equilibrium. The focus with adolescents and adults is more likely to be on functional outcomes and performance. Experienced athletes will learn to use hyperactive stretch reflexes and primitive reflexes to better execute sport specific tasks.

- During growth, hypertonicity in the muscles — and consequently, muscle balance around the joints — may change significantly because of inadequate adaptations in muscle length. Training programs should be adapted continuously to accommodate these changing conditions (179). Medical interventions such as Botox injections, a medication which decreases spasticity, may drastically change the functional potential of the individual.

- For athletes with CP, sport-specific fitness testing may be effective in determining fitness/performance areas for improvement and in planning a fitness-related intervention program for addressing the specific sports-specific goals of the athlete (125).

- Good positioning of the head, trunk, and proximal joints of extremities to control persistent primitive reflexes is preferred to strapping. Inexpensive modifications that enable good position such as Velcro gloves to attach the hands to the equipment should be used whenever needed.

- Individuals with CP are more susceptible to overuse injuries because of their higher incidence of inactivity and associated conditions (*i.e.*, hypertonicity, contractures, and joint pain) (1).

THE BOTTOM LINE

- Exercise provides improvements in the health-related components of physical fitness among individuals with CP (*i.e.*, CRF, muscular strength and endurance, and flexibility). The relationships among the FITT principle of Ex R_x and associated short- and long-term functional improvements have yet to be established.

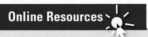
Online Resources

National Institutes of Neurological Disorders and Stroke:
http://www.ninds.nih.gov/disorders/cerebral_palsy/cerebral_palsy.htm

DIABETES MELLITUS

Diabetes mellitus (DM) is a group of metabolic diseases characterized by an elevated blood glucose concentration (*i.e.*, hyperglycemia) as a result of defects in insulin secretion and/or an inability to use insulin. Sustained elevated blood glucose levels place patients at risk for microvascular and macrovascular diseases as well as neuropathies (peripheral and autonomic). Currently, 7% of the United States population has DM, with 1.5 million new cases diagnosed each year (12). Four types of diabetes are recognized based on etiologic origin: Type 1, Type 2, gestational (*i.e.*, diagnosed during pregnancy), and other specific origins (*i.e.*, genetic defects and drug induced); however, most patients have Type 2 (90% of all cases) followed by Type 1 (5%–10% of all cases) (6).

Type 1 DM is most often caused by the autoimmune destruction of the insulin producing β cells of the pancreas, although some cases are idiopathic in origin. The primary characteristics of individuals with Type 1 DM are absolute insulin deficiency and a high propensity for ketoacidosis. Type 2 DM is caused by insulin-resistant skeletal muscle, adipose tissue, and liver combined with an insulin secretory defect. A common feature of Type 2 DM is excess body fat with fat distributed in the upper body (*i.e.*, abdominal or central obesity) (6). Central obesity and insulin resistance often progress to prediabetes.

Prediabetes is a condition characterized by (a) elevated blood glucose in response to dietary carbohydrate, termed *impaired glucose tolerance* (IGT); and/or (b) elevated blood glucose in the fasting state, termed *impaired fasting glucose* (IFG) (see *Table 10.5*). Individuals with prediabetes are at very high risk to develop diabetes as the capacity of the β cells to hypersecrete insulin diminishes over time and becomes insufficient to restrain elevations in blood glucose. It is also increasingly recognized many individuals with DM do not fit neatly into the Type 1 and Type 2 delineations, especially individuals with little or no capacity to secrete insulin but without the obvious presence of antibodies to insulin producing β cells (10).

The fundamental goal for the management of DM is glycemic control using diet, exercise, and, in many cases, medications such as insulin or oral hypoglycemic agents (see *Appendix A*). Intensive treatment to control blood glucose reduces the risk of progression of diabetic complications in adults with Type 1 and Type 2 DM (6). The criteria for diagnosis of DM and prediabetes (12) are presented in *Table 10.5*. Glycosylated hemoglobin (HbA1C) reflects mean blood glucose control over the past 2–3 mo with a general patient goal of <7%. HbA1C may be used as an additional blood chemistry test for patients with DM to provide information on long-term glycemic control (6) (see *Chapter 3*). Although the American Diabetes Association and World Health Organization endorse

TABLE 10.5. Diagnostic Criteria for Diabetes Mellitus (12)

Normal	Prediabetes	Diabetes Mellitus
Fasting plasma glucose <100 mg · dL^{-1} (5.55 mmol · L^{-1})	IFG = Fasting plasma glucose 100 mg · dL^{-1} (5.55 mmol · L^{-1})– 125 mg · dL^{-1} (6.94 mmol · L^{-1})	Symptomatic with casual glucose ≥200 mg · dL^{-1} (11.10 mmol · L^{-1})
	IGT = 2-h plasma glucose 140 mg · dL^{-1} (7.77 mmol · L^{-1})– 199 mg · dL^{-1} (11.04 mmol · L^{-1}) during an OGTT	Fasting plasma glucose ≥126 mg · dL^{-1} (6.99 mmol · L^{-1}) 2-h plasma glucose ≥200 mg · dL^{-1} (11.10 mmol · L^{-1}) during an OGTT

IFG, impaired fasting glucose (at least 8 h); IGT, impaired glucose tolerance; OGTT, oral glucose tolerance test.

using HbA1c >6.5% as a diagnostic tool for diabetes, most diagnoses are still based on elevated fasting glucose.

EXERCISE TESTING

The following are special considerations for exercise testing in individuals with DM:

- When beginning an exercise program of light-to-moderate intensity (*i.e.*, equivalent to noticeable increases in HR and breathing such as walking), exercise testing may not be necessary for individuals with DM or prediabetes who are asymptomatic for cardiovascular disease (CVD) and low risk (<10% risk of cardiac event over a 10-yr period) (252) (see *Tables 2.1* and *2.3*).
- Individuals with diabetes mellitus >35 yr of age; or individuals with Type 1 diabetes mellitus for >15 yr or Type 2 diabetes mellitus for >10 yr, regardless of age, and who want to begin a moderate to vigorous intensity exercise program, should undergo a medically supervised exercise test (GXT) with electrographic (ECG) monitoring.
- If positive or nonspecific ECG changes in response to exercise are noted or nonspecific ST and T wave changes at rest are observed, follow-up testing may be performed (227). However, consider the Detection of Ischemia in Asymptomatic Diabetes (DIAD) trial involving 1,123 individuals with Type 2 DM and no symptoms of coronary artery disease (CAD) found screening with adenosine-stress radionuclide myocardial perfusion imaging for myocardial ischemia over a 4.8 yr follow-up period did not alter rates of cardiac events (273); thus, the cost-effectiveness and diagnostic value of more intensive testing remains in question.
- Silent ischemia in patients with DM often goes undetected (262). Consequently, annual CVD risk factor assessment should be conducted by a health care provider (6).

EXERCISE PRESCRIPTION

The benefits of regular exercise in individuals with Type 2 DM and prediabetes include improved glucose tolerance, increased insulin sensitivity, and decreased HbA1C. In individuals with Type 1 DM and those with Type 2 DM using insulin, regular exercise reduces insulin requirements. Important exercise benefits for individuals with either Type 1 or Type 2 DM or prediabetes include improvement in CVD risk factors (*i.e.*, lipid profiles, blood pressure [BP], body weight, and functional capacity) and well-being (2,6). Regular exercise participation may also prevent or at least delay the transition to Type 2 DM for individuals with prediabetes who are at very high risk for developing DM (132) (see *Table 10.5*).

The FITT principle of Ex R$_x$ for healthy adults generally applies to individuals with DM (see *Chapter 7*). Participating in an exercise program confers benefits that are extremely important to individuals with Type 1 and Type 2 DM. Maximizing the cardiovascular health–related benefits resulting from exercise is a key outcome for both diabetes subtypes. For those with Type 2 DM and pre-diabetes, exercise enhances sensitivity to the insulin increasing cellular uptake of glucose from the blood that facilitates improved control of blood glucose (49). For those with Type 1 DM, greater insulin sensitivity has little impact on pancre-atic function but often lowers requirements for exogenous insulin (50). Healthy weight loss and maintenance of appropriate body weight are often more pressing issues for those with Type 2 DM and prediabetes, but excess body weight and fat can be present in those with Type 1 DM as well, and an exercise program can be useful in either context (see the sections of this chapter on overweight, obesity, and the metabolic syndrome).

FITT RECOMMENDATIONS FOR INDIVIDUALS WITH DIABETES MELLITUS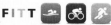

Aerobic, Resistance, and Flexibility Exercise

The aerobic exercise training FITT principle of Ex R_x recommendations for those with DM are the following:

Frequency: 3–7 d · wk^{-1}.

Intensity: 40%–<60% $\dot{V}O_2R$ corresponding to an RPE of 11–13 on a 6–20 scale (27). Better blood glucose control may be achieved at higher exercise intensities (≥60% $\dot{V}O_2R$), so individuals who have been partici-pating in regular exercise may consider raising the exercise intensity to this level of physical exertion.

Time: Individuals with Type 2 DM should engage in a minimum of 150 min · wk^{-1} of exercise undertaken at moderate intensity or greater. Aerobic activity should be performed in bouts of at least 10 min and be spread throughout the week. Moderate intensity exercise totaling 150 min · wk^{-1} is associated with reduced morbidity and mortality in observational studies in all populations. Additional benefits are accrued by increasing to ≥300 min · wk^{-1} of moderate-to-vigorous intensity, physical activity.

Type: Emphasize activities that use large muscle groups in a rhythmic and continuous fashion. Personal interest and desired goals of the exercise program should be considered.

Progression: Because maximizing caloric expenditure will always be a high priority, progressively increase exercise duration (either continuous or accumulated). As individuals improve physical fitness, adding higher intensity physical activity to promote beneficial adaptations and combat boredom may be warranted.

Resistance training should be encouraged for individuals with DM or prediabetes in the absence of contraindications (see *Chapters 2* and *3*), retinopathy, and recent treatments using laser surgery. The recommendations for healthy individuals generally apply to individuals with DM (see *Chapter 7*). Given that many patients may present with comorbidities, it may be necessary to tailor the resistance Ex R_x accordingly.

There is some evidence that a combination of aerobic and resistance training improves blood glucose control more than either modality alone (50). Whether the added benefits are caused by a greater overall caloric expenditure or are specific to the combination of aerobic and resistance training has not yet been resolved.

No more than two consecutive days of physical inactivity per week should be allowed. A greater emphasis should eventually be placed on vigorous intensity exercise if CRF is a primary goal. On the other hand, greater amounts of moderate intensity exercise that result in a caloric EE of $\geq$2,000 kcal $\cdot$ wk^{-1} (>7 hr $\cdot$ wk^{-1}), including daily exercise, may be required if weight loss maintenance is the goal, as is the case for most individuals with Type 2 DM (54) (see this chapter and other relevant ACSM position stands [6,54]).

SPECIAL CONSIDERATIONS

- Hypoglycemia is the most serious problem for individuals with DM who exercise and is mainly a concern for individuals taking insulin or oral hypoglycemic agents that increase insulin secretion (*e.g.*, sulfonylurea drugs) (6) (see *Appendix A*). Hypoglycemia, that is, blood glucose level <70 mg $\cdot$ dL^{-1} (<3.89 mmol $\cdot$ L^{-1}), is relative (6). Rapid drops in blood glucose may occur with exercise and render patients symptomatic even when blood glucose is well above 70 mg $\cdot$ dL^{-1}. Conversely, rapid drops in blood glucose may occur without generating noticeable symptoms. Common symptoms associated with hypoglycemia include shakiness, weakness, abnormal sweating, nervousness, anxiety, tingling of the mouth and fingers, and hunger. Neuroglycopenic symptoms may include headache, visual disturbances, mental dullness, confusion, amnesia, seizures, and coma (3). Importantly, hypoglycemia may be delayed and can occur up to 12 h postexercise.
- Blood glucose monitoring before and for several hours following exercise, especially when beginning or modifying the exercise program, is prudent.
- The timing of exercise should be considered in individuals taking insulin or hypoglycemic agents. For individuals with diabetes using insulin, changing insulin timing, reducing insulin dose, and/or increasing carbohydrate consumption are effective strategies to prevent hypoglycemia both during and after exercise.
- Physical activity combined with oral hypoglycemic agents has not been well studied and little is known about the potential for interactions.

Sulfonylurea drugs, glucagon-like peptide 1 (GLP-1) agonists, and other compounds that enhance insulin secretion probably do increase the risk for hypoglycemia because the effects of insulin and muscle contraction on blood glucose uptake are additive (86). The few data that exist on the common biguanide (*e.g.*, metformin) and thiazolidinedione drugs suggest the interactions are complex and may not be predictable based on individual effects of the drug or exercise alone (226) (see *Appendix A*). Extra blood glucose monitoring is prudent when beginning a program of regular exercise in combination with oral agents to assess whether changes in medication dose are necessary or desirable.

- Adjust carbohydrate intake and/or medications before and after exercise based on blood glucose levels and exercise intensity to prevent hypoglycemia associated with exercise (230).
- For individuals with Type 1 DM using insulin pumps, insulin delivery during exercise can be markedly reduced or the pump can be disconnected depending on the intensity and duration of exercise. Reducing basal delivery rates for up to 12 h postexercise may be necessary to avoid hypoglycemia.
- The use of continuous glucose monitoring can be very useful to detect patterns in blood glucose across multiple days and evaluate both the immediate and delayed effects of exercise (4). Adjustments to insulin dose, oral medications, and/or carbohydrate intake can be fine-tuned using the detailed information provided by continuous glucose monitoring.
- Exercise with a partner or under supervision to reduce the risk of problems associated with hypoglycemic events.
- Hyperglycemia with or without ketosis is a concern for individuals with Type 1 DM who are not in glycemic control. Common symptoms associated with hyperglycemia include polyuria, fatigue, weakness, increased thirst, and acetone breath (3). Individuals who present with hyperglycemia, provided they feel well and have *no* ketone bodies present in either the blood or urine, may exercise; but they should test blood sugar often and refrain from vigorous intensity exercise until they see that blood glucose concentrations are declining (10,230).
- Dehydration resulting from polyuria, a common occurrence of hyperglycemia, may contribute to a compromised thermoregulatory response (259). Thus, a patient with hyperglycemia should be treated as having an elevated risk for heat illness requiring more frequent monitoring of signs and symptoms (see *Chapter 8* and other relevant ACSM positions stands [7,9]).
- Individuals with DM and retinopathy are at risk for retinal detachment and vitreous hemorrhage associated with vigorous intensity exercise. However, risk may be minimized by avoiding activities that dramatically elevate BP. Thus, for those with severe nonproliferative and proliferative diabetic retinopathy, vigorous intensity aerobic and resistance exercise should be avoided (6,230).

- During exercise, autonomic neuropathy may cause chronotropic incompetence (*i.e.*, a blunted BP response), attenuated $\dot{V}O_2$ kinetics, and anhydrosis (*i.e.*, water deprivation) (6,259). In these situations, the following should be considered:
    - Monitor the signs and symptoms of hypoglycemia because of the inability of the individual to recognize them. Also, monitor the signs and symptoms of silent ischemia such as unusual shortness of breath or back pain because of the inability to perceive angina.
    - Monitor BP before and after exercise to manage hypotension and hypertension associated with vigorous intensity exercise (259) (see the section on hypertension in this chapter).
    - The HR and BP responses to exercise may be blunted. RPE should also be used to assess exercise intensity (259).
- Given the likelihood thermoregulation in hot and cold environments is impaired, additional precautions for heat and cold illness are warranted (see *Chapter 8* and other relevant ACSM positions stands [7,9,31]).
- For individuals with peripheral neuropathy, take proper care of the feet to prevent foot ulcers (6). Special precautions should be taken to prevent blisters on the feet. Feet should be kept dry and the use of silica gel or air midsoles as well as polyester or blend socks should be used.
- For individuals with nephropathy (6,11), although protein excretion acutely increases postexercise, there is no evidence vigorous intensity exercise accelerates the rate of progression of kidney disease. Although there are no current exercise intensity restrictions for individuals with diabetic nephropathy, it is prudent to encourage sustainable exercise programming that more likely includes tolerable moderate intensity.
- Most individuals with Type 2 DM and prediabetes are overweight (see the section on overweight and obesity in this chapter and the relevant ACSM position stand [54]).
- Most individuals with prediabetes or either subtype of DM are at high risk for or have CVD (see *Chapter 9*).

THE BOTTOM LINE

- The benefits of regular exercise in individuals with prediabetes and Type 2 DM include improved glucose tolerance and increased insulin sensitivity. Regular exercise reduces insulin requirements in individuals with Type 1 DM. The general FITT principle of Ex R_x generally applies to individuals with DM. Individuals with retinopathy or recent treatments using laser surgery may need to avoid resistance training. Hypoglycemia is the most serious problem for individuals with DM who exercise and is mainly a concern for those taking insulin or oral hypoglycemic agents that increase insulin secretion.

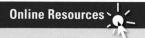

Online Resources

American College of Sports Medicine:
http://www.acsm.org to access the position stand on exercise and Type 2 DM

American Diabetes Association:
http://www.diabetes.org

National Institute of Diabetes and Digestive and Kidney Diseases:
http://www2.niddk.nih.gov/

DYSLIPIDEMIA

Dyslipidemia refers to abnormal blood lipid and lipoprotein concentrations. Dyslipidemia exists when there are elevations in low-density lipoprotein cholesterol (LDL) or triglyceride concentrations or when there is a reduction in high-density lipoprotein cholesterol (HDL). *Table 3.2* provides the National Cholesterol Education Program (NCEP) blood lipid and lipoprotein classification scheme (164). Severe forms of dyslipidemia are usually caused by genetic defects in cholesterol metabolism, but marked dyslipidemia can be "secondary" or caused by other systemic disease. Substantial increases in LDL are often caused by genetic defects related to the hepatic LDL receptor activity but can also be produced by hypothyroidism and the nephritic syndrome. Similarly, some of the highest triglyceride concentrations are produced by insulin resistance and/or DM and marked reductions in HDL are caused by the use of oral anabolic steroids. Dyslipidemia is a major modifiable cause of CVD (164).

Improvements in cholesterol awareness and more effective treatments primarily using statins or hydroxymethylglutaryl-CoA (HMG-CoA) reductase inhibitors are responsible for the decline in the prevalence of elevated blood cholesterol levels in recent years. These improvements have contributed to a 30% decline in CVD (244). Recent clinical trials indicate the added value of cholesterol lowering therapy in high risk individuals (see *Chapters* 2 and 3), individuals with DM, and older individuals with a treatment goal to lower baseline LDL concentrations by 30%–40% (92). Current detection, evaluation, and treatment guidelines for dyslipidemia are available in the NCEP Adult Treatment Panel (ATP) III report (92) (see *Chapter 3*). The NCEP ATP III report recognizes the importance of lifestyle modification in the treatment of dyslipidemia (164). These recommendations include increased physical activity and weight reduction if warranted, but except for the hypertriglyceridemia associated with insulin resistance, most hyperlipidemia requires medication therapy in addition to diet and exercise modification. Nevertheless, exercise is valued for controlling other CVD risk factors and should be a primary component to leading a healthy lifestyle. The ACSM makes the following recommendations regarding exercise testing and training of individuals with dyslipidemia.

EXERCISE TESTING

- Individuals with dyslipidemia should be screened and risk classified prior to exercise testing (see *Chapters* 2 and 3).
- Use caution when testing individuals with dyslipidemia because underlying CVD may be present.
- Standard exercise testing methods and protocols are appropriate for use with individuals with dyslipidemia cleared for exercise testing. Special consideration should be given to the presence of other chronic diseases and health conditions (*e.g.*, metabolic syndrome, obesity, hypertension) that may require modifications to standard exercise testing protocols and modalities (see the sections of this chapter and other relevant ACSM positions stands on these chronic diseases and health conditions [54,183]).

EXERCISE PRESCRIPTION

The FITT principle of Ex R_x for individuals with dyslipidemia without comorbities is very similar to the Ex R_x for healthy adults (87,102) (see *Chapter* 7). A major difference in the FITT principle of Ex R_x for individuals with dyslipidemia compared to healthy adults is that healthy weight maintenance should be emphasized. Accordingly, aerobic exercise becomes the foundation of the Ex R_x. Resistance and flexibility exercises are adjunct to an aerobic training program designed for the treatment of dyslipidemia primarily because these modes of exercise do not substantially contribute to the overall caloric expenditure goals that appear to be beneficial for improvements in blood lipid and lipoprotein concentrations.

FITT RECOMMENDATIONS FOR INDIVIDUALS WITH DYSLIPIDEMIA

FITT

Aerobic Exercise

The FITT principle of Ex R_x recommended for individuals with dylipidemia:

Frequency: ≥5 d · wk^{-1} to maximize caloric expenditure.

Intensity: 40%–75% $\dot{V}O_2R$ or HRR.

Time: 30–60 min · d^{-1}. However, to promote or maintain weight loss, 50–60 min · d^{-1} or more of daily exercise is recommended (54). Performance of intermittent exercise of at least 10 min in duration to accumulate these duration recommendations is an effective alternative to continuous exercise.

Type: The primary mode should be aerobic physical activities that involve the large muscle groups. As part of a balanced exercise program, resistance training and flexibility exercise should be incorporated. Individuals with dyslipidemia without comorbidities may follow the resistance training and flexibility guidelines for healthy adults (see *Chapter* 7).

The FITT recommendations for individuals with dyslipidemia are consistent with the recommendations for healthy weight loss maintenance of >250 min $\cdot$ wk^{-1} (see the sections on overweight and obesity in this chapter and the relevant ACSM position stand [54]).

SPECIAL CONSIDERATIONS

- The FITT principle of Ex R$_x$ may need to be modified should the individuals with dyslipidemia present with other chronic diseases and health conditions such as metabolic syndrome, obesity, and hypertension (see the sections in this chapter and other relevant ACSM position stands on these chronic diseases and health conditions [54,183]).
- Individuals taking lipid-lowering medications that have the potential to cause muscle damage (*i.e.*, HMG-CoA reductase inhibitors or statins and fibric acid) may experience muscle weakness and soreness termed *myalgia* (see *Appendix A*). Physicians should be consulted if an individual experiences unusual or persistent muscle soreness when exercising while taking these medications.

THE BOTTOM LINE

- Dyslipidemia is a major modifiable cause of CVD. Cholesterol-lowering therapy and lifestyle behavioral modifications are important in the management of individuals with dyslipidemia. The FITT principle of Ex R$_x$ for individuals with dyslipidemia without comorbidities is similar to that of healthy adults, although healthy weight maintenance should be emphasized.

Online Resources

National Heart Lung and Blood Institute:
http://www.nhlbi.nih.gov/guidelines/cholesterol/atp4/index.htm

FIBROMYALGIA

Fibromyalgia is a syndrome characterized by widespread chronic nonarticular (soft tissue) musculoskeletal pain. Fibromyalgia affects approximately 2%–4% of the population in the United States (137). Individuals with fibromyalgia do not show signs of inflammation or neurological abnormalities and do not develop joint deformities or joint disease. Therefore, fibromyalgia is not considered a true form of arthritis. Fibromyalgia is primarily diagnosed in women (*i.e.*, seven women for every one man), and its prevalence increases with age.

Signs and symptoms of fibromyalgia include chronic diffuse pain and tenderness, fatigue, sleep disturbance, morning stiffness, and depression. Irritable bowel syndrome, tension headaches, cognitive dysfunction, fine motor weakness, restless leg syndrome, temperature chemical sensitivities, and paresthesia (*i.e.*, burning, prickling, tingling, or itching of the skin with no apparent physical cause) may also be present. Pain has typically been present for many years, but there is no pattern (*i.e.*, fibromyalgia can appear and subside and present in different areas of the body at different times). Fatigue affects approximately 75%–80% of individuals with fibromyalgia and often is linked to poor sleep. Approximately 30% of individuals with fibromyalgia have a diagnosis of depression. Fibromyalgia symptoms may become worse caused by emotional stress, poor sleep, high humidity, physical inactivity, or excessive physical activity (44).

Because of the nature of fibromyalgia, a confirmed diagnosis can be difficult. The 2010 preliminary diagnostic criteria (271) include (a) determining where the individual has pain; (b) the severity of symptoms; (c) if the symptoms have been present at the same level for a minimum of 3 mo; and (d) confirming an individual's pain cannot be attributed to another disorder. Specific areas of the body where pain is assessed are the shoulder girdle, upper and lower arms and legs, hips, jaw, chest, abdomen, upper and lower back, and neck. Level of severity is determined for three symptoms: fatigue, waking unrefreshed, and cognitive symptoms.

Individuals with fibromyalgia have reduced aerobic capacity, muscle function (*i.e.*, strength and endurance), and ROM, as well as overall reductions in physical activity, functional performance (*e.g.*, walking, stair climbing), and physical fitness (29,76). In general, these reductions are caused by the chronic widespread pain that limits the individual's abilities to complete his or her everyday activities, ultimately resulting in continued deconditioning and a loss of physiologic reserve.

Treatment for individuals with fibromyalgia includes medications for pain, sleep, and mood, as well as educational programs, cognitive behavioral therapy, and exercise. Aerobic exercise is beneficial for improving physical function and overall well-being in individuals with fibromyalgia (29). There is also evidence resistance exercise, especially strength training, improves pain, tenderness, depression, and overall well-being (29). In general, exercise improves flexibility, neuromotor function, cardiorespiratory function, functional performance, physical activity levels, pain, and other symptoms of fibromyalgia as well as self-efficacy, depression, anxiety, and quality of life. *Lifestyle physical activity*, defined as accumulating 30 min of moderate intensity, physical activity above one's regular physical activity 5–7 d · wk^{-1}, improves function and reduces pain (79).

Based on the potential for pain and exacerbation of symptoms, an individual's medical history and current health status must be reviewed prior to conducting exercise tests or prescribing an exercise program. Objectively assessing physiologic and functional limitations will allow for the proper exercise testing and most optimal exercise training.

EXERCISE TESTING

Individuals with fibromyalgia can generally participate in symptom-limited exercise testing as described in *Chapter 5*. In this population, the 6-min walk test is also frequently used to measure aerobic performance (29). However, some special precautions should be considered when conducting exercise testing among those with fibromyalgia. These include the following:

- Review symptoms prior to testing to determine the severity and location of pain and the individual's level of fatigue.
- Assess previous and current exercise experience to determine the probability of the individual having an increase in symptoms after testing.
- For individuals with depression, provide high levels of motivation using constant verbal encouragement and possibly rewards for reaching certain intensity levels to have the individual perform to a peak level during testing.
- For individuals with cognitive dysfunction, determine their level of understanding when following through with verbal and written testing and training directions.
- The appropriate testing protocol (see *Chapters 4* and *5*) should be selected based on an individual's symptomatology. Individualize test protocols as needed.
- The order of testing must be considered to allow for adequate rest and recovery of different physiologic systems and/or muscle groups. For example, depending on the most prevalent symptoms (*e.g.*, pain, fatigue) and their locations on the day of testing, endurance testing may be completed before strength testing and alternate between upper and lower extremities.
- Monitor pain and fatigue levels continuously throughout the tests. Visual analog scales (see *Figure 10.1*) are available for these symptoms and easy to administer during exercise. The Fibromyalgia Impact Questionnaire is most often used for individuals with fibromyalgia to assess physical function, general well-being, and symptoms (28).
- Care should be taken to position the individual correctly on the testing or training equipment to allow for the most pain-free exercise possible. This accommodation may require modification to equipment such as adjusting the seat height and types of pedals on a cycle leg ergometer, raising an exercise bench to limit the amount of joint (*e.g.*, hip, knee, back) flexion or extension when getting on or off the equipment, or providing smaller weight increments on standard weight machines.
- If the individual with fibromyalgia has pain in the lower extremities prior to testing, consider a non–weight-bearing type of exercise (*e.g.*, cycle leg ergometry) to achieve a more accurate measurement of CRF, thereby allowing the individual to perform to a higher intensity prior to stopping because of pain.
- Prior to exercise testing and training, educate the individual on the differences between postexercise soreness and fatigue and normal fluctuations in pain and fatigue experienced as a result of fibromyalgia.

EXERCISE PRESCRIPTION

It is important to note the FITT principle of Ex R_x recommendations for individuals with fibromyalgia are based on very limited literature. For this reason, the FITT principle of Ex R_x is generally consistent with the Ex R_x for apparently healthy adults (see *Chapter 7*) with the following considerations:

- Monitor an individual's pain level and location.
- Give appropriate recovery time between exercises within a session and between days of exercise. Exercises should be alternated between different parts of the body or different systems (*e.g.*, musculoskeletal vs. cardiorespiratory).
- Individuals with fibromyalgia are commonly physically inactive because of their symptoms. Prescribe exercise, especially at the beginning, at a physical exertion level that the individual will be able to do or do without undue pain.
- Begin the exercise progression at a low enough level and progress slowly so as to allow for physiologic adaptation without an increase in symptoms (44). In general, this population has poor exercise adherence that is not only because of an increase in symptoms but also because of the mixed and sometimes contradictory information they receive from their various health care providers (212). Individuals with fibromyalgia typically have several different professionals on their health care team (*i.e.*, rheumatologist, primary care physician, clinical exercise physiologist, nurse practitioner, and physical therapist) and may get conflicting advice from several members (212).
- The individual's symptoms always determine the starting point and rate of progression for any type of exercise (27,76,211,242).

FITT RECOMMENDATIONS FOR INDIVIDUALS WITH FIBROMYALGIA F I T T

Aerobic Exercise (29,76)

Frequency: Begin 2–3 d · wk^{-1} and progress to 3–4 d · wk^{-1}.

Intensity: Begin at ≤30% $\dot{V}O_2R$ or HRR and progress to <60% $\dot{V}O_2R$ or HRR.

Time: Begin with 10 min increments and accumulate to a total of at least 30 min · d^{-1} and progress to 60 min · d^{-1}.

Type: Low impact/non–weight-bearing exercise (*e.g.*, water exercise [147], cycling, walking, swimming) initially to minimize pain that may be caused by exercise.

Resistance Exercise

Resistance exercise generally includes muscular strength and endurance to train the muscles for improved performance of functional activities. Resistance training improves muscular strength and endurance in individuals with fibromyalgia, although the level of evidence is less than that for aerobic exercise (129,211,213,242).

Frequency: 2–3 d · wk^{-1}.

Intensity: 50%–80% 1-RM. If the individual cannot complete at least 3 repetitions easily and without pain at 50% 1-RM, it is advised the starting intensity be reduced to a level where no pain is experienced.

Time: If the goal is muscular strength, perform 3–5 repetitions per muscle group, increasing to 2–3 sets. If the goal is muscular endurance, perform 10–20 repetitions per muscle group, increasing to 2–3 sets; or some combination thereof as long as the muscle groups are alternated. Typically, the strength exercises are completed first followed by a 15–20 min rest period before completing endurance exercises (76).

Type: Elastic bands, cuff/ankle weights, and weight machines.

Flexibility Exercise

Simple stretching exercises in combination with other exercises improve functional activities, symptoms, and self-efficacy in individuals with fibromyalgia (120,211), but the evidence is very limited.

Frequency: 1–3 times · wk^{-1}, progress to 5 times · wk^{-1}.

Intensity: Active and gentle ROM stretches for all muscle tendon groups in the pain-free range. The stretch should be held to the point of tightness or slight discomfort.

Time: Initially hold the stretch for 10–30 s. Progress to holding each stretch for up to 60 s.

Type: Elastic bands and unloaded (non–weight-bearing) stretching.

Functional Activity Recommendation

Functional activities (*e.g.*, walking, stair climbing, rising from chair, dancing) are daily activities that can be performed without using specialized equipment. For individuals with symptoms such as pain and fatigue, functional activities are recommended to allow for maintenance of light-to-moderate intensity, physical activity even when symptomatic.

Progression

The rate of progression of the FITT principle of Ex R$_x$ for individuals with fibromyalgia will depend entirely on their symptoms and recovery from or reduction in symptoms on any particular day. They should be educated on how to reduce or avoid certain exercises when their symptoms are exacerbated. Individuals with fibromyalgia should be advised to attempt low levels of exercise during flare ups but listen to their bodies regarding their symptoms in order to minimize the chance of injury.

SPECIAL CONSIDERATIONS

- Teach and have individuals with fibromyalgia demonstrate the correct mechanics for performing each exercise to reduce the potential for injury.
- Teach individuals with fibromyalgia to avoid improper form and exercising when they are excessively fatigued because these factors can lead to long-term exacerbation of symptoms.
- Consider lesser amounts of exercise if symptoms increase during or after exercise. Good judgment should be used to determine which aspect of the FITT principle of Ex R$_x$ needs to be adjusted.
- Avoid the use of free weights for individuals with fibromyalgia when they are fatigued or experiencing excessive pain.
- Individuals with fibromyalgia should exercise in a temperature and humidity controlled room to prevent exacerbation of symptoms.
- Consider group exercise classes because they have been shown to provide a social support system for individuals with fibromyalgia for reducing physical and emotional stress. In addition, they assist in promoting exercise adherence (212).
- Consider including complementary therapies such as tai chi (265) and yoga because they have been shown to reduce symptoms in individuals with fibromyalgia.

THE BOTTOM LINE

- In general, the FITT principle of Ex R$_x$ for healthy adults generally applies to individuals with fibromyalgia. However, it is recommended that symptoms, especially pain and fatigue, are closely monitored because they are tightly linked to the ability to exercise effectively. Including appropriate rest and recovery as part of the Ex R$_x$ is important. In addition, progression should be slower regarding intensity and time (duration) than for healthy individuals so as to minimize the exacerbation of symptoms and promote long-term exercise adherence.

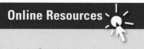

Online Resources

Arthritis Foundation:
http://www.arthritis.org

National Fibromyalgia Association:
http://www.FMaware.org

HUMAN IMMUNODEFICIENCY VIRUS

Broad use of antiretroviral therapy (ART) by industrialized countries to reduce the viral load of human immunodeficiency virus (HIV) has significantly increased life expectancy following diagnosis of HIV infection (263).

ART dramatically reduces the prevalence of the wasting syndrome and immunosuppression. However, ART is associated with metabolic and anthropomorphic health conditions including dyslipidemia, abnormal distribution of body fat (*i.e.*, abdominal obesity and subcutaneous fat loss), and insulin resistance (15). Emerging data suggest an association of HIV infection, cardiac dysfunction, and an increased risk of CVD among individuals living with HIV. With the migration of HIV infection into predominantly minority and lower socioeconomic classes, individuals with HIV are now beginning therapy with higher body mass index (BMI) and reduced muscle strength and mass. They are also more likely to have personal and environmental conditions that predispose them to high visceral fat and obesity (169,229). It is unclear how the aging process will interact with HIV status, sociodemographic characteristics, chronic disease risk, and the extended life expectancy associated with ART use. In addition to standard pharmacological interventions for HIV, physical activity and dietary counseling are treatment options. Additional treatment options include anabolic steroids, growth hormone, and growth factors (272).

Aerobic and resistance exercise provide important health benefits for individuals with HIV/acquired immunodeficiency syndrome (AIDS) (100). Exercise training enhances functional aerobic capacity, cardiorespiratory and muscular endurance, and general well-being. Additionally, physical activity can reduce body fat and indices of metabolic dysfunction. Although there are less data on effects of resistance training, progressive resistance exercise increases lean tissue mass and improves muscular strength. There is also evidence of enhanced mood and psychological status with regular exercise training. Of importance, there is no evidence to suggest regular participation in an exercise program will suppress immune function of asymptomatic or symptomatic individuals with HIV (100,101).

EXERCISE TESTING

The increased prevalence of cardiovascular pathophysiology, metabolic disorders, and the complex medication routines of individuals with HIV/AIDS require physician consultation before exercise testing. The following list of issues should be considered with exercise testing:

- Exercise testing should be postponed in individuals with acute infections.
- Variability of results will be higher for individuals with HIV than in a healthy population.
- When conducting cardiopulmonary exercise tests, infection control measures should be employed (123). Although HIV is not transmitted through saliva, a high rate of oral infections necessitates thorough sterilization of reusable equipment and supplies when disposables are not available.
- The increased prevalence of cardiovascular impairments and particularly cardiac dysfunction requires monitoring of BP and the ECG.
- Because of the high prevalence of peripheral neuropathies, testing should be adjusted if necessary to the appropriate exercise type, intensity, and ROM.

- Typical limitations to stress testing by stage of disease include the following:
  - Asymptomatic — normal GXT with reduced exercise capacity likely related to sedentary lifestyle.
  - Symptomatic — reduced exercise time, peak oxygen consumption ($\dot{V}O_{2peak}$), and ventilatory threshold (VT)
  - AIDS will dramatically reduce exercise time and $\dot{V}O_{2peak}$. Reduced exercise time will likely preclude reaching VT, and achieving $\dot{V}O_{2peak}$ will potentially produce abnormal nervous and endocrine responses

EXERCISE PRESCRIPTION

The chronic disease and health conditions associated with HIV infection suggest health benefits would be gained by regular participation in a program of combined aerobic and resistance exercise. Indeed, numerous clinical studies have shown participation in habitual physical activity results in physical and mental health benefits among this population (98,99). The varied presentation of individuals with HIV requires a flexible approach. Notably, no clinical study of the effects of physical activity on symptomatology of HIV infection has shown an immunosuppressive effect. Further, data indicate individuals living with HIV adapt readily to exercise training, with some studies showing more robust responses than would be expected in a healthy population (101). Therefore, the general FITT principle of Ex R_x is consistent with that for apparently healthy adults (see *Chapter 7*), but the management of CVD risk should be emphasized. However, health/fitness, clinical exercise, and health care professionals should be mindful of the potentially rapid change in health status of this population, particularly the high incidence of acute infections, and should adjust the FITT principle of Ex R_x accordingly.

FITT RECOMMENDATIONS FOR INDIVIDUALS WITH HUMAN IMMUNODEFICIENCY VIRUS   F I T T

Aerobic, Resistance, and Flexibility Exercise

Frequency: Aerobic exercise 3–5 d · wk^{-1}; resistance exercise 2–3 d · wk^{-1}.

Intensity: Aerobic exercise 40%–<60% $\dot{V}O_2R$ or HRR. Resistance exercise 8–10 repetitions at approximately 60% 1-RM.

Time: Aerobic exercise, begin with 10 min and progress to 30–60 min · d^{-1}. Resistance exercise, approximately 30 min to complete 2–3 sets of 10–12 exercises that target major muscle groups. Flexibility activities should be incorporated into exercise sessions following the guidelines for healthy adults (see *Chapter 7*).

Type: Modality will vary with the health status and interests of the individual. Presence of osteopenia will require weight-bearing physical activities. Contact and high-risk (*e.g.*, skateboarding, rock climbing) sports are not recommended because of risk of bleeding.

Progression: Aerobic and resistance exercise programs for this population should be initiated at a low volume and intensity. Because of virus and drug side effects, progression will likely occur at a slower rate than in healthy populations. However, the long-term goals for asymptomatic individuals with HIV/AIDS should be to achieve the ACSM FITT principle of Ex R_x recommendations for aerobic and resistance exercise for healthy adults with appropriate modifications for symptomatic individuals with HIV/AIDS.

SPECIAL CONSIDERATIONS

- There are no currently established guidelines regarding contraindications for exercise for individuals with HIV/AIDS. For asymptomatic individuals with HIV/AIDS, *ACSM Guidelines* for healthy individuals should generally apply (see *Chapter 7*). The FITT principle of Ex R_x should be adjusted accordingly based on the individual's current health status.
- Supervised exercise, whether in the community or at home, is recommended for symptomatic individuals with HIV/AIDS or those with diagnosed comorbidities.
- Individuals with HIV/AIDS should report increased general feelings of fatigue or perceived effort during activity, lower gastrointestinal distress, and shortness of breath if they occur.
- Minor increases in feelings of fatigue should not preclude participation but dizziness, swollen joints, or vomiting should. The high incidence of peripheral neuropathy may require adjustment of exercise type, intensity, and ROM.
- Regularly monitoring the health/fitness benefits related to physical activity and CVD risk factors is critical for clinical management and continued exercise participation.

THE BOTTOM LINE

- Aerobic and resistance exercises provide important health benefits for individuals with HIV/AIDS. No clinical study has demonstrated an immunosuppressive effect of exercise in this population. With exercise testing and Ex R_x, it is important to be mindful of the potential rapid changes in health status. The exercise program should be initiated at a lower volume and intensity, and progression will likely occur at a slower rate than in healthy populations.

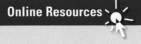

Online Resources

Centers for Disease Control:
http://www.cdc.gov/hiv/

HYPERTENSION

Approximately 76 million Americans have *hypertension* defined as having a resting systolic blood pressure (SBP) ≥140 mm Hg and/or diastolic blood pressure (DBP) ≥90 mm Hg, taking antihypertensive medication, or being told by a physician or other health care professional on at least two occasions that an individual has high BP (see *Chapter 3 Table 3.1*) (224). Hypertension leads to an increased risk of CVD, stroke, heart failure, peripheral artery disease (PAD), and chronic kidney disease (CKD) (183,224). BP readings as low as 115/75 mm Hg are associated with a higher than desirable risk of ischemic heart disease and stroke. The risk of CVD doubles for each incremental increase in SBP of 20 mm Hg or DBP of 10 mm Hg (35,214). The underlying cause of hypertension is not known in approximately 90% of the cases (*i.e.*, essential hypertension). In the other 5%–10% of cases, hypertension is secondary to a variety of known diseases including CKD, coarctation of the aorta, Cushing syndrome, and pheochromocytoma (35).

Recommended lifestyle changes include smoking cessation, weight management, reduced sodium intake, moderation of alcohol consumption, an overall healthy dietary pattern consistent with the Dietary Approaches to Stop Hypertension diet, and participation in habitual physical activity (35,214). There are a variety of medications that are effective in the treatment of hypertension (see *Appendix A*). Most patients may need to be on at least two medications to achieve targeted BP levels (35,214).

EXERCISE TESTING

Recommendations regarding exercise testing for individuals with hypertension vary depending on their BP level and the presence of other CVD risk factors, target organ disease, or clinical CVD (183) (see *Chapter 2 Figures 2.3 and 2.4* and *Chapter 3 Table 3.1*). Recommendations include the following:

- Individuals with hypertension whose BP is not controlled (*i.e.*, resting SBP ≥140 mm Hg and/or DBP ≥90 mm Hg) should consult with their physician prior to initiating an exercise program. When medical evaluation and management is taking place, the majority of these individuals may begin light-to-moderate intensity (<40%–<60% $\dot{V}O_2R$) exercise programs such as walking without consulting their physician.
- Individuals with hypertension in the high risk category (see *Chapters 2 and 3*) should have a medical evaluation before exercise testing. The extent of the evaluation will vary depending on the exercise intensity to be performed and the clinical status of the individual being tested.
- Individuals with hypertension in the high risk category (see *Chapters 2 and 3*) or with target organ disease (*e.g.*, left ventricular hypertrophy, retinopathy) who plan to perform moderate (40%–<60% $\dot{V}O_2R$) to vigorous intensity exercise (≥60% $\dot{V}O_2R$) should have a medically supervised symptom-limited exercise test.

- Resting SBP ≥200 mm Hg and/or DBP ≥110 mm Hg are relative contraindications to exercise testing (see *Chapter 3 Box 3.5*).
- If the exercise test is for nondiagnostic purposes, individuals may take their prescribed medications at the recommended time. When exercise testing is performed for the specific purpose of designing the Ex R_x, it is preferred individuals take their usual antihypertensive medications as recommended. When testing is for diagnostic purposes, BP medication may be withheld before testing with physician approval.
- Individuals on β-blockers will have an attenuated HR response to exercise and reduced maximal exercise capacity. Individuals on diuretic therapy may experience hypokalemia and other electrolyte imbalances, cardiac dysrhythmias, or potentially a false-positive exercise test (see *Appendix A*).
- The exercise test should generally be stopped with SBP >250 mm Hg and/or DBP >115 mm Hg.

EXERCISE PRESCRIPTION

Aerobic exercise training leads to reductions in resting BP of 5–7 mm Hg in individuals with hypertension (183). Exercise training also lowers BP at fixed submaximal exercise workloads. Emphasis should be placed on aerobic activities; however, these may be supplemented with moderate intensity resistance training. Flexibility exercise should be performed after a thorough warm-up and/or during the cool-down period following the guidelines for healthy adults (see *Chapter 7*).

In individuals with hypertension, the following Ex R_x is recommended.

FITT RECOMMENDATIONS FOR INDIVIDUALS WITH HYPERTENSION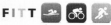

Aerobic and Resistance Exercise

Frequency: Aerobic exercise on most, preferably all days of the week; resistance exercise 2–3 d · wk⁻¹.

Intensity: Moderate intensity, aerobic exercise (*i.e.*, 40%–<60% $\dot{V}O_2R$ or HRR; RPE 11–13 on a 6–20 scale) supplemented by resistance training at 60%–80% 1-RM.

Time: 30–60 min · d⁻¹ of continuous or intermittent aerobic exercise. If intermittent, use a minimum of 10 min bouts accumulated to total 30–60 min · d⁻¹ of exercise. Resistance training should consist of at least one set of 8–12 repetitions for each of the major muscle groups.

Type: Emphasis should be placed on aerobic activities such as walking, jogging, cycling, and swimming. Resistance training using either machine weights or free weights may supplement aerobic training. Such training programs should consist of 8–10 different exercises targeting the major muscle groups (see *Chapter 7*).

Progression: The FITT principle of Ex R_x relating to progression for healthy adults, generally apply to those with hypertension. However, consideration should be given to the level of BP control, recent changes in antihypertensive drug therapy, medication-related adverse effects, and the presence of target organ disease and/or other comorbidities, and adjustments should be made accordingly. Progression should be gradual, avoiding large increases in any of the FITT components of the Ex R_x, especially intensity for most individuals with hypertension.

SPECIAL CONSIDERATIONS

- Patients with uncontrolled severe hypertension (*i.e.*, resting SBP ≥180 mm Hg and/or DBP ≥110 mm Hg) should add exercise training to their treatment plan only after first being evaluated by their physician and being prescribed appropriate antihypertensive medication.
- For individuals with documented CVD such as ischemic heart disease, heart failure, or stroke, vigorous intensity exercise training is best initiated in reha-bilitation centers under medical supervision (see *Chapter 9*).
- Resting SBP >200 mm Hg and/or DBP >110 mm Hg, is a relative contrain-dication to exercise testing. When exercising, it appears prudent to maintain SBP ≤220 mm Hg and/or DBP ≤105 mm Hg.
- β-Blockers and diuretics may adversely affect thermoregulatory function. β-Blockers may also increase the predisposition to hypoglycemia in certain individuals (especially patients with DM who take insulin or insulin secre-tagogues) and mask some of the manifestations of hypoglycemia (particu-larly tachycardia). In these situations, educate patients about the signs and symptoms of heat intolerance (7,9) and hypoglycemia, and the precautions that should be taken to avoid these situations (see the section on DM in this chapter and *Appendix A*).
- β-Blockers, particularly the nonselective types, may reduce submaximal and maximal exercise capacity primarily in patients without myocardial ischemia (see *Appendix A*). Using perceived exertion to monitor exercise intensity is especially beneficial in these individuals (see *Chapters 4* and *7*).
- Antihypertensive medications such as α-blockers, calcium channel blockers, and vasodilators may lead to sudden excessive reductions in postexercise BP. Extend and carefully monitor the cool-down period in these individuals.
- Individuals with hypertension are often overweight or obese. Ex R_x for these individuals should focus on increasing caloric expenditure coupled with reducing caloric intake to facilitate weight reduction (see the section on overweight and obesity in this chapter and the relevant ACSM position stand [54]).

- A majority of older individuals will have hypertension. Older individuals experience similar exercise induced BP reductions as younger individuals (see *Chapter 8* and the relevant ACSM position stand [8]).
- The BP-lowering effects of aerobic exercise are immediate, a physiologic response referred to as *postexercise hypotension*. To enhance exercise adherence, educate these individuals about the acute or immediate BP-lowering effects of exercise, although investigation is limited that education about BP effects of acute exercise will improve adherence.
- For individuals with documented episodes of ischemia during exercise, the exercise intensity should be set below the ischemic threshold (≤ 10 beats $\cdot$ min^{-1}).
- Avoid the Valsalva maneuver during resistance training.

THE BOTTOM LINE

- Recommendations regarding exercise testing for individuals with hypertension vary depending on their BP level and the presence of other CVD risk factors, target organ disease, or CVD, as well as the intensity of the exercise program. Patients with uncontrolled severe hypertension (*i.e.*, resting SBP ≥ 180 mm Hg and/or DBP ≥ 110 mm Hg) should add exercise training to their treatment plan only after first being evaluated by their physician and being prescribed appropriate antihypertensive medication. Although vigorous intensity aerobic exercise (*i.e.*, $\geq 60\%$ $\dot{V}O_2R$) is not necessarily contraindicated in patients with hypertension, moderate intensity aerobic exercise (*i.e.*, 40%–$<60\%$ $\dot{V}O_2R$) is generally recommended in preference to vigorous intensity aerobic exercise to optimize the benefit to risk ratio.

Online Resources

American College of Sports Medicine:
http://www.acsm.org to access the position stand on exercise and hypertension

American Heart Association:
http://www.american heart.org

National Heart Lung and Blood Institute:
http://www.nhlbi.nih.gov/hbp

INTELLECTUAL DISABILITY AND DOWN SYNDROME

Intellectual disability (ID) (older terminology referred to ID as *mental retardation*) is the most common developmental disorder in the Unites States with an estimated prevalence of 3% of the total population (66). ID is defined as (a) significant subaverage intelligence (*i.e.*, two standard deviations below the mean or an IQ <70 for mild ID and <35 for severe/profound ID); (b) having limitations in two or more adaptive skills areas such as communication, self-care, home living, social skills, community use, self-direction, health and safety, functional academics, leisure and work, and the level of care the individual requires (66); and (c) evident before 18 yr. Over 90% of all individuals with ID are classified with mild ID (17,69). The cause of ID is often not known, but genetic disorders, birth trauma, infectious disease, and maternal factors contribute, in addition to behavioral and societal factors including maternal drug and alcohol use, malnutrition, and poverty (17). The most commonly identified cause is fetal alcohol syndrome followed by Down syndrome (DS) or trisomy 21 (17,134).

Most individuals with ID live in the community either at home or in group homes. Furthermore, although mortality is much higher in individuals with ID than in the general population, life expectancy has been increasing rapidly in this population approaching that of the general population (181). Thus, it is highly likely that health/fitness and clinical exercise professionals will encounter individuals with ID in need of both exercise testing and training. Although there are many subpopulations of individuals with ID with their own unique attributes and considerations, the existing literature has focused on two main subpopulations — those with and without DS. Cardiovascular and pulmonary disorders are the most common medical problems in individuals with ID except for individuals with DS (103,210). For individuals with DS, infections, leukemia, and early development of Alzheimer disease are the most frequent causes of mortality and morbidity. However, as in individuals with ID but without DS, life expectancy for individuals with DS has also been increasing to ~60 yr with case reports of individuals living into their 80s (20).

In general, individuals with ID are perceived to have low levels of physical fitness and physical activity and high levels of obesity compared to the general population (20). However, supporting data are inconsistent, and these perceptions may only apply to individuals with DS and not to individuals with ID but without DS (20).

EXERCISE TESTING

Individuals with DS are unique as their response to exercise is clearly different from individuals without DS. Thus, concerns and considerations for exercise testing and Ex R_x are often different for individuals with and without DS. Exercise testing in general appears to be fairly safe in individuals with ID, and safety related to cardiovascular complications may not differ from the general population (68). However, although reports of exercise complications are rare or nonexistent, there is no scientific evidence either for or against the safety of exercise testing in individuals with ID. Concerns have been raised regarding validity and reliability of exercise testing in this population, but individualized treadmill laboratory tests appear to be reliable and valid, as do tests using the Schwinn Airdyne (see *Box 10.1*) (69). However, only a few field tests are valid for estimating CRF in this population (see *Box 10.1*) (69). It is recommended individuals with ID receive a full health-related physical fitness assessment including CRF, muscle strength and endurance, and body composition (see *Chapter 4*).

BOX 10.1	**Fitness Tests Recommendations for Individuals with Intellectual Disability (69)**

	Recommended	**Not Recommended**
Cardiorespiratory fitness	• Walking treadmill protocols with individualized walking speeds • Schwinn Airdyne using both arms and legs with 25-W stages • 20-m shuttle run • Rockport 1-mi walk	• Treadmill running protocols • Cycle ergometry • Arm ergometry • 1–1.5-mi runs
Muscular strength and endurance	• 1-RM using weight machines • Isokinetic testing • Isometric maximal voluntary contraction	• 1-RM using free weights • Push-ups • Flexed arm hang
Anthropometrics and body composition	• Body mass index • Waist circumference • Skinfolds • Air plethysmography • DEXA	
Flexibility	• Sit and reach • Joint-specific goniometry	

1-RM, one repetition maximum; DEXA, dual energy X-ray.

Nevertheless, the following general points should be considered in order to ensure appropriate test outcomes (67,73):

- Preparticipation health screening should follow general *ACSM Guidelines* (see *Chapter 2*), with the exception of individuals with DS. Because up to 50% of individuals with DS also have congenital heart disease and there is a high incidence of atlantoaxial instability (*i.e.*, excessive movement of the joint between C1 and C2 usually caused by ligament laxity in DS), a careful history and physical evaluation of these individuals is needed. In addition, physician supervision of preparticipation health screening exercise tests is also recommended for these individuals regardless of age.
- Familiarization with test procedures and personnel is usually required. Test validity and reliability have only been demonstrated following appropriate familiarization. The amount of familiarization will depend on the level of understanding and motivation of the individual being tested. Demonstration and practice is usually preferred. Thus, several visits to the test facility may be required.

TABLE 10.6. Formulas for Predicting $\dot{V}O_{2max}$ from Field Test Performance in Individuals with Intellectual Disability

20-m shuttle run (72):

$\dot{V}O_{2max}$ (mL · kg^{-1} · min^{-1}) = 0.35 (number of 20-m laps) − 0.59 (BMI) − 4.5 (gender: 1 = boys, 2 = girls) + 50.8

600-yard run/walk (72):

$\dot{V}O_{2max}$ (mL · kg^{-1} · min^{-1}) = −5.24 (600-yard run time in min) − 0.37 (BMI) − 4.61 (gender: 1 = boys, 2 = girls) + 73.64

1-mi Rockport Walk Fitness Test (240):

$\dot{V}O_{2max}$ (L · min^{-1}) = −0.18 (walk time in min) + 0.03 (body weight in kg) + 2.90

BMI, body mass index; $\dot{V}O_{2max}$, maximal oxygen consumption.

- Provide an environment in which the participant feels valued and like a participating member. Give simple, one-step instructions and reinforce them verbally and regularly. Provide safety features to ensure participants do not fall or have a fear of falling.
- Select appropriate tests (see *Box 10.1*) and individualize test protocols as needed. Only some tests of CRF have been shown to be valid and reliable in individuals with ID, whereas others have been shown to be of poor value because of poor reliability or questionable validity. Apply the population-specific formulas in *Table 10.6* when using CRF field tests.
- CRF field tests are reliable but not valid for individual prediction of aerobic capacity in individuals with DS.
- Because maximal heart rate (HR$_{max}$) is different in individuals with ID, especially in individuals with DS, the standard formula of 220 − age to predict HR$_{max}$ should never be used. It is recommended that the following population-specific formula be used as a guide during exercise testing but should not be used for Ex R$_x$ (71): HR$_{max}$ = 210 − 0.56 (age) − 15.5 (DS); (insert 1 for no DS and 2 for DS into the equation).
- Individuals with ID but without DS may not differ from their peers without disabilities except in muscle strength, which is low in this population (69).
- Conversely, individuals with DS exhibit low levels of aerobic capacity and muscle strength and are often overweight and obese (20,42).

EXERCISE PRESCRIPTION

The FITT principle of Ex R$_x$ for individuals with ID is very similar to an Ex R$_x$ for healthy adults (102). However, because physical activity levels are low and body weight is often greater than desired, especially in individuals with DS, a focus on daily physical activity and caloric expenditure is desirable (68). The aerobic exercise training recommendations that follow are consistent with achieving an EE of ≥2,000 kcal · wk^{-1}. However, it is likely that several months of participation is needed before this EE can be achieved.

FITT RECOMMENDATIONS FOR INDIVIDUALS WITH INTELLECTUAL DISABILITY   FITT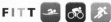

Aerobic Exercise

Frequency: 3–7 d · wk^{-1} is encouraged to maximize caloric expenditure but 3–4 d · wk^{-1} should include moderate and vigorous intensity exercise, whereas light intensity, physical activity should be emphasized on the remaining days.

Intensity: 40%–80% $\dot{V}O_2R$ or HRR; RPE may not be an appropriate indicator of intensity in this population.

Time: 30–60 min · d^{-1}. To promote or maintain weight loss, as much daily activity as tolerated is recommended. Use of intermittent exercise bouts of 10–15 min in duration to accumulate these duration recommendations may be an attractive alternative to continuous exercise.

Type: Walking is recommended as a primary activity, especially in the beginning of the program. Progression to running with use of intermittent runs is recommended. Swimming and combined arm/leg ergometry are also effective. Because muscle strength is low in individuals with ID, a focus on muscle strength exercise is desirable (68).

Resistance Exercise

Frequency: 2–3 d · wk^{-1}.

Intensity: Begin with 12 repetitions at 15–20-RM for 1–2 wk; progress to 8–12-RM (75%–80% of 1-RM).

Time: 2–3 sets with 1–2 min rest between sets.

Type: Use machines targeting 6–8 major muscle groups. Closely supervise the program for the first 3 mo.

SPECIAL CONSIDERATIONS FOR INDIVIDUALS WITH INTELLECTUAL DISABILITY

- Most individuals with ID require more encouragement during both exercise testing and training than individuals without ID. Motivation can be a problem. Asking if they are tired will automatically yield an answer of "yes" in most individuals with ID, regardless of exercise intensity or amount of work performed. For this reason, this question should be avoided. Instead, ask or suggest, "you don't look tired, you can keep going can't you?"
- Many individuals with ID are on various types of medications. These include such medications as antidepressants, anticonvulsants, hypnotics, neuroleptics, and thyroid replacement (see *Appendix A*).
- Many individuals with ID have motor control problems and poor coordination creating balance and gait problems. Thus, most individuals with ID need to use the handrail during treadmill testing. Exercise activities that do not require substantial motor coordination should be chosen or attention to

correctly performing complex movements should be minimized (*e.g.*, if using dance movements, allow each individual to just do what they can).

- Most individuals with ID have a short attention span. Plan exercise testing and programming accordingly.
- Provide appropriate familiarization and practice before actual testing because individuals with ID are often not able to adequately perform exercise tests or exercise training.
- During exercise testing and training, careful supervision is required. Some individuals with ID will eventually be able to perform exercise training in an unsupervised setting but most will require supervised exercise sessions.
- Careful spotting and supervision is needed during the beginning phases of resistance exercise training even when using machines.
- Because individuals with ID have limited attention span and limited exposure to exercise, varied activities are suggested to maximize enjoyment and adherence. Consider using music and simple games as part of the exercise training program. Also consider encouraging participation in sports programs such as Special Olympics.
- Individualize exercise training as much as possible. Large group-based programs are likely to be less effective.

SPECIAL CONSIDERATIONS FOR INDIVIDUALS WITH DOWN SYNDROME

- Individuals with DS have very low levels of aerobic capacity and muscle strength, often at levels approximately 50% of the level expected based on age and sex.
- Individuals with DS are often obese, and severe obesity is not uncommon (see the section on overweight and obesity in this chapter and the relevant ACSM position stand [54]).
- Almost all individuals with DS have low HR_{max} likely caused by reduced catecholamine response to exercise (70).
- The likelihood of congenital heart disease is high in individuals with DS.
- It is not unusual for individuals with DS to have atlantoaxial instability. Thus, activities involving hyperflexion or hyperextension of the neck are contraindicated.
- Many individuals with DS exhibit skeletal muscle hypotonia coupled with excessive joint laxity. Increasing muscle strength, especially around major joints (*e.g.*, knee), is a priority. Also, caution should be used regarding involvement in contact sports.
- Physical characteristics such as short stature, limbs, and digits commonly coupled with malformations of feet and toes, and small mouth and nasal cavities with a large protruding tongue may negatively impact exercise performance.

THE BOTTOM LINE

- Individuals with and without DS have different responses to exercise, and individuals with DS often exhibit a greater number of special considerations such as congenital heart disease, atlantoaxial instability, low levels of physical fitness, and reduced HR_{max}. Exercise testing is generally safe but should be conducted with physician supervision for individuals with congenital heart disease and atlantoaxial instability. Exercise tests need to be carefully selected because some tests are not valid and reliable in this population. The FITT principle of Ex R_x is very similar to individuals without disabilities but supervision is recommended. Issues with attention span, motivation, and behavior may also be present, and the FITT principle of Ex R_x should be appropriately adjusted.

Online Resources

American Association for Physical Activity and Recreation/Adapted Physical Education and Activity:
http://www.aahperd.org/aapar/careers/adapted-physical-education.cfm

American Association on Intellectual and Developmental Disabilities:
http://www.aamr.org

National Association for Down Syndrome:
http:// www.nads.org

National Center on Physical Activity and Disability (NCPAD):
http://www.ncpad.org

National Consortium for Physical Education and Recreation for Individuals with Disabilities:
http://www.ncperid.org

National Down Syndrome Society:
http://www.ndss.org

KIDNEY DISEASE

Individuals are diagnosed with CKD if they have kidney damage evidenced by microalbuminuria or have a glomerular filtration rate <60 mL $\cdot$ min^{-1} $\cdot$ 1.73 m^{-2} for ≥ 3 mo (166). Based on National Kidney Foundation's Kidney Disease Outcomes Quality Initiative (K/DOQI) *Guidelines*, CKD is divided into five stages primarily depending on the glomerular filtration rate of the individual and the presence of kidney damage (166) (see *Table 10.7*). Approximately 23 million Americans have CKD, and the prevalence of the disease is estimated to be 11.5% (139). Hypertension, DM, and CVD are very common in the CKD population with the prevalence of these comorbidities rising incrementally from stage 1 to stage

TABLE 10.7. Stages of Chronic Kidney Disease (166)

Stage	Description	GFR (mL · min⁻¹ · 1.73 m⁻²)
1	Kidney damage with normal or ↑ GFR	≥90
2	Kidney damage with mild ↓ GFR	60–89
3	Moderate ↓ GFR	30–59
4	Severe ↓ GFR	15–29
5	Kidney failure	<15 (or dialysis)

GFR, glomerular filtration rate.

5 CKD (254). When individuals progress to stage 5 CKD (*i.e.*, glomerular filtration rate <15 mL $\cdot$ min^{-1} $\cdot$ 1.73 m^{-2}) their treatment options include renal replacement therapy (hemodialysis or peritoneal dialysis) or kidney transplantation.

EXERCISE TESTING

Because CVD is the major cause of death in individuals with CKD, diagnostic exercise testing is indicated. Exercise testing is included in the pretransplantation workup for kidney recipients (140). However, some authorities believe diagnostic testing for patients with end-stage renal disease (*i.e.*, stage 5 CKD) is not warranted because their performance on a symptom-limited exercise test is affected by muscle fatigue, and such testing may act as an unnecessary barrier to their participation in a training program (177). Exercise testing of individuals with CKD should be supervised by trained medical personnel, with the use of standard test termination criteria and test termination methods (see *Chapter 5*).

Most research on patients with CKD has been done on individuals classified with stage 5 CKD. Current evidence suggests these individuals tend to have low functional capacities with values that are approximately 60%–70% of those seen in healthy age and sex-matched controls (175). $\dot{V}O_{2peak}$ ranges between 17–28.6 mL $\cdot$ kg^{-1} $\cdot$ min^{-1} (175), and can be increased with training by approximately 17% but never reach the values achieved by age and sex-matched controls (119). This reduced functional capacity is thought to be related to several factors including a sedentary lifestyle, cardiac dysfunction, anemia, and musculoskeletal dysfunction. The following exercise testing considerations should be noted:

- Medical clearance should be obtained from both the patient's primary care physician and nephrologist.
- Individuals with CKD are likely to be on multiple medications including those that are commonly used in the treatment of hypertension and DM (see *Appendix A*).
- When performing a graded exercise test on individuals with stage 1–4 CKD, standard testing procedures should be followed (see *Chapter 5*). However, in patients receiving maintenance hemodialysis, testing should be scheduled for nondialysis days and BP should be monitored in the arm that does not contain the arteriovenous fistula (177).
- Patients receiving continuous ambulatory peritoneal dialysis should be tested without dialysate fluid in their abdomen (177). Standard procedures are used to test patients that are transplant recipients.
- Both treadmill and cycle leg ergometry protocols have been used to test individuals with kidney diseases, with the treadmill being more popular. Because of the low functional capacity in this population, more conservative treadmill protocols such as the modified Bruce protocol, Balke, Naughton, or branching protocols are appropriate (176) (see *Chapter 5*). If cycle leg ergometry is used, initial warm-up work rates should be 20–25 W with the work rate increased by 10–30 W increments every 1–3 min (38,260).
- In patients receiving maintenance hemodialysis, peak heart rate (HR$_{peak}$) is approximately 75% of age-predicted maximum (178). Because HR may not

always be a reliable indicator of exercise intensity in patients with CKD, RPE should always be monitored (see *Chapter 4*).

- Isotonic strength testing should be done using a 3-RM or higher load (*e.g.*, 10–12-RM) because 1-RM testing is generally thought to be contraindicated in patients with CKD because of the fear of spontaneous avulsion fractures (25,119,177,215).
- Muscular strength and endurance can be safely assessed using isokinetic dynamometers employing angular velocities ranging from 60 degrees to 180 degrees · s^{-1} is recommended (52,105,176).
- As a result of the very low functional capacities of individuals with CKD, with an estimated 50% not being able to perform symptom-limited testing, traditional exercise tests may not always yield the most valuable information (175). Consequently, a variety of physical performance tests that have been used in other populations (*e.g.*, older adults) can be used (see *Chapter 8*). Tests can be chosen to assess CRF, muscular strength, balance, and flexibility (174,175).

EXERCISE PRESCRIPTION

The ideal FITT principle of Ex R_x for individuals with CKD has not been fully developed, but based on the research that has been done, programs for these patients should consist of a combination of aerobic and resistance training (37,119). It seems prudent to modify the recommendations for the general population; initially using light-to-moderate intensities and gradually progressing over time based on individual tolerance. Medically cleared recipients of kidney transplants can initiate exercise training as early as 8 d following the transplant operation (156,175).

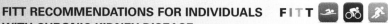

FITT RECOMMENDATIONS FOR INDIVIDUALS   F I T T
WITH CHRONIC KIDNEY DISEASE
Aerobic, Resistance, and Flexibility Exercise

The following FITT principle of Ex R_x is recommended for individuals with CKD:

Frequency: Aerobic exercise 3–5 d · wk^{-1}; resistance exercise 2–3 d · wk^{-1}.

Intensity: Moderate intensity, aerobic exercise (40%–<60% $\dot{V}O_2R$, RPE 11–13 on a scale of 6–20); resistance exercise, 70%–75% 1-RM.

Time: Aerobic exercise 20–60 min of continuous activity; however, if this amount cannot be tolerated, 3–5 min bouts of intermittent exercise aiming to accumulate 20–60 min · d^{-1} is recommended; Resistance training, a minimum of 1 set of 10–15 repetitions. Choose 8–10 different exercises to work the major muscle groups. Flexibility exercise should be performed following the guidelines for healthy adults (see *Chapter 7*).

Type: Walking, cycling, and swimming are recommended aerobic activities. Use either machine weights or free weights for resistance exercise.

SPECIAL CONSIDERATIONS

- Individuals with CKD should be gradually progressed to a greater exercise volume over time. Depending on the clinical status and functional capacity of the individual, the initial intensity selected for training should be light (*i.e.*, 30%–<40% $\dot{V}O_2R$) and for as little as 10–15 min of continuous activity or whatever amount the individual can tolerate. The duration of the physical activity should be increased by 3–5 min increments weekly until the individual can complete 30 min of continuous activity before increasing the intensity.
- The clinical status of the individual is important to consider. The progression may need to be slowed if the individual has a medical setback.
- Some individuals with CKD are unable to do continuous exercise and therefore should perform intermittent exercise with intervals as short as 3 min interspersed with 3 min of rest (*i.e.*, 1:1 work-to-rest ratio). As the individual adapts to training, the duration of the work interval can be increased, whereas the rest interval can be decreased. Initially, a total exercise time of 15 min can be used, and this can be increased within tolerance to achieve up 20–60 min of continuous activity.
- Individuals with CKD performing resistance exercise should be asked to perform at least 1 set of 10 repetitions at 70% 1-RM twice per week. Consider adding a second set when the individual can easily complete 15 repetitions at a specific weight.
- Hemodialysis.
  - Exercise can be performed on nondialysis days and should *not* be done immediately postdialysis.
  - If exercise is done during dialysis, exercise should be attempted during the first half of the treatment to avoid hypotensive episodes.
  - Place great emphasis on the RPE because HR is unreliable.
  - Patients may exercise the arm with the arteriovenous access as long as they do not directly rest weight on that area (119). Measure BP in the arm that does not contain the fistula.
- Peritoneal Dialysis.
  - Patients on continuous ambulatory peritoneal dialysis may attempt exercising with fluid in their abdomen; however, if this produces discomfort then they should be encouraged to drain the fluid before exercising (119).
- Recipients of Kidney Transplants.
  - During periods of rejection, the FITT principle of Ex R_x should be reduced but exercise can still be continued (174).

THE BOTTOM LINE

- Individuals with CKD tend to be very deconditioned depending on their age and disease status. Based on current evidence, exercise is safe for these individuals if performed at moderate intensity and if progression occurs gradually. Exercise testing should be done under medical supervision and may involve the use of functional tests rather than the traditional GXT.

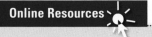

Online Resources

National Institute of Diabetes and Digestive and Kidney Diseases:
http://www2.niddk.nih.gov/

National Kidney Foundation:
http://www.kidney.org/

United States Renal Data System:
http://www.usrds.org/atlas.htm

METABOLIC SYNDROME

The *metabolic syndrome* is characterized by a constellation of risk factors that are associated with increased incidence of CVD, DM, and stroke. A consensus on the definition of the metabolic syndrome has been somewhat controversial; however, the criteria set by the NCEP ATP III *Guidelines* are most commonly used for diagnosis (164). Typically, individuals with the metabolic syndrome are overweight/obese and have elevated plasma triglycerides, hypertension, and elevated plasma glucose. Diagnosis is made when at least three of the risk factors shown in *Table 3.3* are present. At this time, it is underdetermined whether the metabolic syndrome represents a distinct pathophysiologic condition or disease (83). Nonetheless, the metabolic syndrome as a clinical entity is useful in clinical and health/fitness settings.

Although the primary cause is debatable, the root causes of the metabolic syndrome are overweight/obesity, physical inactivity, insulin resistance, and genetic factors. Age-adjusted prevalence data from the National Health and Nutrition Examination Survey (NHANES) 2003–2006 indicates 34% of adults in the United States meet the criteria for the metabolic syndrome (59), an increase compared with the prevalence of 27% in NHANES 1999–2000 (81). The International Diabetes Federation (IDF) proposed a new definition for the metabolic syndrome in 2005 (113) that was based on the presence of abdominal adiposity and two additional CVD risk factors shown in *Table 3.3*. When the metabolic syndrome classifications are compared, the NCEP and IDF definitions provide the same classification of 93% of individuals having the metabolic syndrome (80), indicating their compatibility.

The treatment guidelines for the metabolic syndrome recommended by NCEP ATPIII focus on three interventions including weight control, physical activity, and treatment of the associated CVD risk factors that may include pharmacotherapy (164) (see *Chapter 3*). The IDF *Guidelines* for primary intervention include (113) (a) moderate restriction in energy intake to achieve a 5%–10% weight loss within 1 yr; (b) moderate increases in physical activity consistent with the consensus public health recommendations of 30 min of moderate intensity, physical activity on most days of the week (102,250); and (c) change in dietary intake composition that may require changes in macronutrient composition consistent with modifying specified CVD risk factors.

The IDF secondary intervention includes pharmacotherapy for associated CVD risk factors (49,113).

EXERCISE TESTING

- Special consideration should be given to associated CVD risk factors as outlined in *Chapters* 2 and 3 on exercise testing and in this chapter for individuals with dyslipidemia, hypertension, and hyperglycemia.
- Because many individuals with the metabolic syndrome are either overweight or obese, exercise testing considerations specific to those individuals should be followed (see the section on overweight and obesity in this chapter and the relevant ACSM position stand [54]).
- The potential for low exercise capacity in individuals who are overweight or obese may necessitate a low initial workload (*i.e.*, 2–3 metabolic equivalents [METs]) and small increments per testing stage (0.5–1.0 MET).
- Because of the potential presence of elevated BP, strict adherence to protocols for assessing BP before and during exercise testing should be followed (183) (see *Chapters* 3 and 5).

EXERCISE PRESCRIPTION/SPECIAL CONSIDERATIONS

The FITT principle of Ex R_x is consistent with the recommendations for healthy adults regarding aerobic, resistance, and flexibility exercise (see *Chapter* 7). Similarly, the minimal dose of physical activity to improve health/fitness outcomes is consistent with the consensus public health recommendations of 150 min · wk^{-1} or 30 min of physical activity on most days of the week (102,249). For these reasons and because of the impact of the clustering of chronic diseases and health conditions that accompany the metabolic syndrome, the following FITT principle of Ex R_x and special considerations are combined in this section:

- Individuals with the metabolic syndrome will likely present with multiple CVD and DM risk factors (*i.e.*, dyslipidemia, hypertension, obesity, and hyperglycemia). Special consideration should be given to the FITT principle of Ex R_x recommendations based on the presence of these associated CVD risk factors and the goals of the participant and/or health care provider (see other sections of this chapter on the FITT principle Ex R_x for these other chronic diseases and health conditions as well as relevant ACSM position stands [6,54,183]).
- To reduce risk factors associated with CVD and DM, initial exercise training should be performed at a moderate intensity (*i.e.*, 40%–<60% $\dot{V}O_2R$ or HRR) and when appropriate, progress to a more vigorous intensity (*i.e.*, ≥60% $\dot{V}O_2R$ or HRR), totaling a minimum of 150 min · wk^{-1} or 30 min · d^{-1} most days of the week to allow for optimal health/fitness improvements.
- To reduce body weight, most individuals with the metabolic syndrome may benefit by gradually increasing their physical activity levels to approximately

300 min · wk⁻¹ or 50–60 min on 5 d · wk⁻¹ when appropriate (54,216,251). This amount of physical activity may be accumulated in multiple daily bouts of at least 10 min in duration or through increases in other forms of moderate intensity lifestyle physical activities. For some individuals to promote or maintain weight loss, progression of 60–90 min · d⁻¹ may be necessary (see the Ex R$_x$ recommendations for those with overweight and obesity in this chapter and the relevant ACSM position stand [54]).

THE BOTTOM LINE

- The prevalence of the metabolic syndrome in the United States is increasing. Many individuals with the metabolic syndrome are overweight or obese and present with multiple CVD and DM risk factors. Special consideration should be given to exercise testing and the FITT principle of Ex R$_x$ based on the clustering of these chronic diseases and health conditions. The goal of the Ex R$_x$ is to reduce the risk factors associated with CVD and DM and reduce body weight.

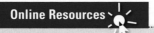

Online Resources

American College of Sports Medicine:
http://www.acsm.org to access relevant position stands to the metabolic syndrome

American Heart Association:
http://www.heart.org

MULTIPLE SCLEROSIS

Multiple sclerosis (MS) is a chronic inflammatory demyelinating disease of the central nervous system (CNS) that currently affects an estimated 2.1 million individuals worldwide (167). The onset of MS usually occurs between 20 and 50 yr and affects women at a rate two to three times more than men. Initial symptoms often include transient neurological deficits such as numbness or weakness and blurred or double vision. Although the exact cause of MS is still unknown, most researchers believe it involves an autoimmune response that is influenced by a combination of environmental, infectious, and genetic factors. During an exacerbation, activated T cells cross the blood–brain barrier precipitating an autoimmune attack on myelin in the CNS. Following the initial inflammatory response, damaged myelin forms scarlike plaques that can impair nerve conduction and transmission (167). This can lead to a wide variety of symptoms; the most common of which include visual disturbances, weakness, sensory loss, fatigue, pain, coordination deficits, bowel or bladder dysfunction, and cognitive and emotional changes (144,225).

The disease course of MS is highly variable from individual to individual and within a given individual over time. However, several distinct disease courses are now recognized as well as the relative frequency of each including (a) *relapsing remitting MS* (RRMS; 85%) characterized by periodic exacerbations followed by full or partial recovery of deficits; (b) *primary progressive MS* (PPMS; 10%) characterized by continuous disease progression from onset with little or no plateaus or improvements; and (c) *progressive relapsing MS* (PRMS; 5%) characterized by a progression from onset with distinct relapses superimposed on the steady progression (144). For the 85% of individuals who have an initial disease course of RRMS, many will eventually (10–25 yr later) develop a *secondary progressive MS* (SPMS) disease course, which is characterized by a slow but steady decline in function. The level of disability related to the progression of MS is commonly documented using the Kurtzke Expanded Disability Status Scale (EDSS), which ranges from 0 to 10. EDSS scores from 0 to 2.5 are indicative of no to minimal disability, 3–5.5 moderate disability and ambulatory without device, 6–7 significant disability but still ambulatory with a device, 7.5–9 essentially chairbound or bedbound, and 10 death because of MS (135).

With respect to CRF, individuals with MS generally have lower maximal aerobic capacity than age- and sex-matched adults without MS. Furthermore, aerobic capacity continues to decrease with increasing levels of disability (189,191). HR and BP responses to GXT are generally linear with respect to work rate but tend to be blunted compared to healthy controls (189). This attenuation of HR and BP may be a result of cardiovascular dysautonomia (236). Following 3–6 mo of progressive aerobic training, individuals with MS who have mild-to-moderate disability have consistently demonstrated improvements in $\dot{V}O_{2peak}$, functional capacity, lung function, and delayed onset of fatigue (162,184,190).

Decreased muscle performance is also a common impairment associated with MS. Individuals with MS have lower isometric and isokinetic force production as well as total work of the quadriceps muscle when compared to age- and sex-matched norms (47,136,190). Changes in muscle performance appear to be associated with central (neural drive and conduction) and peripheral (decreased oxidative capacity) factors associated with the disease process as well as the secondary effects of disuse atrophy (124,199). Although limited, current research demonstrates individuals with MS can improve strength and function with progressive resistance training with greater gains being realized by individuals with less disability because of MS (268).

EXERCISE TESTING

- Generalized fatigue is common in individuals with MS. Because fatigue generally worsens throughout the day, performing exercise testing earlier in the day is likely to yield a more accurate and consistent response.
- Avoid testing during an acute exacerbation of MS symptoms.
- Problems with balance and coordination may require use of an upright or recumbent cycle leg ergometer. When using a cycle leg ergometer, the use

of foot straps may be needed to prevent the foot from falling off the pedal because of weakness and/or spasticity.

- A recumbent stepping ergometer (*e.g.*, NuStep) that allows for the use of upper and lower extremities may be advantageous because it distributes work to all extremities, thus minimizing the potential influence of local muscle fatigue on maximal aerobic testing.
- Depending on the disability and physical fitness level of the individual, use a continuous or discontinuous protocol of 3–5 min stages increasing work rate for each stage from 12 to 25 W.
- Heat sensitivity is common in individuals with MS so it is important to use a fan or other cooling strategies during testing.
- Assessment of joint ROM and flexibility is important because increased tone and spasticity can lead to contracture formation.
- Isokinetic dynamometry can be used to accurately evaluate muscle performance. However, use of an 8–10-RM or functional testing (*e.g.*, 30 s sit-to-stand test) can also be used to measure muscular strength and endurance in the clinical or community setting.
- Use physical performance tests as needed to assess endurance (6-min walk test) (see *Chapter 4*), strength (5 repetition sit-to-stand), gait (walking speed) (see *Chapter 8*), and balance (Berg Balance Scale [23], and Dynamic Gait Index [107]).

EXERCISE PRESCRIPTION

For individuals with minimal disability (EDSS 0–2.5), the FITT principle of Ex R$_x$ is generally consistent with those outlined in *Chapter 7* for healthy adults. As MS symptoms and level of disability increase, the following modifications outlined may be required.

FITT RECOMMENDATIONS FOR INDIVIDUALS WITH MULTIPLE SCLEROSIS   F I T T

Aerobic Exercise

Frequency: 3–5 d · wk^{-1}.

Intensity: 40%–70% $\dot{V}O_2R$ or HRR; RPE 11–14.

Time: Increase exercise time initially to a minimum of 10 min before increasing intensity. Progress to 20–60 min. In individuals with excessive fatigue, begin with lower intensity and discontinuous bouts of exercise.

Resistance Exercise

Frequency: 2 d · wk^{-1}.

Intensity: 60%–80% 1-RM.

Time: 1–2 sets of 8–15 repetitions. When strengthening weaker muscle groups or easily fatigued individuals, increase rest time (*e.g.*, 2–5 min) between sets and exercises as needed to allow for full muscle recovery. Focus on large antigravity muscle groups and minimize total number of exercises performed.

Flexibility Exercise

Frequency: 5–7 d · wk^{-1}, 1–2 times · d^{-1}.

Intensity: Stretch to the point of feeling tightness or mild discomfort.

Time: Hold static stretch 30–60 s, 2–4 repetitions.

SPECIAL CONSIDERATIONS

- In spastic muscles, increase the frequency and time of flexibility exercises. Muscles and joints with significant tightness or contracture may require longer duration (several minutes to several hours), and lower load positional stretching to achieve lasting improvements.
- Whenever possible, incorporate functional activities (*e.g.*, stairs, sit-to-stand) into the exercise program to promote optimal carryover.
- Use RPE in addition to HR to evaluate exercise intensity. With individuals who have significant paresis, consider assessing RPE of the extremities separately using the 6–20 scale (27) to evaluate effects of local muscle fatigue on exercise tolerance.
- During an acute exacerbation of MS symptoms, decrease the FITT of the Ex R$_x$ to the level of tolerance. If the exacerbation is severe, focus on maintaining functional mobility and/or focus on activities such as aerobic exercises and flexibility.
- Commonly used disease-modifying medications such as Avonex, Betaseron, Rebif, and Copaxone can have transient side effects such as flu-like symptoms and localized irritation at the injection site. Take medication side effects into consideration with exercise testing and scheduling.
- Systemic fatigue is common in MS but tends to improve with increased physical fitness. It is important to help the individual understand the difference between more general centrally mediated MS fatigue and temporary peripheral exercise-related fatigue. Tracking the effects of fatigue may be helpful using an instrument such as the Modified Fatigue Impact Scale (168).
- Heat sensitivity is common in MS. Use of fans, evaporative cooling garments, and cooling vests can increase exercise tolerance and reduce symptoms of fatigue.
- HR and BP responses may be blunted because of dysautonomia so that HR may not be a valid indicator of exercise intensity. RPE can be used in addition to HR to evaluate exercise intensity (see *Chapters 4* and *7*).
- Some individuals may restrict their daily fluid intake because of bladder control problems. They should be counseled to increase fluid intake with increased physical activity levels to prevent dehydration.

- Many individuals with MS have some level of cognitive deficit that may affect their understanding of testing and training instructions. They may also have short-term memory loss that requires written instructions and frequent verbal cueing and reinforcement.
- Watch for signs and symptoms of the *Uhthoff Phenomenon*. Uhthoff phenomenon typically involves a transient (<24 h) worsening of neurological symptoms, most commonly visual impairment associated with exercise and elevation of body temperature. Symptoms can be minimized by using cooling strategies and adjusting exercise time and intensity as appropriate.

THE BOTTOM LINE

- Individuals with MS generally have a lower $\dot{V}O_{2peak}$ compared to a healthy population. Fatigue is common in individuals with MS but can be improved with exercise training in individuals who have mild-to-moderate disability. The HR response to exercise may be blunted; RPE can be used in addition to HR to evaluate exercise intensity.

Online Resources

National Center on Physical Activity and Disability:
http://www.ncpad.org

National Institute for Neurological Disorders and Stroke:
http://www.ninds.nih.gov/multiple_sclerosis/multiple_sclerosis.htm

National MS Society:
http://www.nationalmssociety.org

OSTEOPOROSIS

Osteoporosis is a skeletal disease that is characterized by low bone mineral density (BMD) and changes in the microarchitecture of bone that increase susceptibility to fracture. The burden of osteoporosis on society and the individual is significant. More than 10 million individuals in the United States ≥50 yr have osteoporosis, and another 34 million are at risk (253). Hip fractures, in particular, are associated with increased risk of disability and death. The 2007 official position of the International Society of Clinical Densitometry, which has been endorsed by the American Association of Clinical Endocrinologists, the American Society for Bone and Mineral Research, the Endocrine Society, the North American Menopause Society, and the National Osteoporosis Foundation, defines osteoporosis in postmenopausal women and in men ≥50 yr as a BMD T-score of the lumbar spine, total hip, or femoral neck of ≤−2.5 (18). However, it is important to recognize that osteoporotic fractures may occur at BMD levels above this threshold, particularly in the elderly.

Physical activity may reduce the risk for osteoporotic fractures by enhancing the peak bone mass achieved during growth and development, by slowing the rate of bone loss with aging, and/or by reducing the risk of falls via benefits on muscle strength and balance (21,133,206,253). Accordingly, physical activity plays a prominent role in primary and secondary prevention of osteoporosis (253). Physical activity is inversely associated with risk of hip and spine fracture, and exercise training can increase or slow the decrease in spine and hip BMD (186).

EXERCISE TESTING

There are no special considerations for exercise testing of individuals at risk for osteoporosis regarding when a test is clinically indicated beyond those for the general population. However, when exercise tests are performed in individuals with osteoporosis, the following issues should be considered:

- Use of cycle leg ergometry as an alternative to treadmill exercise testing to assess CRF may be indicated in patients with severe vertebral osteoporosis for whom walking is painful.
- Vertebral compression fractures leading to a loss of height and spinal deformation can compromise ventilatory capacity and result in a forward shift in the center of gravity. The latter may affect balance during treadmill walking necessitating handrail support or an alternative modality.
- Maximal muscle strength testing may be contraindicated in patients with severe osteoporosis, although there are no established guidelines for contraindications for maximal muscle strength testing.

EXERCISE PRESCRIPTION

The FITT principle of Ex R_x for individuals with osteoporosis are categorized into two types of populations: (a) individuals at risk for osteoporosis defined as having ≥ 1 risk factor for osteoporosis (e.g., current low bone mass, age, being female) (253); and (b) individuals with osteoporosis.

FITT RECOMMENDATIONS FOR INDIVIDUALS AT RISK FOR AND WITH OSTEOPOROSIS   FITT

Aerobic and Resistance Exercise

Individuals at Risk for Osteoporosis

In individuals *at risk* for osteoporosis, the following FITT principles of Ex R_x are recommended to help *preserve bone health*:

Frequency: Weight-bearing aerobic activities 3–5 d · wk^{-1} and resistance exercise 2–3 d · wk^{-1}.

Intensity: Aerobic: Moderate (*e.g.*, 40%–<60% $\dot{V}O_2R$ or HRR) to vigorous $\geq 60\%$ ($\dot{V}O_2R$ or HRR) intensity; resistance: moderate (*e.g.*, 60%–80%

1-RM, 8–12 repetitions with exercises involving each major muscle group) to vigorous (*e.g.,* 80%–90% 1-RM, 5–6 repetitions with exercises involving each major muscle group) intensity in terms of bone loading forces.

Time: 30–60 min · d^{-1} of a combination of weight-bearing aerobic and resistance activities.

Type: Weight-bearing aerobic activities (*e.g.,* tennis, stair climbing/descending, walking with intermittent jogging), activities that involve jumping (*e.g.,* volleyball, basketball), and resistance exercise (*e.g.,* weight lifting).

Individuals with Osteoporosis

In individuals *with osteoporosis,* the following FITT principle of Ex R_x is recommended to help *prevent disease progression:*

Frequency: Weight-bearing aerobic activities 3–5 d · wk^{-1} and resistance exercise 2–3 d · wk^{-1}.

Intensity: Moderate intensity (*i.e.,* 40%–<60% $\dot{V}O_2R$ or HRR) for weight-bearing aerobic activities and moderate intensity (*e.g.,* 60%–80% 1-RM, 8–12 repetitions of exercises involving each major muscle group) in terms of bone loading forces, although some individuals may be able to tolerate more intense exercise.

Time: 30–60 min · d^{-1} of a combination of weight-bearing aerobic and resistance activities.

Type: Weight-bearing aerobic activities (*e.g.,* stair climbing/descending, walking, other activities as tolerated) and resistance exercise (*e.g.,* weight lifting).

SPECIAL CONSIDERATIONS

- It is difficult to quantify exercise intensity in terms of bone loading forces. However, the magnitude of bone loading force generally increases in parallel with exercise intensity quantified by conventional methods (*e.g.,* %HR_{max} or %1-RM).
- There are currently no established guidelines regarding contraindications for exercise for individuals with osteoporosis. The general recommendation is to prescribe moderate intensity exercise that does not cause or exacerbate pain. Exercises that involve explosive movements or high-impact loading should be avoided. Exercises that cause twisting, bending, or compression of the spine should also be avoided.
- BMD of the spine may appear *normal* or *increased* after osteoporotic compression fractures have occurred or in individuals with osteoarthritis of the spine. Hip BMD is a more reliable indicator of risk for osteoporosis than spine BMD (141).
- For older women and men at increased risk for falls, the Ex R_x should also include activities that improve balance (see *Chapter 8* and the relevant ACSM position stand [8]).

- In light of the rapid and profound effects of immobilization and bed rest on bone loss and poor prognosis for recovery of mineral after remobilization, even the frailest elderly should remain as physically active as his or her health permits to preserve musculoskeletal integrity.

THE BOTTOM LINE

- Physical activity plays an important role in the primary and secondary prevention of osteoporosis by enhancing peak bone mass during growth, slowing the rate of bone loss with aging, and preventing falls. Weight-bearing aerobic and resistance exercise are essential to individuals at risk for and with osteoporosis. It is difficult to quantify the magnitude of bone loading forces, but they generally increase in parallel with exercise intensity.

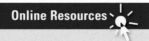

Online Resources

American College of Sports Medicine:
http://www.acsm.org to access the position stand on osteoporosis

National Osteoporosis Foundation:
http://www.nof.org

OVERWEIGHT AND OBESITY

Overweight and *obesity* are characterized by excess body weight with BMI commonly used as the criterion to define these conditions. Recent estimates indicate that more than 68% of adults are classified as overweight (BMI $\geq$25 kg $\cdot$ m^{-2}), 32% as obese (BMI $\geq$30 kg $\cdot$ m^{-2}), and 5% extremely obese (BMI $\geq$40 kg $\cdot$ m^{-2}) (77). Obesity is also an increasing concern in youth with ~14%–18% of children and adolescents classified as overweight, defined as $\geq$95th percentile of BMI for age and sex (173). Overweight and obesity are linked to numerous chronic diseases including CVD, DM, many forms of cancer, and numerous musculoskeletal problems (36). It is estimated obesity-related conditions account for ~7% of total health care costs in the United States, and the direct and indirect costs of obesity are in excess of $113.9 billion annually (245).

The management of body weight is dependent on energy balance that is determined by energy intake and EE. For an individual who is overweight or obese to reduce body weight, EE must exceed energy intake. A weight loss of 5%–10% provides significant health benefits (36), and these benefits are more likely to be sustained through the maintenance of weight loss and/or participation in habitual physical activity (241). Weight loss maintenance is challenging with weight regain averaging approximately 33%–50% of initial weight loss within 1 yr of terminating treatment (270).

Lifestyle interventions for weight loss that combine reductions in energy intake with increases in EE through exercise and other forms of physical activity typically result in an initial 9%–10% reduction in body weight (270). However, physical activity appears to have a modest impact on the magnitude of weight loss observed across the initial weight loss intervention compared with reductions in energy intake (36). The level of impact of exercise on weight loss further decreases when energy intake is reduced to levels that are insufficient to meet the resting metabolic rate (54). Thus, the combination of moderate reductions in energy intake with adequate levels of physical activity maximizes weight loss in individuals with overweight and obesity (36,115). Physical activity appears necessary for most individuals to prevent weight regain (36,115,216,251). However, the literature is absent of well-designed, randomized controlled trials with supervised exercise, known EE of exercise, and energy balance measures upon which to provide evidence-based recommendations for quantity and quality of exercise to prevent weight regain (54).

Based on the existent scientific evidence and practical clinical guidelines (54), the ACSM makes the following recommendations regarding exercise testing and training for individuals with overweight and obesity.

EXERCISE TESTING

- The presence of other comorbidities (e.g., dyslipidemia, hypertension, hyperinsulinemia, hyperglycemia) may increase the risk classification for individuals with overweight and obesity, resulting in the need for additional medical screening before exercise testing and/or appropriate medical supervision during exercise testing (see *Chapters* 2 and 3).
- The timing of medications to treat comorbidities relative to exercise testing should be considered.
- The presence of musculoskeletal and/or orthopedic conditions may require modifications to the exercise testing procedure that may necessitate the need for leg or arm ergometry.
- The potential for low exercise capacity in individuals with overweight and obesity may necessitate a low initial workload (i.e., 2–3 METs) and small increments per testing stage of 0.5–1.0 MET.
- Because of the ease of test administration, consider a cycle leg ergometer (with an oversized seat) versus a treadmill.
- Exercise equipment must be adequate to meet the weight specification of individuals with overweight and obesity for safety and calibration purposes.
- Adults with overweight and obesity may have difficulty achieving traditional physiologic criteria indicative of maximal exercise testing so that standard termination criteria may not apply to these individuals (see *Chapter* 5).
- The appropriate cuff size should be used to measure BP in individuals who are overweight and obese to minimize the potential for inaccurate measurement.

EXERCISE PRESCRIPTION

FITT RECOMMENDATIONS FOR INDIVIDUALS WITH OVERWEIGHT AND OBESITY   FITT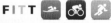

Aerobic, Resistance, and Flexibility Exercise

Frequency: $\geq$5 d $\cdot$ wk^{-1} to maximize caloric expenditure.

Intensity: Moderate-to-vigorous intensity aerobic activity should be encouraged. Initial exercise training intensity should be moderate (*i.e.*, 40%–<60% $\dot{V}O_2R$ or HRR). Eventual progression to more vigorous exercise intensity (*i.e.*, $\geq$60% $\dot{V}O_2R$ or HRR) may result in further health/fitness benefits.

Time: A minimum of 30 min $\cdot$ d^{-1} (*i.e.*, 150 min $\cdot$ wk^{-1}) progressing to 60 min $\cdot$ d^{-1} (*i.e.*, 300 min $\cdot$ wk^{-1}) of moderate intensity, aerobic activity. Incorporating more vigorous intensity exercise into the total volume of exercise may provide additional health benefits. However, vigorous intensity exercise should be encouraged in individuals who are both capable and willing to exercise at a higher than moderate intensity levels of physical exertion with recognition that vigorous intensity exercise is associated with the potential for greater injuries (182). Accumulation of intermittent exercise of at least 10 min is an effective alternative to continuous exercise and may be a particularly useful way to initiate exercise (116).

Type: The primary mode of exercise should be aerobic physical activities that involve the large muscle groups. As part of a balanced exercise program, resistance training and flexibility exercise should be incorporated (see *Chapter 7* on the FITT principle Ex R$_x$ recommendations for resistance training and flexibility).

SPECIAL CONSIDERATIONS

Weight Loss Maintenance

Clear evidence from correctly designed studies is lacking for the amount of physical activity that may be required to prevent weight regain. However, there is literature that suggests it may take more than the consensus public health recommendation for physical activity of 150 min $\cdot$ wk^{-1} or 30 min of physical activity on most days of the week (54,102,250) to prevent weight regain. For these reasons, the following special considerations should be noted:

- Adults with overweight and obesity may benefit from progression to approximately >250 min $\cdot$ wk^{-1} because this magnitude of physical activity may enhance long-term weight loss maintenance (54,115,216,251).
- Adequate amounts of physical activity should be performed on 5–7 d $\cdot$ wk^{-1}.
- The duration of moderate-to-vigorous intensity, physical activity should initially progress to at least 30 min $\cdot$ d^{-1} (102,250) and when appropriate progress to >250 min $\cdot$ wk^{-1} to enhance long-term weight management (54).

- Individuals with overweight and obesity may accumulate this amount of physical activity in multiple daily bouts of at least 10 min in duration or through increases in other forms of moderate intensity lifestyle physical activities. Accumulation of intermittent exercise may increase the volume of physical activity achieved by previously sedentary individuals and may enhance the likelihood of adoption and maintenance of physical activity (145).

- The addition of resistance exercise to energy restriction does not appear to prevent the loss of fat-free mass or the observed reduction in resting EE (55). However, resistance exercise may enhance muscular strength and physical function in individuals with overweight and obesity. Moreover, there may be additional health benefits of participating in resistance exercise such as improvements in CVD and DM risk factors and other chronic disease risk factors (55,243) (see *Chapter 7* for additional information on the FITT principle of Ex R$_x$ recommendations for resistance training).

WEIGHT LOSS PROGRAM RECOMMENDATIONS (115)

- Target a minimal reduction in body weight of at least 5%–10% of initial body weight over 3–6 mo.

- Incorporate opportunities to enhance communication between health care professionals, dietitians, and health/fitness and clinical exercise professionals and individuals with overweight and obesity following the initial weight loss period.

- Target changing eating and exercise behaviors because sustained changes in both behaviors result in significant long-term weight loss.

- Target reducing current energy intake by 500–1,000 kcal · d^{-1} to achieve weight loss. This reduced energy intake should be combined with a reduction in dietary fat to <30% of total energy intake.

- Progressively increase to a minimum of 150 min · wk^{-1} of moderate intensity, physical activity to optimize health/fitness benefits for adults with overweight and obesity.

- Progress to greater amounts of physical activity (*i.e.*, >250 min · wk^{-1}) to promote long-term weight control.

- Include resistance exercise as a supplement to the combination of aerobic exercise and modest reductions in energy intake to lose weight.

- Incorporate behavioral modification strategies to facilitate the adoption and maintenance of the desired changes in behavior (see *Chapter 11*).

BARIATRIC SURGERY

Surgery for weight loss may be indicated for individuals with a BMI ≥40 kg · m^{-2} or those with comorbid risk factors and BMI ≥30 kg · m^{-2}. Comprehensive treatment following surgery includes exercise; however, this has not been studied systematically. Exercise will likely facilitate the achievement and maintenance of energy balance postsurgery. A multicenter National Institutes of Health–sponsored trial is underway (*i.e.*, Longitudinal Assessment of Bariatric

Surgery or "LABS") (143). When the results are published, they will provide the most comprehensive findings for exercise and bariatric surgery to date (128). Individuals with severe obesity do not perform a great deal of exercise; and in similar fashion with the general population, the amount of exercise is inversely related to weight (114,128). Likewise, the achievement of a minimum of 150 min · wk^{-1} has been associated with greater postoperative weight loss at 6 and 12 mo (61). Once individuals are cleared for exercise by their physician after surgery, a progressive exercise program should follow the FITT principle of Ex R$_x$ for healthy adults (see *Chapter* 7). Because of the weight placed on joints and probable history of previous low levels of exercise, intermittent exercise or non–weight-bearing exercise may initially contribute to a successful exercise program. Subsequently, continuous exercise and weight-bearing exercise such as walking can make up a greater portion of the exercise program. Because the goal of exercise postbariatric surgery is the prevention of weight regain, the ACSM recommends ≥250 min · wk^{-1} of moderate-to-vigorous intensity exercise (54).

THE BOTTOM LINE

- Weight management relies on the relative contributions of energy intake and expenditure or "energy balance." To achieve weight loss, reduce current energy intake by 500–1,000 kcal · d^{-1}, progressively increase to a minimum of 150 min · wk^{-1} of moderate intensity, physical activity to optimize health/fitness benefits for overweight and obese adults, and progress to greater amounts of exercise (*i.e.*, >250 min · wk^{-1}) of physical activity to promote long-term weight control.

Online Resources

American College of Sports Medicine:
http://www.acsm.org to access the position stand on overweight and obesity

National Heart, Lung, and Blood Institute. Clinical guidelines on the identification, evaluation, and treatment of overweight and obesity in adults; The evidence report: National Institutes of Health, 1998:
http://www.nhlbi.nih.gov/guidelines/obesity/ob_home.htm

Physical Activity Guidelines Advisory Committee Report to the Secretary of Health and Human Services, 2008:
http:www.health.gov/PAGuidelines/committeereport.aspx

PARKINSON DISEASE

Parkinson disease (PD) is one of the most common neurodegenerative diseases. More than 1.5 million individuals in the United States are believed to have PD, and 70,000 new cases are diagnosed each year (97). It is estimated 6 million

BOX 10.2	**Common Movement Disorders in Individuals with Parkinson Disease (160)**
Bradykinesia	Reduced movement speed and amplitude; at the extreme, it is known as *hypokinesia*, which refers to "poverty" of movement
Akinesia	Difficulty initiating movements
Episodes of freezing	Motor blocks/sudden inability to move during the execution of a movement sequence
Impaired balance and postural instability	Difficulty maintaining upright stance with narrow base of support in response to a perturbation to the center of mass or with eyes closed; difficulty maintaining stability in sitting or when transferring from one position to another; can manifest as frequent falling
Dyskinesia	Overreactivity of muscles; wriggling/writhing movements
Tremor	Rhythmic activity alternating in antagonistic muscles, resembling a pill-rolling movement; usually resting tremor
Rigidity	Muscular stiffness throughout the range of passive movement in both extensor and flexor muscle groups in a given limb
Adaptive responses	Reduced activity, muscle weakness, reduced muscle length, contractures, deformity, reduced aerobic capacity

individuals worldwide are currently living with PD (247). *PD is a chronic, progressive neurological disorder characterized clinically by symptoms consisting of resting tremor, bradykinesia, rigidity, postural instability, and gait abnormalities* (see *Box 10.2*). PD is the result of damage to the dopaminergic nigrostriatal pathway, which results in a reduction in the neurotransmitter dopamine. The cause of PD is unknown; however, genetics and the environment are thought to be factors. Aging, autoimmune responses, and mitochondrial dysfunction may also contribute to the disease process (193).

The severity of PD can be classified as (a) *early disease*, characterized by minor symptoms of tremor or stiffness; (b) *moderate disease*, characterized by mild-to-moderate tremor and limited movement; and (c) *advanced disease*, characterized by significant limitations in activity regardless of treatment or medication (193). The progression of symptoms is described more comprehensively by the Hoehn and Yahr scale (108) (see *Table 10. 8*).

The symptoms of PD affect movement, and individuals with moderate and severe PD may have difficulty performing ADL. Resting tremors are often evident but can be suppressed by voluntary activity, sleep, and complete relaxation of axial muscles. Stress and anxiety increase resting tremors. Rigidity makes

TABLE 10.8. The Hoehn and Yahr Staging Scale of Parkinson Disease (108)

Stage 0.0 = No signs of disease
Stage 1.0 = Unilateral disease
Stage 2.0 = Bilateral disease, without impairment of balance
Stage 2.5 = Mild bilateral disease, with recovery on pull test
Stage 3.0 = Mild-to-moderate bilateral disease; some postural instability; physical independent
Stage 4.0 = Severe disability; still able to walk or stand unassisted
Stage 5.0 = Wheelchair bound or bedridden unless aided

movement difficult and may increase EE. This increases the patient's perception of effort on movement and may be related to feelings of fatigue, especially postexercise fatigue. Bradykinesia and akinesia are characterized by a reduction or inability to initiate and perform purposeful movements. Postural instability or impaired balance is a serious problem in PD that leads to increased episodes of falling and exposes individuals with PD to the serious consequences of falls. Generally, patients with PD demonstrate slowed, short-stepped, shuffling walk with decreased arm swing and forward-stooped posture. Difficulties and slowness in performing turning, getting up, transfer, and ADL are common. Other problems including excessive salivation or drooling, soft, slurred speech, and small handwriting also impact quality of life.

Drug therapy is the primary intervention for the treatment of symptoms related to PD. Levodopa remains the mainstay of treatment for PD and is the single most effective drug available to treat all cardinal features of the disease. Despite its significant benefit, the effectiveness is limited to an average of approximately 10 yr. Long-term use is associated with motor complications including motor fluctuations and dyskinesias in about 50% of patients within 5 yr (185, 237). Other side effects include nausea, sedation, orthostatic hypotension, and psychiatric symptoms (especially hallucinations). Levodopa is now always combined with carbidopa to prevent systemic adverse effects (198). Other adjunctive drug groups are catechol-O-methyltransferase inhibitors, monoamine oxidase B inhibitors (selegiline, rasagiline), amantadine, anticholinergics, and dopamine agonists. These drugs are used as a monotherapy or adjunct therapy to provide symptomatic relief in PD.

Individuals with severe PD may undergo surgical treatment. *Deep brain stimulation* (DBS) is an electrical stimulation of the deep brain nuclei. The internal globus pallidus and subthalamic nucleus are two main stimulation targets in PD. It is the surgical intervention of choice when motor complications are inadequately managed with the medications. The stimulation is adjustable and reversible. Improvement in motor function after either stimulation target is similar (78). DBS is more effective than medical therapy in advanced PD in improving dyskinesia, motor function, and quality of life (266).

Exercise is a crucial adjunct treatment in PD management. Regular exercise will decrease or delay secondary sequelae affecting musculoskeletal and cardiorespiratory systems that occur as a result of reduced physical activity. Because PD is a chronic progressive disease, sustained exercise is necessary to maintain benefits. Evidence demonstrates exercise improves gait performance, quality of life, reduces disease severity, and improves aerobic capacity in individuals with PD (24,106,219). Exercise might also play a neuroprotective role in individuals with PD.

EXERCISE TESTING

Most individuals with PD have impaired mobility and problems with gait, balance, and functional ability, which vary from individual to individual. These impairments are often accompanied by low levels of physical fitness (*e.g.*, CRF, muscular strength and endurance, flexibility). The following are special considerations in performing exercise testing for individuals with PD:

- Tests of balance, gait, general mobility, ROM, flexibility, and muscular strength are recommended before exercise testing is performed. Results of the tests can guide how to safely exercise test the individual with PD.
- Fall history should also be recorded. Patients with PD with more than one fall in the previous year are likely to fall again within the next 3 mo (126).
- Manual muscle testing, arm curl tests, weight machines, dynamometers, and chair rise tests (89) can be used for strength evaluation.
- Flexibility can be measured by using goniometry, the sit-and-reach test, and the back scratch test (202).
- The 6-min walk test can be used to assess CRF (63).
- The Timed Get Up and Go test (146) and chair sit-to-stand test (228) can be used to measure functional mobility. Gait observation can be done during the 10-m walk test at a comfortable walking speed (127,218).
- Balance evaluation and physical limitations of the individual should be used in making decisions regarding testing modes for test validity and safety. Clinical balance tests include the Functional Reach test (57), the Get Up and Go test (146,148,149), tandem stance (180), single limb stance (233), and pull tests (163,180,233). Static and dynamic balance evaluation of sitting and standing should be performed prior to the exercise test for safety.
- Decisions regarding exercise testing protocols may be influenced by the severity of PD (see *Table 10.8*) or physical limitations of the individual. Use of a cycle leg ergometer alone or combined with arm ergometry may be more suitable for individuals with severe gait and balance impairment or with a history of falls (192) because they reduce fear of falling on a treadmill and increase confidence during the test. However, use of leg/arm ergometers may preclude individuals with PD from achieving a maximum cardiorespiratory response because of early muscular fatigue before the maximal cardiorespiratory levels are attained (267). Treadmill protocols can be used safely in individuals with a mild stage of PD (Hoehn and Yahr [HY] stage 1–2) (267). Submaximal tests may be most appropriate in advanced cases (HY stage ≥3) or with severe mobility impairment.
- Individuals with very advanced PD (HY stage ≥4) and those unable to perform a GXT for various reasons, such as inability to stand without falling,

severe stooped posture, and deconditioning, may require a radionuclide stress test or stress echocardiography.

- For an individual who is deconditioned, demonstrates lower extremity weakness, or has a history of falling, care and precautions should be taken, especially at the final stages of the treadmill protocol when fatigue occurs and the individual's walking may deteriorate. A gait belt should be worn and an individual should stand by close to the subject to guard during the treadmill test.

- Use of symptom-limited exercise testing is strongly recommended. Symptoms include fatigue, shortness of breath, abnormal BP responses, and deteriorations in general appearance. Monitoring physical exertion levels during testing by using a scale such as the Borg perceived exertion scale (26) is recommended.

- Individuals with PD may experience orthostatic hypotension because of the severity of PD and medications (234). Antiparkinsonian medication intake should be noted prior to performing the exercise test. Different medications have different adverse effects (see *Table 10.9*).

- Issues to consider when conducting a GXT in individuals with PD include conducting the test during peak medication effect when an individual has optimal mobility, providing practice walking on a treadmill prior to testing, and using the modified Bruce protocol (see *Chapter 5*). These factors allow individuals with PD the opportunity to achieve maximal exercise (267). Although the Bruce protocol is the most commonly used protocol for exercise testing on a treadmill (122), it is an aggressive protocol that may be too strenuous for individuals with PD (267).

TABLE 10.9. Antiparkinsonian Medications (118,198,234)

Drug	Adverse Effects
Levodopa	Nausea, hypotension, and diaphoresis
Rasagiline	Weight loss, vomiting, anorexia, balance difficulty
Oral selegiline	Nausea, dizziness, sleep disorder, impaired cognition, orthostatic hypotension
Selegiline	Dizziness, dyskinesias, hallucinations, headache, dyspepsia
Bromocriptine	Nausea, hypotension, hallucinations, psychosis, peripheral edema, pulmonary fibrosis, sudden onset of sleep
Pergolide	Nausea, hypotension, hallucinations, psychosis, peripheral edema, pulmonary fibrosis, sudden onset of sleep, restrictive valvular heart disease
Cabergoline	Nausea, hypotension, hallucinations, psychosis, peripheral edema, pulmonary fibrosis, sudden onset of sleep, dyskinesia
Lisuride	Nausea, headaches, tiredness, dizziness, drowsiness, sweating, dry mouth, vomiting, sudden decreases in blood pressure (BP), nightmares, hallucinations, paranoid reactions, states of confusion, weight gain, sleep disorders
Pramipexole	Nausea, hypotension, hallucinations, psychosis, peripheral edema, sudden onset of sleep
Ropinirole	Nausea, hypotension, hallucinations, psychosis, peripheral edema, sudden onset of sleep
Tolcapone	Diarrhea, dyskinesia, liver toxicity (monitoring required)
Entacapone	Exacerbation of levodopa side effects, diarrhea, discolored urine
Amantadine	Cognitive dysfunction, hallucinations, peripheral edema, skin rash, anticholinergic effects

- For individuals with DBS, the signal from the DBS pulse generator interferes with the ECG recording. It is possible to perform the test when the DBS is deactivated; however, without the stimulation, the patient will be at a compromised mobile state and will not be able to achieve maximal tolerance. Potential risks when the DBS is deactivated are physical discomfort, tremor, cramping, and emotional symptoms (*e.g.*, nervousness, anxiety, pain). Clinicians should consult with a neurologist prior to performing the exercise test in these patients. Deactivation of the DBS should be done by a trained clinician or neurologist. HR monitoring can be used when DBS is not activated. RPE should be used to monitor during exercise testing.
- In addition to the aforementioned concerns, standard procedures, contraindications to exercise testing, recommended monitoring intervals, and standard termination criteria are used to exercise test individuals with PD (see *Chapter 5*).

EXERCISE PRESCRIPTION

Individualized programming should be used when prescribing exercise for individuals with PD. The main goal of exercise is to delay disability, prevent secondary complications, and improve quality of life as PD progresses. The FITT principle of Ex R$_x$ should address flexibility, CRF, muscle strength, functional training, and motor control. Because PD is a chronic and progressive disorder, an exercise program should be prescribed early when the individual is first diagnosed and continued on a regular, long-term basis. The Ex R$_x$ should be reviewed and revised as PD progresses because different physical problems occur at different stages of the disease.

Four key health outcomes of an exercise program designed for individuals with PD are improved (a) gait; (b) transfers; (c) balance; and (d) joint mobility and muscle power to improve functional capacity (126). However, it is important to note the FITT principle of Ex R$_x$ recommendations for individuals with PD are based on a very limited literature.

FITT RECOMMENDATIONS FOR INDIVIDUALS WITH PARKINSON DISEASE   F I T T

Aerobic Exercise

The FITT principle of Ex R$_x$ for healthy adults generally applies to those with PD (207); however, the limitations imposed by the disease process should be assessed and the Ex R$_x$ should be tailored accordingly.

Frequency: 3 d · wk^{-1}.

Intensity: 40%–<60% $\dot{V}O_2R$ or HRR or RPE of 11–13 on a scale of 6–20 (27).

Time: 30 min of continuous or accumulated exercise.

Type: Aerobic activities such as walking, cycling, swimming, or dancing. Dance provides cardiorespiratory and neuromotor exercise. Tango dancing and waltz/foxtrot improves endurance in PD more than tai chi or no exercise (95). However, the selection of the exercise type is dependent on the individual's clinical presentation of PD severity. A stationary bicycle, recumbent bicycle, or arm ergometer are safer modes for individuals with more advanced PD.

Resistance Exercise

It is important to note that the FITT principle of Ex R_x recommendations for resistance training in individuals with PD are based on a very limited literature. In general, resistance training increases strength in individuals with PD, but the majority of interventions has been conservative (64). After a resistance training program, strength improvements are similar in individuals with PD compared to neurologically normal controls (217). Therefore, recommendations for resistance exercise in neurologically healthy, older adults may be applied to individuals with PD (217).

Frequency: 2–3 d $\cdot$ wk^{-1}.

Intensity: 40%–50% of 1-RM for individuals with PD beginning to improve strength; 60%–70% 1-RM for more advanced exercisers.

Time: $\geq$1 set of 8–12 repetitions; 10–15 repetitions in adults with PD starting an exercise program.

Type: Emphasize extensor muscles of the trunk and hip to prevent faulty posture, and on all major muscles of lower extremities to maintain mobility.

Flexibility Exercise

Frequency: 1–7 d $\cdot$ wk^{-1}.

Intensity: Full extension, flexion, rotation, or stretch to the point of slight discomfort.

Time: Perform flexibility exercises for each major muscle–tendon unit. Hold stretches for 10–30 s.

Type: Slow static stretches for all major muscle groups should be performed. Flexibility and ROM exercises should be emphasized for the upper extremities and trunk as well as all major joints in all severity stages of the disease (192). Spinal mobility and axial rotation exercises are recommended for all severity stages (218). Neck flexibility exercises should be emphasized as neck rigidity is correlated with posture, gait, balance, and functional mobility (84).

RECOMMENDATIONS FOR NEUROMOTOR EXERCISE FOR INDIVIDUALS WITH PARKINSON DISEASE

Balance impairment and falls are major problems in individuals with PD. Balance training is a crucial exercise in all individuals with PD. A recent systemic review reported physical activity and exercise improved postural instability and balance performance in individuals with mild-to-moderate PD (51). Static, dynamic, and balance training during functional activities should be included. Clinicians should take steps to ensure the individual's safety (*e.g.*, using a gait belt and nearby rails or parallel bars and removing clutter on the floor) when using physical activities that challenge balance. Training programs may include a variety of challenging physical activities (*e.g.*, stepping in all directions, step up and down, reaching forward and sideways, obstacles, turning around, walking with suitable step length, standing up and sitting down) (131,160). Tai chi, tango, and waltz are other forms of exercise to improve balance in PD (58,94).

SPECIAL CONSIDERATIONS

- Incorporate functional exercises such as the sit-to-stand, step-ups, turning over, and getting out of bed as tolerated to improve neuromotor control, balance, and maintenance of ADL.
- Individuals with PD also suffer from autonomic nervous system dysfunction including cardiovascular dysfunction, especially in advanced stages. Orthostatic hypotension, cardiac arrhythmias, sweating disturbances, HR, and BP should be observed carefully during exercise.
- Some medications used to treat PD further impair autonomic nervous system functions (93) (see *Table 10.9*). Levodopa/carbidopa may produce exercise bradycardia and transient peak dose tachycardia and dyskinesia. Caution should be used in testing and training an individual who has had a recent change in medications because the response may be unpredictable (194). Several nonmotor symptoms may burden exercise performance (34,188) (see *Box 10.3*).
- The outcome of exercise training varies significantly among individuals with PD because of the complexity and progressive nature of the disease (193).
- Cognitive decline and dementia are common nonmotor symptoms in PD and burden the training and progression (234).
- Incorporate and emphasize fall prevention/reduction and education into the exercise program. Instruction on how to break falls should be given and practiced to prevent serious injuries. Most falls in PD occur during multiple tasks or long and complex movement (159,161).
- Avoid using dual tasking or multitasking with novice exercisers. Individuals with PD have difficulty in paying full attention to all tasks. One activ-

BOX 10.3	Nonmotor Symptoms in Parkinson Disease (34,189)

Domains	Symptoms
Cardiovascular	Symptomatic orthostasis; fainting; light-headedness
Sleep/fatigue	Sleep disorders; excessive daytime sleepiness; insomnia; fatigue; lack of energy; restless legs
Mood/cognition	Apathy; depression; loss of motivation; loss of interest; anxiety syndromes and panic attacks; cognitive decline
Perceptual problems/ hallucinations	Hallucinations; delusion; double vision
Attention/memory	Difficulty in concentration; forgetfulness; memory loss
Gastrointestinal	Drooling; swallowing; choking; constipation
Urinary	Incontinence; excessive urination at night; increased frequency of urination
Sexual function	Altered interest in sex; problems having sex
Miscellaneous	Pain; loss of smell/taste and appetite/weight; excessive sweating; fluctuating response to medication

ity should be completed before commencing of the next activity (127). Multitasking may better prepare an individual with PD for responding to a balance perturbation (231) and can be incorporated into training when they perform well in a single task.

- Although no reports exist suggesting resistive exercise may exacerbate symptoms of PD, considerable attention must be paid to the development and management of fatigue (88).

THE BOTTOM LINE

- The symptoms of PD include resting tremors, slow movement, rigidity, postural instability, and gait abnormalities. Prior to conducting an exercise test, balance, gait, mobility, ROM, muscular strength, and fall history should be assessed to guide the selection of the testing protocol. Limited research has been conducted regarding the most effective Ex R_x for individuals with PD. In general, the FITT principle of Ex R_x for healthy adults applies to those with PD but may require tailoring because of limitations imposed by the disease process. Balance training should be emphasized in all individuals with PD.

Online Resources

American Parkinson Disease Association:
http://www.apdaparkinson.org/userND/index.asp

Davis Phinney Foundation:
http://www.davisphinneyfoundation.org/site/c.mvKWLaMOIqG/b.5109589/k.BFE6/Home.htm

Michael J. Fox Foundation for Parkinson's Research:
http://www.michaeljfox.org

National Institute of Neurological Disorders and Stroke:
http://www.ninds.nih.gov/parkinsons_disease/parkinsons_disease.htm

National Parkinson Foundation:
http://www.parkinson.org/

WE MOVE:
http://www.wemove.org/

PULMONARY DISEASES

Chronic pulmonary diseases are significant causes of morbidity and mortality. Individuals with these diseases are increasingly referred to pulmonary rehabilitation of which exercise is the cornerstone. The majority of the research supporting exercise as an adjunct treatment for patients with chronic respiratory disease has been done in individuals with chronic obstructive pulmonary disease (COPD). However, evidence is now accumulating that shows exercise is of benefit to those with other respiratory diseases. A list of respiratory diseases in which exercise is of potential benefit is shown in *Box 10.4.*

ASTHMA

Asthma is a chronic inflammatory disorder of the airways that is characterized by episodes of bronchial hyperresponsiveness, airflow obstruction, and recurring wheeze, dyspnea, chest tightness, and coughing that occur particularly at night or early morning and are variable and often reversible (90). Asthma symptoms can be provoked or worsened by exercise, which may contribute to reduced participation in sports and physical activity and ultimately to deconditioning and lower CRF. With deconditioning, the downward cycle continues with asthma symptoms being triggered by less intense physical activity and subsequent worsening of exercise tolerance.

Although pharmacologic treatment should prevent exercise-induced bronchoconstriction and associated symptoms, individuals with moderate-to-severe persistent asthma may be referred to pulmonary rehabilitation programs to improve exercise tolerance. Systematic review (195) of exercise training studies indicates the primary exercise-related benefits are increased CRF, work capacity, and decreased exertional dyspnea with little or no effect on resting pulmonary

BOX 10.4	Patients with Pulmonary Disease Benefitting from Pulmonary Rehabilitation and Exercise

- Chronic obstructive pulmonary disease (COPD) — a mostly irreversible airflow limitation consisting of
  - Bronchitis — a chronic productive cough for 3 mo in each of two successive years in a patient in whom other causes of productive chronic cough have been excluded.
  - Emphysema — the presence of permanent enlargement of the airspaces distal to the terminal bronchioles, accompanied by destruction of their walls and without obvious fibrosis.
- Asthma — airway obstruction because of inflammation and bronchospasm that is mostly reversible.
- Cystic fibrosis — a genetic disease causing excessive, thick mucus that obstructs the airways (and other ducts) and promotes recurrent and ultimately chronic respiratory infection.
- Bronchiectasis — abnormal chronic enlargement of the airways with impaired mucus clearance.
- Pulmonary fibrosis — scarring and thickening of the parenchyma of the lungs.
- Lung cancer — one of the deadliest cancers with cigarette smoking being a common etiology.

function. Several recent randomized controlled trials suggest exercise training may also reduce airway inflammation, severity of asthma, number of days with symptoms, number of visits to the emergency department, and symptoms of anxiety and depression, and also improve health-related quality of life (65,153,154,246,264).

EXERCISE TESTING

- Assessment of physiologic function should include cardiopulmonary capacity, pulmonary function (preexercise and postexercise), and oxyhemoglobin saturation via noninvasive methods.
- The mode of exercise testing is typically a motor-driven treadmill or an electronically braked cycle leg ergometer.
- Age-appropriate (i.e., child, adult, and older adult) standard progressive maximal testing protocols may be used (see *Chapter 5*).
- Administration of an inhaled bronchodilator (i.e., β_2-agonists) (see *Appendix A*) prior to testing may be indicated to prevent exercise-induced bronchoconstriction, thus providing optimal assessment of cardiopulmonary capacity.
- Assessment of exercise-induced bronchoconstriction should be assessed via vigorous intensity exercise (i.e., 80% of predicted HR_{max} or 40%–60% of measured or estimated maximal voluntary ventilation) lasting 4–6 min on a motor-driven treadmill or an electronically braked cycle leg ergometer

and may be facilitated by inhalation of cold, dry air. The testing should be accompanied by spirometry performed prior to and 5, 10, 15, and 20 min following the exercise challenge (13,43). Use of age-predicted HR_{max} for setting exercise intensity or for estimation of $\dot{V}O_{2peak}$ may not be appropriate because of possible ventilatory limitation to exercise.

- Evidence of oxyhemoglobin desaturation ≤80% should be used as test termination criteria in addition to standard criteria (13).
- Measurement of exertional dyspnea may also be useful by adapting the Borg CR10 Scale to determine dyspnea versus its intended purpose (see *Figure 9.1*) (171). Patients and clients should be instructed to relate the wording on the scale to their level of breathlessness. Patients and clients should be informed that 0 or nothing at all corresponds to no discomfort with your breathing, whereas 10 or maximal corresponds to the most severe discomfort with your breathing that you have ever experienced or could imagine experiencing.
- 6-min walk testing may be used in individuals with moderate-to-severe persistent asthma when other testing equipment is not available (16).

EXERCISE PRESCRIPTION

The following Ex R_x for aerobic exercise is suitable for all levels of disease severity (mild-to-severe persistent) (195).

FITT RECOMMENDATIONS FOR INDIVIDUALS WITH ASTHMA

FITT

Aerobic Exercise

Frequency: At least 2–3 d · wk^{-1} (65,153,154,195).

Intensity: Approximately at the ventilatory anaerobic threshold or at least 60% $\dot{V}O_{2peak}$ determined from progressive exercise testing with measurement of expired gases (153,195) or 80% of maximal walking speed determined from the 6-min walk test (246).

Time: At least 20–30 min · d^{-1} (65,153,195,246).

Type: Aerobic activities using large muscle groups such as walking, running, or cycling. Swimming (preferably in a nonchlorinated pool) is less asthmogenic, and therefore a better tolerated form of exercise.

Progression: After the first month, if the Ex R_x is well tolerated, greater health/fitness benefits may be gained by increasing the intensity to approximately 70% $\dot{V}O_{2peak}$, the time of each exercise session to 40 min · d^{-1}, and frequency to 5 d · wk^{-1}.

Resistance Exercise

The Ex R_x for resistance training and flexibility should follow the same FITT principles of Ex R_x for healthy adults (see *Chapter 7*).

SPECIAL CONSIDERATIONS

- Individuals experiencing exacerbations of their asthma should not exercise until symptoms and airway function have improved.
- Use of short-acting bronchodilators may be necessary before or after exercise to prevent or treat exercise-induced bronchoconstriction (see *Appendix A*).
- Individuals on prolonged treatment with oral corticosteroids may experience peripheral muscle wasting and may benefit from strength training as presented in *Chapter 7*.
- Exercise in cold environments or those with airborne allergens or pollutants should be limited to avoid triggering bronchoconstriction in susceptible individuals. Exercise-induced bronchoconstriction can also be triggered by prolonged exercise durations or high intensity exercise sessions.
- There is insufficient evidence supporting individuals with asthma have clinical benefit from inspiratory muscle training in individuals with asthma (196).

CHRONIC OBSTRUCTIVE PULMONARY DISEASE

COPD is defined by the Global Initiative for Chronic Obstructive Lung Disease (GOLD) program as a preventable and treatable disease with some significant extrapulmonary effects that are characterized by an airflow limitation that is not fully reversible (see *Box 10.4*) (91). COPD consists of chronic bronchitis and/or emphysema, and patients may be staged into one of four disease severities based on the results of pulmonary function tests (see *Table 10.10*). Dyspnea or shortness of breath with exertion is a cardinal symptom of COPD resulting in physical activity limitations. Consequently, deconditioning occurs causing COPD patients to experience dyspnea at even lower levels of physical exertion further limiting their activity. This adverse downward spiral can lead to eventual functional impairment and disability. Exercise is an effective and potent intervention that lessens the development of functional impairment and disability in all patients with COPD regardless of disease severity (171,201). The beneficial effects of exercise occur mainly through adaptations in the musculoskeletal and cardiovascular systems that in turn reduce stress on the pulmonary system during exercise (232).

TABLE 10.10. Global Initiative for Chronic Obstructive Lung Disease (GOLD) Classification of Disease Severity in Patients with Chronic Obstructive Pulmonary Disease Based on the $FEV_{1.0}$ Obtained from Pulmonary Function Tests (91)

Disease Severity	Postbronchodilator FEV_1/FVC	Postbronchodilator FEV_1%
Mild	<0.70	$FEV_{1.0} \geq 80\%$ of predicted
Moderate	<0.70	$50\% \leq FEV_{1.0} < 80\%$ of predicted
Severe	<0.70	$30\% \leq FEV_{1.0} < 50\%$ of predicted
Very severe	<0.70	$FEV_{1.0} < 30\%$ of predicted or $FEV_{1.0} < 50\%$ of predicted with respiratory failure

$FEV_{1.0}$, forced expiratory volume in 1 s; FVC, forced vital capacity.

EXERCISE TESTING

- Assessment of physiologic function should include CRF, pulmonary function, and determination of arterial blood gases or arterial oxyhemoglobin saturation (SaO_2) via direct or indirect methods.
- Perceptions of dyspnea should be measured during exercise testing using the Borg CR10 Scale (see *Figure 9.1*).
- Modifications of traditional protocols (*e.g.*, smaller increments, slower progression) may be warranted depending on functional limitations and the early onset of dyspnea. Additionally, it is now recommended the duration of the GXT be between 5 and 9 min in patients with severe and very severe disease (22).
- The measurement of flow volume loops using commercially available instruments may help identify individuals with dynamic hyperinflation and increased dyspnea because of expiratory airflow limitations. Use of bronchodilator therapy may be beneficial for such individuals (172).
- Submaximal exercise testing may be used depending on the reason for the test and the clinical status of the patient. However, it should be noted individuals with pulmonary disease may have ventilatory limitations to exercise; thus, prediction of $\dot{V}O_{2peak}$ based on age-predicted HR_{max} may not be appropriate. In recent years, the 6-min walk test has become popular for assessing functional exercise capacity in individuals with more severe pulmonary disease and in settings that lack exercise testing equipment (16).
- In addition to standard termination criteria, exercise testing may be terminated because of severe arterial oxyhemoglobin desaturation (*i.e.*, SaO_2 ≤80%) (13).
- The exercise testing mode is typically walking or stationary cycling. Walking protocols may be more suitable for individuals with severe disease who may lack the muscle strength to overcome the increasing resistance of cycle leg ergometers. Furthermore, if arm ergometry is used, upper extremity aerobic exercise may result in increased dyspnea that may limit the intensity and duration of the activity.

EXERCISE PRESCRIPTION

Because individuals with COPD are typically older adults, the FITT principle of Ex R_x presented in *Chapter 8* for older adults generally applies. For detailed guidelines for the FITT principle of Ex R_x for individuals with COPD, see the following resources (171,201,232).

FITT RECOMMENDATIONS FOR INDIVIDUALS WITH CHRONIC OBSTRUCTIVE PULMONARY DISEASE

F I T T

Aerobic Exercise

Frequency: At least 3–5 d · wk^{-1}.

Intensity: For patients with COPD, vigorous (60%–80% of peak work rates) and light (30%–<40% of peak work rates) intensities have been recommended (171,201). Light intensity training results in improvements in symptoms, health-related quality of life, and performance of ADL, whereas vigorous intensity training has been shown to result in greater physiologic improvements (*e.g.*, reduced minute ventilation and HR at a given workload). Because of these greater physiologic improvements, high intensity training can be encouraged if tolerated. However, it should be recognized that some patients may not be able to exercise at these intensities, and light intensity exercise is recommended for such patients. Intensity may be based on a dyspnea rating of between 4 and 6 on the Borg CR10 Scale (see *Figure 9.1*) (171).

Time: Individuals with moderate or severe COPD may be able to exercise only at a specified intensity for a few minutes at the start of the training program. Intermittent exercise may also be used for the initial training sessions until the individual tolerates exercise at sustained higher intensities and durations of activity. Shorter periods of vigorous intensity exercise separated by periods of rest (*i.e.*, interval training) have been used with those with COPD and shown to result in lower symptom scores despite high training work rates (261).

Type: Walking and/or cycling.

Resistance and Flexibility Exercise

Resistance and flexibility training should be encouraged for individuals with COPD. The Ex R_x for resistance and flexibility training with pulmonary patients should follow the same FITT principle of Ex R_x for healthy adults and/or older adults (see *Chapters 7* and *8*).

SPECIAL CONSIDERATIONS

- Pulmonary diseases and their treatments not only affect the lungs but skeletal muscles as well (232). Resistance training of skeletal muscle should be an integral part of Ex R_x for individuals with COPD. The Ex R_x for resistance training with pulmonary patients should follow the same FITT principle of Ex R_x for healthy adults and older adults (see *Chapters 7* and *8*, respectively).
- Because individuals with COPD may experience greater dyspnea while performing ADL involving the upper extremities, it may be beneficial for these individuals to focus on the muscles of the shoulder girdle when performing resistance exercises.
- Inspiratory muscle weakness is a contributor to exercise intolerance and dyspnea in those with COPD. In patients receiving optimal medical therapy who still present with inspiratory muscle weakness and breathlessness, inspiratory muscle training is recommended. Training of the inspiratory muscles

increases respiratory muscle strength and endurance and may lead to improvements in exercise tolerance (171,201).

- The guidelines for *inspiratory muscle training* are the following:
  - **Frequency:** A minimum of 4–5 d · wk^{-1}.
  - **Intensity:** 30% of maximal inspiratory pressure measured at functional residual capacity.
  - **Time:** 30 min · d^{-1} or two 15 min sessions · d^{-1}.
  - **Type:** Three types of inspiratory muscle training have been used in patients with COPD. These are inspiratory resistive training, threshold loading, and normocapnic hyperpnea. There are no data to suggest that one method is superior to the other (171).

- Regardless of the prescribed exercise intensity, the health/fitness, clinical exercise, or health care professional should closely monitor initial exercise sessions and adjust intensity and duration according to individual responses and tolerance. In many cases, the presence of symptoms, particularly dyspnea/breathlessness, supersedes objective methods of Ex R$_x$.

- The traditional method for monitoring the exercise intensity is HR as discussed in *Chapter 7*. As previously mentioned, an alternative approach to HR is using the dyspnea rating obtained from a GXT test as a "target" intensity for exercise training (111). Most patients with COPD accurately and reliably produce a dyspnea rating obtained from an incremental exercise test as a target to regulate/monitor exercise intensity. A dyspnea rating between 4 and 6 on a scale of 0–10 is the recommended exercise intensity (see *Figure 9.1*) (171).

- Unlike most healthy individuals and individuals with CVD, patients with moderate-to-severe COPD may exhibit oxyhemoglobin desaturation with exercise. Therefore, a measure of blood oxygenation, either the partial pressure of arterial oxygen (P$_a$O$_2$) or %SaO$_2$, should be made during the initial GXT. In addition, oximetry is recommended for the initial exercise training sessions to evaluate possible exercise-induced oxyhemoglobin desaturation and to identify the workload at which desaturation occurred.

- Based on the recommendations of the Nocturnal Oxygen Therapy Trial (40), supplemental oxygen (O$_2$) is indicated for patients with a P$_a$O$_2$ ≤55 mm Hg or a %SaO$_2$ ≤88% while breathing room air. These same guidelines apply when considering supplemental oxygen during exercise. Additionally, there is evidence to suggest the administration of supplemental O$_2$ to those who do not experience exercise-induced hypoxemia may lead to greater gains in exercise endurance (201).

- In selected patients with severe COPD, using noninvasive positive pressure ventilation as an adjunct to exercise training produces modest gains in exercise performance. Because of the difficulty administering such an intervention, it is only recommended in those patients with advanced disease (171,201).

- Individuals suffering from acute exacerbations of their pulmonary disease should limit exercise until symptoms have subsided.

THE BOTTOM LINE

- Exercise training is beneficial for improving CRF and exercise tolerance in individuals with asthma, and growing evidence suggests training may reduce inflammation and disease severity and improve health-related quality of life. COPD is a treatable disease characterized by nonreversible airflow limitation. In addition to its damage to the lungs, the disease has significant extrapulmonary effects. These extrapulmonary effects should be considered when using exercise as a treatment for COPD.

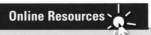

Online Resources

American Lung Association:
http://www.lungusa.org/lung-disease/copd/

Expert Panel Report 3 (EPR3) American Thoracic Society (41):
http://www.thoracic.org/clinical/copd-guidelines/index.php

EPR3: Guidelines for the Diagnosis and Management of Asthma (62):
http://www.nhlbi.nih.gov/guidelines/asthma/asthgdln.htm

Global Initiative for Asthma:
http://www.ginasthma.org

Global Initiative for Chronic Obstructive Lung Disease:
http://www.goldcopd.com/guidelinesresources.asp?l1=2&l2=0

SPINAL CORD INJURY

Spinal cord injury (SCI) results in a complete or incomplete loss of somatic, sensory, and autonomic functions below the lesion level. Lesions in the cervical (C) region typically result in tetraplegia, whereas lesions in the thoracic (T), lumbar (L), and sacral (S) regions lead to paraplegia. Approximately 50% of those with SCI have tetraplegia, and 80% are men (235). SCI of traumatic origin often occurs at an early age. Individuals with SCI have a high risk for the development of secondary complications (*e.g.*, shoulder pain, urinary tract infections, skin pressure ulcers, osteopenia, chronic pain, problematic spasticity, depression, CVD, obesity, Type 2 DM). Proper exercise and physical activity reduce the prevalence of secondary complications and improve the quality of life for individuals with SCI.

The SCI level has a direct impact on physical function and metabolic and cardiorespiratory responses to exercise. It is crucial to take into account the SCI lesion level when exercise testing and prescribing exercise for those with SCI. Those with complete SCI lesions from:

- L2–S2 lack voluntary control of the bladder, bowels, and sexual function; however, the upper extremities and trunk usually have normal function.

- T6–L2 have respiratory and motor control that depends on the functional capacity of the abdominal muscles (*i.e.*, minimal control at T6 to maximal control at L2).
- T1–T6 can experience autonomic dysreflexia (*i.e.*, an uncoordinated, spinally mediated reflex response called the *mass reflex*), poor thermoregulation, and orthostatic hypotension. In instances in which there is no sympathetic innervation to the heart, HR_{peak} is limited to ~115–130 beats $\cdot$ min^{-1}. Breathing capacity is further diminished by intercostal muscle paralysis; however, arm function is normal.
- C5–C8 are tetraplegic. Those with C8 lesions have voluntary control of the shoulder, elbow, and wrist but decreased hand function; whereas those with C5 lesions rely on the biceps brachii and shoulder muscles for self-care and mobility.
- C4 require artificial support for breathing.

EXERCISE TESTING

When exercise testing individuals with SCI, consider the following issues.

- Initially, a functional assessment should be taken including trunk ROM, wheelchair mobility, transfer ability, and upper and lower extremity involvement. This assessment will facilitate the choice of exercise testing equipment, protocols, and adaptations.
- Consider the purposes of the exercise test, the level of SCI, and the physical fitness level of the participant to optimize equipment and protocol selection.
- Voluntary arm ergometry is the easiest to perform and is norm referenced for the assessment of CRF (96). This form of exercise testing, however, is not wheelchair propulsion sport specific, and the equipment may not be accurate in the lower work rate ranges needed for quadriplegics (*i.e.*, 0–25 W).
- If available, a stationary wheelchair roller system and motor-driven treadmill should be used with the participant's properly adjusted wheelchair. Motor-driven treadmill protocols allow for realistic simulation of external conditions such as slope and speed alterations (257).
- Incremental exercise tests for the assessment of CRF in the laboratory should begin at 0 W with incremental increases of 5–10 W per stage among tetraplegics. Depending on function and fitness, individuals with paraplegia can begin at 20–40 W with incremental increases of 10–25 W per stage.
- For sport-specific indoor CRF assessments in the field, an incremental test adapted from the Léger and Boucher shuttle test around a predetermined rectangular court is recommended. Floor surface characteristics and wheelchair user interface should be standardized (138,257).
- After maximal effort exercise in individuals with tetraplegia, it may be necessary to treat postexercise hypotension and exhaustion with rest, recumbency, leg elevation, and fluid ingestion.
- There are no special considerations for the assessment of muscular strength regarding the exercise testing mode beyond those for the general population

with the exception of the lesion level, which will determine residual motor function, need for stabilization, and accessibility of testing equipment.

- Individuals with SCI requiring a wheelchair for mobility may develop joint contractures because of muscle spasticity and their position in the wheelchair (*i.e.*, tight hip flexors, hip adductors, and knee flexors) and excessive wheelchair pushing and manual transfers (*i.e.*, anterior chest and shoulder). Therefore, intensive sport-specific training must be complemented with an upper extremity stretching (*e.g.*, the prime movers) and strengthening (*e.g.*, the antagonists) program to promote muscular balance around the joints.

EXERCISE PRESCRIPTION/SPECIAL CONSIDERATIONS

The FITT principle of Ex R_x recommendations for the general population should be applied (see *Chapter 7*) (88,102). For this reason and because of the impact of SCI on neuromotor, cardiorespiratory, and metabolic function, the following FITT principle of Ex R_x recommendations and special considerations are combined in this section:

- Participants should empty their bowels and bladder or urinary bag before exercising because autonomic dysreflexia can be triggered by a full bladder or bowel distension.
- Skin pressure sores should be avoided at all times and potential risk areas should be checked on a regular basis.
- Decreased cardiovascular performance may be found in individuals with complete SCIs above T6, particularly among those with complete tetraplegia who have no cardiac sympathetic innervation with HR_{peak} limited to ~115–130 beats $\cdot$ min^{-1}. Individuals with high spinal lesions may reach their peak HR, cardiac output ($\dot{Q}$), and $\dot{V}O_2$ at lower exercise levels than those with paraplegia with lesion levels below T5 to T6 (110).
- During exercise, autonomic dysreflexia results in an increased release of catecholamines that increases HR, $\dot{V}O_2$, BP, and exercise capacity (220). BP may be elevated to excessively high levels (*i.e.*, SBP 250–300 mm Hg and/or DBP 200–220 mm Hg). In these situations, immediate emergency responses is needed (*i.e.*, stopping exercise, sitting upright to decrease BP, and identifying and removing the irritating stimulus such as a catheter, leg bag, tight clothing, or braces). If the symptoms (*i.e.*, headache, piloerection, flushing, gooseflesh, shivering, sweating above the lesion level, nasal congestion, and bradycardia) persist, medical attention should be sought. In competition, athletes with a resting SBP ≥180 mm Hg should not be allowed to start the event.
- Novice unfit but healthy participants with SCI will probably experience muscular fatigue before achieving substantial central cardiovascular stimulus. Initially, the exercise sessions should consist of short bouts of 5–10 min of moderate intensity (*i.e.*, 40%–<60% $\dot{V}O_2R$) alternated with active recovery periods of 5 min.

As a starting point and on the basis of proven efficacy and specificity to daily activity patterns, Rimaud et al. (203) has recommended interval wheelchair ergometry training at $\geq 70\%$ HR_{peak} for 30 min $\cdot$ session^{-1}, 3 sessions $\cdot$ wk^{-1}.

- Individuals with tetraplegia who have a very small active musculature will also experience muscular fatigue before exhausting central cardiorespiratory capacity. Aerobic exercise programs should start with 5–10 min bouts of moderate intensity (i.e., 40%–<60% $\dot{V}O_2R$), alternated with 5 min active recovery periods. As exercise tolerance improves, training can progress to 10–20 min bouts of vigorous intensity (i.e., ≥ 60 $\dot{V}O_2R$) alternated with 5 min active recovery periods.

- Individuals with higher SCI levels, especially those with tetraplegia, may benefit from use of lower body positive pressure by applying compressive stockings, an elastic abdominal binder, or electrical stimulation to leg muscles. Beneficial hemodynamic effects may include maintenance of BP, lower HR, and higher stroke volume during arm work to compensate for blood pooling below the lesion. Electrical stimulation of paralyzed lower limb muscles can increase venous return and $\dot{Q}$. These responses usually occur only in individuals with spastic paralysis above T12 who have substantial sensory loss and respond to the stimulation with sustainable static or dynamic contractions.

- Muscular strength training sessions from a seated position in the wheelchair should be complemented with nonwheelchair exercise bouts to involve all trunk stabilizing muscles. However, transfers (e.g., from wheelchair to the exercise apparatus) should be limited because they result in a significant hemodynamic load and increase the glenohumeral contact forces, and the risk of repetitive strain injuries such as shoulder impingement syndrome and rotator cuff strain/tear, especially in individuals with tetraplegia (256). Special attention should be given to shoulder muscle imbalance and the prevention of repetitive strain injuries. The prime movers of wheelchair propulsion should be lengthened (i.e., muscles of the anterior shoulder and chest) and antagonists should be strengthened (i.e., muscles of the posterior shoulder, scapula, and upper back [74]).

- *Tenodesis* (i.e., active wrist extensor driven finger flexion) allows functional grasp in individuals with tetraplegia who do not have use of the hand muscles. To retain the tenodesis effect, these individuals should never stretch the finger flexor muscles (i.e., maximal and simultaneous extension of wrist and fingers).

- Individuals with SCI tend to endure higher core temperatures during endurance exercise than their able-bodied counterparts. Despite this enhanced thermoregulatory drive, they generally have lower sweat rates. The following factors reduce heat tolerance and should be avoided: lack of acclimatization, dehydration, glycogen depletion, sleep loss, alcohol, and infectious disease. During training and competition, the use of light clothing, ice vests, protective sunscreen cream, and mist spray are recommended (7,9).

THE BOTTOM LINE

- Proper exercise and physical activity reduce the prevalence of secondary complications associated with SCI and improve quality of life. The level of the SCI lesion must be taken into account for exercise testing and the FITT principle of Ex R_x. Individuals with SCI have compromised thermoregulatory responses to exercise so caution must be taken, especially during endurance exercise.

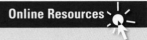

Online Resources

National Spinal Cord Injury Association:
http://www.spinalcord.org

INDIVIDUALS WITH MULTIPLE CHRONIC DISEASES AND HEALTH CONDITIONS

The aging and increasing prevalence of overweight and obesity in the population make it increasingly likely health/fitness, clinical exercise, and health care professionals will be designing Ex R_x for clients and patients with multiple chronic diseases and health conditions. The focus of the *Guidelines* has traditionally been on Ex R_x for healthy and special populations with one chronic disease or health condition. This final section of this chapter presents guidelines for prescribing exercise for individuals with multiple comorbidities.

PREPARTICIPATION HEALTH SCREENING

Exercise training is generally safe for the majority of individuals with multiple diseases and chronic conditions wishing to participate in a light-to-moderate intensity exercise programs (see *Chapters 1* and *2*). For individuals with multiple comorbidities that fall into the high risk category as designated in *Table 2.3*, referral to a health care provider is recommended prior to participating in an exercise program (see *Figure 2.4*). Individuals with multiple CVD risk factors (see *Table 2.2* and *Figure 2.3*) that do not fall into the high risk category should be encouraged to consult with their physician prior to initiating a vigorous intensity exercise program as part of good medical care and should progress gradually with their exercise program of any exercise intensity.

EXERCISE TESTING

Exercise stress testing is recommended only for the highest risk individuals including those with diagnosed CVD, symptoms suggestive of new or changing CVD, DM and additional CVD risk factors (see *Table 2.2*), end-stage renal disease, and specified lung disease (see *Table 2.3*). Nonetheless, the information gathered from an exercise test may be useful in establishing a safe and effective Ex R_x for low- to moderate-risk individuals. Recommending an exercise test for low- to moderate-risk individuals should not be viewed as inappropriate if the purpose of the test is to design an effective Ex R_x. The *Guidelines* also recommends health/fitness, clinical exercise, and health care professionals consult with their medical colleagues when there are questions about clients and patients with known disease and health conditions that may limit their participation in exercise programs.

EXERCISE PRESCRIPTION

In general, the FITT principle of Ex R_x for individuals with multiple diseases and health conditions will follow the recommendations for healthy adults (see *Chapter 7*). *Table 10.11* summarizes the aerobic exercise FIT (*i.e.*, frequency, intensity, and time) principle of Ex R_x recommendations for special populations with one chronic disease, health condition, or CVD risk factor as discussed in this chapter. However, the challenge is determining the specifics of the FITT principle of Ex R_x that should be recommended for the client or patient that presents with multiple chronic diseases, health conditions, and/or CVD risk factors, especially when there is variability in the exercise dose that can most favorably impact a particular disease, health condition, or CVD risk factor (*e.g.*, BP requires lower doses of exercise to improve than does HDL, abdominal adiposity, or bone density).

SPECIAL CONSIDERATIONS

- A large body of scientific evidence supports the role of physical activity in delaying premature mortality and reducing the risks of many chronic diseases and health conditions. There is also clear evidence for a dose-response relationship between physical activity and health. Thus, any amount of physical activity should be encouraged.

TABLE 10.11. Summary of the Aerobic Exercise Frequency, Intensity, and Type Recommendations for a Single Disease, Health Condition, or Cardiovascular Disease (CVD) Risk Factor[a]

Condition	Frequency	Intensity	Time
Arthritis	3–5 d · wk^{-1}	40%–<60% HRR or $\dot{V}O_2R$	20–30 min · d^{-1}
Patients with CVD	4–7 d · wk^{-1}	40%–80% HRR or $\dot{V}O_2R$	20–60 min · d^{-1}
Dyslipidemia	≥5 d · wk^{-1}	40%–75% HRR or $\dot{V}O_2R$	30–60 min · d^{-1}
Hypertension	≥5 d · wk^{-1}	40%–<60% HRR or $\dot{V}O_2R$	30–60 min · d^{-1}
Obesity	≥5 d · wk^{-1}	40%–<60% HRR or $\dot{V}O_2R$	30–60 min · d^{-1}
Osteoporosis	3–5 d · wk^{-1}	40%–<60% HRR or $\dot{V}O_2R$	30–60 min · d^{-1}
Type 2 diabetes	3–7 d · wk^{-1}	50%–80% HRR or $\dot{V}O_2R$	20–60 min · d^{-1}

[a]Moderate intensity resistance exercise is generally recommended 2–3 d · wk^{-1} in addition to the amount of aerobic exercise specified previously for each chronic disease, health condition, and CVD risk factor (see *Chapter 7*).
HRR, heart rate reserve; $\dot{V}O_2R$, maximal oxygen consumption reserve.

- Begin with the FITT principle of Ex R_x for the single disease and health condition that confers the greatest risk and/or is the most limiting regarding ADL, quality of life, and/or starting or maintaining an exercise program. Also consider client and patient preference and goals.
- Alternatively, begin with the FITT that is the most conservative FITT prescribed for the multiple diseases, health conditions, and/or CVD risk factors the client and patient presents with as listed in *Table 10.11*.
- Know the magnitude and time course of response of the various health outcome(s) that can be expected as a result of the FITT principle of Ex R_x that is prescribed in order to progress the client and patient safely and appropriately.
- Frequently monitor signs and symptoms to ensure safety and proper adaptation and progression.

REFERENCES

1. Ahlborg L, Andersson C, Julin P. Whole-body vibration training compared with resistance training: effect on spasticity, muscle strength and motor performance in adults with cerebral palsy. *J Rehabil Med*. 2006;38(5):302–8.
2. Albright A, Franz M, Hornsby G, et al. American College of Sports Medicine position stand. Exercise and type 2 diabetes. *Med Sci Sports Exerc*. 2000;32(7):1345–60.
3. Albright AL. Diabetes. In: Ehrman JK, editor. *Clinical Exercise Physiology*. Champaign: Human Kinetics; 2003. p. 191–210.
4. Allen NA, Fain JA, Braun B, Chipkin SR. Continuous glucose monitoring counseling improves physical activity behaviors of individuals with type 2 diabetes: a randomized clinical trial. *Diabetes Res Clin Pract*. 2008;80(3):371–9.
5. American Cancer Society. *Cancer Facts and Figures 2010* [Internet]. Atlanta (GA): American Cancer Society; [cited 2011 Feb 15]. Available from: http://www.cancer.org/acs/groups/content/@nho/documents/document/acspc-024113.pdf
6. American College of Sports Medicine, American Diabetes Association. Exercise and type 2 diabetes: American College of Sports Medicine and the American Diabetes Association: joint position statement. Exercise and type 2 diabetes. *Med Sci Sports Exerc*. 2010;42(12):2282–303.
7. American College of Sports Medicine, Armstrong LE, Casa DJ, et al. American College of Sports Medicine position stand. Exertional heat illness during training and competition. *Med Sci Sports Exerc*. 2007;39(3):556–72.
8. American College of Sports Medicine, Chodzko-Zajko WJ, Proctor DN, et al. American College of Sports Medicine position stand. Exercise and physical activity for older adults. *Med Sci Sports Exerc*. 2009;41(7):1510–30.
9. American College of Sports Medicine, Sawka MN, Burke LM, et al. American College of Sports Medicine position stand. Exercise and fluid replacement. *Med Sci Sports Exerc*. 2007;39(2):377–90.
10. American Diabetes Association. Diagnosis and classification of diabetes mellitus. *Diabetes Care*. 2010; 33 Suppl 1:S62–9.
11. American Diabetes Association. Standards of medical care in diabetes—2007. *Diabetes Care*. 2007; 30 Suppl 1:S4–41.
12. American Diabetes Association. Standards of medical care in diabetes—2012. *Diabetes Care*. 2012; 35 Suppl 1:S11–63.
13. American Thoracic Society, American College of Chest Physicians. ATS/ACCP Statement on cardiopulmonary exercise testing. *Am J Respir Crit Care Med*. 2003;167(2):211–77.
14. Anandacoomarasamy A, Caterson I, Sambrook P, Fransen M, March L. The impact of obesity on the musculoskeletal system. *Int J Obes (Lond)*. 2008;32(2):211–22.
15. Anuurad E, Semrad A, Berglund L. Human immunodeficiency virus and highly active antiretroviral therapy-associated metabolic disorders and risk factors for cardiovascular disease. *Metab Syndr Relat Disord*. 2009;7(5):401–10.
16. ATS Committee on Proficiency Standards for Clinical Pulmonary Function Laboratories. ATS statement: guidelines for the six-minute walk test. *Am J Respir Crit Care Med*. 2002;166(1):111–7.
17. Auxter D, Pyfer J, Huettig C. *Principles and Methods of Adapted Physical Education and Recreation*. 9th ed. Boston (MA): McGraw-Hill; 2001. 718 p.

18. Baim S, Leonard MB, Bianchi ML, et al. Official positions of the International Society for Clinical Densitometry and executive summary of the 2007 ISCD Pediatric Position Development Conference. *J Clin Densitom.* 2008;11(1):6–21.

19. Bartlett DJ, Hanna SE, Avery L, Stevenson RD, Galuppi B. Correlates of decline in gross motor capacity in adolescents with cerebral palsy in Gross Motor Function Classification System levels III to V: an exploratory study. *Dev Med Child Neurol.* 2010;52(7):e155–60.

20. Baynard T, Pitetti KH, Guerra M, Unnithan VB, Fernhall B. Age-related changes in aerobic capacity in individuals with mental retardation: a 20-yr review. *Med Sci Sports Exerc.* 2008;40(11):1984–9.

21. Beck BR, Snow CM. Bone health across the lifespan—exercising our options. *Exerc Sport Sci Rev.* 2003;31(3):117–22.

22. Benzo RP, Paramesh S, Patel SA, Slivka WA, Sciurba FC. Optimal protocol selection for cardio-pulmonary exercise testing in severe COPD. *Chest.* 2007;132(5):1500–5.

23. Berg K, Wood-Dauphinee S, Williams JI, Gayton D. Measuring balance in the elderly: preliminary development of an instrument. *Physiother Can.* 1989;41(6):304–11.

24. Bergen JL, Toole T, Elliott RG,3rd, Wallace B, Robinson K, Maitland CG. Aerobic exercise intervention improves aerobic capacity and movement initiation in Parkinson's disease patients. *NeuroRehabilitation.* 2002;17(2):161–8.

25. Bhole R, Flynn JC, Marbury TC. Quadriceps tendon ruptures in uremia. *Clin Orthop Relat Res.* 1985;(195):200–6.

26. Borg GA. Psychophysical bases of perceived exertion. *Med Sci Sports Exerc.* 1982;14(5):377–81.

27. Borg GA. Scaling pain and related subjective somatic symptoms. In: Borg GA, editor. *Borg's Perceived Exertion and Pain Scales.* Champaign: Human Kinetics; 1998. p. 63–7.

28. Burckhardt CS, Clark SR, Bennett RM. The fibromyalgia impact questionnaire: development and validation. *J Rheumatol.* 1991;18(5):728–33.

29. Busch AJ, Barber KA, Overend TJ, Peloso PM, Schachter CL. Exercise for treating fibromyalgia syndrome. *Cochrane Database Syst Rev.* 2007;(4):CD003786.

30. Butler JM, Scianni A, Ada L. Effect of cardiorespiratory training on aerobic fitness and carryover to activity in children with cerebral palsy: a systematic review. *Int J Rehabil Res.* 2010;33(2):97–103.

31. Castellani JW, Young AJ, Ducharme MB, et al. American College of Sports Medicine position stand: prevention of cold injuries during exercise. *Med Sci Sports Exerc.* 2006;38(11):2012–29.

32. Centers for Disease Control and Prevention. Prevalence of doctor-diagnosed arthritis and arthritis-attributable activity limitation—United States, 2007–2009. *MMWR Morb Mortal Wkly Rep.* 2010; 59(39):1261–5.

33. Cerebral Palsy International Sports & Recreation Association. *Classification and Sports Rules Manual.* 9th ed. Nottingham, England: CPISRA; 2006.

34. Chaudhuri KR, Martinez-Martin P, Brown RG, et al. The metric properties of a novel non-motor symptoms scale for Parkinson's disease: results from an international pilot study. *Mov Disord.* 2007;22(13):1901–11.

35. Chobanian AV, Bakris GL, Black HR, et al. Seventh report of the Joint National Committee on prevention, detection, evaluation, and treatment of high blood pressure. *Hypertension.* 2003;42(6): 1206–52.

36. Clinical Guidelines on the Identification, Evaluation, and Treatment of Overweight and Obesity in Adults—The Evidence Report. National Institutes of Health. *Obes Res.* 1998;6 Suppl 2:51S–209S.

37. Clyne N, Ekholm J, Jogestrand T, Lins LE, Pehrsson SK. Effects of exercise training in predialytic uremic patients. *Nephron.* 1991;59(1):84–9.

38. Clyne N, Jogestrand T, Lins LE, Pehrsson SK. Factors influencing physical working capacity in renal transplant patients. *Scand J Urol Nephrol.* 1989;23(2):145–50.

39. Colberg SR, Sigal RJ, Fernhall B, et al. Exercise and type 2 diabetes: the American College of Sports Medicine and the American Diabetes Association: joint position statement executive summary. *Diabetes Care.* 2010;33(12):2692–6.

40. Continuous or nocturnal oxygen therapy in hypoxemic chronic obstructive lung disease: a clinical trial. Nocturnal Oxygen Therapy Trial Group. *Ann Intern Med.* 1980;93(3):391–8.

41. *COPD Guidelines (2004)* [Internet]. New York (NY): American Thoracic Society; [cited 2011 Mar 11]. Available from: http://www.thoracic.org/clinical/copd-guidelines/index.php

42. Cowley PM, Ploutz-Snyder LL, Baynard T, et al. Physical fitness predicts functional tasks in indi-viduals with Down syndrome. *Med Sci Sports Exerc.* 2010;42(2):388–93.

43. Crapo RO, Casaburi R, Coates AL, et al. Guidelines for methacholine and exercise challenge testing-1999. This official statement of the American Thoracic Society was adopted by the ATS Board of Directors, July 1999. *Am J Respir Crit Care Med.* 2000;161(1):309–29.

44. Dadabhoy D, Clauw DJ. Musculoskeletal signs and symptoms. E. The Fibromyalgia Syndrome. In: Klippel JH, editor. *Primer on the Rheumatic Diseases.* 13th ed. New York: Springer; 2008. p. 87–93.

45. Damiano DL. Activity, activity, activity: rethinking our physical therapy approach to cerebral palsy. *Phys Ther*. 2006;86(11):1534–40.

46. Darrah J, Wessel J, Nearingburg P, O'Connor M. Evaluation of a community fitness program for adolescents with cerebral palsy. *Ped Phys Ther*. 1999;11(1):18–23.

47. de Haan A, de Ruiter CJ, van Der Woude LH, Jongen PJH. Contractile properties and fatigue of quadriceps muscles in multiple sclerosis. *Muscle Nerve*. 2000;23(10):1534–41.

48. de Jong Z, Munneke M, Zwinderman AH, et al. Is a long-term high-intensity exercise program effective and safe in patients with rheumatoid arthritis? Results of a randomized controlled trial. *Arthritis Rheum*. 2003;48(9):2415–24.

49. Dela F, Larsen JJ, Mikines KJ, Ploug T, Petersen LN, Galbo H. Insulin-stimulated muscle glucose clearance in patients with NIDDM. Effects of one-legged physical training. *Diabetes*. 1995;44(9):1010–20.

50. D'hooge R, Hellinckx T, Van Laethem C, et al. Influence of combined aerobic and resistance training on metabolic control, cardiovascular fitness and quality of life in adolescents with type 1 diabetes: a randomized controlled trial. *Clin Rehabil*. 2011;25(4):349–59.

51. Dibble LE, Addison O, Papa E. The effects of exercise on balance in persons with Parkinson's disease: a systematic review across the disability spectrum. *J Neurol Phys Ther*. 2009;33(1):14–26.

52. Diesel W, Noakes TD, Swanepoel C, Lambert M. Isokinetic muscle strength predicts maximum exercise tolerance in renal patients on chronic hemodialysis. *Am J Kidney Dis*. 1990;16(2):109–14.

53. Dodd KJ, Taylor NF, Damiano DL. A systematic review of the effectiveness of strength-training programs for people with cerebral palsy. *Arch Phys Med Rehabil*. 2002;83(8):1157–64.

54. Donnelly JE, Blair SN, Jakicic JM, et al. American College of Sports Medicine Position Stand. Appropriate physical activity intervention strategies for weight loss and prevention of weight regain for adults. *Med Sci Sports Exerc*. 2009;41(2):459–71.

55. Donnelly JE, Jakicic JM, Pronk NP, et al. Is resistance exercise effective for weight management? *Evid Based Prev Med*. 2004;1(1):21–9.

56. Doyle C, Kushi LH, Byers T, et al. Nutrition and physical activity during and after cancer treatment: an American Cancer Society guide for informed choices. *CA Cancer J Clin*. 2006;56(6):323–53.

57. Duncan PW, Weiner DK, Chandler J, Studenski S. Functional reach: a new clinical measure of balance. *J Gerontol*. 1990;45(6):M192–7.

58. Earhart GM. Dance as therapy for individuals with Parkinson disease. *Eur J Phys Rehabil Med*. 2009; 45(2):231–8.

59. Ervin RB. Prevalence of metabolic syndrome among adults 20 years of age and over, by sex, age, race and ethnicity, and body mass index: United States, 2003–2006. *Natl Health Stat Report*. 2009;13(13):1–7.

60. Ettinger WH,Jr, Burns R, Messier SP, et al. A randomized trial comparing aerobic exercise and resistance exercise with a health education program in older adults with knee osteoarthritis. The Fitness Arthritis and Seniors Trial (FAST). *JAMA*. 1997;277(1):25–31.

61. Evans RK, Bond DS, Wolfe LG, et al. Participation in 150 min/wk of moderate or higher intensity physical activity yields greater weight loss after gastric bypass surgery. *Surg Obes Relat Dis*. 2007; 3(5):526–30.

62. *Expert Panel Report 3 (EPR3): Guidelines for the Diagnosis and Management of Asthma* [Internet]. Bethesda (MD): National Institutes of Health; National Heart, Lung, and Blood Institute; [cited 2011 Mar 11]. Available from: http://www.nhlbi.nih.gov/guidelines/asthma/asthgdln.htm

63. Falvo MJ, Earhart GM. Six-minute walk distance in persons with Parkinson disease: a hierarchical regression model. *Arch Phys Med Rehabil*. 2009;90(6):1004–8.

64. Falvo MJ, Schilling BK, Earhart GM. Parkinson's disease and resistive exercise: rationale, review, and recommendations. *Mov Disord*. 2008;23(1):1–11.

65. Fanelli A, Cabral AL, Neder JA, Martins MA, Carvalho CR. Exercise training on disease control and quality of life in asthmatic children. *Med Sci Sports Exerc*. 2007;39(9):1474–80.

66. Fernhall B. Mental retardation. In: American College of Sports Medicine, editor. *ACSM's Exercise Management for Persons with Chronic Diseases and Disabilities*. Champaign: Human Kinetics; 1997, p. 221–226.

67. Fernhall B. Mental retardation. In: American College of Sports Medicine, editor. *ACSM's Exercise Management for Persons with Chronic Diseases and Disabilities*. 2nd ed. Champaign: Human Kinetics; 2003. p. 304–310.

68. Fernhall B. Mental retardation. In: LeMura LM, Von Duvillard SP, editors. *Clinical Exercise Physiology: Application and Physiological Principles*. Baltimore: Lippincott Williams & Wilkins; 2004. p. 304–310.

69. Fernhall B. The young athlete with a mental disability. In: Hebestreit H, Bar-Or O, IOC Medical Commission, International Federation of Sports Medicine, editors. *The Young Athlete*. Malden: Blackwell Pub; 2008. p. 403–12.

70. Fernhall B, Baynard T, Collier SR, et al. Catecholamine response to maximal exercise in persons with Down syndrome. *Am J Cardiol.* 2009;103(5):724–6.
71. Fernhall B, McCubbin JA, Pitetti KH, et al. Prediction of maximal heart rate in individuals with mental retardation. *Med Sci Sports Exerc.* 2001;33(10):1655–60.
72. Fernhall B, Pitetti KH, Vukovich MD, et al. Validation of cardiovascular fitness field tests in children with mental retardation. *Am J Ment Retard.* 1998;102(6):602–12.
73. Fernhall B, Tymeson G. Graded exercise testing of mentally retarded adults: a study of feasibility. *Arch Phys Med Rehabil.* 1987;68(6):363–5.
74. Figoni SF. Overuse shoulder problems after spinal cord injury: a conceptual model of risk and protective factors. *Clin Kinesiol.* 2009;63(2):12–22.
75. Finckh A, Iversen M, Liang MH. The exercise prescription in rheumatoid arthritis: primum non nocere. *Arthritis Rheum.* 2003;48(9):2393–5.
76. Fisher NM. Osteoarthritis, rheumatoid arthritis, and fibromyalgia. In: Myers J, Nieman DC, American College of Sports Medicine, editors. *ACSM's Resources for Clinical Exercise Physiology: Musculoskeletal, Neuromuscular, Neoplastic, Immunologic, and Hematologic Conditions.* 2nd ed. Baltimore: Lippincott Williams & Wilkins; 2010. p. 132–43.
77. Flegal KM, Carroll MD, Ogden CL, Curtin LR. Prevalence and trends in obesity among US adults, 1999–2008. *JAMA.* 2010;303(3):235–41.
78. Follett KA, Weaver FM, Stern M, et al. Pallidal versus subthalamic deep-brain stimulation for Parkinson's disease. *N Engl J Med.* 2010;362(22):2077–91.
79. Fontaine KR, Conn L, Clauw DJ. Effects of lifestyle physical activity on perceived symptoms and physical function in adults with fibromyalgia: results of a randomized trial. *Arthritis Res Ther.* 2010;12(2):R55.
80. Ford ES. Prevalence of the metabolic syndrome defined by the International Diabetes Federation among adults in the U.S. *Diabetes Care.* 2005;28(11):2745–9.
81. Ford ES, Giles WH, Mokdad AH. Increasing prevalence of the metabolic syndrome among U.S. adults. *Diabetes Care.* 2004;27(10):2444–9.
82. Fowler EG, Knutson LM, Demuth SK, et al. Pediatric endurance and limb strengthening (PEDALS) for children with cerebral palsy using stationary cycling: a randomized controlled trial. *Phys Ther.* 2010;90(3):367–81.
83. Franks PW, Olsson T. Metabolic syndrome and early death: getting to the heart of the problem. *Hypertension.* 2007;49(1):10–2.
84. Franzen E, Paquette C, Gurfinkel VS, Cordo PJ, Nutt JG, Horak FB. Reduced performance in balance, walking and turning tasks is associated with increased neck tone in Parkinson's disease. *Exp Neurol.* 2009;219(2):430–8.
85. *From Cancer Patient to Survivor: Lost in Transition* [Internet]. Washington (DC): National Academies Press; [cited 2011 Mar 11]. Available from: http://www.nap.edu/catalog.php?record_id=11468#toc
86. Gao J, Ren J, Gulve EA, Holloszy JO. Additive effect of contractions and insulin on GLUT-4 translocation into the sarcolemma. *J Appl Physiol.* 1994;77(4):1597–601.
87. Garber CE, Blissmer B, Deschenes MR, et al. American College of Sports Medicine position stand. The quantity and quality of exercise for developing and maintaining cardiorespiratory, musculo-skeletal, and neuromotor fitness in apparently healthy adults: guidance for prescribing exercise. *Med Sci Sports Exerc.* 2011;43(7):1334–559.
88. Garber CE, Friedman JH. Effects of fatigue on physical activity and function in patients with Parkinson's disease. *Neurology.* 2003;60(7):1119–24.
89. Gill TM, Williams CS, Tinetti ME. Assessing risk for the onset of functional dependence among older adults: the role of physical performance. *J Am Geriatr Soc.* 1995;43(6):603–9.
90. *GINA Report, Global Strategy for Asthma Management and Prevention Report* [Internet]. Global Initiative for Asthma; [cited 2010 Dec 22]. Available from: http://www.ginasthma.org
91. *Global Strategy for the Diagnosis, Management and Prevention of Chronic Obstructive Pulmonary Disease* [Internet]. Medical Communications Resources, Inc.; [cited 2012 Jan 7]. Available from: http://www.goldcopd.com/download.asp?intId=>554
92. Grundy SM, Cleeman JI, Merz CN, et al. Implications of recent clinical trials for the National Cholesterol Education Program Adult Treatment Panel III Guidelines. *J Am Coll Cardiol.* 2004;44(3):720–32.
93. Haapaniemi TH, Kallio MA, Korpelainen JT, et al. Levodopa, bromocriptine and selegiline modify cardiovascular responses in Parkinson's disease. *J Neurol.* 2000;247(11):868–74.
94. Hackney ME, Earhart GM. Effects of dance on gait and balance in Parkinson's disease: a comparison of partnered and nonpartnered dance movement. *Neurorehabil Neural Repair.* 2010;24(4):384–92.
95. Hackney ME, Earhart GM. Effects of dance on movement control in Parkinson's disease: a comparison of Argentine tango and American ballroom. *J Rehabil Med.* 2009;41(6):475–81.

96. Haisma JA, van der Woude LH, Stam HJ, Bergen MP, Sluis TA, Bussmann JB. Physical capacity in wheelchair-dependent persons with a spinal cord injury: a critical review of the literature. *Spinal Cord*. 2006;44(11):642–52.

97. Hampton T. Parkinson disease registry launched. *JAMA*. 2005;293(2):149.

98. Hand GA, Jaggers JR, Lyerly GW, Dudgeon WD. Physical activity for CVD prevention in patients with HIV/AIDS. *Curr Cardiovasc Risk Rep*. 2009;3(4):288–95.

99. Hand GA, Lyerly GW, Dudgeon WD. Acquired immune deficiency syndrome (AIDS). In: Durstine JL, American College of Sports Medicine, ACSM's exercise management for persons with chronic diseases and disabilities, editors. *ACSM's Exercise Management for Persons with Chronic Diseases and Disabilities*. 3rd ed. Champaign: Human Kinetics; 2009. p. 219–25.

100. Hand GA, Lyerly GW, Jaggers JR, Dudgeon WD. Impact of aerobic and resistance exercise on the health of HIV-infected persons. *Am J Lifestyle Med*. 2009;3(6):489–99.

101. Hand GA, Phillips KD, Dudgeon WD, William LG, Durstine LJ, Burgess SE. Moderate intensity exercise training reverses functional aerobic impairment in HIV-infected individuals. *AIDS Care*. 2008;20(9):1066–74.

102. Haskell WL, Lee IM, Pate RR, et al. Physical activity and public health: updated recommendation for adults from the American College of Sports Medicine and the American Heart Association. *Med Sci Sports Exerc*. 2007;39(8):1423–34.

103. Hayden MF. Mortality among people with mental retardation living in the United States: research review and policy application. *Ment Retard*. 1998;36(5):345–59.

104. Hazes JM, van den Ende CH. How vigorously should we exercise our rheumatoid arthritis patients? *Ann Rheum Dis*. 1996;55(12):861–2.

105. Headley S, Germain M, Mailloux P, et al. Resistance training improves strength and functional measures in patients with end-stage renal disease. *Am J Kidney Dis*. 2002;40(2):355–64.

106. Herman T, Giladi N, Gruendlinger L, Hausdorff JM. Six weeks of intensive treadmill training improves gait and quality of life in patients with Parkinson's disease: a pilot study. *Arch Phys Med Rehabil*. 2007;88(9):1154–8.

107. Herman T, Inbar-Borovsky N, Brozgol M, Giladi N, Hausdorff JM. The Dynamic Gait Index in healthy older adults: the role of stair climbing, fear of falling and gender. *Gait Posture*. 2009; 29(2):237–41.

108. Hoehn MM, Yahr MD. Parkinsonism: onset, progression and mortality. *Neurology*. 1967;17(5):427–42.

109. Hootman JM, Helmick CG. Projections of US prevalence of arthritis and associated activity limitations. *Arthritis Rheum*. 2006;54(1):226–9.

110. Hopman MT, Oeseburg B, Binkhorst RA. Cardiovascular responses in persons with paraplegia to prolonged arm exercise and thermal stress. *Med Sci Sports Exerc*. 1993;25(5):577–83.

111. Horowitz MB, Littenberg B, Mahler DA. Dyspnea ratings for prescribing exercise intensity in patients with COPD. *Chest*. 1996;109(5):1169–75.

112. Hurley BF, Roth SM. Strength training in the elderly: effects on risk factors for age-related diseases. *Sports Med*. 2000;30(4):249–68.

113. *The IDF Consensus Worldwide Definition of the Metabolic Syndrome. 2006* [Internet]. Brussels, Belgium: International Diabetes Federation; [cited 2008 Jul 23]. Available from: http://www.idf.org/webdata/docs/IDF_Meta_def_final.pdf

114. Jacobi D, Ciangura C, Couet C, Oppert JM. Physical activity and weight loss following bariatric surgery. *Obes Rev*. 2011;12(5):366–77

115. Jakicic JM, Clark K, Coleman E, et al. American College of Sports Medicine position stand. Appropriate intervention strategies for weight loss and prevention of weight regain for adults. *Med Sci Sports Exerc*. 2001;33(12):2145–56.

116. Jakicic JM, Winters C, Lang W, Wing RR. Effects of intermittent exercise and use of home exercise equipment on adherence, weight loss, and fitness in overweight women: a randomized trial. *JAMA*. 1999;282(16):1554–60.

117. Jan MH, Lin JJ, Liau JJ, Lin YF, Lin DH. Investigation of clinical effects of high- and low-resistance training for patients with knee osteoarthritis: a randomized controlled trial. *Phys Ther*. 2008; 88(4):427–36.

118. Jankovic J, Stacy M. Medical management of levodopa-associated motor complications in patients with Parkinson's disease. *CNS Drugs*. 2007;21(8):677–92.

119. Johansen KL. Exercise and chronic kidney disease: current recommendations. *Sports Med*. 2005; 35(6):485–99.

120. Jones KD, Burckhardt CS, Clark SR, Bennett RM, Potempa KM. A randomized controlled trial of muscle strengthening versus flexibility training in fibromyalgia. *J Rheumatol*. 2002;29(5):1041–8.

121. Jones LW, Eves ND, Peppercorn J. Pre-exercise screening and prescription guidelines for cancer patients. *Lancet Oncol*. 2010;11(10):914–6.

122. Kaminsky LA, American College of Sports Medicine. *ACSM's Resource Manual for Guidelines for Exercise Testing and Prescription.* 5th ed. Baltimore (MD): Lippincott Williams & Wilkins; 2005. 749 p.

123. Kendrick AH, Johns DP, Leeming JP. Infection control of lung function equipment: a practical approach. *Respir Med.* 2003;97(11):1163–79.

124. Kent-Braun JA, Sharma KR, Weiner MW, Miller RG. Effects of exercise on muscle activation and metabolism in multiple sclerosis. *Muscle Nerve.* 1994;17(10):1162–9.

125. Kenyon LK, Sleeper MD, Tovin MM. Sport-specific fitness testing and intervention for an adolescent with cerebral palsy: a case report. *Pediatr Phys Ther.* 2010;22(2):234–40.

126. Keus SH, Bloem BR, Hendriks EJ, Bredero-Cohen AB, Munneke M, Practice Recommendations Development Group. Evidence-based analysis of physical therapy in Parkinson's disease with recommendations for practice and research. *Mov Disord.* 2007;22(4):451–60; quiz 600.

127. Keus SHJ, Hendriks HJM, Bloem BR, et al. KNGF Guidelines for physical therapy in Parkinson's disease. *Ned Tijdschr Fysiother.* 2004;114(Suppl 3):5–86.

128. King WC, Belle SH, Eid GM, et al. Physical activity levels of patients undergoing bariatric surgery in the Longitudinal Assessment of Bariatric Surgery study. *Surg Obes Relat Dis.* 2008;4(6):721–8.

129. Kingsley JD, McMillan V, Figueroa A. The effects of 12 weeks of resistance exercise training on disease severity and autonomic modulation at rest and after acute leg resistance exercise in women with fibromyalgia. *Arch Phys Med Rehabil.* 2010;91(10):1551–7.

130. Klippel JH. *Primer on the Rheumatic Diseases.* 13th ed. New York (NY): Springer; 2008. 721 p.

131. Kloos AD, Heiss DG. Exercise for impaired balance. In: Kisner C, Colby LA, editors. *Therapeutic Exercise: Foundations and Techniques.* 5th ed. Philadelphia: F.A. Davis; 2007. p. 251–72.

132. Knowler WC, Barrett-Connor E, Fowler SE, et al. Reduction in the incidence of type 2 diabetes with lifestyle intervention or metformin. *N Engl J Med.* 2002;346(6):393–403.

133. Kohrt WM, Bloomfield SA, Little KD, Nelson ME, Yingling VR, American College of Sports Medicine. American College of Sports Medicine position stand: physical activity and bone health. *Med Sci Sports Exerc.* 2004;36(11):1985–96.

134. Krebs P. Mental retardation. In: Winnick JP, editor. *Adapted Physical Education and Sport.* Champaign: Human Kinetics; 1990. p. 153–76.

135. Kurtzke JF. Rating neurologic impairment in multiple sclerosis: an expanded disability status scale (EDSS). *Neurology.* 1983;33(11):1444.

136. Lambert CP, Archer RL, Evans WJ. Muscle strength and fatigue during isokinetic exercise in individuals with multiple sclerosis. *Med Sci Sports Exerc.* 2001;33(10):1613–9.

137. Lawrence RC, Felson DT, Helmick CG, et al. Estimates of the prevalence of arthritis and other rheumatic conditions in the United States. Part II. *Arthritis Rheum.* 2008;58(1):26–35.

138. Leger L, Boucher R. An indirect continuous running multistage field test: the Universite de Montreal track test. *Can J Appl Sport Sci.* 1980;5(2):77–84.

139. Levey AS, Tangri N, Stevens LA. Classification of chronic kidney disease: a step forward. *Ann Intern Med.* 2011;154(1):65–7.

140. Lin K, Stewart D, Cooper S, Davis CL. Pre-transplant cardiac testing for kidney-pancreas transplant candidates and association with cardiac outcomes. *Clin Transplant.* 2001;15(4):269–75.

141. Liu G, Peacock M, Eilam O, Dorulla G, Braunstein E, Johnston CC. Effect of osteoarthritis in the lumbar spine and hip on bone mineral density and diagnosis of osteoporosis in elderly men and women. *Osteoporos Int.* 1997;7(6):564–9.

142. Lockette KF, Keyes AM. *Conditioning with Physical Disabilities.* Champaign (IL): Human Kinetics; 1994. 272 p.

143. *Longitudinal Assessment of Bariatric Surgery* [Internet]. University of Pittsburgh, Epidemiology Data Center; [cited 2012 Jan 7]. Available from: http://www.edc.gsph.pitt.edu/labs/

144. Lublin FD, Reingold SC, National Multiple Sclerosis Society (USA) Advisory Committee on Clinical Trials of New Agents in Multiple Sclerosis. Defining the clinical course of multiple sclerosis: results of an international survey. *Neurology.* 1996;46(4):907–11.

145. Macfarlane DJ, Taylor LH, Cuddihy TF. Very short intermittent vs continuous bouts of activity in sedentary adults. *Prev Med.* 2006;43(4):332–6.

146. Mak MK, Pang MY. Balance confidence and functional mobility are independently associated with falls in people with Parkinson's disease. *J Neurol.* 2009;256(5):742–9.

147. Mannerkorpi K, Nordeman L, Ericsson A, Arndorw M, GAU Study Group. Pool exercise for patients with fibromyalgia or chronic widespread pain: a randomized controlled trial and subgroup analyses. *J Rehabil Med.* 2009;41(9):751–60.

148. Mathias S, Nayak US, Isaacs B. Balance in elderly patients: the "get-up and go" test. *Arch Phys Med Rehabil.* 1986;67(6):387–9.

149. Matinolli M, Korpelainen JT, Korpelainen R, Sotaniemi KA, Matinolli VM, Myllyla VV. Mobility and balance in Parkinson's disease: a population-based study. *Eur J Neurol.* 2009;16(1):105–11.

150. McNeely ML, Courneya KS. Exercise programs for cancer-related fatigue: evidence and clinical guidelines. *J Natl Compr Canc Netw.* 2010;8(8):945–53.

151. McNeely ML, Peddle C, Parliament M, Courneya KS. Cancer rehabilitation: recommendations for integrating exercise programming in the clinical practice setting. *Curr Cancer Ther Rev.* 2006; 2(4):351–60.

152. The medical and psychological concerns of cancer survivors after treatment. In: Hewitt M, Greenfield S, Stovall E, editors. *From Cancer Patient to Survivor: Lost in Transition.* Washington: National Academies Press; 2006. p. 66–186.

153. Mendes FA, Almeida FM, Cukier A, et al. Effects of aerobic training on airway inflammation in asthmatic patients. *Med Sci Sports Exerc.* 2011;43(2):197–203.

154. Mendes FA, Goncalves RC, Nunes MP, et al. Effects of aerobic training on psychosocial morbidity and symptoms in patients with asthma: a randomized clinical trial. *Chest.* 2010;138(2):331–7.

155. Messier SP. Arthritic diseases and conditions. In: Kaminsky LA, editor. *ACSM's Resource Manual for Guidelines for Exercise Testing and Prescription.* 5th ed. Baltimore: Lippincott Williams & Wilkins; 2006. p. 500–13.

156. Miller TD, Squires RW, Gau GT, Ilstrup DM, Frohnert PP, Sterioff S. Graded exercise testing and training after renal transplantation: a preliminary study. *Mayo Clin Proc.* 1987;62(9):773–7.

157. Minor MA, Kay DR. Arthritis. In: American College of Sports Medicine, editor. *ACSM's Exercise Management for Persons with Chronic Diseases and Disabilities.* 2nd ed. Champaign: Human Kinetics; 2003. p. 210–16.

158. Mockford M, Caulton JM. Systematic review of progressive strength training in children and adolescents with cerebral palsy who are ambulatory. *Pediatr Phys Ther.* 2008;20(4):318–33.

159. Morris ME. Locomotor training in people with Parkinson disease. *Phys Ther.* 2006;86(10): 1426–35.

160. Morris ME. Movement disorders in people with Parkinson disease: a model for physical therapy. *Phys Ther.* 2000;80(6):578–97.

161. Morris ME, Martin CL, Schenkman ML. Striding out with Parkinson disease: evidence-based physical therapy for gait disorders. *Phys Ther.* 2010;90(2):280–8.

162. Mostert S, Kesselring J. Effects of a short-term exercise training program on aerobic fitness, fatigue, health perception and activity level of subjects with multiple sclerosis. *Mult Scler;* 2002;8(2):161–8.

163. Munhoz RP, Li JY, Kurtinecz M, et al. Evaluation of the pull test technique in assessing postural instability in Parkinson's disease. *Neurology.* 2004;62(1):125–7.

164. National Cholesterol Education Program (NCEP) Expert Panel on Detection, Evaluation, and Treatment of High Blood Cholesterol in Adults (Adult Treatment Panel III). Third Report of the National Cholesterol Education Program (NCEP) Expert Panel on Detection, Evaluation, and Treatment of High Blood Cholesterol in Adults (Adult Treatment Panel III) final report. *Circulation.* 2002;106(25):3143–421.

165. National Coalition for Cancer Survivorship Web site [Internet]. Silver Spring (MD): National Coalition for Cancer Survivorship; [cited 2011 Feb 14]. Available from: http://www.canceradvocacy.org/about/org/history.html

166. National Kidney Foundation. K/DOQI clinical practice guidelines for chronic kidney disease: evaluation, classification, and stratification. *Am J Kidney Dis.* 2002;39(2 Suppl 1):S1–266.

167. National Multiple Sclerosis Society Web site [Internet]. New York (NY): National Multiple Sclerosis Society; [cited 2010 Oct 18]. Available from: http://www.nationalmssociety.org/index.aspx

168. National Multiple Sclerosis Society. *Clinical Study Measures: Modified Fatigue Impact Scale (MFIS)* [Internet]. New York (NY): National Multiple Sclerosis Society; [cited 2011 Feb 6]. Available from: http://www.nationalmssociety.org/for-professionals/researchers/clinical-study-measures/mfis/index .aspx

169. Needle RH, Trotter RT,2nd, Singer M, et al. Rapid assessment of the HIV/AIDS crisis in racial and ethnic minority communities: an approach for timely community interventions. *Am J Public Health.* 2003;93(6):970–9.

170. Ness KK, Wall MM, Oakes JM, Robison LL, Gurney JG. Physical performance limitations and participation restrictions among cancer survivors: a population-based study. *Ann Epidemiol.* 2006; 16(3):197–205.

171. Nici L, Donner C, Wouters E, et al. American Thoracic Society/European Respiratory Society statement on pulmonary rehabilitation. *Am J Respir Crit Care Med.* 2006;173(12):1390–413.

172. O'Donnell DE, Laveneziana P, Ora J, Webb KA, Lam YM, Ofir D. Evaluation of acute bronchodilator reversibility in patients with symptoms of GOLD stage I COPD. *Thorax.* 2009;64(3):216–23.

173. Ogden CL, Carroll MD, Curtin LR, Lamb MM, Flegal KM. Prevalence of high body mass index in US children and adolescents, 2007–2008. *JAMA.* 2010;303(3):242–9.

174. Painter PL. Exercise after renal transplantation. *Adv Ren Replace Ther.* 1999;6:159–64.

175. Painter PL. Physical functioning in end-stage renal disease patients: update 2005. *Hemodial Int.* 2005;9(3):218–35.
176. Painter PL, Hector L, Ray K, et al. A randomized trial of exercise training after renal transplantation. *Transplantation.* 2002;74(1):42–8.
177. Painter PL, Krasnoff JB. End-stage metabolic disease: renal failure and liver failure. In: Durstine JL, editor. *ACSM's Exercise Management for Persons with Chronic Diseases and Disabilities.* 2nd ed. Champaign: Human Kinetics; 2003. p. 126–32.
178. Painter P, Moore GE. The impact of recombinant human erythropoietin on exercise capacity in hemodialysis patients. *Adv Ren Replace Ther.* 1994;1(1):55–65.
179. Palisano RJ, Snider LM, Orlin MN. Recent advances in physical and occupational therapy for children with cerebral palsy. *Semin Pediatr Neurol.* 2004;11(1):66–77.
180. Pastor MA, Day BL, Marsden CD. Vestibular induced postural responses in Parkinson's disease. *Brain.* 1993;116(Pt 5):1177–90.
181. Perkins EA, Moran JA. Aging adults with intellectual disabilities. *JAMA.* 2010;304(1):91–2.
182. Perri MG, Anton SD, Durning PE, et al. Adherence to exercise prescriptions: effects of prescribing moderate versus higher levels of intensity and frequency. *Health Psychol.* 2002;21(5):452–8.
183. Pescatello LS, Franklin BA, Fagard R, et al. American College of Sports Medicine position stand. Exercise and hypertension. *Med Sci Sports Exerc.* 2004;36(3):533–53.
184. Petajan JH, Gappmaier E, White AT, Spencer MK, Mino L, Hicks RW. Impact of aerobic training on fitness and quality of life in multiple sclerosis. *Ann Neurol.* 1996;39(4):432–41.
185. Pezzoli G, Zini M. Levodopa in Parkinson's disease: from the past to the future. *Expert Opin Pharmacother.* 2010;11(4):627–35.
186. *Physical Activity Guidelines Advisory Committee Report, 2008* [Internet]. Washington (DC): U.S. Department of Health and Human Services; [cited 2011 Jan 6]. Available from: http://www.health .gov/paguidelines/Report/pdf/CommitteeReport.pdf
187. Pitetti K, Fernandez J, Lanciault M. Feasibility of an exercise program for adults with cerebral palsy a pilot study. *Adapt Phys Act Q.* 1991; 8(4):333–41.
188. Politis M, Wu K, Molloy S, G Bain P, Chaudhuri KR, Piccini P. Parkinson's disease symptoms: the patient's perspective. *Mov Disord.* 2010;25(11):1646–51.
189. Ponichtera-Mulcare JA, Glaser RM, Mathews T, Camaione D. Maximal aerobic exercise in persons with MS. *Clin Kinesiol.* 1983;46(4):12–21.
190. Ponichtera-Mulcare JA, Mathews T, Barrett PJ, Gupta SC. Changes in aerobic fitness of patients with multiple sclerosis during a 6-month training program. *Sports Med Train Rehabil.* 1997;7(3): 265–72.
191. Ponichtera-Mulcare JA, Mathews T, Glaser RM, Mathrews T, Gupta SC. Maximal aerobic exercise of individuals with MS using three modes of ergometry. *Clin Kinesiol.* 1995;49:4–13.
192. Protas EJ, Stanley RK. Parkinson's disease. In: Myers J, Herbert WG, Humphrey RH, editors. *ACSM's Resources for Clinical Exercise Physiology: Musculoskeletal, Neuromuscular, Neoplastic, Immunologic, and Hematologic Conditions.* Baltimore: Lippincott Williams & Wilkins; 2002. p. 38–47.
193. Protas EJ, Stanley RK. Parkinson's disease. In: Myers J, Nieman DC, American College of Sports Medicine, editors. *ACSM's Resources for Clinical Exercise Physiology: Musculoskeletal, Neuromuscular, Neoplastic, Immunologic, and Hematologic Conditions.* 2nd ed. Baltimore: Lippincott Williams & Wilkins; 2010. p. 44–57.
194. Protas EJ, Stanley RK, Jankovic J. Parkinson's disease. In: American College of Sports Medicine, editor. *ACSM's Exercise Management for Persons with Chronic Diseases and Disabilities.* Champaign: Human Kinetics; 1997. p. 212–18.
195. Ram FS, Robinson SM, Black PN, Picot J. Physical training for asthma. *Cochrane Database Syst Rev.* 2005;(4):CD001116.
196. Ram FS, Wellington SR, Barnes NC. Inspiratory muscle training for asthma. *Cochrane Database Syst Rev.* 2003;(4):CD003792.
197. Reid S, Hamer P, Alderson J, Lloyd D. Neuromuscular adaptations to eccentric strength training in children and adolescents with cerebral palsy. *Dev Med Child Neurol.* 2010;52(4):358–63.
198. Rezak M. Current pharmacotherapeutic treatment options in Parkinson's disease. *Dis Mon.* 2007; 53(4):214–22.
199. Rice CL, Vollmer TL, Bigland-Ritchie B. Neuromuscular responses of patients with multiple sclerosis. *Muscle Nerve.* 1992;15(10):1123–32.
200. Richmond J, Hunter D, Irrgang J, et al. American Academy of Orthopaedic Surgeons clinical practice guideline on the treatment of osteoarthritis (OA) of the knee. *J Bone Joint Surg Am.* 2010;92(4): 990–3.
201. Ries AL, Bauldoff GS, Carlin BW, et al. Pulmonary Rehabilitation: Joint ACCP/AACVPR Evidence-Based Clinical Practice Guidelines. *Chest.* 2007;131(5 Suppl):4S–42S.

202. Rikli RE, Jones CJ. *Senior Fitness Test Manual*. Champaign (IL): Human Kinetics; 2001. 161 p.
203. Rimaud D, Calmels P, Devillard X. Training programs in spinal cord injury. *Ann Readapt Med Phys*. 2005;48(5):259–69.
204. Rimmer JH. Physical fitness levels of persons with cerebral palsy. *Dev Med Child Neurol*. 2001; 43(3):208–12.
205. Ritter PL, Gonzalez VM, Laurent DD, Lorig KR. Measurement of pain using the visual numeric scale. *J Rheumatol*. 2006;33(3):574–80.
206. Robertson MC, Campbell AJ, Gardner MM, Devlin N. Preventing injuries in older people by preventing falls: a meta-analysis of individual-level data. *J Am Geriatr Soc*. 2002;50(5):905–11.
207. Robertson RJ, Goss FL, Dube J, et al. Validation of the adult OMNI scale of perceived exertion for cycle ergometer exercise. *Med Sci Sports Exerc*. 2004;36(1):102–8.
208. Roddy E, Zhang W, Doherty M. Aerobic walking or strengthening exercise for osteoarthritis of the knee? A systematic review. *Ann Rheum Dis*. 2005;64(4):544–8.
209. Rogers A, Furler BL, Brinks S, Darrah J. A systematic review of the effectiveness of aerobic exercise interventions for children with cerebral palsy: an AACPDM evidence report. *Dev Med Child Neurol*. 2008;50(11):808–14.
210. Roizen NJ, Patterson D. Down's syndrome. *Lancet*. 2003;361(9365):1281–9.
211. Rooks DS. Fibromyalgia treatment update. *Curr Opin Rheumatol*. 2007;19(2):111–7.
212. Rooks DS. Talking to patients with fibromyalgia about physical activity and exercise. *Curr Opin Rheumatol*. 2008;20(2):208–12.
213. Rooks DS, Silverman CB, Kantrowitz FG. The effects of progressive strength training and aerobic exercise on muscle strength and cardiovascular fitness in women with fibromyalgia: a pilot study. *Arthritis Rheum*. 2002;47(1):22–8.
214. Rosendorff C, Black HR, Cannon CP, et al. Treatment of hypertension in the prevention and management of ischemic heart disease: a scientific statement from the American Heart Association Council for High Blood Pressure Research and the Councils on Clinical Cardiology and Epidemiology and Prevention. *Circulation*. 2007;115(21):2761–88.
215. Ryuzaki M, Konishi K, Kasuga A, et al. Spontaneous rupture of the quadriceps tendon in patients on maintenance hemodialysis—report of three cases with clinicopathological observations. *Clin Nephrol*. 1989;32(3):144–8.
216. Saris WH, Blair SN, van Baak MA, et al. How much physical activity is enough to prevent unhealthy weight gain? Outcome of the IASO 1st Stock Conference and consensus statement. *Obes Rev*. 2003;4(2):101–14.
217. Scandalis TA, Bosak A, Berliner JC, Helman LL, Wells MR. Resistance training and gait function in patients with Parkinson's disease. *Am J Phys Med Rehabil*. 2001;80(1):38–43; quiz 44–6.
218. Schenkman M, Cutson TM, Kuchibhatla M, et al. Exercise to improve spinal flexibility and function for people with Parkinson's disease: a randomized, controlled trial. *J Am Geriatr Soc*. 1998; 46(10):1207–16.
219. Schenkman M, Hall D, Kumar R, Kohrt WM. Endurance exercise training to improve economy of movement of people with Parkinson disease: three case reports. *Phys Ther*. 2008;88(1):63–76.
220. Schmid A, Schmidt-Trucksass A, Huonker M, et al. Catecholamines response of high performance wheelchair athletes at rest and during exercise with autonomic dysreflexia. *Int J Sports Med*. 2001;22(1):2–7.
221. Schmitz KH, Courneya KS, Matthews C, et al. American College of Sports Medicine roundtable on exercise guidelines for cancer survivors. *Med Sci Sports Exerc*. 2010;42(7):1409–26.
222. Schneider CM, Dennehy CA, Roozeboom M, Carter SD. A model program: exercise intervention for cancer rehabilitation. *Integr Cancer Ther*. 2002;1(1):76–82; discussion 82.
223. Scholtes VA, Becher JG, Comuth A, Dekkers H, Van Dijk L, Dallmeijer AJ. Effectiveness of functional progressive resistance exercise strength training on muscle strength and mobility in children with cerebral palsy: a randomized controlled trial. *Dev Med Child Neurol*. 2010;52(6):e107–13.
224. *The Seventh Report of the Joint National Committee on Prevention, Detection, Evaluation, and Treatment of High Blood Pressure* [Internet]: Bethesda (MD): U.S. Department of Health and Human Services, National High Blood Pressure Education Program; 2004 [cited 2012 Jan 7]. Available from: http://www.ncbi.nlm.nih.gov.ezproxy.lib.uconn.edu/books/bv.fcgi?rid=hbp7.TOC
225. Shapiro R. *Managing the Symptoms of Multiple Sclerosis*. 4th ed. New York (NY): Demos Medical Publishers; 2003. 192 p.
226. Sharoff CG, Hagobian TA, Malin SK, et al. Combining short-term metformin treatment and one bout of exercise does not increase insulin action in insulin-resistant individuals. *Am J Physiol Endocrinol Metab*. 2010;298(4):E815–23.
227. Sharples L, Hughes V, Crean A, et al. Cost-effectiveness of functional cardiac testing in the diagnosis and management of coronary artery disease: a randomised controlled trial. The CECaT trial. *Health Technol Assess*. 2007;11(49):iii–iv, ix–115.

228. Shrier I. Flexibility versus stretching. *Br J Sports Med*. 2001;35(5):364.
229. Sidney S, Lewis CE, Hill JO, et al. Association of total and central adiposity measures with fasting insulin in a biracial population of young adults with normal glucose tolerance: the CARDIA study. *Obes Res*. 1999;7(3):265–72.
230. Sigal RJ, Kenny GP, Wasserman DH, Castaneda-Sceppa C, White RD. Physical activity/exercise and type 2 diabetes: a consensus statement from the American Diabetes Association. *Diabetes Care*. 2006;29(6):1433–8.
231. Silsupadol P, Shumway-Cook A, Lugade V, et al. Effects of single-task versus dual-task training on balance performance in older adults: a double-blind, randomized controlled trial. *Arch Phys Med Rehabil*. 2009;90(3):381–7.
232. Skeletal muscle dysfunction in chronic obstructive pulmonary disease. A statement of the American Thoracic Society and European Respiratory Society. *Am J Respir Crit Care Med*. 1999; 159(4 Pt 2):S1–40.
233. Smithson F, Morris ME, Iansek R. Performance on clinical tests of balance in Parkinson's disease. *Phys Ther*. 1998;78(6):577–92.
234. Stacy M. Medical treatment of Parkinson disease. *Neurol Clin*. 2009;27(3):605–31, v.
235. Steadward R. Musculoskeletal and neurological disabilities: implications for fitness appraisal, programming, and counselling. *Can J Appl Physiol*. 1998;23(2):131–65.
236. Sterman AB, Coyle PK, Panasci DJ, Grimson R. Disseminated abnormalities of cardiovascular autonomic functions in multiple sclerosis. *Neurology*. 1985;35(11):1665.
237. Stoessl AJ. Continuous dopaminergic therapy in Parkinson disease: time to stride back? *Ann Neurol*. 2010;68(1):3–5.
238. Stone PC, Minton O. Cancer-related fatigue. *Eur J Cancer*. 2008;44(8):1097–104.
239. Svien LR, Berg P, Stephenson C. Issues in aging with cerebral palsy. *Top Geriatr Rehabil*. 2008; 24(1):26–40.
240. Teo-Koh SM, McCubbin JA. Relationship between peak VO$_2$ and 1-mile walk test performance of adolescent males with mental retardation. *Pediatr Exerc Sci*. 1999;11(2):144–57.
241. Thomas TR, Warner SO, Dellsperger KC, et al. Exercise and the metabolic syndrome with weight regain. *J Appl Physiol*. 2010;109(1):3–10.
242. Tomas-Carus P, Gusi N, Hakkinen A, Hakkinen K, Raimundo A, Ortega-Alonso A. Improvements of muscle strength predicted benefits in HRQOL and postural balance in women with fibromyalgia: an 8-month randomized controlled trial. *Rheumatology (Oxford)*. 2009;48(9):1147–51.
243. Tresierras MA, Balady GJ. Resistance training in the treatment of diabetes and obesity: mechanisms and outcomes. *J Cardiopulm Rehabil Prev*. 2009;29(2):67–75.
244. Troosters T, Casaburi R, Gosselink R, Decramer M. Pulmonary rehabilitation in chronic obstructive pulmonary disease. *Am J Respir Crit Care Med*. 2005;172(1):19–38.
245. Tsai AG, Williamson DF, Glick HA. Direct medical cost of overweight and obesity in the USA: a quantitative systematic review. *Obes Rev*. 2011;12(1):50–61.
246. Turner S, Eastwood P, Cook A, Jenkins S. Improvements in symptoms and quality of life following exercise training in older adults with moderate/severe persistent asthma. *Respiration*. 2011; 81(4):302–10.
247. Twelves D, Perkins KS, Counsell C. Systematic review of incidence studies of Parkinson's disease. *Mov Disord*. 2003;18(1):19–31.
248. Unnithan VB, Clifford C, Bar-Or O. Evaluation by exercise testing of the child with cerebral palsy. *Sports Med*. 1998;26(4):239–51.
249. U.S. Department of Health and Human Services. *2008 Physical Activity Guidelines for Americans* [Internet]. Washington (DC): U.S. Department of Health and Human Services; 2008 [cited 2011 Jan 6] 78 p. Available from: http://www.health.gov/paguidelines/pdf/paguide.pdf
250. U.S. Department of Health and Human Services. *Physical Activity and Health: A Report of the Surgeon General*. Atlanta, GA: U.S. Department of Health and Human Services, Public Health Service, Centers for Disease Control and Prevention, National Center for Chronic Disease Prevention and Health Promotion; 1996. 278 p. Available from: U.S. GPO, Washington.
251. U.S. Department of Health and Human Services, United States Department of Agriculture, United States Dietary Guidelines Advisory Committee. *Dietary Guidelines for Americans, 2005*. 6th ed. Washington (DC): G.P.O; 2005. 71 p.
252. U.S. Preventive Services Task Force. Screening for coronary heart disease: recommendation statement. *Ann Intern Med*. 2004;140(7):569–72.
253. U.S. Public Health Service, Office of the Surgeon General. *Bone Health and Osteoporosis: A Report of the Surgeon General*. Rockville (MD): U.S. Department of Health and Human Services, Public Health Service, Office of the Surgeon General; 2004. 404 p.
254. *U.S. Renal Data System. USRDS 2009 Annual Data Report: Atlas of Chronic Kidney Disease and End-Stage Renal Disease in the United States* [Internet]. Bethesda (MD): National Institutes of Health,

National Institute of Diabetes and Digestive and Kidney Diseases; [cited 2012 Jun 9]. Available from: http://www.usrds.org/atlas09.aspx

255. van den Ende CH, Hazes JM, le Cessie S, et al. Comparison of high and low intensity training in well controlled rheumatoid arthritis. Results of a randomised clinical trial. *Ann Rheum Dis.* 1996;55(11):798–805.

256. van Drongelen S, van der Woude LH, Janssen TW, Angenot EL, Chadwick EK, Veeger DH. Glenohumeral contact forces and muscle forces evaluated in wheelchair-related activities of daily living in able-bodied subjects versus subjects with paraplegia and tetraplegia. *Arch Phys Med Rehabil.* 2005;86(7):1434–40.

257. Vanlandewijck Y, Theisen D, Daly D. Wheelchair propulsion biomechanics: implications for wheelchair sports. *Sports Med.* 2001;31(5):339–67.

258. Verschuren O, Takken T. Aerobic capacity in children and adolescents with cerebral palsy. *Res Dev Disabil.* 2010;31(6):1352–7.

259. Vinik A, Erbas T. Neuropathy. In: Ruderman N, editor. *Handbook of Exercise in Diabetes.* 2nd ed. Alexandria: American Diabetes Association; 2002. p. 463–496.

260. Violan MA, Pomes T, Maldonado S, et al. Exercise capacity in hemodialysis and renal transplant patients. *Transplant Proc.* 2002;34(1):417–8.

261. Vogiatzis I, Nanas S, Roussos C. Interval training as an alternative modality to continuous exercise in patients with COPD. *Eur Respir J.* 2002;20(1):12–9.

262. Wackers FJ, Young LH, Inzucchi SE, et al. Detection of silent myocardial ischemia in asymptomatic diabetic subjects: the DIAD study. *Diabetes Care.* 2004;27(8):1954–61.

263. Walensky RP, Paltiel AD, Losina E, et al. The survival benefits of AIDS treatment in the United States. *J Infect Dis.* 2006;194(1):11–9.

264. Wang JS, Hung WP. The effects of a swimming intervention for children with asthma. *Respirology.* 2009;14(6):838–42.

265. Wang C, Schmid CH, Rones R, et al. A randomized trial of tai chi for fibromyalgia. *N Engl J Med.* 2010;363(8):743–54.

266. Weaver FM, Follett K, Stern M, et al. Bilateral deep brain stimulation vs best medical therapy for patients with advanced Parkinson disease: a randomized controlled trial. *JAMA.* 2009;301(1):63–73.

267. Werner WG, DiFrancisco-Donoghue J, Lamberg EM. Cardiovascular response to treadmill testing in Parkinson disease. *J Neurol Phys Ther.* 2006;30(2):68–73.

268. White LJ, McCoy SC, Castellano V, et al. Resistance training improves strength and functional capacity in persons with multiple sclerosis. *Mult Scler.* 2004;10(6):668–74.

269. Wiart L, Darrah J, Kembhavi G. Stretching with children with cerebral palsy: what do we know and where are we going? *Pediatr Phys Ther.* 2008;20(2):173–8.

270. Wing RR. Behavioral weight control. In: Wadden TA, editor. *Handbook of Obesity Treatment.* New York: Guilford Press; 2002. p. 301–16.

271. Wolfe F, Clauw DJ, Fitzcharles MA, et al. The American College of Rheumatology preliminary diagnostic criteria for fibromyalgia and measurement of symptom severity. *Arthritis Care Res (Hoboken).* 2010;62(5):600–10.

272. Yarasheski KE, Roubenoff R. Exercise treatment for HIV-associated metabolic and anthropomorphic complications. *Exerc Sport Sci Rev.* 2001;29(4):170–4.

273. Young LH, Wackers FJ, Chyun DA, et al. Cardiac outcomes after screening for asymptomatic coronary artery disease in patients with type 2 diabetes: the DIAD study: a randomized controlled trial. *JAMA.* 2009;301(15):1547–55.

274. Zhang W, Nuki G, Moskowitz RW, et al. OARSI recommendations for the management of hip and knee osteoarthritis: part III: changes in evidence following systematic cumulative update of research published through January 2009. *Osteoarthritis Cartilage.* 2010;18(4):476–99.

11

Behavioral Theories and Strategies for Promoting Exercise

The purpose of this chapter is to provide health/fitness, public health, clinical exercise, and health care professionals a basic understanding of how to assist individuals to adopt and adhere to the exercise prescription (Ex R_x) recommendations that are made in the *Guidelines*. *Chapter 1* of the *Guidelines* focuses on the public health recommendations for a physically active lifestyle, yet most of the public remains unaware of these recommendations (10). Furthermore, (a) most adults in the United States do not engage in these recommended amounts of physical activity (53); (b) even for individuals who choose to enroll in an exercise program, greater than 50% will drop out within the first 6 mo (25); and (c) simply providing knowledge and promoting awareness of Ex R_x recommendations may be insufficient to produce behavior change (44). These significant obstacles highlight the need for health/fitness, public health, clinical exercise, and health care professionals to better understand behavior adoption and maintenance strategies for a physically active lifestyle.

Research has identified basic determinants and barriers to engaging in regular physical activity. Numerous demographic factors (*e.g.*, age, gender, socioeconomic status, education, ethnicity) are consistently related to the likelihood that an individual will exercise on a regular basis (53). These factors are not amenable to intervention, although they do suggest who might benefit most from the exercise intervention. This chapter will focus on (a) the role that modifiable factors such as attitudes toward exercise have on the Ex R_x; and (b) basic concepts of the behavioral theories, applications, and strategies that enhance physical activity adoption and maintenance.

EXERCISE PRESCRIPTION

Given the flexibility in the Frequency, Intensity, Time, and Type (*FITT*) principle of Ex R_x for the targeted population, it is important to first understand what impact variations in the Ex R_x might have on adoption or maintenance of a habitually active lifestyle.

FREQUENCY/TIME

Ex R_x recommendations allow for flexibility in the different combinations of frequency and/or time/duration to achieve them. A commonly held belief was that flexibility in terms of the time/duration and exercise volume recommended would allow individuals to overcome the most frequently reported barrier to regular exercise, that is, lack of time (63). However, the lack of any real change in physical activity levels in the United States from 1998–2008 suggests otherwise (13). A review of randomized trials showed that there is no difference in exercise adherence when different combinations of frequency and time are used to achieve the same total volume of physical activity (75). These results should be viewed with caution, however, because the included studies were randomized trials that *assigned* participants to different combinations. Allowing individuals to *self-select* frequency and time may influence adherence to exercise interventions.

INTENSITY

Research on the effects of exercise intensity on adherence suggests that individuals are more likely to adhere to lower intensity programs (29,65). However, a recent review suggests the inverse relationship between intensity and adherence is not particularly strong, and it is possible that such an effect is moderated by prior exercise behavior (75). There is evidence that individuals with more exercise experience fare better with higher intensity programs (65%–75% heart rate reserve [HRR]), whereas those adopting exercise for the first time may be better suited to, and self-select, moderate intensity programs (45%–55% HRR) (6).

TYPE

Although it is recommended that individuals participate in a variety of exercise types (*i.e.*, aerobic, resistance, neuromotor, and flexibility) (3), there have been few systematic tests of the effects of different exercise modalities on adoption and maintenance. Most of the research that has examined adherence has investigated aerobic activity, often with a focus on walking (75). Little is known about the characteristics of those that adopt and maintain resistance training and flexibility-exercise programs. The best data come from mixed modality programs in older adult and middle-aged populations (10,21), which suggest no differences in adherence by exercise type.

Lifestyle approaches to physical activity that commonly have individuals exercising on their own at home have supported greater adherence to home-based programs compared to structured, supervised programs (47,66). However, several studies failed to find beneficial effects of home-based programs on adherence and retention when reinforcers/rewards were used in the supervised programs (see *Box 11.1*) (5,20).

THEORETICAL FOUNDATIONS FOR UNDERSTANDING EXERCISE BEHAVIOR

Theories provide a framework for understanding why individuals want to be physically active and what things may prevent them from being physically

BOX 11.1	FITT Principle of Ex R$_x$ Effects on Adherence

The evidence for the impact of effective FITT effects on adherence is essentially equivocal, with only limited evidence that higher intensity programs may reduce adherence among novice exercisers. However, these results can be viewed positively, as health/fitness, public health, clinical exercise, and health care professionals can take advantage of the flexibility of the current guidelines to develop an Ex R$_x$ geared toward an individual's preferences and goals without undue concern for creating adherence issues. Measures of individual exercise preference and tolerance (31) could be useful for helping identify what level of physical activity is appropriate to prescribe for different individuals.

Ex R$_x$, exercise prescription; FITT, Frequency, Intensity, Time, and Type of exercise.

active. Using appropriate theories can guide health/fitness, public health, clinical exercise, and health care professionals in determining appropriate strategies to assist individuals to adopt and maintain regular physical activity (79). *Table 11.1* outlines common challenges (12,58) that individuals face in both adoption and maintenance that can be better understood and addressed through the application of different behavioral theories. The purpose is not to critique each theory but to provide an understanding of the theories, which will suggest behavior change principles and strategies that can be used to enhance exercise adoption and maintenance.

SOCIAL COGNITIVE THEORY AND SELF-EFFICACY

Social cognitive theory (SCT) is a comprehensive theoretical framework that has been extensively employed in understanding, describing, and changing exercise behavior. SCT is based on the principle of triadic reciprocation; that is, the individual (*e.g.*, emotion, personality, cognition, biology), behavior (*i.e.*, past and current achievement), and environment (*i.e.*, physical, social, and cultural) all interact to influence future behavior (9). It is important to recognize that these are dynamic factors that influence each other differently over time. For example, an individual who begins an exercise program may feel a sense of accomplishment, which makes them exercise even more that then leads them to make their environment more conducive to exercising (*e.g.*, buying home exercise equipment). Conversely, another individual may start an exercise program, work too hard and feel fatigued, lose motivation, and move their exercise equipment to the basement to make their environment less conducive to exercising.

Central to SCT is the concept of *self-efficacy*, which refers to one's beliefs in their capability to successfully complete a course of action such as exercise (9). There are two salient types of self-efficacy when considering exercise behavior

TABLE 11.1. Most Common Exercise Barriers (12), Relevant Theories, and Potential Strategies

Common Problem	Percent Endorsing Barrier	Applicable Theories	Example Strategies
"I don't have enough time"	69%	SCT, TPB, SET	• Discuss modifications to FITT principles • Examine priorities/goals • Brief counseling/motivational interviewing
"I don't have enough energy"	59%	SCT, HBM, SET, TPB	• Discuss modifications to FITT principles • Brief counseling/motivational interviewing • Discuss affect regulation techniques for setting exercise intensity
"I'm just not motivated"	52%	SCT, HBM, TPB, TTM, SET, SDT	• Discuss attitudes and outcome expectations • Determine stage of change and provide stage-tailored counseling • Examine perceived susceptibility and severity • Discuss potentially effective reinforcements
"It costs too much"	37%	HBM, TTM, SET	• Examine exercise alternatives to meet goals • Evaluate exercise opportunities in the environment
"I'm sick or hurt"	36%	TTM	• Discuss maintenance/relapse prevention • Discuss alternative exercises to keep progressing toward goals
"There's nowhere for me to exercise"	30%	SET	• Evaluate exercise opportunities in the environment • Discuss different types of activities for which there are resources
"I feel awkward when I exercise"	29%	SCT, TPB	• Examine self-efficacy • Examine alternative settings • Use strategies such as association/dissociation
"I don't know how to do it"	29%	SCT, HBM, TTM, TPB	• Build task self-efficacy using appropriate strategies
"I might get hurt"	26%	SCT, HBM, TPB	• Evaluate exercise prescription • Determine task-specific self-efficacy
"It's not safe"	24%	SCT, SET	• Evaluate exercise opportunities in the environment
"No one will watch my child if I exercised"	23%	SCT, SET	• Develop social support structures • Examine opportunities for exercise in which childcare may be provided
"There is no one to exercise with me"	21%	SCT, TPB, TTM	• Develop social support and exercise buddy system • Identify different types of activities one can do on your own

FITT, Frequency, Intensity, Time, and Type of exercise; HBM, health belief model; SCT, social cognitive theory; SDT, self-determination theory; SET, social ecological theory; TPB, theory of planned behavior; TTM, transtheoretical model.

(see *Box 11.2*) (54). *Task self-efficacy* refers to an individuals' belief they can actually do the behavior in question, whereas *barriers self-efficacy* refers to whether an individual believes they can regularly exercise in the face of common barriers such as lack of time, poor weather, and feeling tired. The higher the sense of efficacy, the greater the effort, persistence, and resilience an individual will exhibit. Self-efficacy also influences thought patterns and emotional reactions (54). Individuals with low self-efficacy believe things are more difficult

BOX 11.2	Types of Self-Efficacy

Exercise task self-efficacy: Belief in capability to physically complete the task. The measure must be specific to the task — for instance walking, running, weight training.

- Measured by asking the confidence of an individual to engage in incrementally challenging activities (*e.g.*, confidence to walk continuously at a brisk pace for 15 min, 30 min, 45 min)

Exercise barriers self-efficacy: Belief in the capability to exercise regularly in the face of common barriers.

- Measured by asking the confidence of an individual to do a set amount of exercise when faced with common barriers (*e.g.*, time, weather, fatigue)

Practically, when working with individuals, it is important first to establish a high level of task self-efficacy. Unless an individual feels physically able to exercise for at least 30 min, it is not important whether or not they perceive any barriers.

For more information including complete measures and appropriate citations, see Exercise Psychology Lab Measures at http://www.epl.illinois.edu/measures.html.

than they are; a belief that may lead to anxiety, stress, and depression. Individuals high in self-efficacy are optimistic and believe they can overcome challenges.

Outcome expectations, another key concept of SCT, are anticipatory results of a behavior (99). If specific outcomes are valued, then behavior change is more likely to occur (96). For example, if increased muscle strength and size are valued outcomes, then it is more likely that the individual will adhere to a resistance training program, as opposed to a program to increase cardiorespiratory fitness.

Both self-efficacy and positive outcome expectations are necessary for an individual to adopt and maintain a program of regular physical activity; that is, they must feel both confident that they will be able to do the physical activity (*i.e.*, physically capable and capable of overcoming any obstacles/barriers) and feel that the behavior will lead to a valued outcome (9). If a woman believes that engaging in resistance training will result in "bulking up," she may avoid such a program; therefore, a first step would be education to change those outcome expectations. Likewise, an older adult who does not believe she or he can "lift weights" would not even consider enrolling in a program that included resistance training. This individual would have to work on increasing their confidence in their capability to perform resistance training.

Although SCT contains numerous other constructs, such as modeling, the research has consistently focused on self-efficacy and outcome expectations. SCT has successfully been applied in interventions across multiple groups and ages (54,76,95).

TRANSTHEORETICAL MODEL

The Transtheoretical Model (TTM) was developed as a framework for understanding behavior change and is arguably the most popular approach for promoting exercise behavior (71). The popularity of the use of stages of change from the TTM stems from the intuitive appeal that individuals are at different stages of readiness to make behavioral changes, and thus require tailored interventions. The TTM includes five stages of change: (a) precontemplation (*i.e.*, no intention to be regularly active in the next 6 mo); (b) contemplation (*i.e.*, intending to be regularly active in the next 6 mo); (c) preparation (intending to be regularly active in the next 30 d); (d) action (regularly active for <6 mo); and finally (e) maintenance (regularly active for ≥6 mo) (73). As individuals attempt to change their behavior, they may move linearly through these stages, but the TTM allows for the possibility of repeated relapse and successful change after several unsuccessful attempts.

Associated with the five stages of change are the constructs of processes of change, decisional balance, and self-efficacy. The 10 processes of change illustrate the strategies used by individuals in attempting to advance through the five stages of change. The 10 processes can be divided into two second order factors: (a) experiential (*i.e.*, consciousness raising, dramatic relief, self-reevaluation, social reevaluation, and social liberation); and (b) behavioral (*i.e.*, self-liberation, counterconditioning, stimulus control, contingency management, and helping relationship). There are specific processes of change and patterns in decisional balance and self-efficacy that have been shown to be most useful to facilitate progression through each of the stages of change for exercise (27,59) (see *Figure 11.1*).

Decisional balance is an assessment of the relative weighting of the pros and cons of changing exercise behavior. The strong and weak principle suggests that individuals need to increase their pros of exercising twice as much as they decrease the cons of exercising as they progress through the stages (70). Practically, this means that if an individual can only think of a few reasons to exercise, she or he may view the time required for exercise as a major barrier; however, if that same individual can endorse 10 or 15 reasons to exercise, then time may be less of a barrier. Finally, the TTM includes the construct of confidence/self-efficacy that increases across the five stages of change (27).

The TTM highlights different approaches to exercise adoption and maintenance that need to be taken with different individuals. For example, when someone is in an earlier stage of change you are trying to encourage them to consider making an effort to start exercising. Therefore, giving them a trial gym membership might be inappropriate. Rather, the focus should be on educating them on the benefits of exercise and perhaps how they might reduce the perceived cons by realizing they can get benefits from accumulated bouts of moderate intensity, physical activity. However, the trial membership may very well be a great tool for someone in the preparation stage who is ready to start exercising. There is solid evidence that stage-based interventions have been effective in helping individuals make progress toward becoming regularly active. These interventions have been used across various groups and populations (41,87).

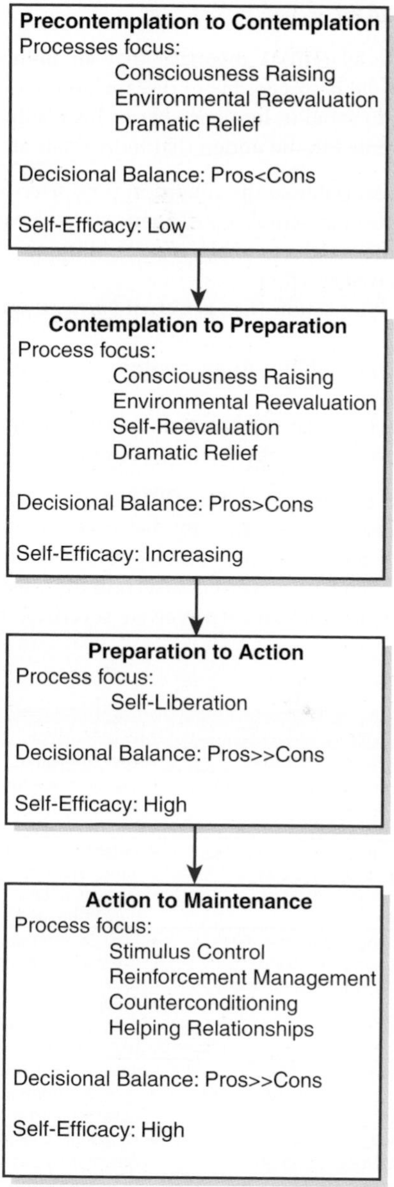

Precontemplation to Contemplation
Processes focus:
    Consciousness Raising
    Environmental Reevaluation
    Dramatic Relief

Decisional Balance: Pros<Cons

Self-Efficacy: Low

Contemplation to Preparation
Process focus:
    Consciousness Raising
    Environmental Reevaluation
    Self-Reevaluation
    Dramatic Relief

Decisional Balance: Pros>Cons

Self-Efficacy: Increasing

Preparation to Action
Process focus:
    Self-Liberation

Decisional Balance: Pros>>Cons

Self-Efficacy: High

Action to Maintenance
Process focus:
    Stimulus Control
    Reinforcement Management
    Counterconditioning
    Helping Relationships

Decisional Balance: Pros>>Cons

Self-Efficacy: High

■ **FIGURE 11.1.** Key Processes and Relationships to Progress through the Stages of Change (27,59).

HEALTH BELIEF MODEL

The Health Belief Model (HBM) theorizes that an individual's beliefs about whether or not she or he is susceptible to disease, and her or his perceptions of the benefits of trying to avoid it, influence her or his readiness to act (78).

The theory is grounded in the notion that individuals are ready to act if they:

- Believe they are susceptible to the condition (*i.e.*, *perceived susceptibility*).
- Believe the condition has serious consequences (*i.e.*, *perceived severity*).
- Believe taking action reduces their susceptibility to the condition or its severity (*i.e.*, *perceived benefits*).
- Believe costs of taking action (*i.e.*, *perceived barriers*) are outweighed by the benefits.
- Are confident in their ability to successfully perform an action (*i.e.*, *self-efficacy*).
- Are exposed to factors that prompt action (*e.g.*, seeing their weight on the scale, a reminder from one's physician to exercise) (*i.e.*, *cues to action*).

Together, the six constructs of the HBM suggest strategies for motivating individuals to change their exercise behavior because of health issues (see *Table 11.2*). For example, an individual would need to feel that they are at risk of having a heart attack (perceived susceptibility), feel that a heart attack would negatively impact their life (perceived severity), believe that starting

TABLE 11.2. Health Belief Model Constructs and Strategies (78)		
Construct	**Exercise-Specific Definition**	**Change Strategy**
Perceived susceptibility	Beliefs about the chances of getting a disease/condition if do not exercise	• Explain risk information based on current activity, family history, other behaviors, etc.
Perceived severity	Beliefs about the seriousness/consequences of disease/condition as a result of inactivity	• Refer individual to medically valid information about disease • Discuss different treatment options, outcomes, and costs
Perceived benefits	Beliefs about the effectiveness of exercising to reduce susceptibility and/or severity	• Provide information on benefits of exercise to preventing/treating condition or disease • Provide information regarding all of the other potential benefits of exercise (*e.g.*, quality of life, mental health)
Perceived barriers	Beliefs about the direct and indirect costs associated with exercise	• Discuss FITT options to minimize burden • Provide information on different low cost activity choices
Cues to action	Factors that activate the change process and get someone to start exercising	• Help individual look for potential cues • Ask them what it would take for them to get started
Self-efficacy	Confidence in ability to exercise	• Assess level of confidence for different types of activity • Use self-efficacy building techniques to enhance exercise confidence

FITT, *F*requency, *I*ntensity, *T*ime, and *T*ype of exercise.

an exercise program would reduce their risk (perceived benefits), feel that the amount of reduction in risk is worth the time and energy they would have to commit to exercise (perceived benefits outweigh perceived barriers), and believe they could exercise on a regular basis (self-efficacy). However, those factors alone are not enough for them to start exercising, they also need some type of prompt (e.g., a friend/relative having a heart attack) to actually begin to exercise (cue to action). Therefore, there is a need to prime individuals to be ready to change and also help devise ways to prompt them into taking action.

Given its obvious focus on health issues for understanding motivation, the HBM may be most suitable for understanding and intervening with populations that are motivated to be physically active primarily for health (36). Thus, the HBM has been applied to cardiac rehabilitation and diabetes mellitus prevention and management (56,86).

SELF-DETERMINATION THEORY

A theory that recently has received an increasing amount of attention related to exercise is the self-determination theory (SDT) (22). The underlying assumption of the SDT is individuals have three primary psychosocial needs that they are trying to satisfy: (a) self-determination or autonomy; (b) demonstration of competence or mastery; and (c) relatedness or ability to experience meaningful social interactions with others. The theory proposes motivation exists on a continuum from amotivation to intrinsic motivation, with amotivation having the lowest levels of self-determination and intrinsic motivation having the highest degree of self-determination. Individuals with amotivation have no desire to engage in exercise, whereas individuals high in intrinsic motivation are interested in engaging in physical activity for the satisfaction, challenge, or pleasure that comes from it. Between amotivation and intrinsic motivation is extrinsic motivation, that is, when individuals engage in a physical activity for reasons that are external to the individual, such as being physically active to make yourself more attractive to other individuals. Those with the highest degree of self-determination have greater intentions to exercise, self-efficacy to overcome barriers to exercise, and physical self-worth (90).

The SDT suggests that the use of rewards to get individuals to start exercising may have limited effectiveness because they promote extrinsic motivation. Rather, programs should be designed to enhance autonomy by promoting choice and incorporating simple, easy exercises initially to enhance feelings of competence and enjoyment. Initial evidence supports interventions focusing on development and promotion of autonomy are effective at enhancing physical activity levels (15,84).

THEORY OF PLANNED BEHAVIOR

The theory of planned behavior (TPB) postulates intention to perform a behavior is the primary determinant of behavior (2). Intentions reflect an individual's probability that she or he will exercise. Unfortunately, intentions do not always

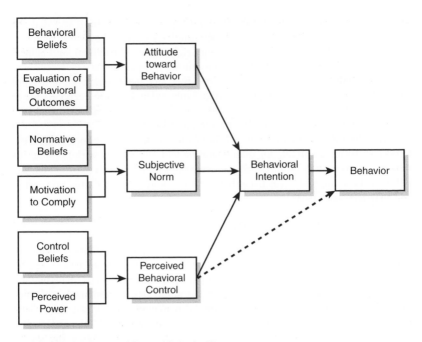

■ **FIGURE 11-2.** Theory of Planned Behavior (2).

translate directly into behavior because of issues related to behavioral control (19). Intentions are determined by an individual's attitudes, subjective norms, and perceived behavioral control. Attitudes are theorized to reflect the affective and evaluative component of the TPB, and therefore, measure an individual's feelings about exercising. Subjective norms are the social component and are measured as the function of an individual's beliefs that others want them to exercise and their motivation to comply with the desires of significant others. *Perceived behavioral control* is defined as the individual's belief about how easy or difficult performance of the behavior is likely to be. Thus, an individual intends to be physically active if they believe exercise would be beneficial, feel good, be valued by individual's opinions that they value, and is within their control (see *Figure 11.2*).

Intentions are the primary predictor of behavior, but there is also a hypothesized direct link (dashed line in *Figure 11.2*) between perceived behavioral control and behavior. This link is proposed to be significant only when perceived control reflects actual control of a nonvolitional behavior. For example, an individual perceives low control over her or his exercise behavior when the weather is poor. That individual may have high overall intentions to exercise, but when rain threatens, the perception of control is directly relevant to the actual situation and the individual may not exercise. There is clear evidence of the ability of the

TPB to predict exercise intentions and behavior (11), and limited evidence that interventions based on the TPB are effective at increasing physical activity levels (45), although one large study found an intensive intervention to be no more effective than brief advice (48).

The formation of implementation intentions may enhance the link between exercise intentions and behavior. Implementation intentions reflect an individual's specific plans to exercise such as where they will exercise, when they will exercise, and with whom they will exercise. They are analogous to the setting of specific strategies that will be discussed in the goal setting process. Evidence has supported that the addition of implementation intentions improves exercise behavior outcomes beyond standard motivational interventions (7,22).

SOCIAL ECOLOGICAL

Social ecological models are important because they consider the impact of and connections between individuals and their environments. The explicit recognition of relations between an individual and their physical environment is a defining feature of ecological models (81). The foundation of this work is that multiple levels of factors influence health behaviors including intrapersonal factors, social environment factors, physical environments, and policies (see *Table 11.3*). For example, aspects of the natural environment can impact exercise behaviors (*e.g.*, weather, geography) but so too can aspects of the built environment (*e.g.*, access to parks). Importantly, environmental factors influence behavior not only directly but also indirectly through an individual's perceptions. This type of approach highlights the fact that multilevel interventions may be most effective or even necessary (81). Targeting aspects of the individual are important, but if a physical environment is not conducive to changing one's lifestyle, then the exercise intervention will not be successful. For example, telling an individual to walk around the block three times per week may be ineffective if the individual feels their neighborhood is unsafe. Alternatively, changing the physical environment (*e.g.*, adding walking trails) without considering individual exerciser characteristics (*e.g.*, an older adult with little/no mobility) will not induce behavior change.

THEORETICAL STRATEGIES AND APPROACHES TO CHANGE BEHAVIOR/INCREASE ADHERENCE

Individualized, theory-based, tailored behavioral programs enhance the adoption and maintenance of exercise (44). Behavioral programs should be tailored to the individual's motivations and circumstances and typically include different strategies to enhance theoretical constructs (44). There are also strategies that are suggested by several theories such as building self-efficacy, brief counseling techniques, stage counseling, group leader strategies, goal setting, use of reinforcements, social support, relapse prevention, affect regulation, and associative/dissociative strategies that are discussed in the sections that follow, and may enhance adoption and maintenance of regular exercise.

TABLE 11.3. Levels of Social Ecological Model and Potential Exercise Intervention Strategies

Social Ecological Level	Components	Potential Change Strategies
Intrapersonal	• Knowledge, attitudes, behaviors, beliefs, perceived barriers, motivation, enjoyment • Skills and self-efficacy • Demographics (age, sex, education, and socioeconomic and employment status)	• Focus on changing individuals knowledge, skills, attitudes • Use theories and approaches such as the transtheoretical model, theory of planned behavior, and self-determination theory
Social environment	• Family, spouse, or partner • Peers • Schools, workplaces, and community organizations • Access to social support • Influence of health professionals • Community norms • Cultural background	• Use community education, support groups, and peer programs • Implement workplace incentives • Social marketing campaigns may promote positive community attitudes and awareness to participation in physical activity
Physical environment	• Natural factors such as weather or geography • Availability and access to exercise facilities • Aesthetics or perceived qualities of facilities or the natural environment • Safety such as crime rates and traffic • Community design • Public transportation options	• Creation of walking trails or parks • Implement changes to the physical environment first if possible. For example, encouraging individuals to walk will be ineffective in communities where there are no or poorly maintained walking paths or where safety is an issue.
Policy	• Urban planning policies • Education policies such as physical education classes • Health policies • Environmental policies • Workplace policies	• Align physical activity participation with priorities such as reducing reliance on fossil fuels and the reduction of greenhouse gas emissions • Emphasize importance of regular physical education • Require workplaces to provide support for exercise

BUILDING SELF-EFFICACY

Self-efficacy is a central component of most of the theories previously discussed (*i.e.*, SCT, TTM, HBM, and TPB). Individuals draw upon sources of efficacy information to increase exercise behavior. Strategies to increase self-efficacy include experiencing successful completion of tasks (*i.e.*, mastery experiences/performance accomplishments), hearing and seeing others' experiences and successful application of strategies (*i.e.*, modeling/vicarious experiences), social persuasion (*i.e.*, having other individuals tell you that you can do the behavior), and reduction of stress and physical/emotional arousal. *Table 11.4* outlines several strategies that can be used to enhance an individual's sense of self-efficacy in both individual and group settings.

TABLE 11.4. Individual and Group Strategies for Enhancing Self-Efficacy

Source of Self-Efficacy Information	Individual Setting	Group Setting
Mastery experiences/ performance accomplishments	• Use moderately difficult tasks • Use exercise logs to track progress • Allow input into exercise programs	• Use cooperative activities so everyone gets involved as is vital to success • Track and monitor individuals within the group
Social modeling/ vicarious experiences	• Demonstrate all skills and tasks • Use videos to model behaviors • Discuss "success" stories of individuals with similar backgrounds and characteristics	• Attend a fitness facility with individuals like yourself (*e.g.*, all women's fitness club) • Have appropriate group exercise leaders that individuals can identify with
Social persuasion	• Give frequent feedback (*e.g.*, encouragement, compliments) • Make feedback contingent on performance	• Use buddy groups to encourage participation and adherence • Use appropriate frequent verbal and nonverbal feedback and encouragement
Reduction of stress and physical/ emotional arousal	• Provide education about the effects of exercise on the body to alleviate misinterpretation of physiologic cues • Make a point to discuss how exercise makes the individual feel	• Choose a comfortable setting to minimize stress from outside observers • Allow some self-pacing in activity so everyone can be challenged without creating excessive anxiety and arousal

BRIEF COUNSELING AND MOTIVATIONAL INTERVIEWING

A promising area for increasing exercise adoption is through the use of brief counseling, often conducted by health care professionals (57,100). These brief counseling approaches can be based upon any of the theories previously discussed. Numerous medical associations have adopted the position that primary care providers should make physical activity counseling a part of every routine patient visit (42). However, effective counseling programs need to incorporate more than simply asking about physical activity levels and advising the patient to increase their behavior by incorporating established counseling strategies and techniques. See *Box 11.3* for some examples of effective counseling strategies to increase physical activity levels (68).

Motivational interviewing is a technique that has gained support as a brief intervention technique that has been successfully used to promote engagement in physical activity (43,64). Motivational interviewing varies from traditional counseling approaches by being client/patient centered so rather than pushing individuals toward a change, the client/patient and counselor work and pull together to achieve the client's/patient's desired outcome (55). *Table 11.5* highlights some of the differences between traditional counseling and a motivational interviewing approach. Motivational interviewing does not espouse a particular theory but can be adapted and used in combination with existing theories to help motivate change and confidence among individuals who are seeking to adopt or maintain an Ex R$_x$.

BOX 11.3	Client-Centered Physical Activity Counseling (Five-A's Model)

ADDRESS AGENDA
- Attend to client's agenda (*e.g.*, "Why did you come to see me today?").
- Express desire to talk about a health behavior (*e.g.*, "I'd like to talk with you about your physical activity.").

ASSESS
- Readiness for change (*e.g.*, "Have you considered changing your exercise habits?").
- Knowledge of risks/problems (*e.g.*, "Do you think there are any risks of exercise?").
- History of risk-related symptoms/illnesses (*e.g.*, "You are concerned about getting too tired if you exercise. Has fatigue been a problem for you?").
- Fears/concerns (*e.g.*, "Do you have any concerns about increasing your physical activity?").
- Feelings about the health behavior (*e.g.*, "How do you feel about exercising more?").
- History of addressing health behavior (*e.g.*, "Have you ever tried to exercise in the past?").
- History of problems during previous attempts to change (*e.g.*, "Tell me about what happened when you were exercising previously. Did you have any problems?").
- History of problems that may interfere with change (*e.g.*, "Is there any reason why you can't begin to exercise now?").
- Reasons for wanting to change behavior (*e.g.*, "Why do you want to start exercising?").
- Reasons for maintaining risk behavior (*e.g.*, "Why do you want to keep things as they are and not exercise?").

ADVISE
- Tell client you strongly advise behavioral change (*e.g.*, "As your exercise professional, I'd strongly recommend that you begin a program of exercise to improve your health.").
- Personalize risk (*e.g.*, "You are worried about having a heart attack. Remaining inactive doubles your risk of having a heart attack.").
- Personalize immediate and long-term benefits of change (*e.g.*, "Exercise will help you to control your high blood pressure and greatly reduce your risk of developing heart disease.").

ASSIST
- Use verbal and nonverbal relationship/facilitation skills (*i.e.*, Use open-ended questions. Avoid prescriptive statements such as "You should . . ." "Make direct eye contact; lean toward the client, etc.").

BOX 11.3	Client-Centered Physical Activity Counseling (Five-A's Model) (*Continued*)

ASSIST (*Continued*)

- Correct misunderstandings; provide information (*e.g.*, "You want to lose 10 lb [4.5 kg] in 6 wk by exercising more. That is not a realistic or healthy goal. Exercise will help you over the long term to maintain a weight loss, but it will have only a small effect, if any, in the short term.").
- Address feelings/provide support (*e.g.*, "I understand you are nervous about starting to exercise. It is hard to get started, but I am confident you can do it.").
- Address barriers to change (*e.g.*, "You mentioned that you have a tight schedule. Let's look at your schedule to see if we can identify some time when you can fit in a short walk.").
- Identify potential resources and support (*e.g.*, "Is your spouse interested in exercising with you? Is there a gym or park near your home?").
- Describe options available for change (*e.g.*, "Based on what you have told me, it seems your choices are to join an exercise class at the Y or to begin walking during your lunch break.").
- Negotiate selection among options (*e.g.*, "Which of these options do you think would be best for you?").
- Provide resources/materials (*e.g.*, "Here is a tip sheet with some simple steps to help you with your walking program.").
- Teach skills/recommend behavior strategies (*e.g.*, "It is hard to begin an exercise program. One thing that can help is to put exercise on your calendar and treat it as an appointment.").
- Refer, when appropriate (*e.g.*, "I think you would enjoy going to a yoga class at _____.").
- Consider a written contract (*e.g.*, "Many individuals find a written contract to be helpful in staying on track with their exercise plans. Is it OK with you if we try that?").
- Identify barriers and solve problems (*e.g.*, "Individuals usually run into challenges that make it hard to exercise. What do you think may be a problem for you? Let's think about strategies to overcome these challenges.").
- Encourage use of supports, coping strategies (*e.g.*, "Bad weather often makes it difficult to walk outside. Can you think of an alternate place to walk? How about another kind of exercise for bad weather days?").

ARRANGE FOLLOW-UP

- Reaffirm plan (*e.g.*, "Now let's be sure we both understand our plan. You plan to visit three gyms near your house to check out the facilities and exercise classes. Is that correct?").
- Schedule follow-up appointment or phone call (*e.g.*, "Let's check in with each other in 2 wk to see how things are going. Can you give me a call in 2 wk?").

Adapted with permission from (69).

TABLE 11.5. Principles of Motivational Interviewing Compared to Advice Giving

	Motivational Interviewing	Advice Giving
Counseling aim	Explore why the individual isn't sure they want to exercise and build their motivation to want to change	Persuade the individual that they need to change and start exercising by providing a specific FITT Ex R_x
Client	Individual who needs help exploring why they are inactive and how and why they might begin exercising; use empathy	Someone who has an increased susceptibility to disease (*e.g.,* diabetes mellitus, CVD) because they are inactive
Information presentation	Neutrally explain discrepancies between current activity and recommended levels and allow client to react	Give the evidence for why being inactive increases their risk for disease and how the Ex R_x will work
Questioning approach	Open-ended questioning to encourage exploration of thoughts and feelings regarding exercise	Leading questions to have them "prove" to themselves the risks of their inactivity and why they should be active
Dealing with resistance	Use reflection to try to acknowledge their point and move on to other areas quickly	Have counterarguments ready and "correct" any misconceptions
Summarizing	Use their language to summarize both the pros and cons of exercising	Summarize the dangers of staying inactive and steps they should take to be active

CVD, cardiovascular disease; Ex R_x, exercise prescription; FITT, *F*requency, *I*ntensity, *T*ime, and *T*ype of exercise.

STAGE OF CHANGE TAILORED COUNSELING

The TTM is predicated on the notion of stages of change, but the key to progressing through the model is the appropriate use of stage specific strategies and the processes of change to help individuals advance that result in "tailoring" interventions. A typical strategy for individuals in the earlier stages is to have her or him do a decisional balance exercise in which they list the pros and cons of exercising, and then are challenged to try and add pros and brainstorm ways to eliminate the cons (or barriers) to exercising (38). *Box 11.4* discusses examples of how one might use specific strategies within each stage to tailor the intervention to an individual in order to help them progress to the next stage. Intervention studies have consistently supported that stage-tailored interventions that include all of the components of the TTM are appropriate for a greater range of the population and are effective at enhancing physical activity levels (41,87).

GROUP LEADER INTERACTIONS

Exercise leaders have an influence on physical activity participation and the psychological benefits that occur as a result of physical activity (32). The exercise leader and group play significant roles in SCT and SDT. An exercise leader with a socially supportive leadership style is one that provides encouragement, verbal reinforcement, praise, and interest in the participant (34). Participants who have an exercise leader that has a socially supportive leadership style report greater

BOX 11.4	Example Strategies to Facilitate Stage Transitions

PRECONTEMPLATION → CONTEMPLATION
- Emphasize the benefits of regular exercise by not focusing on what might happen if they stay inactive but what will happen if they become active
- Discuss how some of the barriers they perceive may be misconceived such as it can be done in shorter and accumulated bouts if they don't have the time
- Have them visualize what they would feel like if they would exercise with an emphasis on short-term, easily achievable benefits of activity such as sleeping better, reducing stress, and having more energy
- Discuss how their inactivity impacts individuals other than themselves such as their spouse and children

CONTEMPLATION → PREPARATION
- Explore potential solutions to their exercise barriers
- Assess level of self-efficacy and begin techniques to build efficacy
- Discuss potential activities that they might be able to do
- Emphasize the importance of even small steps in progressing toward being regularly active

PREPARATION → ACTION
- Help develop an appropriate plan of activity to meet their exercise goals and use a goal setting worksheet to make it a formal commitment
- Use reinforcement to reward steps toward being active
- Teach self-monitoring techniques such as tracking time and distance
- Continue discussion of how to overcome any obstacles they feel are in their way of being active
- Encourage them to help create an environment that helps remind them to be active

ACTION → MAINTENANCE
- Provide positive and contingent feedback on goal progress
- Explore different types of activities they can do to avoid burnout
- Encourage them to work with and even help others become more active
- Discuss relapse prevention strategies
- Discuss potential rewards that can be used to maintain motivation

self-efficacy, more energy, more enjoyment, stronger intentions to exercise, less fatigue, and less concern about embarrassment (37). In addition to the exercise leader, aspects of the exercise group may also influence physical activity participation. One such aspect is that of group cohesion, that is, a dynamic process reflected in the tendency of a group to stick together and remain united in the pursuit of its instrumental objectives and/or satisfaction of member affective needs. Five principles have been successfully used to improve cohesion and lower dropout rates among exercise groups (14,33):

- Distinctiveness, that is, creating a group identity (*e.g.*, group name).
- Positions, that is, giving members of the class responsibilities and roles for the group.
- Group norms, that is, adopt common goals for the group to achieve.
- Sacrifice, that is, individuals in the group may have to give up something for the greater good of the group.
- Interaction and communication, that is, the belief that the more social interactions that are made possible for the group, the greater the cohesion.

COGNITIVE-BEHAVIORAL APPROACHES

Cognitive-behavioral approaches encompass techniques such as behavioral contracting, goal setting, self-monitoring, and reinforcement, which are used to impact constructs in nearly all of the theories previously discussed. Rooted in cognitive behavior therapy, these approaches involve relatively simple techniques for promoting physical activity. Cognitive-behavioral approaches are often integrated with other theories as techniques for promoting behavior changes such as several of the 10 processes of change in the TTM or the sources of self-efficacy in SCT (9). Despite their relatively low complexity, cognitive-behavioral interventions are among the most effective at increasing physical activity levels (26). For example, simply placing signs that encourage individuals to use the stairs instead of the elevator, having individuals create and sign exercise "contracts," and using rewards can be effective short-term strategies to increase physical activity (26,44).

Reinforcement

The use and type of reinforcements individuals receive are important for understanding motivation in SCT and SDT. In stimulus response theory (85), positive reinforcement is believed to be one way to increase a desired behavior such as physical activity. Positive reinforcement can be in several forms. In physical activity programs, there are several extrinsic reinforcers that are often used and are successful in increasing short-term adherence including social reinforcers (*e.g.*, praise), material reinforcers (*e.g.*, T-shirts), activity reinforcers (*e.g.*, playing a game), and special outings (*e.g.*, throwing a party) (60). However, individuals are more likely to adhere to exercise over the long term if they are doing the activity for intrinsic reasons such as for fun, enjoyment, and challenge (80). It may be difficult to give intrinsic reinforcers to participants, but it may be possible to develop an environment that can promote intrinsic motivation. These environments focus on the autonomy of the participant and have been shown to lead to higher levels of physical activity (15). Environments promoting intrinsic motivation focus on (a) providing positive feedback to help the participant increase feelings of competence; (b) acknowledging participant difficulties within the program; and (c) enhancing sense of choice and self-initiation of activities to build feelings of autonomy.

Goal Setting

Goal setting is a powerful tool for behavior change that cuts across numerous theories but must be done as part of an ongoing process to be effective. It requires the client/patient and the health/fitness, public health, clinical exercise, and health care professional to work together to develop, implement, measure, and revise the client's/patient's goals on a consistent basis to provide direction to their efforts, enhance persistence, and learn new strategies (52). *Box 11.5* outlines principles for effective goal setting and provides a sample goal setting sheet. The goal setting sheet allows individuals to describe specific strategies for achieving their goal (*e.g.*, implementation intentions) and has places for the goal setter and a witness to sign because sharing goals and making them public

---

BOX 11.5   SMARTS Principles in Goal Setting (61)

Specific. Goals need to be precise.

Measurable. Goals should be quantifiable rather than subjective.

Action-oriented. Goals should indicate what needs to be done.

Realistic. Goals should be achievable.

Timely. Goals should have some reasonable time constraint.

Self-determined. Goals should be developed primarily by the client/individual.

EXAMPLE OF A GOAL SETTING SHEET

Goal Sheet

Today's Date: _____   Target Goal Date: _____

Goal: _____

Specific Strategies to Achieve Goal:

1)

2)

3)

Signed
Goal setter: _____   Witness: _____

can enhance their effectiveness (52). Finally, it is important for individuals to set both short- and long-term goals that allow for measurement and assessment on a regular basis. In this way, new strategies can be developed if insufficient progress is being made, and goals can be altered if they are not realistic or are too easy (52). Setting proper goals and monitoring them is an important part of numerous physical activity studies and is increasingly popular as technology (e.g., pedometers) makes monitoring goals easier (92). However, because goal setting is incorporated in many theories and interventions, there is limited evidence on its sole contribution to changing exercise behavior (82,83).

SOCIAL SUPPORT

Social support is a powerful motivator to exercise for many individuals and important in SCT, TTM, and TPB; and can come from an instructor, family members, workout partners, coworkers, or neighbors, as well as from health/fitness, public health, clinical exercise, and health care professionals. Social support can be provided to clients/patients in various ways including (a) guidance (i.e., advice and information); (b) reliable alliance (i.e., assurance that others can be counted on in times of stress); (c) reassurance of worth (i.e., recognition of one's competence that individuals in the exercise group or personal trainer believe in their abilities); (d) attachment (i.e., emotional closeness with the personal trainer or at least one other individual in the exercise group); (e) social integration (i.e., a sense of belonging and feeling comfortable in group exercise situations); and (f) opportunity for nurturance (i.e., providing assistance to others in the exercise group) (94).

Providing social support in the form of guidance is most common when working with clients/patients. The basis of working with individuals for behavior change is providing them with information and advice. Individuals beginning an exercise program also need to feel their health/fitness, public health, clinical exercise or health care professional, or fellow exercisers will support them in times of stress or times when continuing to exercise is difficult (32–34). Moreover, individuals beginning an exercise program may have feelings of incompetence. Increasing their confidence through mastery experiences, social modeling, and providing praise are practical ways to increase acknowledgment of one's competence (9).

Implementing ways to increase an individual's attachment and feelings of being part of a group is also important. The exerciser needs to feel comfortable. A method to make exercisers feel comfortable is to establish buddy groups. In group settings, exercisers can benefit from watching others complete their exercise routines, and from instructors and fellow exercisers giving input on proper technique and execution. Creating supportive exercise groups within communities has been linked with greater levels of exercise behavior (44).

ASSOCIATION VERSUS DISASSOCIATION

A long-held belief is that feelings of fatigue and negative affect often accompany the initiation of physical activity programs and can act as a deterrent to continued participation (74). Therefore, any strategies that can be adapted to change these negative feelings may improve exercise adherence. As a result, many have advocated for novice exercisers to engage in cognitive-strategy techniques that decrease discomfort or improve positive affect (51,74). For example, exercisers can engage in dissociation strategies that encourage the individual to block out feelings associated with exertion such as fatigue, sweating, or discomfort, usually by focusing on positive thoughts and enjoyment. In contrast are association strategies where the exerciser focuses on bodily sensations such as respiration, temperature, and fatigue. At light-to-moderate intensities of exercise (*i.e.*, below ventilatory threshold), disassociation techniques may be beneficial to reducing perceptions of effort and increasing affect. However, at higher intensities (*i.e.*, above ventilatory threshold), physiologic cues likely dominate, and therefore disassociation strategies are less effective as individuals cannot "block out" the physiologic stimuli (51). Association techniques may be helpful for the individuals to regulate exercise intensity to avoid potential injury or overexertion. Therefore, both association and disassociation strategies may be important for health/fitness and clinical exercise professionals to understand and use. They also have been shown to have some use in enhancing feelings associated with exercise and increasing exercise behavior (51).

AFFECT REGULATION

Individuals are often advised to pick an exercise activity they enjoy (91). The inherent belief is that individuals are more likely to adopt and maintain a behavior they enjoy (93). Affect regulation is a key component to establishing intrinsic motivation in SDT (49). Positive affective responses to moderate intensity exercise (*i.e.*, 65% of maximal heart rate [HR_{max}]) can be predictive of physical activity participation 6 and 12 mo later (97). This finding is consistent with a body of research repeatedly demonstrating that affective responses are more negative when exercise intensity is greater than ventilatory threshold (39). As a result, it has been proposed that self-ratings of affective valence and ratings of pleasantness/unpleasantness of an experience can be used to as a marker of the transition from aerobic to anaerobic metabolism and may be useful for Ex R_x (31). Specifically, exercisers can use feelings of increasing displeasure to be a sign exercise intensity may be too high, and they should decrease exercise intensity to reduce these feelings. Rose et al. (77) recently examined whether or not ratings of affective valence could be used to regulate exercise intensity. Sedentary women were asked to exercise at a rating of 1 on the feeling scale (40) equivalent to "fairly good" or a rating of 3 equivalent to "good." The exercise intensities were lowest at the "good" level of affect (*i.e.*, 64% HR_{max}) and highest at the "fairly good" rating (*i.e.*, 68% HR_{max}). These intensities are appropriate for achieving health/fitness benefits and suggest that affect may be a useful tool in prescribing exercise intensity.

RELAPSE PREVENTION

All individuals will eventually struggle to meet their exercise goals (72). Therefore, it is an important part of many theories and approaches to develop strategies for helping individuals to overcome setbacks and maintain their physical activity levels (88). Relapse prevention is not the domain of any one theoretical approach but can be implemented across all approaches once individuals adopt and try to maintain exercise (89). Relapse prevention strategies include having individuals brainstorm ways and create plans to stay active when they are outside of their traditional routine (*e.g.*, on vacation, inclement weather), varying their exercise routines to avoid boredom and creating new exercise goals to enhance and maintain motivation. It is also important for individuals not to get discouraged when they miss a session of planned activity. Exercisers need to maintain a high sense of self-efficacy through encouragement and social support that can be accomplished by offering praise when individuals come back after missing a class or session and even reaching out with a phone call when someone has missed a class or two. There is evidence to support relapse prevention as an effective strategy to enhance the maintenance of exercise behavior (35).

SPECIAL POPULATIONS

An important area of exercise promotion is the proper tailoring of interventions to promote exercise behavior across diverse populations that present unique challenges. Proper tailoring requires an understanding of potential unique beliefs, values, environments, and obstacles within a population or individual. Although every individual is clearly unique, the following sections discuss typical issues of some of the more common special groups with whom health/fitness and clinical exercise professionals may work.

CULTURAL DIVERSITY

In order to provide culturally competent care, health/fitness, public health, clinical exercise, and health care professionals' knowledge of cultural beliefs, values, and practices is necessary. Without this knowledge, errors in the FITT Ex R_x recommendations and progression of clients/patients can occur (23). For example, the higher levels of physical inactivity among African Americans compared to other racial/ethnic groups may be caused not only by environmental constraints but also by cultural beliefs (62). A focus group study examining urban African Americans' perceptions of exercise found study participants believed resting during leisure time was as important as exercising (1). These same participants were less likely to recognize exercise as a possible treatment for hypertension. In fact, they were more likely to view physical activity as a cause of high blood pressure.

Perhaps, the most important characteristic of exercise interventions that target different racial/ethnic groups is being culturally sensitive and tailored. One common, erroneous assumption individuals make when culturally tailoring approaches is they only need to translate the materials used in an intervention, such as brochures or public service announcements, into another language (62). Such superficial tailoring is not adequate. There should be an in-depth knowledge and understanding of the population that can be best achieved through meaningful involvement of community members and through research conducted by representatives of the culture. This in-depth understanding of the target population can lead to better, more appropriate recommendations.

For example, in Latino cultures, the family unit is very important. Thus, recommendations for increasing physical activity might incorporate methods to get all family members exercising together (*e.g.*, taking walks with the whole family).

OLDER ADULTS

There are several challenges when working with promoting the adoption and adherence of exercise among older adults (see *Chapter 8*) (4,21). Older adults often lack knowledge about the benefits of physical activity or how to set up a personal physical activity program so that health/fitness and clinical exercise professionals need to provide some initial education (98). Although typically viewed as beneficial, social support is not necessarily positive, especially in older adults (16). Family and friends may exert negative influences by telling them to "take it easy" and "let me do it." The implicit message is they are too old or frail to be physically active (16).

Many of the typical barriers to physical activity are similar among younger and older adults such as lack of time and motivation (21,58); however, there are several barriers that may take on special significance among older adults. These barriers include lack of social support and increased social isolation (21,58). An older adult may rely on another individual for transportation to a physical activity facility. Quite possibly, the largest barrier to exercise participation in older adults is the fear that exercise will cause injury, pain, and discomfort or exacerbate existing conditions (58). These can be very significant and often realistic fears that require careful consideration. When older adults have responsibilities such as being a caregiver, they may be operating with limited energy resources and feel that exercising will simply make them too tired to perform other daily activities (46).

CHILDREN

When working with children (see *Chapter 8*), it is important to recognize they are likely engaging in an exercise program because their parents wish them to, implying an extrinsic motivation, and typically require tangible forms of social support (*e.g.*, transportation, payment of fees) (58). However, to help them maintain exercise behavior over their lifetime, children need help shifting toward a sense of autonomy (90). Therefore, it is important they feel a sense of self-efficacy and behavioral control. It is imperative to work toward establishing a sense of autonomy and intrinsic motivation through the creation of a supportive environment as discussed previously (15).

INDIVIDUALS WITH OBESITY

Excess weight-related concerns are a primary reason why many individuals adopt an exercise program (28). Individuals with obesity may have had negative mastery experiences with exercise in the past and will need to enhance their self-efficacy so that they will believe they can successfully exercise (8,18). They may also be quite deconditioned and perceive even moderate intensity exercise as challenging so that keeping activities fun and at a low enough intensity that they feel positive may be particularly important (30). Health/fitness, public health, clinical exercise, and health care professionals often try to shift motivations toward health, but goals must remain self-determined. Individuals with obesity may need help setting realistic weight loss goals and identifying appropriate levels of physical activity to help them reach those goals (24).

INDIVIDUALS WITH CHRONIC DISEASES AND HEALTH CONDITIONS

A concern when working with individuals with chronic diseases and health conditions (see *Chapters 8–10*) is their ability to do the exercise both from a task self-efficacy perspective as well as in the face of the barriers presented by their condition (*e.g.*, fatigue) (58). Special consideration should be given to ensure activities are chosen to prevent, treat, or control the disease or health condition. Specific behavioral strategies and concerns are often included for a variety of chronic disease and conditions in *Chapter 10* of the *Guidelines* and in the American College of Sports Medicine positions stands (17,50,67).

THE BOTTOM LINE

- Nearly all individuals will struggle with exercise adoption and maintenance, and the health/fitness and clinical exercise professional must be ready to address the common barriers.
- Practitioners can be flexible in modifying the FITT Ex R_x principles to meet client/patient preferences.
- Several behavioral theories can be used to understand and then begin to change exercise behavior including the HBM, SDT, SCT, social ecological model, TPB, and TTM of behavior change.
- There are a variety of different strategies with which health/fitness, public health, clinical exercise, and health care professionals need to be acquainted to optimize client/patient adoption and maintenance.
- Health/fitness, public health, clinical exercise, and health care professionals must be able to adapt approaches to meet the unique needs, concerns, and abilities of their clients/patients.

Online Resources

National Physical Activity Plan:
http://www.physicalactivityplan.org/

The Community Guide to Promoting Physical Activity:
http://www.thecommunityguide.org/pa/index.html

Theory at a Glance:
http://www.cancer.gov/PDF/481f5d53-63df-41bc-bfaf-5aa48ee1da4d/TAAG3.pdf

Transtheoretical Model Overview:
http://www.uri.edu/research/cprc/transtheoretical_model.html

REFERENCES

1. Airhihenbuwa CO, Kumanyika S, Agurs TD, Lowe A. Perceptions and beliefs about exercise, rest, and health among African-Americans. *Am J Health Promot.* 1995;9(6):426–9.
2. Ajzen I. From intentions to actions: a theory of planned behavior. In: Kuhl J, Beckman J, editors. *Action-Control: From Cognition to Behavior.* Heidelberg: Springer; 1985. p. 11–39.
3. American College of Sports Medicine. *ACSM's Resources for Clinical Exercise Physiology: Musculoskeletal, Neuromuscular, Neoplastic, Immunologic, and Hematologic Conditions.* 3rd ed. Baltimore (MD): Lippincott Williams & Wilkins; 2013. 323 p.
4. American College of Sports Medicine, Chodzko-Zajko WJ, Proctor DN, et al. American College of Sports Medicine position stand. Exercise and physical activity for older adults. *Med Sci Sports Exerc.* 2009;41(7):1510–30.
5. Andersen RE, Wadden TA, Bartlett SJ, Zemel B, Verde TJ, Franckowiak SC. Effects of lifestyle activity vs structured aerobic exercise in obese women: a randomized trial. *JAMA.* 1999;281(4):335–40.
6. Anton SD, Perri MG, Riley J,III, et al. Differential predictors of adherence in exercise programs with moderate versus higher levels of intensity and frequency. *J Sport Exercise Psychol.* 2005;27:171–87.
7. Armitage CJ, Sprigg CA. The roles of behavioral and implementation intentions in changing physical activity in young children with low socioeconomic status. *J Sport Exerc Psychol.* 2010;32(3):359–76.
8. Baba R, Iwao N, Koketsu M, Nagashima M, Inasaka H. Risk of obesity enhanced by poor physical activity in high school students. *Pediatr Int.* 2006;48(3):268–73.
9. Bandura A. *Self-Efficacy: The Exercise of Control.* New York (NY): Freeman; 1997. 604 p.
10. Bennett GG, Wolin KY, Puleo EM, Masse LC, Atienza AA. Awareness of national physical activity recommendations for health promotion among US adults. *Med Sci Sports Exerc.* 2009;41(10):1849–55.
11. Blue CL. The predictive capacity of the theory of reasoned action and the theory of planned behavior in exercise research: an integrated literature review. *Res Nurs Health.* 1995;18(2):105–21.
12. Canadian Fitness and Lifestyle Research Institute. *Progress in Prevention* [Internet]. Ottawa (Ontario): Canadian Fitness and Lifestyle Research Institute; [cited 2011 Mar 10]. Available from: http://www.cflri.ca/eng/progress_in_prevention/index.php
13. Carlson SA, Fulton JE, Schoenborn CA, Loustalot F. Trend and prevalence estimates based on the 2008 Physical Activity Guidelines for Americans. *Am J Prev Med.* 2010;39(4):305–13.
14. Carron AV, Spink KS. Team building in an exercise setting. *Sport Psychol.* 1993;7(1):8–18.
15. Chatzisarantis NL, Hagger MS. Effects of an intervention based on self-determination theory on self-reported leisure-time physical activity participation. *Psychol Health.* 2009;24(1):29–48.
16. Chogahara M. A multidimensional scale for assessing positive and negative social influences on physical activity in older adults. *J Gerontol B Psychol Sci Soc Sci.* 1999;54(6):S356–67.
17. Colberg SR, Sigal RJ, Fernhall B, et al. Exercise and type 2 diabetes: the American College of Sports Medicine and the American Diabetes Association: joint position statement. *Diabetes Care.* 2010;33(12):e147–67.
18. Conn VS, Minor MA, Burks KJ. Sedentary older women's limited experience with exercise. *J Community Health Nurs.* 2003;20(4):197–208.
19. Cooke R, Sheeran P. Moderation of cognition-intention and cognition-behaviour relations: a meta-analysis of properties of variables from the theory of planned behaviour. *Br J Soc Psychol.* 2004;43 (Pt 2):159–86.
20. Cox KL, Burke V, Gorely TJ, Beilin LJ, Puddey IB. Controlled comparison of retention and adherence in home- vs center-initiated exercise interventions in women ages 40-65 years: the S.W.E.A.T. study (Sedentary Women Exercise Adherence Trial). *Prev Med.* 2003;36(1):17–29.
21. Cress ME, Buchner DM, Prohaska T, et al. Best practices for physical activity programs and behavior counseling in older adult populations. *J Aging Phys Activity.* 2005;13(1):61–74.
22. Deci EL, Ryan RM. *Intrinsic Motivation and Self-Determination in Human Behavior.* New York (NY): Plenum Publishing; 1985. 371 p.
23. Dein S. ABC of mental health: Mental health in a multiethnic society. *BMJ.* 2007;315:473–9.
24. Delahanty LM, Nathan DM. Implications of the diabetes prevention program and Look AHEAD clinical trials for lifestyle interventions. *J Am Diet Assoc.* 2008;108(4 Suppl 1):S66–72.
25. Dishman RK. *Exercise Adherence: Its Impact on Public Health.* Champaign (IL): Human Kinetics; 1988. 447 p.
26. Dishman RK, Buckworth J. Increasing physical activity: a quantitative synthesis. *Med Sci Sports Exerc.* 1996;28(6):706–19.
27. Dishman RK, Vandenberg RJ, Motl RW, Nigg CR. Using constructs of the transtheoretical model to predict classes of change in regular physical activity: a multi-ethnic longitudinal cohort study. *Ann Behav Med.* 2010;40(2):150–63.
28. Donnelly JE, Blair SN, Jakicic JM, et al. American College of Sports Medicine Position Stand. Appropriate physical activity intervention strategies for weight loss and prevention of weight regain for adults. *Med Sci Sports Exerc.* 2009;41(2):459–71.

29. Duncan GE, Anton SD, Sydeman SJ, et al. Prescribing exercise at varied levels of intensity and frequency: a randomized trial. *Arch Intern Med.* 2005;165(20):2362–9.

30. Ekkekakis P, Lind E. Exercise does not feel the same when you are overweight: the impact of self-selected and imposed intensity on affect and exertion. *Int J Obes (Lond).* 2006;30(4):652–60.

31. Ekkekakis P, Thome J, Petruzzello SJ, Hall EE. The Preference for and Tolerance of the Intensity of Exercise Questionnaire: a psychometric evaluation among college women. *J Sports Sci.* 2008; 26(5):499–510.

32. Estabrooks PA. Sustaining exercise participation through group cohesion. *Exerc Sport Sci Rev.* 2000;28(2):63–7.

33. Estabrooks PA, Carron AV. Group cohesion in older adult exercisers: prediction and intervention effects. *J Behav Med.* 1999;22(6):575–88.

34. Estabrooks PA, Munroe KJ, Fox EH, et al. Leadership in physical activity groups for older adults: a qualitative analysis. *J Aging Phys Activity.* 2004;12(3):232–45.

35. Ferrier S, Blanchard CM, Vallis M, Giacomantonio N. Behavioural interventions to increase the physical activity of cardiac patients: a review. *Eur J Cardiovasc Prev Rehabil.* 2010;18(1):15–32.

36. Fitzpatrick SE, Reddy S, Lommel TS, et al. Physical activity and physical function improved following a community-based intervention in older adults in Georgia senior centers. *J Nutr Elder.* 2008;27(1–2):135–54.

37. Fox LD, Rejeski WJ, Gauvin L. Effects of leadership style and group dynamics on enjoyment of physical activity. *Am J Health Promot.* 2000;14(5):277–83.

38. Griffin JC. *Client-Centered Exercise Prescription.* 2nd ed. Champaign (IL): Human Kinetics; 2006. 339p.

39. Hall EE, Ekkekakis P, Petruzzello SJ. The affective beneficence of vigorous exercise revisited. *Br J Health Psychol.* 2002;7(1):47–66.

40. Hardy CJ, Rejeski WJ. Not what, but how one feels: the measurement of affect during exercise *J Sport Exer Psych.* 1989;11:304–17.

41. Hutchison AJ, Breckon JD, Johnston LH. Physical activity behavior change interventions based on the transtheoretical model: a systematic review. *Health Educ Behav.* 2009;36(5):829–45.

42. Jacobson DM, Strohecker L, Compton MT, Katz DL. Physical activity counseling in the adult primary care setting: position statement of the American College of Preventive Medicine. *Am J Prev Med.* 2005;29(2):158–62.

43. Jones KD, Burckhardt CS, Bennett JA. Motivational interviewing may encourage exercise in persons with fibromyalgia by enhancing self efficacy. *Arthritis Rheum.* 2004;51(5):864–7.

44. Kahn EB, Ramsey LT, Brownson RC, et al. The effectiveness of interventions to increase physical activity. A systematic review. *Am J Prev Med.* 2002;22(4 Suppl):73–107.

45. Kelley K, Abraham C. RCT of a theory-based intervention promoting healthy eating and physical activity amongst out-patients older than 65 years. *Soc Sci Med.* 2004;59(4):787–97.

46. King AC, Brassington G. Enhancing physical and psychological functioning in older family caregivers: the role of regular physical activity. *Ann Behav Med.* 1997;19(2):91–100.

47. King AC, Haskell WL, Young DR, Oka RK, Stefanick ML. Long-term effects of varying intensities and formats of physical activity on participation rates, fitness, and lipoproteins in men and women aged 50 to 65 years. *Circulation.* 1995;91(10):2596–604.

48. Kinmonth AL, Wareham NJ, Hardeman W, et al. Efficacy of a theory-based behavioural intervention to increase physical activity in an at-risk group in primary care (ProActive UK): a randomised trial. *Lancet.* 2008;371(9606):41–8.

49. Kiviniemi MT, Voss-Humke AM, Seifert AL. How do I feel about the behavior? The interplay of affective associations with behaviors and cognitive beliefs as influences on physical activity behavior. *Health Psychol.* 2007;26(2):152–8.

50. Kohrt WM, Bloomfield SA, Little KD, Nelson ME, Yingling VR, American College of Sports Medicine. American College of Sports Medicine Position Stand: physical activity and bone health. *Med Sci Sports Exerc.* 2004;36(11):1985–96.

51. Lind E, Welch AS, Ekkekakis P. Do 'mind over muscle' strategies work? Examining the effects of attentional association and dissociation on exertional, affective and physiological responses to exercise. *Sports Med.* 2009;39(9):743–64.

52. Locke EA, Latham GP. Building a practically useful theory of goal setting and task motivation. A 35-year odyssey. *Am Psychol.* 2002;57(9):705–17.

53. Macera CA, Ham SA, Yore MM, et al. Prevalence of physical activity in the United States: Behavioral Risk Factor Surveillance System, 2001. *Prev Chronic Dis.* 2005;2(2):A17.

54. McAuley E, Blissmer B. Self-efficacy determinants and consequences of physical activity. *Exerc Sport Sci Rev.* 2000;28(2):85–8.

55. Miller WR, Rose GS. Toward a theory of motivational interviewing. *Am Psychol.* 2009;64(6):527–37.

56. Mirotznik J, Feldman L, Stein R. The health belief model and adherence with a community center-based, supervised coronary heart disease exercise program. *J Community Health.* 1995;20(3):233–47.

57. Morgan O. Approaches to increase physical activity: reviewing the evidence for exercise-referral schemes. *Public Health.* 2005;119(5):361–70.

58. Netz Y, Zeev A, Arnon M, Tenenbaum G. Reasons attributed to omitting exercising: a population-based study. *Int J Sport Exerc Psyc.* 2008;6:9–23.

59. Nigg CR, Motl RW, Horwath CC, Wertin KK, Dishman RK. A research agenda to examine the efficacy and relevance of the transtheoretical model for physical activity behavior. *Psychol Sport Exerc.* 2010;12(1):7–12.

60. Noland MP. The effects of self-monitoring and reinforcement on exercise adherence. *Res Q Exerc Sport.* 1989;60(3):216–24.

61. O'Brien K, Nixon S, Tynan AM, Glazier RH. Effectiveness of aerobic exercise in adults living with HIV/AIDS: systematic review. *Med Sci Sports Exerc.* 2004;36(10):1659–66.

62. Pasick R, D'Onofrio C, Otero-Sabogal R. Similarities and differences across cultures: questions to inform a third generation for health promotion research. *Health Educ Q.* 1996;23(S):S142–61.

63. Pate RR, Pratt M, Blair SN, et al. Physical activity and public health. A recommendation from the Centers for Disease Control and Prevention and the American College of Sports Medicine. *JAMA.* 1995;273(5):402–7.

64. Perry CK, Rosenfeld AG, Bennett JA, Potempa K. Heart-to-Heart: promoting walking in rural women through motivational interviewing and group support. *J Cardiovasc Nurs.* 2007;22(4):304–12.

65. Perri MG, Anton SD, Durning PE, et al. Adherence to exercise prescriptions: effects of prescribing moderate versus higher levels of intensity and frequency. *Health Psychol.* 2002;21(5):452–8.

66. Perri MG, Martin AD, Leermakers EA, Sears SF, Notelovitz M. Effects of group-versus home-based exercise in the treatment of obesity. *J Consult Clin Psychol.* 1997;65(2):278–85.

67. Pescatello LS, Franklin BA, Fagard R, et al. American College of Sports Medicine position stand. Exercise and hypertension. *Med Sci Sports Exerc.* 2004;36(3):533–53.

68. Pinto BM, Goldstein MG, Ashba J, Sciamanna CN, Jette A. Randomized controlled trial of physical activity counseling for older primary care patients. *Am J Prev Med.* 2005;29(4):247–55.

69. Pinto BM, Goldstein MG, Marcus BH. Activity counseling by primary care physicians. *Prev Med.* 1998;27(4):506–13.

70. Prochaska JO. Strong and weak principles for progressing from precontemplation to action on the basis of twelve problem behaviors. *Health Psychol.* 1994;13(1):47–51.

71. Prochaska JO, DiClemente CC, Norcross JC. In search of how people change. Applications to addictive behaviors. *Am Psychol.* 1992;47(9):1102–14.

72. Pulmonary rehabilitation: joint ACCP/AACVPR evidence-based guidelines. ACCP/AACVPR Pulmonary Rehabilitation Guidelines Panel. American College of Chest Physicians. American Association of Cardiovascular and Pulmonary Rehabilitation. *Chest.* 1997;112(5):1363–96.

73. Reed GR, Velicer WF, Prochaska JO, Rossi JS, Marcus BH. What makes a good staging algorithm: examples from regular exercise. *Am J Heal Promot.* 1997;12(1):57–66.

74. Rejeski WJ, Kenney EA. *Fitness Motivation: Preventing Participant Dropout.* Champaign (IL): Human Kinetics; 1988. 168 p.

75. Rhodes RE, Warburton DE, Murray H. Characteristics of physical activity guidelines and their effect on adherence: a review of randomized trials. *Sports Med.* 2009;39(5):355–75.

76. Rogers LQ, Hopkins-Price P, Vicari S, et al. A randomized trial to increase physical activity in breast cancer survivors. *Med Sci Sports Exerc.* 2009;41(4):935–46.

77. Rose EA, Parfitt G. Can the feeling scale be used to regulate exercise intensity? *Med Sci Sports Exerc.* 2008;40(10):1852–60.

78. Rosenstock IM, Strecher VJ, Becker MH. Social learning theory and the Health Belief Model. *Health Educ Q.* 1988;15(2):175–83.

79. Rothman A. "Is there nothing more practical than a good theory?": Why innovations and advances in health behavior change will arise if interventions are used to test and refine theory. *Int J Behav Nutr Phys Activ.* 2004;1(1):11.

80. Ryan RM, Frederick CM, Lepes D, Rubio N, Sheldon KM. Intrinsic motivation and exercise adherence. *Int J Sport Psyc.* 1997;28:335–54.

81. Sallis JF, Owen N. Ecological models of health behavior. In: Glanz K, Rimer BK, Lewis FM, editors. *Health Behavior and Health Education: Theory, Research, and Practice, Third Edition.* San Francisco: Jossey-Bass; 2002. p. 462–84.

82. Shilts MK, Horowitz M, Townsend MS. Goal setting as a strategy for dietary and physical activity behavior change: a review of the literature. *Am J Health Promot.* 2004;19(2):81–93.

83. Shilts MK, Horowitz M, Townsend MS. Guided goal setting: effectiveness in a dietary and physical activity intervention with low-income adolescents. *Int J Adolesc Med Health.* 2009;21(1):111–22.

84. Silva MN, Vieira PN, Coutinho SR, et al. Using self-determination theory to promote physical activity and weight control: a randomized controlled trial in women. *J Behav Med.* 2010;33(2):110–22.

85. Skinner BF. *Science and Human Behavior*. New York (NY): MacMillan; 1953. 461 p.

86. Speer EM, Reddy S, Lommel TS, et al. Diabetes self-management behaviors and A1c improved following a community-based intervention in older adults in Georgia senior centers. *J Nutr Elder*. 2008;27(1–2):179–200.

87. Spencer L, Adams TB, Malone S, Roy L, Yost E. Applying the transtheoretical model to exercise: a systematic and comprehensive review of the literature. *Health Promot Pract*. 2006;7(4):428–43.

88. Stetson BA, Beacham AO, Frommelt SJ, et al. Exercise slips in high-risk situations and activity patterns in long-term exercisers: an application of the relapse prevention model. *Ann Behav Med*. 2005;30(1):25–35.

89. Stevens VJ, Funk KL, Brantley PJ, et al. Design and implementation of an interactive website to support long-term maintenance of weight loss. *J Med Internet Res*. 2008;10(1):e1.

90. Thogersen-Ntoumani C, Ntoumanis N. The role of self-determined motivation in the understanding of exercise-related behaviours, cognitions and physical self-evaluations. *J Sports Sci*. 2006;24(4):393–404.

91. U.S. Department of Health and Human Services. *Physical Activity and Health: A Report of the Surgeon General*. Atlanta, GA: US Department of Health and Human Services, Public Health Service, CDC, National Center for Chronic Disease Prevention and Health Promotion; 1996. 278 p.

92. van den Berg MH, Schoones JW, Vliet Vlieland TP. Internet-based physical activity interventions: a systematic review of the literature. *J Med Internet Res*. 2007;9(3):e26.

93. Wankel LM. The importance of enjoyment to adherence and psychological benefits from physical activity. *Int J Sport Psychol*. 1993;24(2):151–69.

94. Weiss RS. The provisions of social relationships. In: Rubin Z, editor. *Doing Unto Others*. Englewood Cliffs: Prentice-Hall; 1974. p. 17–26.

95. Wilcox S, Dowda M, Leviton LC, et al. Active for life: final results from the translation of two physical activity programs. *Am J Prev Med*. 2008;35(4):340–51.

96. Williams DM, Anderson ES, Winett RA. A review of the outcome expectancy construct in physical activity research. *Ann Behav Med*. 2005;29(1):70–9.

97. Williams DM, Dunsiger S, Ciccolo JT, Lewis BA, Albrecht AE, Marcus BH. Acute affective response to a moderate-intensity exercise stimulus predicts physical activity participation 6 and 12 months later. *Psychol Sport Exerc*. 2008;9(3):231–45.

98. Winett RA, Williams DM, Davy BM. Initiating and maintaining resistance training in older adults: a social cognitive theory-based approach. *Br J Sports Med*. 2009;43(2):114–9.

99. Wojcicki TR, White SM, McAuley E. Assessing outcome expectations in older adults: the multidimensional outcome expectations for exercise scale. *J Gerontol B Psychol Sci Soc Sci*. 2009;64(1):33–40.

100. Writing Group for the Activity Counseling Trial Research Group. Effects of physical activity counseling in primary care: the Activity Counseling Trial: a randomized controlled trial. *JAMA*. 2001;286(6):677–87.

Common Medications

LIST OF COMMON MEDICATIONS

The first section of *Appendix A* is a listing of common medications with their indication for use along with their drug and brand name that health/fitness, public health, clinical exercise, and health care professionals are likely to encounter among their clients/patients that are about to be or are physically active. This listing is not inclusive and is only meant as a reference guide. For a more detailed informational listing, the reader is referred to the American Hospital Formulary Service (AHFS) Drug Information from which the following brief listings were obtained (1).

I. CARDIOVASCULAR

β-Blockers

Indications: Hypertension (HTN), angina, arrhythmias including supraventricular tachycardia, atrial fibrillation, acute myocardial infarction (MI), migraine headaches, anxiety, and heart failure (HF) because of systolic dysfunction.

Drug Name	Brand Name[a]
Acebutolol[a,b]	Sectral[b]
Atenolol[a]	Tenormin
Betaxolol[a]	Kerlone
Bisoprolol[a]	Zebeta
Carvedilol[c]	Coreg
Esmolol	Brevibloc
Labetalol[c]	Normodyne, Trandate
Metoprolol Succinate, Metoprolol Tartrate[b]	Toprol XL, Lopressor SR
Nadolol[c]	Corgard
Nebivolol	Bystolic
Penbutolol[c]	Levatol[b]
Pindolol[b,c]	Visken[b]
Propranolol[c]	Inderal
Sotalol[c]	Betapace
Timolol[c]	Blocadren

[a]Cardioselective.
[b]β-Blockers with intrinsic sympathomimetic activity.
[c]Noncardioselective.

Angiotensin-Converting Enzyme Inhibitors (ACE-I)

Indications: HTN, coronary artery disease, and HF caused by systolic dysfunction, diabetes mellitus, chronic kidney disease, and cerebrovascular disease.

Drug Name	Brand Name	Combination ACE-I + HCTZ[a]	ACE-I + CCB[b]
Benazepril	Lotensin	Lotensin Hct	Lotrel (+ amlodipine)
Captopril	Capoten	Capozide	
Enalapril	Vasotec	Vaseretic	Lexxel (+ felodipine)
Fosinopril	Monopril		
Lisinopril	Zestril, Prinivil	Prinzide, Zestoretic	
Moexipril	Univasc	Uniretic	
Perindopril	Aceon		
Quinapril	Accupril	Accuretic	
Ramipril	Altace		
Trandolapril	Mavik		Tarka (+ verapamil)

[a]HCTZ, hydrochlorothiazide, a thiazide diuretic for use in HTN and HF.
[b]CCB, calcium channel blocker for use in HTN, HF, and angina.

Angiotensin II Receptor Blockers (ARBs)

Indications: HTN, diabetic nephropathy, and HF.

Drug Name	Brand Name	Combination ARB + HCTZ[a]
Candesartan	Atacand	Atacand HCT
Eprosartan	Teveten	Teveten HCT
Irbesartan	Avapro	Avalide
Losartan	Cozaar	Hyzaar
Olmesartan	Benicar	
Telmisartan	Micardis	Micardis HCT
Valsartan	Diovan	Diovan HCT

[a]ARB + HCTZ for use in HTN, HF, and angina.

Calcium Channel Blockers (CCB)

Dihydropyridines

Indications: HTN, isolated systolic HTN, angina, diabetes mellitus, and ischemic heart disease.

Drug Name	Brand Name
Amlodipine	Norvasc
Felodipine	Plendil
Isradipine	DynaCirc, DynaCirc CR
Nicardipine	Cardene, Cardene SR
Nifedipine long acting	Adalat, Procardia XL
Nimodipine	Nimotop
Nisoldipine	Sular

Nondihydropyridines

Indication: Angina, HTN, paroxysmal supraventricular tachycardia, and arrhythmia.

Drug Name	Brand Name
Diltiazem	Cardizem
Diltiazem, extended-release	Cardizem CD or LA, Cartia XT, Dilacor XR, Tiazac
Verapamil	Calan
Verapamil, controlled- and extended-release	Calan SR, Isoptin SR, Covera HS, Verelan PM, Verelan
Verapamil + trandolapril	Tarka

Diuretics

Indications: Edema, HTN, HF, and certain kidney disorders.

Drug Name	Brand Name	Combined with HCTZ
Thiazides		
Bendroflumethiazide	Naturein	
Chlorothiazide	Diuril	
Chlorthalidone	Hygroton (combined with atenolol is Tenoretic)	
Hydrochlorothiazide (HCTZ)	Microzide, Hydrodiuril, Oretic	
Indapamide	Lozol	
Methylclothiazide	Enduron	
Metolazone	Mykron, Zaroxolyn	
Polythiazide	Renese	
Loop Diuretics		
Bumetanide	Bumex	
Ethacrynic acid	Edecrin	
Furosemide	Lasix	
Torsemide	Demadex	
Potassium-Sparing Diuretics		**Combined with HCTZ**
Amiloride	Midamor	Moduretic, Hydro-ride
Triamterene	Dyrenium	Dyazide, Maxzide
Aldosterone Receptor Blockers		
Eplerenone	Inspra	
Spironolactone	Aldactone	

II. VASODILATING AGENTS

Nitrates and Nitrites

Indications: Angina, acute MI, HF, low cardiac output syndromes, and HTN.

Drug Name	Brand Name
Amyl nitrite (inhaled)	Amyl Nitrite
Isosorbide mononitrate	Ismo, Imdur, Monoket
Isosorbide dinitrate	Dilatrate, Isordil
Isosorbide dinitrate + hydralazine HCl	BiDil
Nitroglycerin, capsules ER	Nitro-Time, Nitroglycerin Slocaps
Nitroglycerin, lingual (spray)	Nitrolingual Pumpspray
Nitroglycerin, sublingual	Nitrostat, NitroQuick, Nitrotab
Nitroglycerin, topical ointment	Nitro-Bid
Nitroglycerin, transdermal	Minitran, Nitro-Dur, Nitrek, Deponit
Nitroglycerin, transmucosal (buccal)	Nitrogard

α-Blockers

Indications: HTN and benign prostatic hyperplasia.

Drug Name	Brand Name
Doxazosin	Cardura
Prazosin	Minipress
Tamsulosin	Flomax
Terazosin	Hytrin

Central α-Agonists

Indication: HTN.

Drug Name	Brand Name
Clonidine	Catapres, Catapres-TTS patch
Guanabenz	Wytensin
Guanfacine	Tenex
Methyldopa	Aldomet

Direct Vasodilators

Indications: HTN, hair loss, and HF.

Drug Name	Brand Name
Diazoxide	Hyperstat
Hydralazine	Apresoline
Minoxidil	Loniten
Sodium nitroprusside	Nipride

Peripheral Adrenergic Inhibitors

Indications: HTN and psychotic disorder.

Drug Name	Brand Name
Reserpine	Serpasil

III. OTHERS

Cardiac Glycosides

Indications: HF in the setting of dilated cardiomyopathy and increasing atrioventricular (AV) block to slow ventricular response with atrial fibrillation.

Drug Name	Brand Name
Amrinone	Inocor
Digoxin	Lanoxin
Milrinone	Primacor

Antiarrhythmic Agents

Indications: Specific for individual drugs but generally includes suppression of atrial fibrillation and maintenance of normal sinus rhythm, serious ventricular arrhythmias in certain clinical settings, and increase in AV nodal block to slow ventricular response in atrial fibrillation.

Drug Name	Brand Name
Class I	
IA	
Disopyramide	Norpace
Procainamide	Pronestyl, Procan SR
Quinidine	Quinora, Quinidex, Quinaglute, Quinalan, Cardioquin
IB	
Lidocaine	Xylocaine, Xylocard
Mexiletine	Mexitil
Phenytoin	Dilantin
Tocainide	Tonocard
IC	
Flecainide	Tambocor
Moricizine	Ethmozine
Propafenone	Rythmol
Class II	
β-Blockers	
Atenolol	Tenormin
Bisoprolol	Zebeta
Esmolol	Brevibloc

(continued)

Drug Name	Brand Name
Metoprolol	Lopressor SR, Toprol XL
Propranolol	Inderal
Timolol	Blocadren
Class III	
Amiodarone	Cordarone, Pacerone
Bretylium	Bretylol
Dofetilide	Tikosyn
Dronedarone	Multaq
Ibutilide	Covert (IV)
Sotalol	Betapace
Class IV	
Diltiazem	Progor, Cardizem
Verapamil	Isoptin, Calan, Covera

IV. ANTILIPEMIC AGENTS

Indications: Elevated total blood cholesterol, low-density lipoproteins (LDL), and triglycerides; low high-density lipoproteins (HDL); and metabolic syndrome.

Drug Name	Brand Name
Bile Acid Sequestrants	
Cholestyramine	Questran, Cholybar, Prevalite
Colesevelam	Welchol
Colestipol	Colestid
Fibric Acid Sequestrants	
Clofibrate	Atromid
Fenofibrate	Tricor, Lofibra
Gemfibrozil	Lopid
HMG-CoA Reductase Inhibitors (Statins)	
Atorvastatin	Lipitor
Fluvastatin	Lescol
Lovastatin	Mevacor
Lovastatin + Niacin	Advicor
Pravastatin	Pravachol
Rosuvastatin	Crestor
Simvastatin	Zocor
Statin + CCB[a]	
Atorvastatin + Amlodipine	Caduet
Nicotinic Acid	
Niacin (vitamin B$_6$)	Niaspan, Nicobid, Slo-Niacin
Cholesterol Absorption Inhibitor	
Ezetimibe	Zetia, Vytorin (with Simvastatin)

[a]CCB, calcium channel blocker.

V. BLOOD MODIFIERS

Anticoagulants

Indications: Treatment and prophylaxis of thromboembolic disorders. To prevent blood clots, heart attack, stroke, and intermittent claudication; or vascular death in patients with established peripheral arterial disease, or acute ST-segment elevation with myocardial infarction.

Drug Name	Brand Name
Coumadin	Warfarin
Dabigatran (thrombin inhibitor)	Pradaxa
Enoxaparin (LMWH)	Lovenox
Fondaparinux (LMWH)	Arixtra
Heparin	Calciparine
Warfarin	Coumadin

LMWH, Low-molecular weight heparin.

Antiplatelet

Indications: Antiplatelet drugs reduce platelet aggregation and are used to prevent further thromboembolic events in patients who have suffered MI, ischemic stroke, transient ischemic attacks, or unstable angina; and for primary prevention for patients at risk of a thromboembolic event. Some are also used for the prevention of reocclusion or restenosis following angioplasty and bypass procedures.

Drug Name	Brand Name
Aspirin (COX-I inhibitor)	None
Cilostazol (PDE inhibitor)	Pletal
Clopidogrel (ADP-R inhibitor)	Plavix
Dipyridamole (adenosine reuptake inhibitor)	Persantine, Aggrenox
Pentoxifylline	Trental
Prasugrel (ADP-R inhibitor)	Effient
Ticlopidine (ADP-R inhibitor)	Ticlid

ADPR, adenosine diphosphate-ribose; COX-I, cyclooxygenase inhibitor; PDE, phosphodiesterase.

VI. RESPIRATORY

Inhaled Corticosteroids

Indications: Asthma, nasal polyp, and rhinitis.

Drug Name	Brand Name
Beclomethasone	Beclovent, Qvar
Budesonide	Pulmicort
Ciclesonide	Alvesco
Flunisolide	AeroBid
Fluticasone	Flovent
Mometasone	Asmanex
Triamcinolone	Azmacort

Bronchodilators

Anticholinergics (Acetylcholine Receptor Antagonist)

Indications: Anticholinergic or antimuscarinic medications are used for the management of obstructive pulmonary disease and acute asthma exacerbations. They prevent wheezing, shortness of breath, and troubled breathing caused by asthma, chronic bronchitis, emphysema, and other lung diseases.

Drug Name	Brand Name	Combined with Sympathomimetic (β_2-Receptor Agonists)
Glycopyrrolate	Robinul	
Ipratropium	Atrovent	(+ Albuterol) Combivent
Tiotropium	Spiriva	

Sympathomimetics (β_2-Receptor Agonists)

Indications: Relief of asthma symptoms and in the management of chronic obstructive pulmonary disease. They prevent wheezing, shortness of breath, and trouble breathing caused by asthma, chronic bronchitis, emphysema, and other lung diseases.

Drug Name	Brand Name	Combined with Steroid
Albuterol	Proventil, Ventolin	
Formoterol (LA)	Foradil	(+ Budesonide) Symbicort (+ Mometasone) Dulera
Isoproterenol	Medihaler-Iso	
Levalbuterol	Xopenex	
Metaproterenol	Alupent	
Pirbuterol	Maxair	
Salmeterol (LA)	Serevent	(+ Fluticasone) Advair
Terbutaline	Brethine, Brethaire, Bricanyl	

Xanthine Derivatives

Indications: Combination therapy in asthma and chronic obstructive pulmonary disease.

Drug Name	Brand Name
Aminophylline	Phyllocontin, Truphylline
Caffeine	None
Theophylline	Theo-Dur, Uniphyl

Leukotriene Inhibitors and Antagonists

Indications: Asthma, exercise-induced asthma, and rhinitis.

Drug Name	Brand Name
Montelukast	Singulair
Zafirlukast	Accolate
Zileuton	Zyflo

Mast Cell Stabilizers

Indications: To prevent wheezing, shortness of breath, and troubled breathing caused by asthma, chronic bronchitis, emphysema, and other lung diseases.

Drug Name	Brand Name
Cromolyn (inhaled)	Intal
Nedocromil	Tilade
Omalizumab	Xolair

VII. COUGH/COLD PRODUCTS

Antihistamines

First Generation

Indications: Allergy, anaphylaxis (adjunctive), insomnia, motion sickness, pruritis of skin, rhinitis, sedation, and urticaria (hives).

Drug Name	Brand Name
Brompheniramine	Lodrane, Bidhist; combinations available with pseudoephedrine and phenylephrine
Carbinoxamine	Palgic
Chlorpheniramine	Teldrin, Aller-Chlor, Chlor-Trimeton, Chlo-Amine; combinations available with pseudoephedrine and phenylephrine
Clemastine	Dayhist, Tavist
Cyproheptadine	Cyproheptadine
Diphenhydramine	Benadryl, Nytol; combinations available with acetaminophen (APAP), pseudoephedrine, and phenylephrine
Doxylamine	Aldex, Unisom SleepTabs
Promethazine	Phenergan; with phenylephrine: Prometh VC Syrup
Triprolidine	Zymine, Zymine-D (with pseudoephedrine)

Second Generation

Indications: Allergic rhinitis and urticaria (hives).

Drug Name	Brand Name
Acrivastine	Semprex-D (with pseudoephedrine)
Cetirizine	Zyrtec, Zyrtec-D (with pseudoephedrine)
Desloratadine	Clarinex, Clarinex-D (with pseudoephedrine)
Fexofenadine	Allegra, Allegra-D (with pseudoephedrine)
Levocetirizine	Xyzal
Loratadine	Claritin, Claritin-D (with pseudoephedrine), Alavert, Alavert-D (with pseudoephedrine)

Sympathomimetic/Adrenergic Agonists

Indications: Allergic rhinitis and nasal congestion.

Drug Name	Brand Name
Phenylephrine	Sudafed PE; Preparation H (topical); many combinations
Pseudoephedrine	Sudafed; many combinations

Expectorant

Indication: Abnormal sputum (thin secretions/mucus).

Drug Name	Brand Name
Guaifenesin	Robitussin, Mucinex; many combinations

Antitussives

Indications: Cough and pain.

Drug Name	Brand Name
Benzonatate	Tessalon Perles
Codeine	Codeine; many combinations
Dextromethorphan	Robitussin Cough Gels, Robitussin Pediatric Cough Suppressant; many combinations
Hydrocodone	Many combinations

VIII. HORMONAL

Human Growth Hormone

Indications: Cachexia associated with acquired immunodeficiency syndrome (AIDS), growth hormone deficiency, and short bowel syndrome.

Drug Name	Brand Name
Somatropin	Genotropin, Nutropin, Humatrope, Omnitrope
Mecasermin (IV)	Increlex

Adrenals — Corticosteroids

Indications: Adrenocortical insufficiency, adrenogenital syndrome, hypercalcemia, thyroiditis, rheumatic disorders, collagen diseases, dermatologic diseases, allergic conditions, occular disorders, respiratory diseases (*e.g.*, asthma, chronic obstructive pulmonary disorders), hematologic disorders, gastrointestinal diseases (*e.g.*, ulcerative colitis, Crohn disease), and liver disease among others.

Drug Name	Brand Name
Beclomethasone	QVAR, Beclovent
Betamethasone	Celestone, Diprosone
Budesonide	Entocort EC, Pulmicort
Ciclesonide	Alvesco
Cortisone	Cortisone
Dexamethasone	Decadron
Fludrocortisone	Florinef
Flunisolide	AeroBid
Fluticasone	Flovent, with salmeterol: Advair
Hydrocortisone	Cortef, Hydrocortone
Methylprednisolone	Medrol, Solu-Medrol, Depo-Medrol
Mometasone	Asmanex
Prednisolone	Orapred, Prelone, Pediapred
Prednisone	Sterapred, Prednisone Intensol
Triamcinolone	Aristocort, Aristospan, Tac, Kenalog, Azmacort

Androgenic-Anabolic

Indications: Hypogonadism in males, catabolic and wasting disorders, endometriosis, hereditary angioedema, fibrocystic breast disease, and precocious puberty.

Drug Name	Brand Name
Danazol	Danocrine
Fluoxymesterone	Halotestin, Androxy
Methyltestosterone	Android, Testred, Virilon
Oxandrolone	Oxandrin
Testosterone	Striant ER, AndroGel, Androderm

Contraceptives

Drug Name	Brand Name
Estrogen–progestin combinations	Oral: Yaz, Alesse, Loestrin, Yasmin, Microgestin Fe, Sprintec, Ortho-Cyclen, Ortho Tri-Cyclen
Transdermal	Ortho Evra
Vaginal ring	NuvaRing
Intrauterine	Mirena
Progestins: etonogestrel	Parenteral implant: Implanon
Progestins: levonorgestrel	Oral: Next Choice, Plan B One Step
Progestins: norethindrone	Oral: Micronor, Nor-QD

Thyroid Agents

Indications: Hypothyroidism and pituitary thyroid-stimulating hormone suppression.

Drug Name	Brand Name
Levothyroxine	Levothroid, Synthroid, Levoxyl
Liothyronine	Cytomel
Liotrix	Thyrolar
Thyroid	Armour

Antidiabetic

Indication: Management of Type 2 diabetes mellitus.

CLASS: α-Glucosidase Inhibitors (slows absorption of carbohydrates in the gastrointestinal tract)

Drug Name	Brand Name	Combination
Acarbose	Precose/Glucobay	
Miglitol	Glyset	

CLASS: Amylin Analogue (mimics amylin, a hormone secreted with insulin to inhibit glucose, for postprandial glycemic control)

Drug Name	Brand Name	Combination
Pramlintide	Symlin	

CLASS: Biguanides (decreases sugar production by liver and decreases insulin resistance)

Drug Name	Brand Name	Combination
Metformin	Glucophage	

CLASS: Dipeptidylpeptidase-4 Inhibitors (enhances insulin release by preventing breakdown of glucagon-like peptide 1 [GLP-1] that is a potent antihyperglycemic hormone)

Drug Name	Brand Name	Combination
Saxagliptin	Onglyza	
Sitagliptin	Januvia	(+ Metformin) Janumet

CLASS: Glucagon-like Peptide 1 Receptor Agonists (activate GLP-1 that is a potent antihyperglycemic hormone that stimulates insulin release)

Drug Name	Brand Name	Combination
Exenatide	Byetta	

CLASS: Meglitinides (short-acting stimulation of β-cells to produce more insulin)

Drug Name	Brand Name	Combination
Nateglinide	Starlix	
Repaglinide	Prandin, Gluconorm	(+ Metformin) Prandimet

CLASS: Sulfonylureas (stimulate β-cells to produce more insulin)

Drug Name	Brand Name	Combination
Chlorpropamide – 1st gen.	Diabinese	
Glimepiride	Amaryl	
Glipizide	Glucotrol	(+ Metformin) Metaglip
Glyburide	DiaBeta, Glynase, Micronase	(+ Metformin) Glucovance
Tolazamide — 1st gen.	Tolinase	
Tolbutamide — 1st gen.	Orinase	

CLASS: Thiazolidinediones (improves sensitivity of insulin receptors in muscle, liver, and fat cells)

Drug Name	Brand Name	Combination
Pioglitazone	Actos	(+ Metformin) Actoplus Met (+ Glimepiride) Duetact
Rosiglitazone	Avandia	(+ Metformin) Avandamet (+ Glimepiride) Avandaryl

CLASS: Insulin

Rapid-Acting	Intermediate-Acting	Intermediate- and Rapid-Acting Combination	Long-Acting
Humalog	Humulin L	Humalog Mix	Humulin U
Humulin R	Humulin N	Humalog 50/50	Lantus injection
Novolin R	Iletin II Lente	Humalog 70/30	Levemir
Iletin II R	Iletin II NPH	Novolin 70/30	
	Novolin L		
	Nivalin N		

IX. CENTRAL NERVOUS SYSTEM

Antidepressants

Indication: Depression.

Drug Name	Brand Name
Amitriptyline	Elavil (TCA)
Amoxapine (TCA)	Asendin
Bupropion	Wellbutrin, Zyban
Citalopram (SSRI)	Celexa
Clomipramine (TCA)	Anafranil
Desipramine (TCA)	Norpramin
Desvenlafaxine (SNRI)	Pristiq
Doxepin (TCA)	Adapin, Sinequan
Duloxetine (SNRI)	Cymbalta
Escitalopram (SSRI)	Lexapro
Fluoxetine (SSRI)	Prozac; Fluoxetine + Olanzepine = Symbyax
Fluvoxamine (SSRI)	Luvox
Imipramine (TCA)	Tofranil
Isocarboxazid (MAO-I)	Marplan
Maprotiline (TeCA)	Ludiomil
Mirtazapine (TeCA)	Remeron
Nefazodone	Serzone (Brand d/c 2004)
Nortriptyline (second-generation TCA)	Pamelor, Aventyl
Paroxetine (SSRI)	Paxil
Phenelzine (MAO-I)	Nardil
Protriptyline (TCA)	Vivactil
Selegiline (MAO-I)	Anipryl
Sertraline (SSRI)	Zoloft
Tranylcypromine (MAO-I)	Parnate
Trazodone (SARI)	Desyrel
Trimipramine (TCA)	Surmontil
Venlafaxine (SNRI)	Effexor

MAO-I, monoamine oxidase inhibitor; SARI, serotonin antagonist reuptake inhibitor; SNRI, serotonin-norepinephrine reuptake inhibitor; SSRI, selective serotonin reuptake inhibitor; TCA, tricyclic antidepressant; TeCA, tetracyclic antidepressant.

Antipsychotics

Indications: Behavioral syndrome, bipolar disorder, Gilles de la Tourette syndrome, hyperactive behavior, psychotic disorder, and schizophrenia.

Drug Name	Brand Name
Aripiprazole (atypical)	Abilify
Chlorpromazine (typical)	Thorazine
Clozapine (atypical)	Clozaril, FazaClo
Fluphenazine (typical)	Permitil, Prolixin
Haloperidol (typical)	Haldol
Iloperidone	Fanapt
Lithium	Eskalith (CR), Lithobid
Loxapine (typical)	Loxitane
Mesoridazine (phenothiazine)	Serentil
Olanzapine (atypical)	Zyprexa
Paliperidone (atypical)	Invega
Perphenazine (typical)	Trilafon
Pimozide	Orap
Promazine	Sparine
Quetiapine (atypical)	Seroquel
Risperidone (atypical)	Risperdal
Thioridazine (typical)	Mellaril
Thiothixene (typical)	Navane
Triflupromazine	Vesprin
Valproic Acid	Depakote (ER), Depakene
Ziprasidone	Geodon

Antianxiety

Indications: Anxiety and panic disorder.

Drug Name	Brand Name	
Alprazolam	Xanax	
Buspirone	Buspar	
Chlordiazepoxide	Libritabs, Librium	(+ Clidinium) Librax
Clonazepam	Klonopin	
Clorazepate	Tranxene	
Diazepam	Valium	
Lorazepam	Ativan	
Meprobamate	Equanil, Miltown, Meprospan	
Oxazepam	Serax	

Sedative-Hypnotics

Indications: General anesthesia, insomnia, and sedation.

Drug Name	Brand Name
Amobarbital	Amytal
Butabarbital	Butisol
Chloral Hydrate	Somnote, Aquachloral, Supprettes
Dexmedetomidine	Precedex
Estazolam	ProSom
Eszopiclone	Lunesta, Lunestar
Flurazepam	Dalmane
Fospropofol	Lusedra
Propofol	Diprivan
Quazepam	Doral, Dormalin
Ramelteon	Rozerem
Secobarbital	Seconal
Temazepam	Restoril
Triazolam	Halcion
Zaleplon	Sonata
Zolpidem	Ambien

Stimulants

Indications: Attention deficit hyperactivity disorder, narcolepsy, obstructive sleep apnea, and shift work sleep disorder.

Drug Name	Brand Name
Amphetamine salts	Adderall (XR)
Armodafinil	Nuvigil
Caffeine	None
Dexmethylphenidate	Focalin (XR)
Dextroamphetamine	Dexedrine, Dextrostat
Lisdexamfetamine	Vyvanse
Methamphetamine	Desoxyn
Methylphenidate	Concerta, Ritalin (LA, SR)
Modafinil	Provigil

Nicotine Replacement Therapy

Indication: Smoking cessation assistance.

Drug Name	Brand Name
Nicotine	Solution: Nicotrol NS Inhalant: Nicotrol Inhaler Transdermal: Nicotrol Step 1,2,3; NicoDerm CQ Step 1,2,3
Nicotine Polacrilex	Lozenges: Commit Chewing gum: Nicorette, Nicorette DS

Nonsteroidal Anti-inflammatory Drugs (NSAIDS)

Indications: Fever, headache, juvenile rheumatoid arthritis, migraine, osteo-arthritis, pain, primary dysmenorrhea, and rheumatoid arthritis.

Drug Name	Brand Name
Celecoxib	Celebrex
Diclofenac	Cataflam, Voltaren
Diflunisal	Dolobid
Etodolac	Lodine
Fenoprofen	Nalfon, Naprofen
Flurbiprofen	Ansaid
Ibuprofen	Advil, Motrin, Nuprin
Indomethacin	Indocid, Indocin
Ketoprofen	Actron, Orudis, Oruvail
Ketorolac	Toradol
Meclofenamate	Meclomen
Mefenamic acid	Ponstel
Meloxicam	Mobic
Nabumetone	Relafen
Naproxen	Aleve, Naprosyn
Oxaprozin	Daypro
Piroxicam	Feldene
Sulindac	Clinoril
Tolmetin	Tolectin

Opioids

Opiate Agonists

Indications: Pain, chronic nonmalignant pain, MI, delirium, acute pulmonary edema, preoperative sedation, cough, and opiate dependence.

Drug Name	Brand Name
Codeine	Codeine; with acetaminophen (APAP), pseudoephedrine, and phenylephrine: Tylenol with Codeine no. 3 and no. 4
Fentanyl	Duragesic; Actiq, Fentora
Hydrocodone	Lorcet, Hydrocet; with APAP: Lortab, Vicodin; with Ibuprofen: Vicoprofen
Hydromorphone	Dilaudid
Levorphanol	Levo-Dromoran
Meperidine	Demerol
Methadone	Dolophine, Intensol, Methadose
Morphine	Avinza, MSContin, Oramorph SR,
Opium	None
Oxycodone	OxyIR, OxyContin, Roxicodone; with APAP: Percocet; with aspirin (ASA) Percodan
Oxymorphone	Opana (ER)
Propoxyphene	Darvon Pulvules
Remifentanil	Ultiva (IV)
Sufentanil	Sufenta (IV)
Tapentadol	Nucynta
Tramadol	Ultram (ER)

Opiate Partial Agonists (Pain and Opiate Dependence)

Indications: General anesthesia (adjunctive) and pain.

Drug Name	Brand Name
Buprenorphine	Suboxone (sublingual tablet), Subutex, Buprenex
Butorphanol	Stadol
Nalbuphine	Nubain
Pentazocine	With naloxone: Talwin NX; with acetaminophen (APAP), pseudoephedrine, and phenylephrine: Talacen

Analgesics and Antipyretics

Indications: Dysmenorrhea, fever, headache, and pain.

Drug Name	Brand Name
Acetaminophen	Tylenol
Salicylamide	BC Powder

X. UNCLASSIFIED

Antigout

Indication: To treat or prevent gout or treat hyperuricemia (excess uric acid in the blood).

Drug Name	Brand Name
Allopurinol	Zyloprim
Colchicine	Colcrys
Probenecid	Benemid

THE EFFECT OF COMMON MEDICATIONS ON THE RESPONSE TO EXERCISE

The second section of *Appendix A* contains *Table A.1* that lists the common medications with available published data regarding their influence on the response to exercise; specifically hemodynamics, the electrocardiogram (ECG), and exercise capacity. Exercise data are presented by drug category and then by specific drug if information is available. The influence of common medications during rest and/or exercise is presented with the directional relationships when they were specified in the literature. *Exercise capacity* is a generic term that often was used and not defined by a specific measure in the literature. In instances in which measures of exercise capacity were reported, they are listed, that is, maximal oxygen consumption ($\dot{V}O_{2max}$), endurance, performance, and tolerance, often times with no clear distinctions among them provided by the author.

Table A.1 is not intended to be inclusive as that would require an evidence-based meta-analysis of the literature that is beyond the scope of the *Guidelines*.

TABLE A.1. Effects of Medications on Hemodynamics, the Electrocardiogram (ECG), and Exercise Capacity				
Medications	**Cardiac Output (Q̇)**	**Heart Rate (HR)**	**Blood Pressure (BP)**	**ECG Changes**	**Exercise Capacity**
I. Cardiovascular Medications					
Beta-Blockers (BB)	↓ or ↔ Exercise (3)	↓ Rest and exercise ↓ Rest less by intrinsic sympathomimetic activity (ISA) + BB ↓ Exercise less by cardioselective BB (3)	↓ Rest and exercise	↓ Rest ↓ Ischemia during exercise	↓ V̇O$_{2max}$ acute administration, and ↑ chronic administration (3)
Angiotensin-Converting Enzyme Inhibitors (ACE-I)	↔ Exercise (3)	↔ Exercise (3)	↓ Rest and exercise (3)		↔ Performance (3); ↑ tolerance patients with congestive heart failure (CHF) (4)
Captopril		↔ Exercise	↓ Rest and exercise		
Angiotensin II Receptor Blockers (ARB) **Calcium Channel Blockers (CCB)**		↓ or ↔ Rest and exercise	↓ Rest and exercise		↔
Nondihydropyridines (non-DHP)	↔ Exercise (3)		↓ Exercise (3)		↔ Performance and endurance; responses can be variable (3)
Diltiazem		↓ Exercise patients with hypertension (3)			
Verapamil		↓ Exercise patients with hypertension (3)			
Dihydropyridine		↔ Exercise (3)	↓ Exercise (greater vs. non-DHP) (3)		↔ Performance and endurance; responses can be variable (3)
Nifedipine	↔ Exercise (3) ↓ Stroke volume (3)	↔ Exercise (3)			

(continued)

TABLE A.1. Effects of Medications on Hemodynamics, the Electrocardiogram (ECG), and Exercise Capacity (Continued)

Medications	Cardiac Output ($\dot{Q}$)	Heart Rate (HR)	Blood Pressure (BP)	ECG Changes	Exercise Capacity
II. Vasodilating Agents					
Nitrates	↔ Exercise (3)	↑ Rest ↑ or ↔ Exercise	↓ Rest ↓ or ↔ Exercise	↑ Rest HR ↑ or ↔ Exercise HR ↓ Exercise ischemia	↑ Patients with angina (4) ↔ Patients without angina ↑ or ↔ Patients with CHF
α-Blockers	↔ Exercise (3)	↔ Exercise (3)	↓ Exercise systolic BP (SBP) (not diastolic BP [DBP]) (3)	↓ Exercise ischemia	↔ Performance (3)
Prazosin	↔ Exercise (3)	↑ Exercise acute administration ↔ Exercise chronic administration (3)			
Doxazosin	↑ Exercise at 50% $\dot{V}O_{2max}$	↑ Exercise at 75% $\dot{V}O_{2max}$ ↔ Exercise up to 50% $\dot{V}O_{2max}$ (3)			
Central α-Agonist	↔ Exercise (3)	↓ Exercise (3)	↓ Exercise (3)		
Clonidine	↔	↓ Exercise (3)	↓ BP regular exercisers (3) ↔ During exercise SBP		Blunts the sympathetic response to exercise; consider avoiding if exercising (3)
Guanabenz		↔ Exercise			
III. Others					
Cardiac Glycosides					
Digitalis		↓ Patients with atrial fibrillation and possibly CHF Not significantly altered in patients with sinus rhythm	↔ Rest and exercise	Rest may produce nonspecific ST-T wave changes During exercise may produce ST-segment depression	↑ Patients with atrial fibrillation or CHF

Antiarrhythmic Agents				
All antiarrhythmic agents may cause new or worsened arrhythmias (*i.e.*, proarrhythmic effect)				
Class I				
Quinidine	↑ or ↔ Rest and exercise	↓ or ↔ Rest	↑ or ↔ Rest HR; Exercise may result in false-negative test results	↔
Disopyramide		↔ Exercise	Rest may prolong QRS and QT intervals	
Procainamide	↔ Rest and exercise	↔ Rest and exercise	Rest may prolong QRS and QT intervals; Exercise may result in false positive test results	↔
Tocainide	↔ Rest and exercise	↔ Rest and exercise	↔ Rest and exercise	↔
Moricizine	↔ Rest and exercise	↔ Rest and exercise	Rest may prolong QRS and QT intervals; ↔ Exercise	↔
Propafenone	↓ Rest; ↓ or ↔ Exercise	↔ Rest and exercise	↓ Rest HR; ↓ or ↔ Exercise HR	↔
Class II				
β-Blockers (see Class I)				
Class III				
Amiodarone	↓ Rest and exercise (4)	↔ Rest; ↑ Exercise	↓ Rest HR	↔ or ↑ (4)
Sotalol	↔ (4)		↔ Exercise	
Class IV				
CCB (see Class III)				

(continued)

TABLE A.1. Effects of Medications on Hemodynamics, the Electrocardiogram (ECG), and Exercise Capacity *(Continued)*

Medications	Cardiac Output ($\dot{Q}$)	Heart Rate (HR)	Blood Pressure (BP)	ECG Changes	Exercise Capacity
IV. Antilipemic Agents					↔ Performance (3)
V. Blood Modifiers					
Anticoagulants		↔ Rest and exercise	↔ Rest and exercise	↔ Rest and exercise	↔
Antiplatelet		↔ Rest and exercise	↔ Rest and exercise	↔ Rest and exercise	↔
VI. Respiratory					
Inhaled Corticosteroids		↔ Rest and exercise (3)	↔ Exercise (3)	↔ Exercise (3)	↔
Bronchodilators		↔ Rest and exercise	↔ Rest and exercise	↔ Rest and exercise	↔ $\dot{V}O_{2max}$ patients limited by bronchospasm
Anticholinergics		↔ Rest and exercise	↔	↑ or ↔ HR	
Sympathomimetics (β_2-Receptor Agonists)		↔ Rest and exercise (3)	↔		↔ Performance or $\dot{V}O_{2max}$ (3)
— Albuterol		May ↑ exercise (3)			↔ Performance and $\dot{V}O_{2max}$ (3)
Pseudoephedrine		↔ Rest and exercise (3) May ↑ exercise (3)	↔ Exercise May ↑ exercise SBP (3)	May produce premature ventricular contractions (PVC) (3)	↔ Performance (3)
Xanthine Derivatives				Rest and exercise may produce PVCs	
— Theophylline		↑ Rest ↔ Exercise (3)			↔ Performance and $\dot{V}O_{2max}$ (3)
— Caffeine	↔ (3)	↑ Resting ↑ or ↔ Exercise (3)	↑ Exercise (3)		↑ Endurance (3)
Mast Cell Stabilizers		↔ Rest and exercise	↔	↔	↔ $\dot{V}O_{2max}$ (3)
Antihistamines		↑ Rest ↔ Exercise (3)			↔ Performance and endurance (3)
VII. Hormonal					
Human Growth Hormone		↔ Rest and exercise	↔	↔	↑ Performance and $\dot{V}O_{2max}$ (3)
Androgenic-Anabolic		↔ Rest and exercise (3)	↑ DBP (3)		↔ or ↑ Performance and $\dot{V}O_{2max}$ (3)

Medication	Heart Rate	Blood Pressure	ECG	Exercise Capacity
Thyroid Agents	↑ Rest and exercise	↑ Rest and exercise	↑ HR May provoke arrhythmias	↔ Unless angina worsens during exercise
Levothyroxine				↑ Cardiopulmonary reserve ↔ Recovery and performance (2)
VIII. Central Nervous System				
Antidepressants	↑ or ↔ Rest and exercise	↓ or ↔ Rest and exercise	Variable rest	
Antipsychotics				
— Lithium	↔ Rest and exercise	↔ Rest and exercise		
Antianxiety	↑ or ↔ Rest and exercise	↓ or ↔ Rest and exercise	Variable rest	
Stimulants	↑ (3)	↑ (3)		↑ or ↔ Endurance and performance
Nicotine Replacement Therapy	↔	↔		↔ or ↓
Nonsteroidal Anti-inflammatory Drugs (NSAIDS)				↔ or ↑ Performance dose related (3)
Opioids				↔
Analgesics and Antipyretics				↔ Performance (3)
IX. Unclassified				
Antigout	↔ Rest and exercise	↔ Rest and exercise	↔ Rest and exercise	↔
Alcohol	↔ Rest and exercise	Rest and exercise Chronic use may have role in ↑ BP ↑ BP after acute ingestion (3)	Rest and exercise may provoke arrhythmias	↓ Performance and $\dot{V}O_{2max}$ (3)
Marijuana				↓

↑, increased; ↓, decreased; ↔, not changed.

Thus, *Table A.1* serves as a reference guide for health/fitness, public health, clinical exercise, and health care professionals. It is important to note exercise may impact the pharmacokinetic (*i.e.*, what the body does to the medication) and pharmacodynamic (*i.e.*, what the medication does to the body) properties of a medication, necessitating a change in (a) dose; (b) dosing interval; (c) length of time the patient or client takes the medication; and/or (d) the exercise prescription.

The primary sources used to extract the information in *Table A.1* were *Pharmacology in Exercise and Sports* (4) and *Sport and Exercise Pharmacology* (3). In addition, a literature search by generic drug name or class and exercise response and/or capacity was done using MEDLINE and Google Scholar on February 23, 2011.

THE BOTTOM LINE

Health/fitness, public health, clinical exercise, and health care professionals should be aware of the influence medications may have on the response to exercise (*i.e.*, hemodynamic, ECG, and exercise). In some cases, exercise may impact the pharmacokinetic (*i.e.*, what the body does to the medication) and pharmacodynamic (*i.e.*, what the medication does to the body) properties of a medication, necessitating a change in (a) dose; (b) dosing interval; (c) length of time the patient or client takes the medication; and/or (d) the exercise prescription.

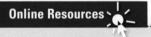

Online Resources

The American Hospital Formulary Service (AHFS) Drug Information:
http://www.ahfsdruginformation.com

MICROMEDEX 2.0 (unbiased, referenced information about medications):
http://www.micromedex.com/

REFERENCES

1. American Society of Health-System Pharmacists. *AHFS Drug Information 2010*. Bethesda (MD): American Society of Health-System Pharmacists; 2010. 3824 p.
2. Mainenti MRM, Teixeira PFS, Oliveira FP, Vaisman M. Effect of hormone replacement on exercise cardiopulmonary reserve and recovery performance in subclinical hypothyroidism. *Braz J Med Biol Res*. 2010;43(11):1095–101.
3. Reents S. *Sport and Exercise Pharmacology*. Champaign (IL): Human Kinetics; 2000. 347 p.
4. Somani SM, editor. *Pharmacology in Exercise and Sports*. Boca Raton (FL): CRC Press; 1996. 359 p.

B

Emergency Risk Management[1]

Having a well-thought-out emergency response system in place at all types of exercise settings is critical to providing a safe environment for participants and represents a fundamental practice in risk management. Emergency policies, procedures, and practices for health/fitness facilities and clinical exercise testing laboratories have been previously described in detail in recommendations published by the American College of Sports Medicine (ACSM) and American Heart Association (AHA) (2,3,5,8) (see *Box B.1*). The types of settings in which exercise takes place vary markedly from rooms that are essentially hotel amenities to medically supervised clinical exercise centers. Such facilities often serve different purposes and clientele, may or may not have organized program offerings, and may or may not have qualified health/fitness, clinical exercise, or health care professionals trained in emergency preparedness. *Appendix B* provides an overview of emergency risk management for exercise settings typically overseen by qualified health/fitness, clinical exercise, or health care professionals trained in emergency preparedness (see *Appendix D*).

The following ACSM standards on emergency response risk management are highlighted:

1. Facilities offering exercise services must have written emergency response system policies and procedures that must be reviewed and rehearsed regularly and include documentation of these activities. These policies enable staff to handle basic first-aid situations and emergency cardiac events.
   - The emergency response system must be fully documented (*e.g.*, staff training, emergency instructions) and the documents kept in an area that can be easily accessed by the staff.
   - The emergency response system should identify a local coordinator (*e.g.*, a staff person that is responsible for the overall level of emergency readiness).
   - Exercise facilities should use local health care or medical personnel to help them develop their emergency response program.
   - The emergency response system must address the major emergency situations that might occur. Among those situations are medical emergencies

---

[1]This appendix is adapted with permission from (8).

BOX B.1	ACSM and AHA Emergency Risk Management Comprehensive Resources

The fourth edition of the *ACSM's Health/Fitness Facility Standards and Guidelines* (8) provides the most comprehensive information published to date on developing an emergency response system for the nonclinical or health/fitness exercise setting, and the reader is referred to this textbook for more detailed information regarding these types of settings. Additional information on matters of preparing emergency policies, procedures, and practices specific to clinical, research, health/fitness, or other exercise settings can be found in the contents of the joint ACSM/AHA publications (2,3). Emergency procedures specific to the clinical exercise testing setting have been described by the AHA (5).

....
ACSM, American College of Sports Medicine; AHA, American Heart Association.

that are reasonably foreseeable with the onset of moderate or more intense exercise such as hypoglycemia, sudden cardiac arrest (SCA), heart attack, stroke, heat illness, and common orthopedic injuries. The response system must also address other foreseeable emergencies not necessarily associated with physical activity such as fires or chemical accidents.

- The emergency response system must provide explicit steps or instructions on how each emergency situation will be handled, and the roles each staff member or responder plays in an emergency. In addition, the emergency response system needs to provide locations for all emergency equipment, the location for all emergency exits, and accessible telephones for calling 911 as well as other contact information and steps necessary for contacting the local emergency medical services (EMS).
- The emergency response system must be physically reviewed and rehearsed at least four times per year with notations maintained in a logbook that indicate when the rehearsals were performed and who participated.
- The emergency response system must address the availability of first-aid kits and other medical equipment within the facility.

2. Exercise facilities in the health/fitness or community setting must have as part of their written emergency response system a public access defibrillation program.
   - Every site with automated external defibrillators (AEDs) should strive to get the response time from collapse caused by cardiac arrest to defibrillation to ≤3 min (*e.g.*, AEDs located throughout the facility so that the walk to retrieve an AED is ≤1.5 min).
   - The Food and Drug Administration (FDA) requires that a physician *prescribe* an AED before it can be purchased. The AHA strongly recommends that a physician, licensed to practice medicine in the community in

which the facility is located, should provide the oversight of the facility's emergency system and AEDs.

- The emergency and AED plan should be coordinated with the local EMS provider.
- A skills and practice session with the AED is recommended every 3–6 mo for most exercise settings.
- The AED should be monitored and maintained according to the manufacturer's specifications on a daily, weekly, and monthly basis, and all related information should be carefully documented and maintained as part of the facility's emergency response system records. Most contemporary AEDs provide this function through an automated process.

3. Exercise facilities must have in place a written system for sharing information with users and employees or independent contractors regarding the handling of potentially hazardous materials including the handling of bodily fluids by the facility's staff in accordance with the standards of the Occupational Safety and Health Administration (OSHA). These standards include the following:

- Provide appropriate training for staff on the handling of bodily fluids.
- Store all chemicals and agents in proper locations. Ensure these materials are stored off the floor and in an area that is off-limits to users. These areas should also have locks to prevent accidental or inappropriate entry.
- Provide regular training to workers in the handling of hazardous materials.
- Post the appropriate signage to warn users that they may be exposed to these hazardous agents.

Other key points regarding medical emergency plans and special circumstances such as clinical exercise testing or participation are the following:

- All personnel involved with exercise testing and supervision should be trained in basic cardiopulmonary resuscitation (CPR) and preferably advanced cardiac life support (ACLS).
- There should be a physician immediately available at all times when maximal sign or symptom-limited exercise testing is performed on high-risk individuals.
- Telephone numbers for emergency assistance should be posted clearly on or near all telephones. Emergency communication devices must be readily available and working properly.
  - Designated personnel should be assigned to the regular maintenance (i.e., monthly and/or as determined by hospital and/or facility protocol) of the emergency equipment and regular surveillance of all pharmacological substances.
  - Incident reports should be clearly documented including the event time and date, witnesses present, and a detailed report of the medical emergency care provided. Copies of all documentation should be preserved on site maintaining the injured personnel's confidentiality, and a corresponding follow-up postincident report is highly recommended.

- If a medical emergency occurs during exercise testing and/or training in the clinical exercise setting, the nearest available physician and/or other trained CPR provider should be solicited along with the medical emergency response team and/or paramedic (*i.e.*, if exercise is conducted outside of the hospital setting). In the medical exercise setting, the physician or lead medical responder should decide whether to evacuate the patient to the emergency department based on whether the medical emergency is life threatening or not. If a physician is not available and there is any likelihood of decompensation, then transportation to the emergency department should be made immediately.

SPECIAL CIRCUMSTANCES: EMERGENCY EQUIPMENT AND DRUGS

Records should be kept documenting proper functioning of medical emergency equipment such as a defibrillator, AED, oxygen supply, and suction (*i.e.*, daily for all days of operations). All malfunctioning medical emergency equipment should be locked or removed immediately with operations suspended until repaired and/or replaced. In addition, expiration dates for pharmacological agents and other supportive supplies (*e.g.*, intravenous equipment, intravenous fluids) should be kept on file and readily available for review.

Emergency equipment and drugs should be available in any area where maximal exercise testing is performed on high-risk individuals such as in hospital-based exercise programs. Only personnel authorized by law and policy to use certain medical emergency equipment (*e.g.*, defibrillators, syringes, needles) and dispense drugs can lawfully do so. It is expected that such personnel be immediately available during maximal exercise testing of individuals with known cardiovascular disease in the clinical exercise setting. For more details, the reader is referred to guidelines on clinical exercise laboratories published by the AHA (5).

ADDITIONAL INFORMATION ON AUTOMATED EXTERNAL DEFIBRILLATORS

AEDs are computerized, sophisticated devices that provide voice and visual cues to guide lay and health care providers to safely defibrillate pulseless ventricular tachycardia/fibrillation (VF) SCA. Early defibrillation plays a critical role for successful survival of SCA for the following reasons:

1. VF is the most frequent SCA witnessed.
2. Electrical defibrillation is the treatment for VF.
3. With delayed electrical defibrillation, the probability of success diminishes rapidly.
4. VF deteriorates to asystole within minutes.

According to the AHA 2010 Guidelines for CPR and Emergency Cardiovascular Care Guidelines, "rescuers must be able to rapidly integrate CPR with use of the AED" (4). Three key components must occur within the initial moments of a cardiac arrest and include the following:

1. Activation of the EMS.
2. CPR.
3. Operation of an AED.

AUTOMATED EXTERNAL DEFIBRILLATOR GENERAL GUIDELINES

Because delays in CPR or defibrillation reduces SCA survival, the AHA urges the placement and use of AEDs in medical and nonmedical settings (*e.g.*, airports, airplanes, casinos, health/fitness facilities) (4). In hospital settings, CPR and an AED should be used immediately for cardiac arrest incidents. For out-of-hospital events when an AED is available, the AED should be used as soon as possible. Survival rate is improved when AED use is proceeded by CPR (4).

For more detailed explanations on the expanding role of AEDs and management of various cardiovascular emergencies, refer to the 2010 AHA Guidelines for Cardiopulmonary Resuscitation and Emergency Cardiovascular Care (4) or any AHA subsequent updates.

THE BOTTOM LINE

- Having a well-thought-out emergency response system in any exercise setting is critical to providing a safe environment for participants and represents a fundamental practice in risk management.
- Facilities offering exercise services must have written emergency response system policies and procedures that must be reviewed and rehearsed regularly and include documentation of these activities. These policies must enable staff to handle basic first-aid situations and emergency cardiac events.
- The emergency response system must provide explicit steps or instructions on how each emergency situation will be handled and the roles each staff member or responder has in an emergency.
- Exercise facilities must have as part of their written emergency response system a public access defibrillation program.

It is essential to recognize that emergency equipment alone does not save lives. All exercise facilities and settings should have written emergency policies and procedures. These policies and procedures should be practiced regularly throughout the year by designated staff members that are trained in CPR and can function as first responders during hours of operation; and staff should be trained to recognize and respond to cardiac arrest and coordinate their emergency plan with local EMS.

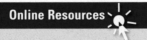

Online Resources

The following links provide additional information on emergency risk management. The reader will find sample plans for medical incidents/nonemergency situations and use of AEDs in the exercise setting; however, specific plans must be customized according to individual program needs and local standards. The ACSM recommends particular attention to local, state, and federal laws governing emergency risk management policies and procedures.

AED Implementation Guide (PDF) (1):
http://www.americanheart.org/presenter.jhtml?identifier=3027225AHA

OSHA: Emergency Action Plans (6):
http://www.osha.gov/pls/oshaweb/owadisp.show_document?p_id=9726&p_table=STANDARDS

Public Access Defibrillator Guidelines (7):
http://www.foh.dhhs.gov/whatwedo/AED/HHSAED.ASP

All links last accessed December 22, 2010.

REFERENCES

1. AED Implementation Guide [Internet]. Dallas (TX): American Heart Association; [cited 2010 Dec 21]. Available from: http://www.americanheart.org/presenter.jhtml?identifier=3027225AHA
2. Balady GJ, Chaitman B, Driscoll D, et al. Recommendations for cardiovascular screening, staffing, and emergency policies at health/fitness facilities. *Circulation.* 1998;97(22):2283–93.
3. Balady GJ, Chaitman B, Foster C, et al. Automated external defibrillators in health/fitness facilities: supplement to the AHA/ACSM Recommendations for Cardiovascular Screening, Staffing, and Emergency Policies at Health/Fitness Facilities. *Circulation.* 2002;105(9):1147–50.
4. Field JM, Hazinski MF, Sayre MR, et al. Part 1: executive summary: 2010 American Heart Association Guidelines for Cardiopulmonary Resuscitation and Emergency Cardiovascular Care. *Circulation.* 2010; 122(18 Suppl 3):S640–56.
5. Myers J, Arena R, Franklin B, et al. Recommendations for clinical exercise laboratories: a scientific statement from the American Heart Association. *Circulation.* 2009;119(24):3144–61.
6. Occupational Safety and Health Administration. *Emergency Action Plans* [Internet]. Washington (DC): U.S. Department of Labor, Occupational Safety and Health Administration; [cited 2010 Dec 21]. Available from: http://www.osha.gov/pls/oshaweb/owadisp.show_document?p_id=9726&p_table=STANDARDS
7. Public Access Defibrillation Guidelines [Internet]. Washington (DC): Office of Public Health and Science, Office of the Secretary, HHS and Office of Governmentwide Policy, GSA; [cited 2010 Dec 21]. Available from: http://www.foh.dhhs.gov/whatwedo/AED/HHSAED.ASP
8. Tharrett SJ, Peterson JA, American College of Sports Medicine. *ACSM's Health/Fitness Facility Standards and Guidelines.* 4th ed. Champaign (IL): Human Kinetics; 2012. 256 p.

C

Electrocardiogram Interpretation

The tables in *Appendix C* provide a quick reference source for electrocardiogram (ECG) recording and interpretation. Each of these tables should be used as part of the overall clinical profile when making diagnostic decisions about an individual.

TABLE C.1. Limb and Augmented Lead Electrode Placement[a]

Lead	Electrode Placement	Heart Surface Viewed
Lead I	Left arm (+), right arm (−)	Lateral
Lead II	Left leg (+), right arm (−)	Inferior
Lead III	Left leg (+), left arm (−)	Inferior
aVR	Right arm (+)	None
aVL	Left arm (+)	Lateral
aVF	Left leg (+)	Inferior

[a]Exercise modifications: The limb leads are positioned over the left and right infraclavicular region for the arm leads, and over the left and right lower quadrants of the abdomen for the leg leads. This ECG configuration minimizes motion artifacts during exercise. However, torso-placed limb leads should be noted for all ECG tracings to avoid misdiagnosis of an ECG tracing. The most common changes observed are produced by right axis deviation and standing that may obscure or produce Q waves inferiorly or anteriorly and T wave or frontal QRS axis changes even in normal people (2,4).

TABLE C.2. Precordial (Chest Lead) Electrode Placement

Lead	Electrode Placement	Heart Surface Viewed
V_1	Fourth intercostal space just to the right of the sternal border	Septum
V_2	Fourth intercostal space just to the left of the sternal border	Septum
V_3	At the midpoint of a straight line between V_2 and V_4	Anterior
V_4	On the midclavicular line in the fifth intercostal space	Anterior
V_5	On the anterior axillary line and on a horizontal plane through V_4	Lateral
V_6	On the midaxillary line and on a horizontal plane through V_4 and V_5	Lateral

Adapted from (3).

TABLE C.3. Electrocardiogram Interpretation Steps

1.	Check for correct calibration (1 mV = 10 mm) and paper speed (25 mm · s^{-1}).
2.	Verify the heart rate and determine the heart rhythm.
3.	Measure intervals (PR, QRS, QT).
4.	Determine the mean QRS axis and mean T wave axis in the limb leads.
5.	Look for morphologic abnormalities of the P wave, QRS complex, ST-segment, T wave, and U wave (*e.g.*, chamber enlargement, conduction delays, infarction, repolarization changes).
6.	Interpret the present ECG.
7.	Compare the present ECG with previous available ECGs.
8.	Offer conclusion, clinical correlation, and recommendations.

TABLE C.4. Resting Electrocardiogram: Normal Limits

Parameter	Normal Limits	Abnormal if:	Possible Interpretation(s)[a]
Heart rate	60–100 beats · min^{-1}	<60 beats · min^{-1}	Bradycardia
		>100 beats · min^{-1}	Tachycardia
P wave	<0.11 s	Broad and notched (>0.11 s) in leads I, II, aVL, V_4–V_6, and inverted in V_1	Left atrial hypertrophy
	<2.5 mm tall	Peaked (<2.5 mm tall) in leads II, III, and aVF and upright in V_1	Right atrial hypertrophy
		Peaked and broad in leads I, II, III, aVL, aVF, V4–V6, and bi-phasic in V_1	Combined atrial hypertrophy
PR interval	0.12–0.20 s	<0.12 s	Preexcitation (*i.e.*, W-P-W or L-G-L)
		>0.20 s	First-degree AV block
QRS duration	Up to 0.10 s	If ≥0.11 s	Conduction abnormality (*i.e.*, incomplete or complete bundle branch block, W-P-W, IVCD, or electronic pacer)
QT interval	Rate dependent	QTc long	Drug effects, electrolyte abnormalities, or ischemia
	Normal QT = $K\sqrt{RR}$, where K = 0.37 for men and children and 0.40 for women	QTc short	Digitalis effect, hypercalcemia, or hypermagnesia
QRS axis	−30 to +110 degrees	<−30 degrees	Left axis deviation (*i.e.*, chamber enlargement, hemiblock, or myocardial infarction)
		>+110 degrees	Right axis deviation (*i.e.*, RVH, pulmonary disease, or myocardial infarction)
		Indeterminate	All limb leads transitional
T wave	Upright in leads I, II, and V_5–V_6; inverted in aVR; flat, inverted, or diphasic in III, V_1–V_2	Upright, inverted, or biphasic alone or with ST-segment changes	Can be a normal variant; ischemia or caused by physiologic conditions (posture changes, respiration, drugs)
T axis	Generally same direction as QRS axis	The T axis (vector) is typically deviated away from the area of "mischief" (*i.e.*, ischemia, bundle branch block, or hypertrophy)	Chamber enlargement, ischemia, drug effects, or electrolyte disturbances
ST-segment	Generally at isoelectric line (PR-segment) or within 1 mm	Elevation of ST-segment	Normal variant (early repolarization), injury, ischemia, pericarditis, or electrolyte abnormality
	The ST may be elevated up to 1–2 mm in leads V_1–V_4 (5)	Depression of ST-segment 80 ms after the J-point	Injury, ischemia, electrolyte abnormality, drug effects, or normal variant

TABLE C.4. Resting Electrocardiogram: Normal Limits (*Continued*)

Parameter	Normal Limits	Abnormal if:	Possible Interpretation(s)[a]
Q wave	<0.04 s and <25% of R wave amplitude (exceptions lead III and V_1)	>0.04 s and/or >25% of R wave amplitude except lead III and V_1	Myocardial infarction or pseudoinfarction (as from chamber enlargement, conduction abnormalities, W-P-W, COPD, or cardiomyopathy)
Transition zone	Usually between V_2–V_4	Before V_2	Counterclockwise rotation (early transition)
		After V_4	Clockwise rotation (late transition)

[a]If supported by other electrocardiograms and related clinical criteria.

AV, atrioventricular; COPD, chronic obstructive pulmonary disease; IVCD, intraventricular conduction delay; L-G-L, Lown-Ganong-Levine syndrome; QTc, QT corrected for heart rate; RVH, right ventricular hypertrophy; W-P-W, Wolff-Parkinson-White syndrome.

TABLE C.5. Estes Electrocardiogram Criteria for the Determination of Left Ventricular Enlargement

	Points

1. Any of the following
     R or S in limb lead ≥20 mm
     S wave in V1, V2, V3 ≥25 mm
     R wave in V4, V5, V6 ≥25 mm
	3

2. Any ST shift Typical strain ST-T changes	3 1
3. LAD >15 degrees	2
4. QRS interval >0.09 s	1
5. Intrisicoid deflection >0.04 s	1
6. P-terminal force V1 >0.04	3
Total (LVH >5 points, probable LVH >4 points)	13

Adapted with permission from (7).

TABLE C.6. Scott Electrocardiogram Criteria for the Determination of Left Ventricular Hypertrophy

Any one listed below
S in V1 or V2 + R in V5 or V6 ≥35 mm
R in V5 or V6 ≥26 mm
R + S in any V lead ≥45 mm
R in I + S in III ≥25 mm
R in aVL ≥7.5 mm
R in aVF ≥20 mm
S in aVR ≥14 mm

Adapted with permission from (7).

TABLE C.7. Localization of Transmural Infarcts[a] (Location of Diagnostic Q Wave)

Typical ECG Leads	Infarct Location
V_1–V_3	Anteroseptal
V_3–V_4	Localized anterior
V_4–V_6, I, aVL	Anterolateral
V_1–V_6	Extensive anterior
I, aVL	High lateral
II, III, aVF	Inferior
V_1–V_2	Septal or true posterior (R/S >1)
V_1, V_{3R}, V_{4R}	Right ventricular

[a]When diagnostic Q waves are present in the inferior leads and the R wave is greater than the S wave in V_1 or V_2, this can reflect the presence of posterior extension of the inferior myocardial infarction.

V_{3R}, V_{4R}, right precordial leads.

TABLE C.8. Supraventricular versus Ventricular Ectopic Beats[a]

Parameter		Supraventricular (Normal Conduction)	Supraventricular (Aberrant Conduction)	Ventricular
QRS complex	Duration	Up to 0.10 s	≥0.11 s	≥0.11 s
	Configuration	Normal	Widened QRS usually with unchanged initial vector	Widened QRS often with abnormal initial vector
			P wave precedes QRS	QRS usually not preceded by a P wave
P wave		Present or absent but with relationship to QRS	Present or absent but with relationship to QRS	Present or absent but without relationship to QRS
Rhythm		Usually less than compensatory pause	Usually less than compensatory pause	Usually compensatory pause

[a]Numerous ECG criteria exist to try to distinguish premature ventricular contractions (PVCs) from aberrant conduction (1,6). A major clinical problem is the patient with a wide QRS tachycardia. Such tachycardias can be ventricular or supraventricular with aberrant conduction. Typically, ventricular tachycardia is characterized by a significant shift in frontal plane axis. In contrast, a wide QRS (supraventricular tachycardia) maintains proximity to the axis in absence of this arrhythmia. A good rule of thumb is that any wide QRS tachycardia in a patient with heart disease or a history of heart failure is likely to be ventricular tachycardia, especially if atrioventricular (AV) dissociation is identified.

TABLE C.9. Atrioventricular Block

Interpretation	P Wave Relationship to QRS	PR Interval	R–R Interval
First-degree atrioventricular (AV) block	1:1	>0.20 s	Regular or follows P–P interval
Second-degree AV block: Mobitz I (Wenckebach)	>1:1	Progressively lengthens until a P wave fails to conduct	Progressively shortens; pause less than two other cycles
Second-degree AV block: Mobitz II	>1:1	Constant but with sudden dropping of QRS	Regular except for pause, which usually equals two other cycles
Third-degree AV block	None	Variable but P–P interval constant	Usually regular (escape rhythm)

TABLE C.10. Atrioventricular Dissociation[a]

Type of Atrioventricular (AV) Dissociation	Electrophysiology	Example	Significance	Comment
AV dissociation resulting from complete AV block	AV block	Sinus rhythm with complete AV block	Pathologic	Unrelated P wave and QRS complexes P–P interval is shorter than R–R interval
AV dissociation by default causing interference	Slowing of the primary or dominant pacemaker with escape of a subsidiary pacemaker	Sinus bradycardia with junctional escape rhythm	Physiologic	Unrelated P wave and QRS complexes P–P interval is longer than R–R interval
AV dissociation by usurpation	Acceleration of a subsidiary pacemaker usurping control of the ventricles	Sinus rhythm with either AV junctional or ventricular tachycardia	Physiologic	Unrelated P wave and QRS complexes P–P interval is longer than R–R interval
Combination	AV block and interference	Atrial fibrillation with accelerated AV junctional pacemaker and block below this pacemaker	Pathologic	Unrelated P wave and QRS complexes

[a]What is meant by AV *dissociation*? When the atria and ventricles beat independently, their contractions are "dissociated," and AV dissociation exists. Thus, P waves and QRS complexes in the electrocardiogram (ECG) are unrelated. AV dissociation may be complete or incomplete, transient, or permanent. The causes of AV dissociation are block and interference, and both may be present in the same ECG. *Block* is associated with a pathologic state of refractoriness, preventing the primary pacemaker's impulse from reaching the lower chamber. An example of this is sinus rhythm with complete AV block. *Interference* results from slowing of the primary pacemaker or acceleration of a subsidiary pacemaker. The lower chamber's impulse "interferes" with conduction by producing physiologic refractoriness, and AV dissociation results. An example of this is sinus rhythm with AV junctional or ventricular tachycardia and no retrograde conduction into the atria. A clear distinction must be made between block and interference. *Table C.8* describes the four types of AV dissociation.

THE BOTTOM LINE

- *Appendix C* is intended to be a quick guide to ECG interpretation. For more detailed information regarding ECG interpretation the reader is referred to:
  - *ACSM's Resource Manual for Guidelines for Exercise Testing and Prescription*, Seventh Edition (6).
  - *Dubin's Rapid Interpretation of EKG's: An Interactive Course* (1).

REFERENCES

1. Dubin D. *Rapid Interpretation of EKG's: An Interactive Course*. 6th ed. Tampa (FL): Cover Publications; 2000. 368 p.
2. Gamble P, McManus H, Jensen D, Froelicher V. A comparison of the standard 12-lead electrocardiogram to exercise electrode placements. *Chest*. 1984;85(5):616–22.
3. Goldberger AL. *Clinical Electrocardiography: A Simplified Approach*. 7th ed. Philadephia (PA): Mosby Elsevier; 2006. 337 p.
4. Jowett NI, Turner AM, Cole A, Jones PA. Modified electrode placement must be recorded when performing 12-lead electrocardiograms. *Postgrad Med J*. 2005;81(952):122–5.
5. Menown IB, Mackenzie G, Adgey AA. Optimizing the initial 12-lead electrocardiographic diagnosis of acute myocardial infarction. *Eur Heart J*. 2000;21(4):275–83.
6. Swain DP, American College of Sports Medicine. *ACSM's Resource Manual for Guidelines for Exercise Testing and Prescription*. 7th ed. Baltimore (MD): Lippincott Williams & Wilkins; 2014.
7. Wagner GS, Marriott HJL. *Marriott's Practical Electrocardiography*. 9th ed. Baltimore (MD): Williams & Wilkins; 1994. 434 p.

D

American College of Sports Medicine Certifications

Exercise practitioners are becoming increasingly aware of the advantages of maintaining professional credentials. In efforts to ensure quality, reduce liability, and remain competitive, more and more employers are requiring professional certification of their exercise staff. Additionally, in efforts to improve public safety, mandates for certification by state and/or regulatory agencies (*e.g.,* licensure) as well as third party payers now exist. The American College of Sports Medicine (ACSM) offers five primary and three specialty certifications for exercise professionals. These include the following:

Primary Certifications:
- ACSM Certified Group Exercise Instructor^{SM} (GEI)
- ACSM Certified Personal Trainer® (CPT)
- ACSM Certified Health Fitness Specialist^{SM} (HFS)
- ACSM Certified Clinical Exercise Specialist^{SM} (CES)
- ACSM Registered Clinical Exercise Physiologist® (RCEP)*

Specialty Certifications:
- ACSM/NCPAD Certified Inclusive Fitness Trainer^{SM}
  - NCPAD = National Center on Physical Activity and Disability
- ACSM/ACS Certified Cancer Exercise Trainer^{SM}
  - ACS = American Cancer Society
- ACSM/NPAS Physical Activity in Public Health Specialist^{SM}
  - NPAS = National Physical Activity Society

Advances in the exercise profession have been substantial over the past decade. Specific conditions that are considered essential for a formalized profession to exist are now in place (1). These include:

- A standardized system to develop skills.
- A standardized system to validate skills.
- An organized community to advocate for the profession.

The Committee on Accreditation for the Exercise Sciences (CoAES) under the auspices of the Commission on Accreditation of Allied Health Education Programs (CAAHEP) now validates and accredits university curriculum in the exercise sciences (*i.e.,* standardized skills development). The National Commission for Certifying Agencies (NCCA) provides a standardized, independent, and objective third party evaluation of examination design, development, and performance to ensure certification integrity (*i.e.*, skills validation). ACSM and other organizations such as Clinical Exercise Physiology Association (CEPA), a member of the ACSM affiliate societies, have created professional communities that advocate specifically for the interests of exercise and fitness practitioners.

ACSM CERTIFICATION DEVELOPMENT

The process of developing a certification examination begins with a job task analysis (JTA) (2). The purpose of the JTA is to define the major areas of professional practice (*i.e.*, domains), delineate the tasks performed "on-the-job," and identify the knowledge and skills required for safe and competent practice. The domains are subsequently weighted according to the importance and frequency of performance of their respective tasks. The number of examination test items is then determined based on the domain weight. Each examination reflects the content and weights defined by the JTA. By linking the content of the examination to the JTA (*e.g.*, what professionals do), it is possible to ensure that the examination is practice related.

Examination development continues with question writing. Content experts representing academia and practice are selected and trained on examination item writing. This examination writing team is charged with the task of creating test items that are representative of and consistent with the JTA. Each test item is evaluated psychometrically, undergoing extensive testing, editing, and retesting before being included as a scored item on the examination. Finally, passing scores are determined using a criterion-referenced methodology. Passing scores for each examination are associated with a minimum level of mastery necessary for safe and competent practice. Setting passing scores in this manner ensures that qualified candidates will become certified regardless of how other candidates perform on the examination.

The job definition, domains, and tasks from the JTA for ACSM's five primary certifications are listed in the following sections, and the primary population served, the eligibility criteria, and the competencies for these certifications are found in *Table D.1*. The complete JTA including knowledge and skill statements for all eight ACSM certifications can be found online at http://certification.acsm. org/exam-content-outlines. Because every question on each of the certification examinations must refer to a specific knowledge or skill statement within the associated JTA, these documents provide a resource to guide exam preparation.

ACSM'S FIVE PRIMARY CERTIFICATIONS

ACSM CERTIFIED GROUP EXERCISE INSTRUCTOR^{SM}
JOB TASK ANALYSIS

The JTA is intended to serve as a blueprint of the job of a GEI. As one prepares for the examination, it is important to remember that all questions are based on the following outline.

TABLE D.1. American College of Sports Medicine's Certifications at a Glance

Certification	Primary Population Served	Eligibility Criteria	Competencies
ACSM Certified Group Exercise Instructor[SM]	Apparently healthy individuals and those with health challenges who are able to exercise independently	• ≥18 yr • High school diploma or equivalent • Current CPR and AED certifications (must contain a live skills component) — AED not required for those practicing outside of the United States and Canada	• Develops and implements a variety of exercises in group settings and modifies exercise according to need • Leads safe and effective exercise using a variety of leadership techniques to enhance the motor skills related to the domains of physical fitness
ACSM Certified Personal Trainer®	Apparently healthy individuals and those with health challenges who are able to exercise independently	• ≥18 yr • High school diploma or equivalent • Current CPR and AED certifications (must contain a live skills component such as the American Heart Association [AHA] or the American Red Cross) — AED not required for those practicing outside of the United States and Canada	• Identifies health risk factors, performs fitness appraisals and preparticipation health screenings, and develops exercise programs that promote lasting behavior change • Incorporates suitable and innovative activities to improve functional capacity and manages health risk to promote lasting behavior change
ACSM Certified Health Fitness Specialist[SM]	Apparently healthy individuals and those with medically controlled diseases	• Bachelor's degree in an exercise science, exercise physiology, kinesiology, or exercise science based degree (one is eligible to sit for the examination if the candidate is in the last term of their degree program) • Current CPR and AED certifications (must contain a live skills component such as the AHA or the American Red Cross) — AED not required for those practicing outside of the United States and Canada	• Applies knowledge of exercise science including kinesiology, functional anatomy, exercise physiology, nutrition, program administration, psychology, and injury prevention in the health fitness setting • Performs preparticipation health screenings and fitness assessments • Interprets assessment results and develops exercise prescriptions • Performs duties related to fitness management, administration, and program supervision • Incorporates suitable physical activities to improve functional capacity • Applies appropriate behavioral change techniques to effectively educate and counsel on lifestyle modification

(continued)

TABLE D.1. American College of Sports Medicine's Certifications at a Glance (Continued)

Certification	Primary Population Served	Eligibility Criteria	Competencies
ACSM Certified Clinical Exercise Specialist[SM]	Apparently healthy individuals and those with cardiovascular, pulmonary, and metabolic disease	• Bachelor's degree in an exercise science, exercise physiology, kinesiology, or exercise science based degree (one is eligible to sit for the exam if the candidate is in the last term of their degree program) • Minimum of 400 h of clinical experience for graduates from a CAAHEP accredited program or 500 h of clinical experience for graduates from a non-CAAHEP accredited program • Current certification for the AHA BLS for Healthcare Provider or American Red Cross CPR/AED for the Professional Rescuer or equivalent (must contain live skills component) — AED not required for those practicing outside of the United States and Canada	• Applies extensive knowledge of functional anatomy, exercise physiology, pathophysiology, electrocardiography, human behavior/psychology, gerontology, and graded exercise testing in the clinical setting • Provides exercise supervision/leadership and counsels patients on lifestyle modification • Conducts emergency procedures in exercise testing and training settings
ACSM Registered Clinical Exercise Physiologist®	Apparently healthy individuals and those with cardiovascular, pulmonary, metabolic, orthopedic/musculoskeletal, neuromuscular, neoplastic, immunologic, and hematologic disorders	• Graduate degree in clinical exercise physiology with coursework in clinical assessment, exercise testing, exercise prescription, and exercise training (one is eligible to sit for the exam if the candidate is in the last term of their degree program) • Minimum of 600 h of clinical experience (external to classroom/laboratory) working with individuals with chronic disease • Current certification for the AHA BLS for Healthcare Provider or American Red Cross CPR/AED for the Professional Rescuer or equivalent (must contain live skills component) — AED not required for those practicing outside of the United States and Canada	• Performs exercise screening and exercise and fitness testing • Develops exercise prescriptions and supervises exercise programs • Conducts exercise and physical activity education counseling • Conducts measurement and evaluation of exercise and physical activity-related outcomes

AED, automated external defibrillators; BLS, basic life support; CPR, cardiopulmonary resuscitation.

Job Definition

The GEI (a) possesses a minimum of a high school diploma; and (b) works in a group exercise setting with apparently healthy individuals and those with health challenges who are able to exercise independently to enhance quality of life, improve health-related physical fitness, manage health risk, and promote lasting health behavior change. The GEI leads safe and effective exercise programs using a variety of leadership techniques to foster group camaraderie, support, and motivation to enhance muscular strength and endurance, flexibility, cardiorespiratory fitness, body composition, and any of the motor skills related to the domains of health-related physical fitness.

Performance Domains and Associated Job Tasks

The JTA for the GEI certification describes what the professional does on a day-to-day basis. The JTA is divided into domains and associated tasks performed on the job. The percentages listed in this section indicate the number of questions representing each domain on the 100 question GEI examination.

The performance domains are the following:

- Domain I: Participant and Program Assessment — 10%.
- Domain II: Class Design — 25%.
- Domain III: Leadership and Instruction — 55%.
- Domain IV: Legal and Professional Responsibilities — 10%.

Domain I: Participant and Program Assessment

Associated Job Tasks

A. Evaluate and establish participant screening procedures to optimize safety and minimize risk by reviewing assessment protocols based on ACSM standards and guidelines.
B. Administer and review as necessary participants' health risk to determine if preparticipation assessment is needed prior to exercise using Physical Activity Readiness Questionnaire (PAR-Q), ACSM preparticipation health screening, or other appropriate tools.
C. Screen participants as needed for known acute or chronic health conditions to provide recommendations and/or modifications.

Domain II: Class Design

Associated Job Tasks

A. Establish the purpose and determine the objectives of the class based on the needs of participants and facility.
B. Determine class content (i.e., warm-up, stimulus, and cool-down) in order to create an effective workout based on the objectives of the class.

C. Select and sequence appropriate exercises in order to provide a safe workout based on the objectives of the class.

D. Rehearse class content, exercise selection, and sequencing and revise as needed in order to provide a safe and effective workout based on the purpose and objectives of the class.

Domain III: Leadership and Instruction

Associated Job Tasks

A. Prepare to teach by implementing preclass procedures including screening new participants and organizing equipment, music, and room setup.

B. Create a positive exercise environment in order to optimize participant adherence by incorporating effective motivational skills, communication techniques, and behavioral strategies.

C. Demonstrate all exercises using proper form and technique to ensure safe execution in accordance with ACSM standards and guidelines.

D. Incorporate verbal and nonverbal instructional cues in order to optimize communication, safety, and motivation based on industry guidelines.

E. Monitor participants' performance to ensure safe and effective exercise execution using observation and participant feedback techniques in accordance with ACSM standards and guidelines.

F. Modify exercises based on individual and group needs to ensure safety and effectiveness in accordance with ACSM standards and guidelines.

G. Monitor sound levels of vocal and/or audio equipment following industry guidelines.

H. Respond to participants' concerns in order to maintain a professional, equitable, and safe environment by using appropriate conflict management or customer service strategies set forth by facility policy and procedures and industry guidelines.

I. Educate participants in order to enhance knowledge, enjoyment, and adherence by providing health/fitness-related information and resources.

Domain IV: Legal and Professional Responsibilities

Associated Job Tasks

A. Evaluate the class environment (e.g., outdoor, indoor, capacity, flooring, temperature, ventilation, lighting, equipment, acoustics) to minimize risk and optimize safety by following preclass inspection procedures based on established facility and industry standards and guidelines.

B. Promote participants' awareness and accountability by informing them of classroom safety procedures and exercise and intensity options in order to minimize risk.

C. Follow industry accepted professional, ethical, and business standards in order to optimize safety and reduce liability.

D. Respond to emergencies in order to minimize untoward events by following procedures consistent with established standards of care and facility policies.

E. Respect copyrights to protect original and creative work, media, etc., by legally securing copyright material and other intellectual property based on national and international copyright laws.

F. Engage in healthy lifestyle practices in order to be a positive role model for class participants.

G. Select and participate in continuing education programs that enhance knowledge and skills on a continuing basis, maximize effectiveness, and increase professionalism in the field.

ACSM CERTIFIED PERSONAL TRAINER® (CPT) JOB TASK ANALYSIS

The JTA is intended to serve as a blueprint of the job of a CPT. As you prepare for the examination, it is important to remember that all examination questions are based on the following outline.

Job Definition

The CPT (a) possesses a minimum of a high school diploma; and (b) works with apparently healthy individuals and those with health challenges who are able to exercise independently to enhance quality of life, improve health-related physical fitness, performance, manage health risk, and promote lasting health behavior change. The CPT conducts basic preparticipation health screening assessments, submaximal aerobic exercise tests, and muscular strength/endurance, flexibility, and body composition tests. The CPT facilitates motivation and adherence as well as develops and administers programs designed to enhance muscular strength/endurance, flexibility, cardiorespiratory fitness, body composition, and/or any of the motor skill-related components of physical fitness (*i.e.*, balance, coordination, power, agility, speed, and reaction time).

Performance Domains and Associated Job Tasks

The JTA for the CPT certification describes what the professional does on a day-to-day basis. The JTA is divided into domains and associated tasks performed on the job. The percentages listed in this section indicate the number of questions representing each domain on the 150 question CPT examination.

The performance domains are the following:

- Domain I: Initial Client Consultation and Assessment — 26%.
- Domain II: Exercise Programming and Implementation — 27%.
- Domain III: Exercise Leadership and Client Education — 27%.
- Domain IV: Legal, Professional, Business, and Marketing — 20%.

Domain I: Initial Client Consultation and Assessment

Associated Job Tasks

A. Provide instructions and initial documents to the client in order to proceed to the interview.
B. Interview client in order to gather and provide pertinent information to proceed to the fitness testing and program design.
C. Review and analyze client data (*i.e.*, classify risk) to formulate a plan of action and/or conduct physical assessments.
D. Evaluate behavioral readiness to optimize exercise adherence.
E. Assess physical fitness including cardiorespiratory fitness, muscular strength, muscular endurance, flexibility, and anthropometric measures in order to set goals and establish a baseline for program development.
F. Develop a comprehensive (*i.e.*, physical fitness, goals, and behavior) reassessment plan/timeline.

Domain II: Exercise Programming and Implementation

Associated Job Tasks

A. Review assessment results, medical history, and goals to determine appropriate training program.
B. Select exercise modalities to achieve desired adaptations based on goals, medical history, and assessment results.
C. Determine initial frequency, intensity, time (duration), and type (*i.e.*, the FITT principle of exercise prescription [Ex R_x]) of exercise based on goals, medical history, and assessment results.
D. Review proposed program with client; demonstrate and instruct the client to perform exercises safely and effectively.
E. Monitor client technique and response to exercise modifying as necessary.
F. Modify FITT to improve or maintain the client's physical fitness level.
G. Seek client feedback to ensure satisfaction and enjoyment of the program.

Domain III: Leadership and Education Implementation

Associated Job Tasks

A. Create a positive exercise experience in order to optimize participant adherence by applying effective communication techniques, motivation techniques, and behavioral strategies.
B. Educate clients using scientifically sound health/fitness information and resources to enhance client's knowledge base, program enjoyment, adherence, and overall awareness of health/fitness related information.

Domain IV: Legal, Professional, Business, and Marketing

Associated Job Tasks

A. Obtain medical clearance for clients based on ACSM guidelines prior to starting an exercise program.

B. Collaborate with various health care professionals and organizations in order to provide clients with a network of providers that minimizes liability and maximizes program effectiveness.

C. Develop a comprehensive risk management program (including emergency action plan and injury prevention program) to enhance the standard of care and reflect a client-focused mission.

D. Participate in approved continuing education programs on a regular basis to maximize effectiveness, increase professionalism, and enhance knowledge and skills in the field of health/fitness.

E. Adhere to ACSM's Code of Ethics by practicing in a professional manner within the Scope of Practice of a CPT (see ACSM's Code of Ethics for Certified and Registered Professionals at http://certification.acsm.org/faq28-codeofethics).

F. Develop a business plan to establish mission, business, budgetary, and sales objectives.

G. Develop marketing materials and engage in networking/business exchanges to build client base, promote services, and increase resources.

H. Obtain appropriate personal training and liability insurance and follow industry accepted professional, ethical, and business standards in order to optimize safety and to reduce liability.

I. Engage in healthy lifestyle practices in order to be a positive role model for all clients.

J. Respect copyrights to protect original and creative work, media, etc., by legally securing copyright material and other intellectual property based on national and international copyright laws.

K. Safeguard client confidentiality and privacy rights unless formally waived or in emergency situations.

ACSM CERTIFIED HEALTH FITNESS SPECIALIST[SM] JOB TASK ANALYSIS

The JTA is intended to serve as a blueprint of the job of an HFS. As one prepares for the examination, it is important to remember that all examination questions are based on the following outline.

Job Definition

The HFS is a health fitness professional with a minimum of a bachelor's degree in exercise science. The HFS performs preparticipation health screenings, conducts physical fitness assessments, interprets results, develops exercise prescriptions, and applies behavioral and motivational strategies to apparently healthy individuals and individuals with medically controlled diseases and health conditions to support clients in adopting and maintaining healthy lifestyle behaviors. The academic preparation of the HFS also includes fitness management, administration, and supervision. The HFS is typically employed or self-employed in commercial, community, studio, corporate, university, and hospital settings.

Performance Domains and Associated Job Tasks

The JTA for the HFS describes what the professional does on a day-to-day basis. The JTA is divided into domains and associated tasks performed on the job. The following percentages listed in this section indicate the number of questions representing each domain on the 150 question HFS examination.

The performance domains are the following:

- Domain I: Health and Fitness Assessment — 30%.
- Domain II: Exercise Prescription and Implementation (and Ongoing Support) — 30%.
- Domain III: Exercise Counseling and Behavioral Strategies — 15%.
- Domain IV: Legal/Professional — 10%.
- Domain V: Management — 15%.

Domain I: Health and Fitness Assessment

Associated Job Tasks

A. Implement assessment protocols and preparticipation health screening procedures to maximize participant safety and minimize risk.
B. Determine participant's readiness to take part in a health-related physical fitness assessment and exercise program.
C. Select and prepare physical fitness assessments for healthy participants and those with controlled disease.
D. Conduct and interpret cardiorespiratory fitness assessments.
E. Conduct assessments of muscular strength, muscular endurance, and flexibility.
F. Conduct anthropometric and body composition assessments.

Domain II: Exercise Prescription and Implementation

Associated Job Tasks

A. Review preparticipation health screening including self-guided health questionnaires and appraisals, exercise history, and physical fitness assessments.
B. Determine safe and effective exercise programs to achieve desired outcomes and goals.
C. Implement cardiorespiratory Ex R_x using the FITT principle (i.e., Frequency, Intensity, Time, and Type) for apparently healthy participants based on current health status, fitness goals, and availability of time.

D. Implement Ex R$_x$ using the FITT principle for flexibility, muscular strength, and muscular endurance for apparently healthy participants based on current health status, fitness goals, and availability of time.
E. Establish exercise progression guidelines for resistance, aerobic, and flexibility activity to achieve the goals of apparently healthy participants.
F. Implement a weight management program as indicated by personal goals that are supported by preparticipation health screening, health history, and body composition/anthropometrics.
G. Prescribe and implement exercise programs for participants with controlled cardiovascular, pulmonary, and metabolic diseases and other clinical populations.
H. Prescribe and implement exercise programs for healthy and special populations (i.e., older adults, youth, and pregnant women).
I. Modify Ex R$_x$ based on environmental conditions.

Domain III: Exercise Counseling and Behavioral Strategies

Associated Job Tasks

A. Optimize adoption and adherence to exercise programs and other healthy behaviors by applying effective communication techniques.
B. Optimize adoption of and adherence to exercise programs and other healthy behaviors by applying effective behavioral and motivational strategies.
C. Provide educational resources to support clients in the adoption and maintenance of healthy lifestyle behaviors.
D. Provide support within the scope of practice of an HFS and refer to other health professionals as indicated.

Domain IV: Legal/Professional

Associated Job Tasks

A. Create and disseminate risk management guidelines for a health/fitness facility, department, or organization to reduce member, employee, and business risk.
B. Create an effective injury prevention program and ensure that emergency policies and procedures are in place.

Domain V: Management

Associated Job Tasks

A. Manage human resources in accordance with leadership, organization, and management techniques.
B. Manage fiscal resources in accordance with leadership, organization, and management techniques.

C. Establish policies and procedures for the management of health/fitness facilities based on accepted safety and legal guidelines, standards, and regulations.
D. Develop and execute a marketing plan to promote programs, services, and facilities.
E. Use effective communication techniques to develop professional relationships with other allied health professionals (*e.g.*, nutritionists, physical therapists, physicians, nurses).

ACSM CERTIFIED CLINICAL EXERCISE SPECIALIST^{SM} (CES) JOB TASK ANALYSIS

The JTA is intended to serve as a blueprint of the job of the CES. As one prepares for the examination, it is important to remember that all examination questions are based on the following outline.

Job Definition

The CES is an allied health professional with a minimum of a bachelor's degree in exercise science. The CES works with patients and clients challenged with cardiovascular, pulmonary, and metabolic diseases and disorders, as well as with apparently healthy populations in cooperation with other health care professionals to enhance quality of life, manage health risk, and promote lasting health behavior change. The CES conducts preparticipation health screening, maximal and submaximal graded exercise tests, and performs strength, flexibility, and body composition tests. The CES develops and administers programs designed to enhance cardiorespiratory fitness, muscular strength and endurance, balance, and range of motion. The CES educates their clients about testing, exercise program components, and clinical and lifestyle self-care for control of chronic disease and health conditions.

Performance Domains and Associated Job Tasks

The JTA for the CES describes what the professional does on a day-to-day basis. The JTA is divided into domains and associated tasks performed on the job. The percentages listed in this section indicate the number of questions representing each domain on the 100 question CES examination.

The performance domains are the following:

- Domain I: Patient/Client Assessment — 30%.
- Domain II: Exercise Prescription — 30%.
- Domain III: Program Implementation and Ongoing Support — 20%.
- Domain IV: Leadership and Counseling — 15%.
- Domain V: Legal and Professional Considerations — 5%.

Domain I: Patient/Client Assessment

Associated Job Tasks

A. Determine and obtain the necessary physician referral and medical records to assess the potential participant.
B. Perform a preparticipation health screening including review of the participant's medical history and knowledge, their needs and goals, the program's potential benefits, and additional required testing and data.
C. Evaluate the participant's risk to ensure safe participation and determine level of monitoring/supervision in a preventive or rehabilitative exercise program.

Domain II: Exercise Prescription

Associated Job Tasks

A. Develop a clinically appropriate Ex R_x using all available information (*e.g.*, clinical and physiological status, goals, behavioral assessment).
B. Review the Ex R_x and exercise program with the participant including home exercise, compliance, and participant's expectations and goals.
C. Instruct the participant in the safe and effective use of exercise modalities, exercise plan, reporting symptoms, and class organization.

Domain III: Program Implementation and Ongoing Support

Associated Job Tasks

A. Implement the program (*e.g.*, Ex R_x, education, counseling, goals).
B. Continually assess participant feedback, clinical signs and symptoms, and exercise tolerance, and provide feedback to the participant about their exercise, general program participation, and clinical progress.
C. Reassess and update the program (*e.g.*, exercise, education, client goals) based on the participant's progress and feedback.
D. Maintain participant records to document progress and clinical status.

Domain IV: Leadership & Counseling

Associated Job Tasks

A. Educate the participant about performance and progression of aerobic, strength, and flexibility exercise programs.
B. Provide disease management and risk factor reduction education based on the participant's medical history, needs, and goals.
C. Create a positive environment for participant adherence and outcomes by incorporating effective motivational skills, communication techniques, and behavioral strategies.

D. Collaborate and consult with health care professionals to address clinical issues and provide referrals to optimize participant outcomes.

Domain V: Legal and Professional Considerations

Associated Job Tasks

A. Evaluate the exercise environment to minimize risk and optimize safety by following routine inspection procedures based on established facility and industry standards and guidelines.
B. Perform regular inspections of emergency equipment and practice emergency procedures (*e.g.*, crash cart, advanced cardiac life support procedures, activation of emergency medical system).
C. Promote awareness and accountability and minimize risk by informing participants of safety procedures and self-monitoring of exercise and related symptoms.
D. Comply with Health Insurance Portability and Accountability Act (HIPAA) laws and industry accepted professional, ethical, and business standards in order to maintain confidentiality, optimize safety, and reduce liability.
E. Promote a positive image of the program by engaging in healthy lifestyle practices.
F. Select and participate in continuing education programs that enhance knowledge and skills on a continuing basis, maximize effectiveness, and increase professionalism in the field.

ACSM REGISTERED CLINICAL EXERCISE PHYSIOLOGIST® (RCEP) JOB TASK ANALYSIS

The JTA is intended to serve as a blueprint of the job of a RCEP. As one prepares for the examination, it is important to remember that all examination questions are based on the following outline.

Job Definition

The RCEP (a) is an allied health professional with a minimum of a master's degree in exercise science; and (b) works in the application of physical activity and behavioral interventions for those clinical diseases and health conditions that have been shown to provide therapeutic and/or functional benefit. Persons that RCEP services are appropriate for may include, but are not limited to, individuals with cardiovascular, pulmonary, metabolic, orthopedic, musculoskeletal, neuromuscular, neoplastic, immunologic, and hematologic disease. The RCEP provides primary and secondary prevention and rehabilitative strategies designed to improve physical fitness and health in populations ranging across the lifespan.

The RCEP provides exercise screening, exercise and physical fitness testing, exercise prescriptions, exercise and physical activity counseling, exercise supervision, exercise and health education/promotion, and measurement and evaluation of exercise and physical activity-related outcome measures. The RCEP works individually or as part of an interdisciplinary team in a clinical, community, or public health setting. The practice and supervision of the RCEP is guided by published professional guidelines, standards, and applicable state and federal laws and regulations.

Performance Domains and Associated Job Tasks

The JTA for the RCEP describes what the professional does on a day-to-day basis. The JTA is divided into domains and associated tasks performed on the job. The percentages listed in this section indicate the number of questions representing each domain on the 125 question RCEP examination.

The performance domains are the following:

- Domain I: Clinical Assessment — 20%.
- Domain II: Exercise Testing — 20%.
- Domain III: Exercise Prescription — 20%.
- Domain IV: Exercise Training — 20%.
- Domain V: Education and Behavior Change — 10%.
- Domain VI: Program Administration — 5%.
- Domain VII: Legal and Professional Considerations — 5%.

Domain I: Clinical Assessment

Associated Job Tasks

In this domain, chronic disease(s) includes cardiovascular, pulmonary, metabolic, orthopedic/musculoskeletal, neuromuscular, neoplastic, immunologic, and hematologic disorders.

A. Review patient's medical record for information pertinent to the reason for their visit.
B. Interview patient for medical history pertinent to the reason for their visit and reconcile medications.
C. Assess resting vital signs and symptoms.
D. Collect and evaluate clinical and health measurements including, but not limited to ECG, spirometry, or blood glucose.

Domain II: Exercise Testing

Associated Job Tasks

In this domain, chronic disease(s) includes cardiovascular, pulmonary, metabolic, orthopedic/musculoskeletal, neuromuscular, neoplastic, immunologic, and hematologic disorders.

A. Assess appropriateness of and contraindications to symptom-limited, maximal exercise testing and/or other health assessments.
B. Select, administer, and interpret tests to assess muscular strength and/or endurance.
C. Select, administer, and interpret tests to assess flexibility and/or body composition.

D. Select, administer, and interpret submaximal aerobic exercise tests.
E. Select, administer, and interpret functional and balance tests (*e.g.*, Get Up and Go, Berg Balance).
F. Prepare patient for a symptom-limited, maximal exercise test by providing an informed consent and prepping the patient for electrocardiogram (ECG) monitoring.
G. Administer a symptom-limited, maximal exercise test using appropriate protocol and monitoring.
H. Evaluate results from a symptom-limited, maximal exercise test and report in the medical record and to health care providers.
I. Calibrate, troubleshoot, operate, and maintain testing equipment.

Domain III: Exercise Prescription

Associated Job Tasks

In this domain, chronic disease(s) includes cardiovascular, pulmonary, metabolic, orthopedic/musculoskeletal, neuromuscular, neoplastic, immunologic, and hematologic disorders.

A. Evaluate and document exercise goals and motivations of the patient to design an individualized Ex R_x.
B. Determine and document the Ex R_x for exercise training based on the patient's history, available data, and goals and discuss with the patient.
C. Determine the appropriate level of supervision and monitoring needed to provide a safe exercise environment based on risk classification guidelines.
D. Explain exercise intensity and measures to guide exercise intensity (*e.g.*, target heart rate, ratings of perceived exertion, signs/symptoms, ability to carry on a conversation) to the patient.
E. Design a home component for an exercise program to help transition a patient to more independent exercise using appropriate behavioral strategies.
F. Discuss the importance of, barriers to, and strategies to optimize adherence.
G. Regularly evaluate the appropriateness of and modify, as needed, the Ex R_x based on the patient's compliance, signs/symptoms, and physiologic response to the exercise program.

Domain IV: Exercise Training

Associated Job Tasks

In this domain, chronic disease(s) includes cardiovascular, pulmonary, metabolic, orthopedic/musculoskeletal, neuromuscular, neoplastic, immunologic, and hematologic disorders.

A. Meet with patient to discuss exercise training plan, expectations, and goals.
B. Identify, adapt, and instruct patient in appropriate exercise modes in order to reduce risk and maximize the development of cardiorespiratory fitness, strength, and flexibility.

C. Monitor and/or supervise patient during exercise based on their level of risk (*e.g.*, cardiopulmonary risk, fall risk) in order to provide a safe exercise environment.

D. Evaluate patient's contraindications to exercise training to make a risk/reward assessment.

E. Evaluate, document, and report patient's clinical status and response to exercise training in the medical record and to their health care provider.

F. Discuss clinical status and response to exercise training with patients and adapt and/or modify the exercise program as needed in order to prevent injury, maximize adherence, and progress toward desired outcomes.

G. Report new or worsening symptoms and adverse events in the patient's medical record and consult with the health care provider.

Domain V: Education and Behavior Strategies

Associated Job Tasks

In this domain, chronic disease(s) includes cardiovascular, pulmonary, metabolic, orthopedic/musculoskeletal, neuromuscular, neoplastic, immunologic, and hematologic disorders.

A. Evaluate patients to identify those who may benefit from mental health services using industry accepted screening tools.

B. Observe and interact with patients on an ongoing basis to identify recent changes that may benefit from counseling or other mental health services.

C. Assess patient for level of understanding of their disease and/or disability, readiness to adopt behavior change, and learning needs.

D. Conduct group and individual education sessions to teach patients about their disease/disability, secondary prevention, and how to manage their condition.

E. Assess knowledge of and compliance with health behaviors and apply behavior change techniques to encourage the adoption of healthy behaviors.

F. Teach relapse prevention techniques for maintenance of healthy behaviors.

Domain VI: Program Administration

Associated Job Tasks

In this domain, chronic disease(s) includes cardiovascular, pulmonary, metabolic, orthopedic/musculoskeletal, neuromuscular, neoplastic, immunologic, and hematologic disorders.

A. Maintain patient records as an ongoing documentation device to provide continuity of care and to meet legal standards.

B. Develop and/or maintain program evaluation tools and report program outcomes.

C. Develop strategies to improve program outcomes.

D. Develop and maintain relationships with referring physicians and other health care providers to enhance patient care.

E. Recruit, hire, train, motivate, and evaluate staff, students, and volunteers in order to provide effective services within a positive work environment.

F. Manage fiscal resources to provide efficient and effective services.

G. Develop, update, and/or maintain policies and procedures for daily operations, routine care, and adverse events.

H. Develop and maintain a safe environment that promotes positive outcomes and follows current industry recommendations and facility policies.

I. Develop and maintain an atmosphere of caring and support in order to promote patient adherence.

J. Promote the program and enhance its reputation through excellent communication and customer service.

K. Regularly conduct departmental needs assessment and develop/modify programs to accommodate changing environment.

Domain VII: Legal and Professional Considerations

Associated Job Tasks

In this domain, chronic disease(s) includes cardiovascular, pulmonary, metabolic, orthopedic/musculoskeletal, neuromuscular, neoplastic, immunologic, and hematologic disorders.

A. Follow industry accepted professional, ethical, and business standards in order to optimize safety, reduce liability, and protect patient confidentiality.

B. Participate in continuing education and/or professional networks to maintain certification, enhance knowledge, and remain current in the profession.

C. Maintain an environment that promotes ongoing written and verbal communication (*e.g.*, insurance providers, patients) and provides documentation of treatment that meets legal standards.

D. Take action in emergencies consistent with current certification, institutional procedures, and industry guidelines.

E. Inform patients of personal and facility safety procedures in order to minimize risk.

THE BOTTOM LINE

Obtaining professional credentials enhances the career development of health/fitness, clinical exercise, and health care professionals conducting exercise programs and exercise testing and improves the delivery of care to the consumer, client, and patient. ACSM offers high quality professional certifications for a variety of health/fitness, exercise, and health care professionals in corporate, health/fitness, and clinical settings.

Online Resources

American College of Sports Medicine Certifications:
http://certification.acsm.org/get-certified

American College of Sports Medicine Certifications Job Task Analysis:
http://certification.acsm.org/exam-content-outlines

American College of Sports Medicine Code of Ethics for Certified and Registered Professionals:
http://certification.acsm.org/faq28-codeofethics

Clinical Exercise Physiology Association:
http://www.acsm-cepa.org

Commission on Accreditation of Allied Health Education Programs:
http://www.caahep.org

Committee on Accreditation for the Exercise Sciences:
http://www.coaes.org

The National Commission for Certifying Agencies under the National Organization for Competency Assurance:
http://www.noca.org

REFERENCES

1. Costanzo DG. ACSM Certification: The Evolution of the Exercise Professional. *ACSM Health Fitness J.* 2006;10(4):38–9.
2. Paternostro-Bayles M. The role of a job task analysis in the development of professional certifications. *ACSM Health Fitness J.* 2010;14(4):41–2.

Contributing Authors to the Previous Two Editions

CONTRIBUTORS TO THE EIGHTH EDITION

Kelli Allen, PhD
VA Medical Center
Durham, North Carolina

Lawrence E. Armstrong, PhD, FACSM
University of Connecticut
Storrs, Connecticut

Gary J. Balady, MD
Boston University School of Medicine
Boston, Massachusetts

Michael J. Berry, PhD, FACSM
Wake Forest University
Winston-Salem, North Carolina

Craig Broeder, PhD, FACSM
Benedictine University
Lisle, Illinois

John Castellani, PhD, FACSM
U.S. Army Research Institute of
Environmental Medicine
Natick, Massachusetts

Bernard Clark, MD
St. Francis Hospital and Medical Center
Hartford, Connecticut

Dawn P. Coe, PhD
Grand Valley State University
Allendale, Michigan

Michael Deschenes, PhD, FACSM
College of William and Mary
Willamsburg, Virginia

J. Andrew Doyle, PhD
Georgia State University
Atlanta, Georgia

Barry Franklin, PhD, FACSM
William Beaumont Hospital
Royal Oak, Michigan

Charles S. Fulco, ScD
U.S. Army Research Institute of
Environmental Medicine
Natick, Massachusetts

Carol Ewing Garber, PhD, FACSM
Columbia University
New York, New York

Paul M. Gordon, PhD, FACSM
University of Michigan
Ann Arbor, Michigan

Sam Headley, PhD, FACSM
Springfield College
Springfield, Massachusetts

John E. Hodgkin, MD
St. Helena Hospital
St. Helena, California

John M. Jakicic, PhD, FACSM
University of Pittsburgh
Pittsburgh, Pennsylvania

Wendy Kohrt, PhD, FACSM
University of Colorado — Denver
Aurora, Colorado

Timothy R. McConnell, PhD, FACSM
Bloomsburg University
Bloomsburg, Pennsylvania

Kyle McInnis, ScD, FACSM
University of Massachusetts
Boston, Massachusetts

Miriam C. Morey, PhD
VA and Duke Medical Centers
Durham, North Carolina

Stephen Muza, PhD
U.S. Army Research Institute of
Environmental Medicine
Natick, Massachusetts

Jonathan Myers, PhD, FACSM
VA Palo Alto Health Care System/
Stanford University
Palo Alto, California

Patricia A. Nixon, PhD, FACSM
Wake Forest University
Winston-Salem, North Carolina

Jeff Rupp, PhD
Georgia State University
Atlanta, Georgia

Ray Squires, PhD, FACSM
Mayo Clinic
Rochester, Minnesota

Clare Stevinson, PhD
University of Alberta
Edmonton, Canada

Scott Thomas, PhD
University of Toronto
Toronto, Canada

Yves Vanlandewijck, PhD
Katholieke Universiteit Leuven
Leuven, Belgium

CONTRIBUTORS TO THE SEVENTH EDITION

Lawrence E. Armstrong, PhD, FACSM
Professor, Department of Kinesiology
Human Performance Laboratory
University of Connecticut
Storrs, Connecticut

Gary J. Balady, MD
Co-Director, Noninvasive Cardiac Labs
Boston Medical Center
Professor of Medicine
Boston University School of Medicine
Boston, Massachusetts

Michael J. Berry, PhD, FACSM
Professor, Department of Health and
Exercise Science
Wake Forest University
Winston-Salem, North Carolina

Shala E. Davis, PhD, FACSM
Associate Professor, Department of
Movement Studies and Exercise Science
East Stroudsburg University
East Stroudsburg, Pennsylvania

Brenda M. Davy, PhD, RD, LD
Assistant Professor, Department of Human
Nutrition, Foods and Exercise
Virginia Polytechnic Institute and
State University
Blacksburg, Virginia

Kevin P. Davy, PhD, FACSM
Associate Professor, Department of Human
Nutrition, Foods, and Exercise
Virginia Polytechnic Institute and
State University
Blacksburg, Virginia

Barry A. Franklin, PhD, FACSM
Director, Cardiac Rehabilitation and
Exercise Laboratories
Beaumont Rehab and Health Center
William Beaumont Hospital
Royal Oak, Michigan
Professor of Physiology
Wayne State University
Detroit, Michigan

Neil F. Gordon MD, PhD, MPH, FACSM
President, Intervention Center for
Heart Disease Prevention
St. Joseph's/Candler Health System
Savannah, Georgia

I-Min Lee, MD, ScD
Associate Professor, Department of Medicine
Harvard Medical School
Associate Epidemiologist, Department of
Preventive Medicine
Brigham and Women's Hospital
Boston, Massachusetts

Timothy R. McConnell, PhD, FACSM
Assistant Professor Coordinator, Graduate
Student Department of Science and Athletics
Bloomsburg University
Bloomsburg, Pennsylvania

Jonathan N. Myers, PhD, FACSM
Clinical Assistant Professor of Medicine
Department of Cardiology
Stanford University
Palo Alto VA Health Care System
Palo Alto, California

Francis X. Pizza, PhD
Professor
Department of Kinesiology
The University of Toledo
Toledo, Ohio

Thomas W. Rowland, MD, FACSM
Professor, Department of Pediatrics
Tufts University School of Medicine
Boston, Massachusetts
Director, Pediatric Cardiology
Bay State Medical Center
Springfield, Massachusetts

Kerry Stewart, EdD, FACSM
Associate Professor of Medicine
Division of Cardiology
Director, Johns Hopkins Heart Health
Johns Hopkins Bayview Medical Center
Baltimore, Maryland

Paul D. Thompson, MD, FACSM
Director, Preventive Cardiology
Hartford Hospital
Hartford, Connecticut

Janet P. Wallace, PhD, FACSM
Professor and Director of Adult Fitness
Department of Kinesiology
Indiana University
Bloomington, Indiana

Index

Note: Page numbers followed by *b*, *f*, or *t* indicate boxed, figures, or table material.